*A Syllabus of*

# LABORATORY EXAMINATIONS
# IN
# CLINICAL DIAGNOSIS

*A Syllabus of*

# LABORATORY EXAMINATIONS IN CLINICAL DIAGNOSIS

Critical Evaluation of Laboratory Procedures

in the

Study of the Patient

REVISED EDITION

*Edited by*

## LOT B. PAGE, *M.D.*

*Chief of the Hypertension Unit and
Assistant Physician, Massachusetts General Hospital;
Associate in Medicine at the Massachusetts General
Hospital, Harvard Medical School*

*and*

## PERRY J. CULVER, *M.D.*

*Associate Physician, Massachusetts General Hospital;
Member of the American Gastroenterologic Association;
Clinical Associate in Medicine, Harvard Medical School*

HARVARD UNIVERSITY PRESS

*Cambridge, Massachusetts*

*1966*

*To*

PATRICIA PAGE ⁓ KATE CULVER

*and the wives and families
of all who have contributed
to this volume*

# Preface

The first edition of this book grew out of a course in laboratory diagnosis given during the second year at the Harvard Medical School. In the years since its publication, the book has been widely used as a textbook in medical schools and as an aid to performance and interpretation of laboratory procedures in hospitals and offices. Meanwhile, the original editor, Dr. Thomas Hale Ham, has left the Harvard medical community and, with the adoption of an integrated curriculum at Harvard Medical School in 1957, the course in laboratory diagnosis has ceased to exist as a separate subject.

The editors of this revised edition have endeavored to retain the spirit of the original *Syllabus*, and especially to preserve and extend its unique emphasis on the critical interpretation of laboratory procedures in the study of the patient. In the units dealing with hematologic studies, much of the original material has been retained, although the text has been altered somewhat, and a considerable amount of new material has been added. A majority of the units have been completely rewritten. Since the scope of the book is not limited by the requirements of a particular course, the editors have exercised a free choice in selecting additional topics for inclusion. It is hoped that these additions will make the book more useful.

The reasons for including certain tests, for excluding others, and for allotting more space to one procedure than to another, have varied. The emphasis no doubt reflects the bias of the contributors and editors. In general, detailed technical information has been given for procedures that a physician or house officer might be called on to perform himself. Where more specialized procedures are involved, only the principle has been described. Certain procedures are described here in detail chiefly because they are not available in any existing textbook.

There has been an enormous increase, in recent years, in both the number and the availability of laboratory procedures. The rate of growth has been most rapid in the area of biochemical determinations. Many of the new tests represent applications of current research techniques and reflect a deepening knowledge of disease mechanisms. When appropriately used, a wide choice of laboratory procedures can provide the means for improving the precision of diagnostic studies, and for obtaining glimpses of the disordered physiology of disease. On the other hand, the proliferation of laboratory facilities has also increased the opportunity to use them excessively and unwisely. It is for these reasons that a considerable amount of space has been devoted in this book to the physiologic variables that influence laboratory results, and to pathologic physiology of disease as reflected in laboratory data. In recent years, specialized equipment has been developed to facilitate speedy performance of many types of laboratory procedures, and its use is rapidly supplementing the older methods in large laboratories. Recently, fully automatic methods for quantitative chemical determinations and cell counts have been introduced. However, the majority of the procedures described here require equipment that is commonly available in hospital laboratories.

The contributors and critics have given their time and talent generously and deserve full credit for the virtues of this book. Many of the contributors also acted as critics for manuscripts other than their own. The suggestions of the critics were reviewed by the authors and editors, but, since not all of their suggestions have been followed, the editors must accept final responsibility for the shortcomings of the book.

Miss Dorothy W. Bishop has not only typed the manuscripts with unusual accuracy, but has also helped materially in the editorial work and in the many problems involved in bringing the book to its final form. Mr. Joseph D. Elder of Harvard University Press has given us invaluable assistance in all the steps involved in bringing this revised edition of the *Syllabus* to print. The editors are also indebted to Dr. Paul C. Zamecnik and the members of the Executive Committee of the Department of Medicine, Harvard Medical School, for their continued interest and encouragement.

Lot B. Page, M.D.
Perry J. Culver, M.D.

# Preface to the First Edition

The physician is responsible for care of the patient and for prevention of illness. This requires professional evaluation of the person in his environment and the application of knowledge from the humanities and from the preclinical and clinical fields to the care of the patient. Since the physician continuously and humbly searches for the truth, he remains an investigator for life, and, by the intellectual process of distinguishing between fact and theory, he is judging information by a scientific method of thought. Moreover, the use of a scientific method of thought is frequently equivalent to the use of good judgment or of common sense and is quite compatible with the physician's sincere human kindness and sympathy for the patient's welfare.

Diagnosis, prognosis, and treatment are derived from data that are collected and analyzed by the following series of procedures, which constitute objective and subjective methods for investigation of the patient by the physician. (1) At least three different kinds of *data* form the basis of a case study, each obtained in a different manner and each requiring critical analysis for validity, sources of error, and clinical significance in the particular patient. The kinds of information are: (i) data obtained from the history of the patient as a person and as a member of society, and from the history of health or illness; (ii) data obtained by physical examination; (iii) data obtained by laboratory or by special examinations. All subsequent steps represent the *processing* of these data to establish a diagnosis, on which the prognosis and treatment are based. (2) The data are recorded. (3) A summary is prepared, representing a codification of all the important data. (4) From the summary, the data are evaluated and integrated into a preliminary diagnosis. (5) The preliminary diagnosis is analyzed for limitations of its accuracy so that further examinations may be performed as needed. (6) Information is applied to the data of the case to confirm the diagnosis or to continue the study so that a diagnosis may be evolved. (7) An estimate is made of the prognosis. (8) Treatment is based on the diagnosis, the symptoms, and the needs of the individual patient, and is changed as indicated by the progress of the patient.

There remains yet another aspect of the study of a patient, namely, the *presentation* of data to others. Too often the presentation is poorly planned, lacks integration and critical evaluation, and is confused with the procedures used in the collection and the processing of data. When data are presented, the form of presentation may emphasize the person, the environment, the summary, the diagnosis, the symptoms, or the treatment, and may be varied markedly from patient to patient, depending on the individual problem.

Obviously, the results of laboratory examinations represent only one portion of the data. Although certain basic or routine examinations are indicated as screening procedures in the study of each patient, all special examinations are planned critically as suggested by information obtained from the history, the physical examination, and the screening laboratory examinations. In clinical medicine a laboratory procedure begins and ends with a patient. Accordingly, the laboratory examinations described in this *Syllabus* are discussed from the following points of view: clinical value, availability, cost, principle, method, and limitations and interpretations of the test itself and as a diagnostic aid related to the history and physical examination of the patient.

As is noted, laboratory examinations are frequently performed with a degree of *inaccuracy* that may—on occasion—endanger the life of the patient, and they may be ordered and interpreted without critical evaluation of the limits of accuracy of the test, the limits of accuracy required to be of clinical significance, or the diagnostic limitations of the results. Accordingly, these limitations have been described in detail in the *Syllabus*. Suggestions have also been made to aid in the planning of laboratory tests so that the physician may proceed from the simple screening tests to the more complex procedures, evaluating data step by step in the study of a patient. There appears to be no doubt that the responsibility for obtaining laboratory data of reliable quality rests on the physician who is in charge of the patient.

This *Syllabus* and its companion volume, the *Color Atlas,** are intended to serve as teaching aids in the diagnosis and management of the patient, to form a link between preclinical and clinical medicine, and thus to be of assistance to medical students, technicians, and physicians. It is recognized that the *Syllabus* differs radically from many textbooks in the field of clinical diagnosis, and it may be found to suffer from complexity in some parts and oversimplicity in others. It doubtless contains errors and omissions. The critics who reviewed the several units in manuscript aided enormously, but, since not all their suggestions were accepted, they are responsible only for the possible good features of the *Syllabus*.

Thomas Hale Ham, M.D.

---

* A *Color Atlas of Morphologic Hematology with a Guide to Technique and Clinical Diagnosis*, by Geneva A. Daland, edited by Thomas Hale Ham, M.D., color plates by Etta Piotti (Harvard University Press, 1950); A *Color Atlas of Morphologic Hematology with a Guide to Clinical Interpretation* (rev. ed.; Harvard University Press, 1959).

# Contents

xi

CONTENTS

CONTENTS

# Tables

# Figures

# Contributors

IRVING P. ACKERMAN, A.B., M.D.

*Instructor in Medicine, Harvard Medical School; Assistant Physican and Member, Diabetic and Endocrine Group, Massachusetts General Hospital*

RAYMOND D. ADAMS, A.B., M.D., A.M. (hon.)

*Bullard Professor of Neuropathology, Harvard Medical School; Chief, Neurology Service, Massachusetts General Hospital*

ALAN C. AISENBERG, M.D., PH.D.

*Associate in Medicine, Harvard Medical School; Clinical Assistant in Medicine, Massachusetts General Hospital*

WILLIAM H. BAKER, A.B., M.D.

*Clinical Associate in Medicine, Harvard Medical School; Assistant Physician, Massachusetts General Hospital*

EVAN CALKINS, A.B., M.D.

*Assistant Professor of Medicine, Harvard Medical School; Director, Arthritis Unit and Lovett Memorial Laboratories, Massachusetts General Hospital*

B. W. COBBS, JR., A.B., M.D.

*Associate in Medicine (Cardiology), Emory University Medical School; Staff Physician, Grady Hospital, Staff Physician, Emory University Hospital, Atlanta, Georgia*

PERRY J. CULVER, A.B., M.D.

*Clinical Associate in Medicine, Harvard Medical School; Associate Physician, Massachusetts General Hospital*

GENEVA A. DALAND, B.S.

*Research Technologist in Hematology, Thorndike Memorial Laboratory, Boston City Hospital*

LESLIE J. DE GROOT, B.S., M.D.

*Instructor in Medicine, Harvard Medical School; Clinical and Research Fellow in Medicine, Massachusetts General Hospital*

ALLAN J. ERSLEV, M.D.

*Associate Professor of Internal Medicine, Jefferson Medical College; Associate Director, Cardeza Foundation for Hematologic Research, Philadelphia*

CHARLES H. DuTOIT, A.B., M.D. (deceased)

*Associate in Medicine, Harvard Medical School; Associate Physician and Director of Chemistry Laboratory, Massachusetts General Hospital*

PAUL FREMONT–SMITH, M.D.

*Clinical Associate in Medicine, Harvard Medical School; Director, Division of Bacteriology and Infectious Diseases, Peter Bent Brigham Hospital, Boston; Attending Physician, Boston Lying-In Hospital; Visiting Physician, Robert Breck Brigham Hospital, Boston*

# CONTRIBUTORS

## MORTIMER S. GREENBERG, B.A., M.D.

*Instructor in Medicine, Harvard Medical School; Hematologist, Lemuel Shattuck Hospital, Boston; Assisting Physician, 2nd and 4th (Harvard) Medical Services, Boston City Hospital; Associate Physician and Consultant in Hematology, Mount Auburn Hospital, Cambridge, Massachusetts*

## MORTEN GROVE–RASSMUSSEN, M.D.

*Director, Blood Bank, Massachusetts General Hospital*

## PHILIP H. HENNEMAN, A.B., M.D.

*Associate Professor of Medicine and Director, Division of Endocrinology and Metabolism, Seton Hall College of Medicine, New Jersey; Visiting Physician, Jersey City Medical Center*

## JAMES H. JANDL, B.S., M.D.

*Assistant Professor of Medicine, Harvard Medical School; Research Associate, Thorndike Memorial Laboratory, Boston City Hospital*

## ALAN R. JONES, B.S., M.B.

*Research Associate, Department of Pediatrics, Harvard Medical School; Director of Transfusion Service and Research Associate in Hematology, Children's Hospital, Boston; Associate Director, Blood Grouping Laboratory of Boston*

## EDWARD H. KASS, A.B., M.S., PH.D., M.D., M.A. (hon)

*Associate Professor of Bacteriology and Immunology, Harvard Medical School; Associate Physician, Thorndike Memorial Laboratory, Boston City Hospital; Director, Mallory Institute of Pathology; Associate Visiting Physician, 2nd and 4th (Harvard) Medical Services, Boston City Hospital*

## EDMUND M. KLEIN, B.A., M.D.

*Research Associate, Department of Dermatology, Harvard Medical School; Assistant Professor, Department of Medicine, Tufts Medical School; Research Associate, Department of Pathology, Children's Hospital and Children's Cancer Research Foundation, Boston*

## JOHN H. KNOWLES, A.B., M.D.

*Associate in Medicine, Harvard Medical School; Chief of Pulmonary Disease Unit, Massachusetts General Hospital*

## JANET W. McARTHUR, A.B., M.S., M.D.

*Clinical Associate in Medicine (Assigned to Gynecology), Harvard Medical School; Associate Physician, Massachusetts General Hospital*

## JOSEPH M. MILLER, A.B., M.D.

*Instructor in Medicine, Harvard Medical School; Associate in Medicine, Peter Bent Brigham Hospital, Boston*

## MARC P. MOLDAWER, M.D.

*Chief, Division of Endocrinology, Department of Medicine, Baylor University College of Medicine; Attending Physician, Methodist and Jefferson Davis Hospitals, Houston, Texas; Consultant in Endocrinology, Veterans Administration Hospital and Texas Institute for Rehabilitation and Research, Houston, Texas*

## LOT B. PAGE, M.D.

*Instructor in Medicine, Harvard Medical School; Chief, Hypertension Clinic, Acting Director of the Clinical Chemistry Laboratory, and Assistant Physician, Massachusetts General Hospital*

# CONTRIBUTORS

### ALBERT F. PARLOW, PH.D.

*Research Fellow in Physiology in Obstetrics and Gynecology, Harvard Medical School; Research Associate, Vincent Memorial Hospital, Boston*

### MAURICE M. PECHET, B.SC., A.M., PH.D., M.D.

*Research Associate in Medicine, Harvard Medical School; Resident Senior Tutor, Lowell House, Harvard University; Clinical and Research Fellow in Medicine, Massachusetts General Hospital; Junior Consultant in Medicine, Lemuel Shattuck Hospital, Boston*

### ROBERT B. PENNELL, B.S., M.S., PH.D.

*Lecturer in Immunology, Department of Microbiology, Harvard School of Public Health; Senior Investigator and Director of Laboratories, Protein Foundation, Inc., Boston*

### MARIAN W. ROPES, A.B., M.S., M.D.

*Assistant Clinical Professor in Medicine, Harvard Medical School; Associate Physician, Massachusetts General Hospital; Associate Physician, House of the Good Samaritan, Boston; Consultant-Lecturer, Chelsea Naval Hospital, Chelsea, Massachusetts*

### WILLIAM H. SHAFER, M.D.

*Department of Internal Medicine, The Cleveland Clinic Foundation; The Frank E. Bunts Educational Institute, Cleveland, Ohio*

### JOHN T. SHARP, M.D.

*Instructor in Medicine, Harvard Medical School; Assistant in Medicine, Massachusetts General Hospital*

### STEPHEN M. SHEA, M.D., M.SC.

*Assistant Professor of Pathology, University of Toronto*

### LLOYD H. SMITH, A.B., M.D.

*Assistant Professor of Medicine, Harvard Medical School; Assistant Physician, Massachusetts General Hospital*

### YANG WANG, M.B., M.D.

*Instructor in Medicine, University of Minnesota Medical School; University of Minnesota Hospitals, Minneapolis*

# Critics

BENJAMIN ALEXANDER, A.B., M.D.

*Associate Professor of Medicine, Harvard Medical School; Associate Director of the Medical Service and Associate in Medical Research, Beth Israel Hospital, Boston; Consultant in Medicine, Children's Hospital, Boston*

WILLIAM S. BECK, B.S., M.D.

*Assistant Professor of Medicine, Harvard Medical School; Chief of the Hematology Unit and Director of the Clinical Laboratories, Massachusetts General Hospital; Tutor in Biochemical Sciences, Harvard College*

WILLIAM B. CASTLE, M.D., S.M. (hon.), M.D. (hon.), S.D. (hon.)

*George Richards Minot Professor of Medicine and Head of the Department at the Boston City Hospital; Director, Thorndike Memorial Laboratory; Director, 2nd and 4th (Harvard) Medical Services, Boston City Hospital; Visiting Physician, 2nd and 4th (Harvard) Medical Services, Boston City Hospital*

RICHARD A. FIELD, A.B., M.D.

*Associate in Medicine, Harvard Medical School; Program Director, Diabetes Research Unit and Clinic, Massachusetts General Hospital; Investigator, Howard Hughes Medical Institute*

ANNE P. FORBES, A.B., M.D.

*Associate Physician, Massachusetts General Hospital*

FRANK GARDNER, B.S., M.D.

*Assistant Professor of Medicine, Harvard Medical School; Senior Associate in Medicine, Peter Bent Brigham Hospital, Boston*

DAVID GITLIN, B.S., M.D.

*Assistant Professor of Pediatrics, Harvard Medical School; Associate Physician, Children's Hospital, Boston*

KURT J. ISSELBACHER, M.D.

*Assistant Professor of Medicine, Harvard Medical School; Chief, Gastrointestinal Unit, Massachusetts General Hospital*

HENRY JANOWITZ, A.B., M.D., M.S.

*Assistant Clinical Professor of Medicine, Columbia University College of Physicians and Surgeons; Associate Attending Physician for Gastroenterology and Head, Division of Gastroenterology, Department of Medicine, Mount Sinai Hospital, New York*

ALEXANDER LEAF, B.S., M.D.

*Assistant Professor of Medicine at the Massachusetts General Hospital, Harvard Medical School; Chief, Cardio-Renal Unit, Massachusetts General Hospital*

GORDON S. MYERS, B.A., M.D.

*Associate in Medicine, Harvard Medical School; Chief of Cardiac Catheterization Laboratory, Massachusetts General Hospital; Consulting Physician, Massachusetts Eye and Ear Infirmary, Boston; Attendant in Cardiology, West Roxbury Veterans Administration Hospital, Boston*

*A Syllabus of*

# LABORATORY EXAMINATIONS
## IN
## CLINICAL DIAGNOSIS

# *Unit 1*

# Units of Measure and Tables of Normal Values

### Units of Measure

The selection of appropriate units of measure is essential to the development of all quantitative laboratory procedures. Many different kinds of laboratory tests are used in clinical medicine and many different units of measure are required. For certain types of tests, such as bioassays and measurements of enzymatic activity, arbitrary units are necessary. Some specialized tests are performed simultaneously on an unknown and a normal (or "control") sample, and results are expressed as a ratio of the unknown to the control. The definitions of these specialized units of measure are discussed in subsequent units in connection with the tests that use them. For the majority of the clinical laboratory measurements it is possible to express results in one or more of the familiar units of the metric system.

The metric system is too well known to require definition. For convenience, some of the units commonly used in biological and medical sciences are listed in Table 1 together with their equivalent values and abbreviations. There is a slight differ-

Table 1. *Selected units of measure.*

| Unit | Abbreviation | Equivalents | |
|------|:---:|---|---|
| *Length* | | | |
| 1 meter | m | $= 10$ decimeters (dm) $=$ | 100 centimeters |
| 1 centimeter | cm | $= 10^{-2}$ m $=$ | 10 millimeters |
| 1 millimeter | mm | $= 10^{-3}$ m $= 10^{-1}$ cm $=$ | 1000 microns |
| 1 micron | $\mu$ | $= 10^{-6}$ m $= 10^{-4}$ cm $=$ | 1000 millimicrons |
| 1 millimicron | m$\mu$ | $= 10^{-9}$ m $= 10^{-7}$ cm $=$ | 10 angstroms |
| 1 angstrom | Å | $= 10^{-10}$ m $= 10^{-8}$ cm $=$ | 100 micromicrons |
| 1 micromicron | $\mu\mu$ | $= 10^{-12}$ m $= 10^{-10}$ cm | |
| *Area* | | | |
| 1 square meter | m$^2$ | $=$ | 10,000 square centimeters |
| 1 square centimeter | cm$^2$ | $=$ | 100 square millimeters |
| 1 square millimeter | mm$^2$ | | |
| *Volume* | | | |
| 1 liter | L | $=$ | 1000 milliliters |
| 1 cubic millimeter | mm$^3$ | $=$ | $10^9$ cubic microns |
| 1 cubic micron | $\mu^3$ | | |
| *Mass* | | | |
| 1 kilogram | kg | $=$ | 1,000 grams |
| 1 gram | gm | $=$ | 1,000 milligrams |
| 1 milligram | mg | $=$ | 1,000 micrograms |
| 1 microgram | $\mu$g | $=$ | 1,000,000 micromicrograms |
| 1 micromicrogram | $\mu\mu$g | $= 10^{-12}$ gm | |

1

ence between the milliliter and the cubic centimeter ($1 \text{ ml} = 1.000027 \text{ cm}^3$). At atmospheric pressure and at 4°C, the mass of 1 ml of water is equal to exactly 1 gm. The milliliter is therefore the preferable unit of volume, and is used throughout this book. The term "milligrams percent" is usually understood to mean "milligrams per 100 milliliters," although it literally means "milligrams per 100 milligrams" (or parts per 100 parts). Concentrations should be expressed instead in milligrams per 100 ml.

The electrolytes of body fluids are related through molecular and ionic interactions, and the relations between them are clarified by expressing their concentrations in terms of their chemical behavior. Chemical equivalents are now widely employed for expressing the concentrations of the major electrolytes of plasma. However, it is still customary to express the concentrations of most of the constituents of biologic fluids in mass per unit volume (mg/100 ml) rather than in molar concentrations. When knowledge of the interactions among the various solutes of body fluids becomes more complete, many more of these substances will probably be described in terms of their chemical behavior.

### DEFINITIONS

*Millimol* (mM). One mol of a substance is a quantity whose mass in grams is numerically equal to its molecular weight. One millimol is 0.001 of this amount; its mass in milligrams is numerically equal to its molecular weight. Conversion of concentrations can be made as follows:

$$\text{Concentration (mM/L)} = \frac{\text{Concentration (mg/L)}}{\text{Molecular weight}}.$$

The concentration of blood gases can also be expressed in millimols. In the case of carbon dioxide, 1 mM occupies 22.26 ml at standard temperature and pressure. The concentration of the gas in fluid is measured in milliliters per 100 ml (vol-umes percent). Conversion may be made as follows:

$$\text{Concentration } CO_2 \text{ (mM/L)}$$
$$= \frac{\text{Concentration } CO_2 \text{ (vol. percent)}_{\text{S.T.P.}} \times 10}{22.26}.$$

*Milliequivalent* (mEq). For any ion in solution, the equivalent weight is equal to the sum of the atomic weights divided by the valence. A milliequivalent is a quantity whose mass in milligrams is numerically equal to this ratio. For univalent ions, 1 mM is equal to 1 mEq. For divalent ions, 1 mM = 2 mEq. It is evident that a solution containing 1 mM of sodium chloride (58.5 mg) will contain 1 mEq of sodium ion (23 mg) and 1 mEq of chloride ion (35.5 mg).

*Milliosmol* (mOsm). The osmotic pressure of an aqueous solution can be estimated by accurately measuring its freezing point, since an inverse relation exists between the molal concentration of solute and the freezing point of the solution. The results of such a determination can be expressed directly in degrees centigrade, or may be converted into other units such as pressure or molal concentration of solute. The molal concentration is the most convenient unit for medical purposes, because it is comparable to other measurements that are often made on the same fluid. It must be emphasized that the osmotic pressure of a solution depends on the total concentration of osmotically active particles present, regardless of their chemical properties. Biologic fluids such as serum and urine contain a large number of different solutes, all of which contribute to the depression of the freezing point. To take cognizance of this heterogeneity, the term "osmolality" is used rather than molality. This implies that the result is a composite measurement of the molal concentrations of all the solutes present in the solution. Molal, rather than molar, concentrations should be used for dealing with colligative properties of solutions, since in molal solutions the relative quantities of solute and solvent are

2

constant, whereas in molar solutions they are variable.

In homogeneous solutions of nonelectrolytes such as glucose or urea, 1 mol = 1 osmol  (and  1 millimol = 1 milliosmol). In very weak solutions of electrolytes, 1 mM = 2 mEq = 2 mOsm. However, in more concentrated electrolyte solutions, 2 mEq equal somewhat less than 2 mOsm, since, owing to variations in activity, the ions no longer behave as completely dissociated particles. At the concentration of electrolyte normally encountered in serum, 2 mEq = approximately 1.86 mOsm.

The relation of osmolality to specific gravity in the urine is discussed in Unit 19, and the clinical value of serum osmolality measurements, in Unit 21.

### Normal Values

There are serious semantic pitfalls involved in the use of the term "normal." These difficulties are discussed in a clever and illuminating article by Smith,[1] and elsewhere. Nevertheless, standards of reference are inescapable necessities in medicine, since the diagnosis and evaluation of disease depend on recognition of the ways in which sick people differ from the "normal" healthy population. In general, "normal values" for biologic variables (such as blood pressure, serum protein concentration, white-cell count, bleeding time, maximal breathing capacity, and so forth) are established by making measurements on individuals who are not known to have any disease that will affect the variable being measured. The measurement must be made on a group that is large enough in number and sufficiently varied in age, sex, race, body size, and so on to be considered a representative sample of the population as a whole. By constructing a frequency-distribution curve, a graphic description of the data may then be obtained. In the "normal" or theoretical curve (Fig. 1), the values are symmetrically dispersed on each side of the center, and the mean, the mode, and the median all coincide at the central point. In practice, biologic

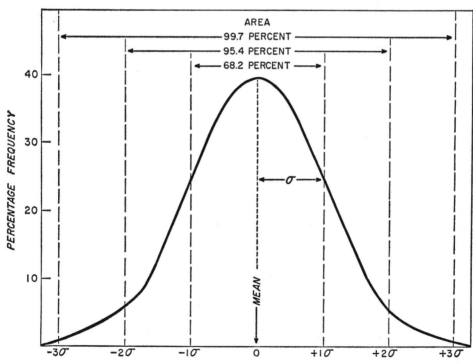

Fig. 1. Theoretical frequency-distribution curve (modified from Smith [1]).

data usually deviate to a greater or lesser extent from this symmetric pattern, and are often asymmetrically distributed about the central area. Several types of frequency distribution occur in nature and can be analyzed by appropriate statistical methods.

The frequency-distribution curve may be narrow or wide. In either case, the degree of dispersion is given by the standard deviation ($\sigma$), since $\pm 1\sigma$ will include 68.2 percent, $\pm 2\sigma$ will include 95.4 percent, and $\pm 3\sigma$ will include 99.7 percent of the values under consideration. Measurements that yield results farther from the mean than $\pm 2\sigma$ will occur by chance in less than 5 percent of instances; measurements that yield results farther from the mean than $\pm 3\sigma$ will occur by chance in less than 1 percent of instances. In the statistical sense, such observations are significant departures from the mean at the 5-percent and at the 1-percent levels, respectively.

When a frequency-distribution curve is constructed from values representing multiple determinations (for example, glucose concentration) made on the same sample of blood or urine, the standard deviation is a measure of the error of the method of measurement. When the frequency-distribution curve is constructed from single determinations made on different individuals or at different times, the dispersion measured by the standard deviation represents a combined effect of the error of the method and the "biologic variation" among different individuals and from one time to another. Usually the biologic variation in the results of a test is much greater than the error due to the method of measurement. Indeed, this must be so if the test or measurement is to have any practical value.

The establishment of standards of reference, or "normal limits," for biologic variables can be reasonably approximated by statistical analysis, cognizance being taken of the expected dispersion in the "normal" population. Nevertheless, the selection of limits is arbitrary and a certain amount of overlap in values between healthy individuals and those with disease is inevitable for many biologic variables. Inasmuch as all the individuals in the population sample used for the establishment of a standard of reference are presumed to be normal, the selection of $\pm 2\sigma$ or even $\pm 3\sigma$ as "limits of normal" will exclude a certain number of healthy individuals from the "normal range." On the other hand, if the limits are set wide enough to include most or all of the normals, a certain number of diseased individuals will be erroneously regarded as normal.

For many measurements, a compromise must be accepted, and values at the extreme ends of the arbitrarily defined normal range must be considered of dubious clinical significance. The statistical approach to the evaluation of laboratory data is discussed further in Unit 2.

In Tables 2 through 6 are given the normal values for many of the tests in use in one large general hospital,[2] together with certain practical considerations in the use of the tests and references to the methods currently employed. The compilation is by no means all-inclusive, and most of these tests, as well as many others, are discussed at greater length in subsequent Units. More detailed tables are available elsewhere.[3]

## REFERENCES

1. H. W. Smith, "Plato and Clementine," *Bull. N. Y. Acad. Med. 23*, 352 (1947).
2. Tables of normal values from the Massachusetts General Hospital, compiled by G. M. Rourke, L. B. Page, M. A. King, W. S. Beck, and L. W. Gaston, adapted from "Normal laboratory values," *New Engl. J. Med. 262*, 84 (1960).
3. F. W. Sunderman and F. Boerner, *Normal Values in Clinical Medicine* (Saunders, Philadelphia, 1949).

Table 2. *Normal blood, plasma, or serum values.*[a]

| Determination | Normal value | Material analyzed | Minimum quantity required [b] (ml) | Note | Method |
|---|---|---|---|---|---|
| Acetone | 0.3–2.0 mg/100 ml | Serum | 2 | | Behre, *J. lab. clin. Med.* *13*, 770 (1928) |
| Alpha amino nitrogen | 3.0–5.5 mg/100 ml | Plasma | 5 | Collect with heparin | Hamilton and Van Slyke, *J. biol. Chem. 150*, 231 (1943) |
| Ammonia | 40–70 µg/100 ml | Blood | | Special processing necessary | McDermott and Adams, *J. clin. Invest. 33*, 1 (1954) |
| Amylase | 4–25 Russell units | Serum | 3 | | Huggins and Russell, *Ann. Surg. 128*, 668 (1948) |
| Ascorbic acid | 0.4–1.5 mg/100 ml | Blood | 7 | Collect with heparin | Roe and Kuether, *J. biol. Chem. 147*, 399 (1943) |
| Ascorbic acid load test | | | | See Table 6 | |
| Bilirubin (van den Bergh test) | One minute: 0.26 mg/100 ml Direct: 0.4 mg/100 ml Total: 1.0 mg/100 ml Indirect is total minus direct | Serum | 5 | | Malloy and Evelyn, *J. biol. Chem. 119*, 481 (1937) |
| Bromsulfalein (BSP) | Less than 5 percent retention | Serum | 3 | Inject 5 mg/kg of dye intravenously; draw blood 45 min after injection | Goebler, *Amer. J. clin. Path. 15*, 452 (1945) |
| BUN | 8–25 mg/100 ml | Serum | 1 | | Skeggs, *Amer. J. clin. Path. 28*, 311 (1957); Marsh, *ibid.*, 681 |
| Calcium | 8.5–10.5 mg/100 ml (Slightly higher in children) | Serum Serum | 5 2 | Do serum protein also Rapid method | Fiske and Logan, *J. biol. Chem. 93*, 211 (1931) Fales, *J. biol. Chem. 204*, 577 (1953) |
| Carbon dioxide content | 26–28 mEq/L 20–26 mEq/L in infants | Serum | 3 | Draw without stasis under oil or in heparinized syringe | Van Slyke and Neill, *J. biol. Chem. 61*, 523 (1924) |
| Carbon dioxide pressure | 35–45 mm Hg | Blood | 5 | Collect and deliver in sealed, heparinized syringe; carbon dioxide determination done on remaining plasma | pH on meter. Carbon dioxide method: see under carbon dioxide content |
| Carotenoids | 1–3 units per ml | Serum | 5 | Vitamin A may be done on same specimen | Josephs, *Bull. Johns Hopk. Hosp. 65*, 112 (1939) |
| Cephalin flocculation | Up to 2+ in 48 hr | Serum | 1 | | Hanger, *J. clin. Invest. 18*, 261 (1939) |
| Chloride | 100–106 mEq/L | Serum | 1 | | Modification of Schales and Schales, *J. biol. Chem. 140*, 879 (1941) |
| Cholesterol | 150–280 mg/100 ml | Serum | 2 | | Bloor, *J. biol. Chem. 24*, 227 (1916) |
| Cholesterol esters | 50–65 percent of cholesterol | Serum | 2 | | Bloor and Knudson, *J. biol. Chem. 27*, 107 (1916) |
| Cholinesterase (pseudocholinesterase) | 0.5 pH units or over/hr for serum 0.7 pH units or over/hr for packed cells | Serum Packed cells | 1 1 | | Michel, *J. lab. clin. Med. 34*, 1564 (1949) |

For values in newborn infants refer to C. A. Smith, *The Physiology of the Newborn Infant* (ed. 3; Thomas, Springfield, 1959). Minimum quantity refers to amount of whole blood required for a single analysis. Micromethods are available for most colorimetric methods.

Table 2. *Normal blood, plasma, or serum values (continued).*

| Determination | Normal value | Material analyzed | Minimum quantity required (ml) | Note | Method |
|---|---|---|---|---|---|
| Congo-red test | More than 60 percent retention in the serum | Serum | 6 | Inject 10 ml of 1 percent Congo-red solution intravenously; draw blood from arm not used for injection 4 and 60 min after injection | Unger *et al., J. clin. I vest. 27*, 111 (1948) |
| Copper | Total: 130–230 $\mu$g/100 ml Free: 4 percent of total Ceruloplasmin is total minus free | Serum | 8 | | Gubler *et al., J. bi Chem. 196*, 209 (195 Gubler, *J. clin. Invest. 3* 405 (1953) |
| Creatinine | 0.7–1.5 mg/100 ml | Serum | 5 | | Peters, *J. biol. Chem. 14* 179 (1942) |
| Cryoglobulins | 0 | Serum | 10 | Collect and transport at 37°C | Barr *et al., Ann. inter Med. 32*, 6 (195 (modified) |
| Glucose | Fasting: 70–100 mg/100 ml | Blood | 2 | Collect with oxalate-fluoride mixture | Folin, *New Engl. J. Me 216*, 727 (1932) Hoffman, *J. biol. Che 120*, 51 (1937) (moc fied for autoanalyzer) |
| Iodine (protein bound or hormonal) | 3.5–8.0 $\mu$g/100 ml | Serum | 12 | Avoid iodide therapy, x-ray contrast media, iodine on skin | Barker, *J. biol. Chem. 17* 715 (1948) |
| Iron | 50–150 $\mu$g/100 ml (higher in males than in females) | Serum | 10 | | Barkan and Walker, *biol. Chem. 135*, (1940) |
| Iron-binding capacity | Serum iron equals approximately 33 percent of capacity | Serum | 12 | Patient must be fasting and serum not icteric | Cartwright and Wintrol *J. clin. Invest. 28*, (1948) |
| Lactic acid | 6–16 mg/100 ml | Blood | 2 | Use special bottles with iodoacetate; draw without stasis; patient must be fasting and at complete rest | Barker and Summerso *J. biol. Chem. 138*, 5 (1941) |
| Lipase | Under 2 units | Serum | 5 | | Comfort and Osterber *J. lab. clin. Med. 2* 271 (1934) |
| Lipid partition: Cholesterol | 150–280 mg/100 ml | Blood | 20 | Done on fasting serum | Comfort and Osterber *J. lab. clin. Med. 2* 271 (1934) |
| Cholesterol esters | 50–65 percent of cholesterol | | | | |
| Phospholipids | 9–16 mg/100 ml as lipid phosphorus | | | | Fiske and Subbarrow, *biol. Chem. 66*, 2 (192 |
| Total fatty acids | 190–420 mg/100 ml | | | | Stoddard and Drury, *biol. Chem. 84*, 7 (1929) |
| Neutral fat | 0–200 mg/100 ml | | | Calculated from above values | |
| Magnesium | 1.5–2.5 mEq/L | Serum | 3 | | Garner, *Biochem. J.* 828 (1946) |
| Nonprotein nitrogen | 15–35 mg/100 ml | Serum | 3 | | Folin, *Lab. Manual Bi Chem.* (ed. 5, 1934), 265 |
| Osmolality | 285–295 mOsm/L | Serum | 5 | In uremia BUN should be done to apply a correction | Crawford and Nicosia, *lab. clin. Med. 40*, 9 (1952) |
| Oxygen saturation (arterial) | 96–100 percent | Blood | 10 | Deliver in sealed heparinized syringe packed in ice | Gordy and Drabkin, *biol. Chem. 227*, 2 (1957) |

Table 2. *Normal blood, plasma, or serum values (continued)*.

| Determination | Normal value | Material analyzed | Minimum quantity required (ml) | Note | Method |
|---|---|---|---|---|---|
| Oxygen content | 15–23 vol percent | Blood | | | |
| Oxygen capacity | 16–24 vol percent | Blood | | Hemoglobin=oxygen capacity divided by 1.34 | Van Slyke and Neill, *J. biol. Chem. 61*, 523 (1924) |
| pH | 7.35–7.45 | Serum | 2 | Collect under oil without stasis; pack in ice; carbon dioxide determination done on same sample; method not suitable if $pCO_2$ elevated | Hastings and Sendroy, *J. biol. Chem. 61*, 695 (1924) |
| Pepsinogen | 100–230 units | Plasma or serum | 2 | | Mirsky, Futterman, Kaplan and Broh-Kahn, *J. lab. clin. Med. 40*, 17 (1952) |
| Phenylalanine | 3–5 mg/100 ml | Serum | 10 | | Armstrong and Tyler, *Clin. Chem. 34*, 565 (1955) |
| Phosphatase (acid) | 0.5–2.0 units, total 0.0–0.7 units, prostatic | Serum | 10 | Must always be drawn just prior to analysis or stored as frozen serum; avoid hemolysis | Fishman and Lerner, *J. biol. Chem. 200*, 89 (1953) |
| Phosphatase (alkaline) | 2.0–4.5 units (infants to 14 units; adolescents to 5 units) | Serum | 3 | | Bodansky, *J. biol. Chem. 101*, 93 (1933) |
| Phosphorus inorganic | 3.0–4.5 mg/100 ml (infants in 1st year up to 6.0 mg/100 ml) | Serum | 1 | Obtain blood in fasting state; serum must be separated promptly from cells | Fiske and Subbarrow, *J. biol. Chem. 66*, 375 (1925) |
| Potassium | 3.5–5.0 mEq/L | Serum | 2 | Serum must be separated promptly from cells (within 1 hr) | Adapted from Berry, Chappell and Barnes, *Indust. Engin. Chem. 18*, 19 (1946) |
| Protein: Total | 6.0–8.0 gm/100 ml | Serum | 1 | Preferably fasting; avoid BSP dye | Lowry and Hastings, *J. biol. Chem. 143*, 257 (1947) |
| Albumin | 4.5–5.5 gm/100 ml | Serum | 3 | | Modified from Gornall, Bardawill and David, |
| Globulin | 1.5–3.0 gm/100 ml | | | Globulin calculated by difference | *J. biol. Chem. 177*, 751 (1949) |
| Paper electrophoresis: Albumin Globulin: Alpha₁ Alpha₂ Beta Gamma | *Percentage of total protein* 45–55 5–8 8–13 11–17 15–25 | Serum | 1 | Quantitated by dye elution and photocolorimetry | Kunkel and Tiselius, *J. gen. Physiol. 35*, 89 (1951) |
| Pyruvic acid | 1.0–2.0 mg/100 ml | Plasma | 2 | Use special iodoacetate tube; avoid stasis | Friedman and Haugen, *J. biol. Chem. 147*, 415 (1943) |
| Sodium | 136–145 mEq/L | Serum | 2 | Flame photometer | Adapted from Berry, Chappell and Barnes, *Indust. Engin. Chem. 18*, 19 (1946) |
| Sulfates | 0.5–1.5 mg/100 ml | Serum | 3 | Avoid hemolysis | Letonoff and Reinhold, *J. biol. Chem. 114*, 147 (1936) |

7

Table 2. *Normal blood, plasma, or serum values* (*continued*).

| Determination | Normal value | Material analyzed | Minimum quantity required (ml) | Note | Method |
|---|---|---|---|---|---|
| Thymol Flocculation Turbidity | Up to 1+ in 24 hr 0–4 units | Serum | 1 | Checked with phosphate buffer of higher molarity to rule out false-positive reaction | Maclagan, *Nature* 154, 670 (1944) |
| Transaminase (SGOT) | 10–40 units | Serum | 1 | | Karmen *et al.*, *J. clin. Invest. 32*, 126 (1955) |
| Urea | 25–52 mg/100 ml | Serum | | *See* BUN (BUN × 2.12 gives urea) | |
| Uric acid | 3.0–6.0 mg/100 ml | Serum | 3 | Must be separated from cells at once, and serum refrigerated | Folin, *J. biol. Chem. 101*, 111 (1933) |
| Vitamin A | 0.3–1.0 units/ml | Serum | 5 | | Josephs, *Bull. John Hopk. Hosp. 65*, 119 (1939) |
| Vitamin A tolerance test | Rise to twice fasting level in 3 to 5 hr | Serum | 5 | Children: 0.1 ml oleopercomorphum/lb body weight Adults: 200,000 units vitamin A (samples taken fasting and at intervals up to 8 hr after test dose) | Josephs, *Bull. John Hopk. Hosp. 65*, 119 (1939) |

Table 3. *Normal urine values.*

| Determination | Normal value | Minimum quantity required | Note | Method |
|---|---|---|---|---|
| Acetone and acetoacetate (quantitative) | 0 | 2 ml | Keep cold | Behre, *J. lab. clin. Med.* *13*, 770 (1928) |
| Alpha amino nitrogen | 64–199 mg/day; not over 1.5 percent of total nitrogen | 24-hr specimen | Preserve with thymol; refrigerate | Hamilton and Van Slyke, *J. biol. Chem. 150*, 231 (1943) |
| Ammonia | 20–70 mEq/L | 24-hr specimen | Collect under toluol | Van Slyke and Cullen, *J. biol. Chem. 24*, 117 (1916) |
| Calcium | Under 150 mg/day | 24-hr specimen | Collect in bottle with 10 ml concentrated HCl | Fiske and Logan, *J. biol. Chem. 93*, 211 (1931) |
| Catechol amines | Epinephrine: under 10 µg/day Norepinephrine: under 100 µg/day | 24-hr specimen | Should be collected with 8 ml concentrated HCl (pH should be between 2.0 and 3.0) | DuToit, *WADC Technical Report* No. 59–175 (1959) |
| Chorionic gonadotropin | 0 | 12-hr concentrated specimen | Volume should not exceed 500 ml | Morris and Hon, *Progr. Gynec. 3*, 142 (1957) |
| Coproporphyrin | 50–250 µg/day Children under 80 lb.: 0–75 µg/day | 24-hr specimen | Collect with 5 gm of sodium carbonate | Schwartz, *J. lab. clin. Med. 37*, 843 (1951) |
| Creatine | Under 100 mg/day or less than 6 percent of creatinine. In pregnancy, up to 12 percent. In children under 1 yr, may equal creatinine; in older children, up to 30 percent of value of creatinine | 24-hr specimen | Preserve with toluol; also order creatinine | Folin, *Lab. Manual Biol. Chem.* (ed. 5, 1933), p. 163 |
| Creatinine | 15–25 mg/kg of body weight per day | 24-hr specimen | Preserve with toluol | Folin, *Lab. Manual Biol. Chem.* (ed. 5, 1933), p. 163 |
| Creatinine clearance | 150–180 L/day per 1.73 $m^2$ of body-surface area | 24-hr specimen | Preserve with toluol | Brod and Sirota, *J. clin. Invest. 27*, 645 (1948) |
| Cystine or cysteine | 0 | 10 ml | Qualitative | Hawk, Oser, and Summerson, *Pract. physiol. Chem.* (ed. 13, 1954), p. 141 |
| Hemoglobin and myoglobin | 0 | Freshly voided sample | Chemical examination with benzidine; spectroscopic examination for differentiation | |
| Homogentisic acid | 0 | Freshly voided sample or 24-hr sample kept cold | Must be refrigerated if not determined at once; test also measures gentisic acid; may therefore be positive in patients on high doses of salicylates | Neuberger, *Biochem. J. 41*, 431 (1947) |
| 5-hydroxyindoleacetic acid | 0 | Freshly voided sample | | Sjoerdsma *et al.*, *J.A.M.A. 159*, 397 (1955) |
| 17-ketosteroids | *Age* *Males* *Females* 10 1–4 mg 1–4 mg 20 6–21 4–16 30 8–26 4–14 50 5–18 3–9 70 2–10 1–7 | 24-hr specimen | Not valid if patient is receiving meprobamate | Vestergaard, *Acta endocri. (Kbh.) 13*, 241 (1953). Normal values taken from Hamburger, *Acta endocri. (Kbh.) 1*, 19 (1948) |
| 11-oxysteroids (17OH) | 2–7 mg/day (women lower than men) | 24-hr specimen | Keep cold; chlorpromazine and related drugs interfere with determination | Peterson *et al.*, *Endocrinology 57*, 594 (1955) |

9

Table 3. *Normal urine values (continued)*.

| Determination | Normal value | Minimum quantity required | Note | Method |
|---|---|---|---|---|
| Lead | To 0.08 $\mu$g/ml or 120 $\mu$g/24 hr | 24-hr specimen | | Bessman and Layne, *lab. clin. Med. 45*, 1 (1955) |
| Phenolsulfon-phthalein (PSP) | At least 25 percent by 15 min; 40 percent by 30 min; 60 percent by 120 min | Total output of urine collected 15, 30, and 120 min after injection | Inject 1 ml (6 mg) intravenously; BSP interferes | Chapman, *New Engl. Med. 214*, 16 (1936) |
| Phenylpyruvic acid | 0 | Freshly voided sample unless quantitation needed | | Kropp and Lang, *Kl. Wschr. 33*, 19 (1955) |
| Phosphorus inorganic | Varies with intake; average 1 gm/day | 24-hr specimen | Collect in bottle with 10 ml concentrated HCl | Fiske and Logan, *J. bi. Chem. 93*, 211 (1931) |
| Pituitary gonadotropins | 5–10 rat units/24 hr for normal men and women; over 25 rat units/24 hr in postmenopausal women | 24-hr specimen | 48-hr specimen preferable if abnormally low value anticipated | Albert, *Fertil. and Ster. 10*, 60 (1959) |
| Porphobilinogen | 0 | 10 ml | Freshly voided specimen | Watson and Schwar. *Proc. Soc. exp. Bi. (N. Y.) 47*, 393 (1941) |
| Pregnancy test | | | *See* chorionic gonadotropin | |
| Protein: Quantitative | 0 | 24-hr specimen | Preserve with toluol; refrigerate | Hawk, Oser, and Su. merson, *Pract. Physi. Chem.* (ed. 13, 195. p. 927 |
| Electrophoresis | 0 | 50 ml | Freshly voided specimen | *See* Protein (Table 2) |
| Sugar: Quantitative | 0 | 24-hr or other timed specimen | Collect with toluol; refrigerate | Somogyi, *J. lab. clin. M. 26*, 1220 (1941) |
| Identification of reducing substances | | 50 ml | Use freshly voided specimen without preservatives | |
| Fructose (quantitative) | 0 | Freshly voided sample | Should be run in conjunction with quantitative total reducing substances or quantitative glucose | Epstein *et al.*, *J. bi. Chem. 178*, 839 (194. |
| Pentose (quantitative) | 0 | Freshly voided sample | | Roe and Rice, *J. bi. Chem. 173*, 507 (194. |
| Titrable acidity | 20–40 mEq/day | 24-hr sample | Collect with toluol; refrigerate | Henderson and Palmer, *biol. Chem. 17*, 3. (1914) |
| Urea clearance | Expressed as percent of normal | Blood and urine; two exactly timed samples of urine | | *See* BUN (Table 2) |
| Urinary pigments | | Freshly voided sample | Work-up includes acid hematins, indoles, porphyrins, melanin, indican, homogentisic acid and phenylpyruvic acid | *See under separate headin.* |
| Urobilinogen | Up to 1.0 Ehrlich unit | 2-hr sample (1–3 p.m.) | | Watson *et al.*, *Amer. clin. Path. 15*, 6 (1944) |

10

Table 4. *Normal hematologic values.*

| Determination | Normal value | Material analyzed | Minimum quantity required [a] (ml) | Note | Method |
|---|---|---|---|---|---|
| Coagulation factors: | | | | | |
| Bleeding time: | | | | | |
| Method I | Below 4½ min | | | | Dukes, *J.A.M.A. 55*, 1185 (1910) |
| Method II | Below 6½ min | | | | Jacobson, *Arch. intern. Med. 92*, 471 (1953) |
| Clotting time | Below 20 min, 4th tube | | 12 | Draw at bedside; use 5 tubes | Lee and White, in Todd and Sanford, *Clin. Diag. by Lab. Methods* (ed. 11, 1948), p. 199 |
| Fibrinogen | 0.15–0.30 gm/100 ml | Plasma | 2 | Collect as for prothrombin content | Cullen and Van Slyke, *J. biol. Chem. 41*, 587 (1920) (modified) |
| Fibrinolysins | 0 | Blood | 2 | Collect as for prothrombin content | Cullen and Van Slyke, *J. biol. Chem. 41*, 587 (1920) (modified) |
| Prothrombin consumption | Over 80 percent prothrombin consumed in 1 hr | Citrated plasma and serum | 2 (citrated) 3 (clotted blood) | Collect in special citrated tube and in clean test tube; note time of drawing; take immediately to laboratory | Stefanini and Crosby, *Blood 5*, 964 (1950) |
| Prothrombin content | 100 percent | Plasma | 2 | Use special oxalate tube; collect rapidly; send to laboratory at once | Quick, *J.A.M.A. 110*, 1658 (1938) |
| Thromboplastin generation test | Controlled with normal plasma | Plasma, serum and platelet | | Special handling of blood necessary | Biggs and Macfarlane, *Human Blood Coagulation* (1957) |
| Cephalin time | 60–70 sec | Plasma | | Special handling of blood necessary | Waaler, *Scand. J. clin. Lab. Invest. 9*, 322 (1957) |
| Antihemophilic globulin assay (AHF) | 50–200 percent | Plasma | | Special handing of blood necessary | Adapted from Waaler, *Scand. J. clin. Lab. Invest. 11* (Supp.), 37 (1959) |
| Plasma thromboplastin component (PTC) assay | 75–125 percent | Plasma | | Special handing of blood necessary | Adapted from Stapp, *Scand. J. clin. Lab. Invest. 10*, 169 (1958) |
| Proaccelerin (Factor V) assay | 75–125 percent | Plasma | | Special handing of blood necessary | Adapted from Owren, *Scand. J. clin. Lab. Invest. 3*, 201 (1951) |
| Specific prothrombin assay | 75–125 percent | Plasma | | Special handing of blood necessary | Owren, *Scand. J. clin. Lab. Invest. 3*, 201 (1951) |
| Stuart factor assay | 75–125 percent | Plasma | | Special handing of blood necessary | Backman, *Thrombosis Diathesis Haemorrhagica* (1958), vol. 2, p. 24 |
| Erythrocyte sedimentation rate: | | | | | |
| Method I | Less than 0.4 mm/min corrected for hematocrit | | 5 | Use heparin as anticoagulant | Rourke and Ernstene, *J. clin. Invest. 8*, 545 (1930) |
| Method II (screening purposes) | Less than 20 mm in 1 hr | | 5 | Use double oxalate or sequestrene tube | Similar to Wintrobe and Landsberg, *Amer. J. med. Sci. 189*, 102 (1935) (differs in use of 4-mm tube) |

[a] Minimum quantity refers to amount of whole blood required for a single analysis.

Table 4. *Normal hematologic values* (*continued*).

| Determination | Normal value | Material analyzed | Minimum quantity required (ml) | Note | Method |
|---|---|---|---|---|---|
| Hematocrit | Males: 42–50 percent Females: 40–48 percent | | 2 | Use double oxalate tube | Wintrobe, *Clin. Hemat* (ed. 4, 1956), p. 366 |
| Hemoglobin: | Males: 13–16 gm/100 ml Females: 12–14 gm/100 ml | Blood | 0.05 | | Wintrobe, *Clin. Hemat* (ed. 4, 1956), p. 366 |
| Electrophoresis for abnormal hemoglobins | 0 | Blood | 5 | Collect with anticoagulant | Singer, *Amer. J. Med. 18* 633 (1955) Chernoff, *New Engl. J Med. 253*, 322 (1955) |
| Fetal hemoglobin (alkali resistant) | Less than 2 percent | Blood | 5 | Collect with anticoagulant | Singer, *Amer. J. Med. 18* 633 (1955) Chernoff, *New Engl. J Med. 253*, 322 (1955) |
| Hemoglobins, met- and sulf- | 0 | Blood | 5 | Use heparinized blood | Michel and Harris, *J. lab clin. Med. 25*, 44 (1940) |
| L.E. (lupus erythematosus) preparation: | | | | | |
| Method I | Negative | Blood | 5 | Use blood in heparin | Hargreaves *et al.*, *Proc Mayo Clin. 24*, 23 (1949) |
| Method II | Negative | Blood | 5 | Use defibrinated blood; Method II more sensitive but positive results in diseases other than lupus may be more frequent | Barnes *et al.*, *J. inves Derm. 14*, 397 (1950) |
| Leukocyte alkaline phosphatase | 15–40 mg phosphorus liberated per hour per $10^{10}$ cells | Isolated blood leukocytes | | Special handling of blood necessary | Beck and Valentine, *J lab. clin. Med. 38*, 3 (1951) |
| Methemalbumin | 0 | Serum | 3 | | Fairley, *Quart. J. Med* (N.S.) *10*, 38 (1941) |
| Osmotic fragility of red cells | Increased if hemolysis occurs in over 0.5 percent NaCl; decreased if hemolysis is incomplete in 0.3 percent NaCl | Blood | 5 | Use heparin as anticoagulant | Dacie, *The Hemolytic Ane mias* (1954), p. 476 |
| Platelet count | 250,000 to 450,000/mm³ | Blood | 0.05 | Use special sequestrene tube | Brecher *et al.*, *Amer. clin. Path. 23*, 15 (195 |
| Red-cell corpuscular values: | | | | | Wintrobe, *Clin. Hema* (ed. 4, 1956), p. 366 |
| Mean corpuscular volume (MCV) | 80–94 $\mu^3$ | | | | (Hematocrit × 10)/red cells ($10^6$/mm³) |
| Mean corpuscular hemoglobin (MCH) | 27–32 $\mu\mu$g | | | | Hemoglobin (gm) × 10 red cells ($10^6$/mm³) |
| Mean corpuscular hemoglobin concentration (MCHC) | 33–38 percent | | | | Hemoglobin (gm) × 10 hematocrit |
| Reticulocyte count | 0.5–1.5 percent of red cells | | | | Brecher, *Amer. J. cli Path. 19*, 895 (1949) |
| Vitamin B$_{12}$ | 200–800 $\mu\mu$g/ml | Serum | | Special handling of blood necessary | Adapted from *Difco Mar ual* (ed. 9, 1953), p. 22 |

Table 5. *Normal cerebrospinal-fluid values.*

| Determination | Normal value | Minimum quantity required (ml) | Note | Method |
|---|---|---|---|---|
| Initial pressure | 70–180 mm of water | | | |
| Cell count | 0–5 mononuclear cells | 0.5 | | |
| Chloride | 120–130 mEq/L | 0.5 | 20 mEq/L higher than serum; obtain serum for comparison | *See* Chloride (Table 2) |
| Protein: | | | | |
| Lumbar | 15–45 mg/100 ml | 1 | | Adapted from Ayer *et al.*, *Arch. Neurol. Psychiat.* *(Chicago)* 26, 1038 (1931) |
| Cisternal | 12–25 mg/100 ml | | | |
| Ventricular | 5–15 mg/100 ml | | | |
| Electrophoresis | Predominantly albumin | 10 | Concentrated by dialysis against polyvinyl pyrrolidone in barbital buffer | *See* Table 2 |
| Glucose | 50–75 mg/100 ml | 0.5 | 20 mg/100 ml less than blood; compare with blood | *See* Glucose (Table 2) |
| Colloidal gold test | 0000000000 | 0.1 | | Wuth and Faupel, *Bull. Johns Hopk. Hosp. 40*, 297 (1927) |
| Bilirubin | 0 | 2 | | Adapted from Malloy and Evelyn, *J. biol. Chem. 119*, 481 (1937) |

Table 6. *Miscellaneous normal values.*

| Determination | Normal value | Minimum quantity required | Note | Method |
|---|---|---|---|---|
| Ascorbic acid load test | 0.2–2.0 mg/hr in control sample<br>29–49 mg/hr after loading | Urine—an approximate 1½-hr sample<br>Urine—2 timed samples of about 2 hr each | Administer 500 mg ascorbic acid orally | Harvard Fatigue Labs, *Laboratory Manual* (1945) |
| Chylous fluid | | Fresh sample | Systematic examination includes pH, presence of fat, etc. | Todd, Sanford, and Wells, *Clin. Diag.* (ed. 12, 1953), p. 624 |
| D-xylose absorption | 5–8 gm/5 hr | Urine—5-hr sample<br>Blood—5 ml 5 hr after ingestion of 25 gm D-xylose | For test directions see Benson *et al.*, *New Engl. J. Med.* 256, 335 (1957) | Roe and Rice, *J. biol Chem.* 173, 507 (1948) |
| Duodenal drainage | | | pH should be in proper range with minimum amount of gastric juice present | |
|   pH | 5.5–7.5 | 1 drop | | |
|   Amylase | Over 1200 Russell units | 1 ml | | Huggins and Russell, *Ann. Surg.* 128, 668 (1948) |
|   Trypsin | Values from 35 to 160 percent "normal" | 1 ml | | Anderson and Early, *Amer. J. Dis. Child.* 63 891 (1942) |
|   Viscosity | 3 min or under | 4 ml | Run ice cold in 34-sec viscosimeter | |
| Renal calculi | | Representative sample | | *See* Calcium, Magnesium Uric acid (Table 2) |
| Stool fat | Less than 5 gm in 24 hr or less than 4 percent of measured fat intake in a 3-day period as determined by carmine marker | 24-hr or 3-day specimen, preferably with carmine markers | | Van de Kramer *et al.*, *J biol. Chem.* 177, 374 (1949) |
| Stool nitrogen | Less than 2 gm/day or 10 percent of urinary nitrogen | 24-hr or 3-day specimen | | Peters and Van Slyke *Quant. Clin. Chem.* (1932), vol. 2, p. 353 |
| Synovial fluid:<br>  Mucin | Type 1 or 2 | 1 ml fresh synovial fluid | Graded as:<br>Type 1 — tight clump<br>Type 2 — soft clump<br>Type 3 — soft clump that breaks up<br>Type 4 — cloudy — no clump | |
|   Glucose | Not less than 20 mg/100 ml lower than simultaneously drawn blood sugar | 1 ml | Collect with oxalate fluoride mixture | *See* Glucose (Table 2) |
| Tubeless gastric analysis:<br>  Diagnex Blue | Positive for free gastric HCl if over 0.6 mg in 2 hr | 1 1-hr pretest urine sample<br>1 2-hr posttest urine sample | | Segal, *Monographs or Therapy* 2, 147 (1957) |

# Unit 2

# The Evaluation of Laboratory Data

The clinical assessment of a patient involves the evaluation of laboratory data and their meaning in the context of all the other clinical findings. An abnormal value is one that lies outside the range of variation due to the distribution of values in the population of healthy individuals. The weight to be attributed to an abnormal value is the problem of the clinician. He may require a test to be repeated, or order other clinical or laboratory examinations. Sometimes qualitative tests alone may be sufficient to answer a clinical question; in other situations, semiquantitative or quantitative tests may be of greater value.

Quantitative laboratory data must be both precise and accurate. *Precision* may be operationally defined as reproducibility and requires that repeated measurements give closely comparable results. *Accuracy* includes the notion of precision with the added concept that the result must give a correct measure of the variable under consideration. For example, in certain chemical determinations, interfering substances or technical errors can produce consistent, as opposed to fluctuating, deviations from the correct result. Such results will be precise, but inaccurate.

The control of accuracy and precision is a particular problem in chemical and bioassay procedures. Each laboratory usually provides its own standardized solutions and biologically active preparations, and there is no easy way to achieve uniform standards of accuracy on an extensive scale. International standards are now available for many pharmacologic agents, and have superseded the use of animal units. International standards for a wide variety of biochemical and other biologic preparations for use on an international scale in diagnostic laboratories are urgently needed. If they were available, it would be possible to establish universal standards of precision and accuracy.

NUMBERS AND DATA. Measurement implies the use of a scale. Depending on the empirical operations, we may be forced to use one or another of several types of scale. Even qualitative tests imply measurement of a sort. For example, it may be recorded that a particular patient belongs to blood group B. This is the most primitive kind of measurement, based on identity, and in Stevens's terms is measurement on a "nominal" scale.[1] A more powerful scale of measurement is one based on order, such as is involved where objects can be ranked—for example, when data are expressed as scores (0 to ++++) or grades. This is called measurement on an "ordinal" scale. The majority of laboratory determinations depend upon the determination of ratios, and give rise to data expressed in terms of a "ratio" scale. Such data include measurements of time, weight, density of color, specific gravity, and so on. Sometimes the units are, in effect, logarithmic, as

15

when serial dilutions are made in serologic tests, or in tests for fibrinolysis, and the result is expressed in terms of the number of tubes showing the effect. Much ingenuity has been expended in finding measurable quantities. The osmotic-fragility test, for example, measures in terms of NaCl concentration a function of the shape of the red cell. In the field of blood coagulation, the concentrations for many factors are expressed in terms of the *time* that elapses between the onset of a reaction and a qualitative end point, the clotting of fibrinogen.

## Statistical Concepts

### STANDARD DEVIATION

The standard deviation, $\sigma$, is used as a measure of the dispersion, or spread, of a set of values, assuming them to be normally distributed. If the dispersion is of a series of determinations upon a single specimen, then $\sigma$ is a measure of the precision of the method. On the other hand, where technical and statistical errors are minimized by multiple estimations upon each individual, $\sigma$ may be used as a measure of the dispersion of values of the factor measured among a population of normal persons. When a single determination is performed on each of a group of normal persons, $\sigma$ is a measure of the dispersion due to both factors combined, that is, error of the method and spread among individuals.

Neither the true value of a mean nor the true value of $\sigma$ is ever determined with absolute accuracy. The value of $\sigma$ can be approximately determined from a sample of the population studied. The following sequence of steps can be used in estimating $\sigma$. First the mean of the observed values ($\bar{x}$) is calculated, according to the formula

$$\bar{x} = \frac{\Sigma x}{n},$$

where $x$ stands for any of the observed values, and $n$ is the total number of observations. The deviation of each observed value, $(x - \bar{x})$, is calculated by subtracting the mean from it; it may be either positive or negative. Each value of $(x - \bar{x})$ is then squared, giving $(x - \bar{x})^2$, and the sum $\Sigma(x - \bar{x})^2$ is obtained. The best estimate of $\sigma$ is then calculated from

$$\sigma = \sqrt{\frac{\Sigma(x - \bar{x})^2}{n - 1}}.$$

A worked example is given in Table 7.

Table 7. *Example of the calculation of the standard deviation from 11 determinations of the red-cell count.*

| Red-cell count, $x$ ($10^6$/mm$^3$) | Deviation from mean, $x - \bar{x}$ | $(x - \bar{x})^2$ |
|---|---|---|
| 3.6 | +0.1 | 0.01 |
| 3.7 | +0.2 | 0.04 |
| 3.2 | −0.3 | 0.09 |
| 3.5 | 0.0 | 0.00 |
| 3.6 | +0.1 | 0.01 |
| 3.2 | −0.3 | 0.09 |
| 3.5 | 0.0 | 0.00 |
| 3.4 | −0.1 | 0.01 |
| 3.6 | +0.1 | 0.01 |
| 3.5 | 0.0 | 0.00 |
| 3.5 | 0.0 | 0.00 |
| $\Sigma x = 38.3$ | | $\Sigma(x - \bar{x})^2 = 0.26$ |

$$n = 11, \quad \bar{x} = \frac{\Sigma x}{n} = \frac{38.3}{11} = 3.5,$$

$$\sigma = \sqrt{\left[\frac{\Sigma(x - \bar{x})^2}{n - 1}\right]} = \sqrt{\left(\frac{0.26}{10}\right)} = \sqrt{0.026}$$

$$= \pm 0.16 \times 10^6/\text{mm}^3$$

The ratio of the estimated standard deviation to the estimated mean is called the coefficient of variation (C.V.) and is expressed as a percentage:

$$\text{C.V.} = \frac{\sigma}{\bar{x}} \, 100 \text{ percent.}$$

The C.V. expresses the dispersion of values about the mean when the mean is expressed as 100 percent. The C.V., like $\sigma$, may describe the dispersion of normal values about a mean, or it may express the precision of a set of determinations upon a sample.

### CONFIDENCE AND FIDUCIAL LIMITS

Since the true value of a mean cannot be absolutely determined, but can only be estimated, it is sometimes desirable to define terms in such a way that no single value is regarded as a best estimate of the mean, but, instead, that the interval within which it probably lies is precisely delimited. A number of logically distinct approaches to this problem have been adopted. One, the theory of "confidence limits," is based on probability statements about the location of the true mean. Another, that of "fiducial limits," is based upon calculations of the probability of obtaining the observed sample from the whole universe of (hypothetically) possible values of the true mean.

When the theories of confidence and fiducial limits were first developed, many statisticians regarded them as equivalent. As Kendall[2] remarks in the papers written between 1930 and 1938 "confidence limits" and "fiducial limits" were often used in the same sense, even in the titles of papers, and they appeared to lead to identical results. In particular, it should be noted that the "fiducial limits" of a certain frequency distribution (the Poisson distribution) tabulated by Garwood,[3] which are used here in the preparation of tables of limits for the differential white-cell count (for small percentages) and for the reticulocyte count in Unit 9, are now classified by Kendall[2] as confidence limits.

The terminology of fiducial limits is commonly used in the pharmacologic literature, owing to the fact that the problem of estimating limits for the *difference of two means*, where the samples may differ not only in means but also in variances, is not amenable to treatment by the theory of confidence limits, and requires the fiducial theory. For this reason, the estimates of precision used in the statistics of biologic assay are stated in terms of fiducial limits.

## Precision and Accuracy of Laboratory Procedures

It is necessary to have some means of determining the accuracy and precision of all types of laboratory measurement. In general, the statistical methods used for this purpose vary with the scale of measurement. Most often, this is a ratio scale of number, color, weight, volume, time, or the like. Where the numbers are very large, as with automatic counting devices, the results can be treated by ordinary statistical methods. With smaller numbers, special statistical treatment is required, as in the red-cell count, the white-cell count, the differential white-cell count, and the reticulocyte count.

In controlling the precision of chemical determinations, the objective is to reject those results in which there is evidence that more than the permitted amount of error has occurred. Otherwise results are taken at face value. The limits within which a chemical determination should vary are narrow. With hematologic counts, however, the limits within which the true value lies are wider. Thus, the result of a chemical determination can be expressed by the single value obtained. The standard deviation from a group of observations will be determined only to establish limits for control charts.

With hematologic counts, results are so imprecise that the result is best expressed in terms of confidence limits within which the true value lies. These limits are quite wide even when they are based on $\pm 2\sigma$. If they were to be based on $\pm 3\sigma$, they would be so wide as to be meaningless. Thus, confidence limits based on $2\sigma$ must be used, even though this means that a 5-percent probability of error is tolerated.

In clinical chemistry, standard solutions of known composition are analyzed, and the standard deviation of the results of many such analyses is used to calculate the limits of permissible variation. Since these methods are quite accurate, limits based on $\pm 3\sigma$ can be used. Results outside of these limits should occur by chance in less than 1 percent of instances.

17

Precision depends upon the reproducibility of results. The term is somewhat ambiguous, inasmuch as the conditions of reproducibility may be variously defined. In general, the standard deviation of a set of values from a set of determinations upon the same material is a measure of the reproducibility of a measurement. A very popular way of estimating $\sigma$ for this purpose is by the routine performance of duplicate measurements on each one of a number of specimens. This is interpreted by means of the formula

$$\sigma = \sqrt{\frac{\Sigma d^2}{2n}},$$

where $d$ is the difference between duplicates and $n$ is the number of specimens.

The method of duplicates as usually employed gives rise to a measure of the reproducibility of results obtained *at the same time by the same analyst.* Day-to-day variations are not detected. Thus the duplicate estimations are not fully independent, for technical reasons.

A different method of estimating $\sigma$ is to perform measurements on several aliquots from one sample. The formula given earlier is used:

$$\sigma = \sqrt{\frac{\Sigma(x - \bar{x})^2}{n - 1}}.$$

Here $(x - \bar{x})$ is the difference between the value for each measurement $x$ and the mean of all the measurements $\bar{x}$ and $n$ is the number of aliquots.

The results obtained will have more validity if the determinations are performed on different days and if the analyst does not treat the sample differently from routine analyses.

Recently, a special statistical method has been applied to the comparison of the precision of two *different* analytic methods, where only *one* estimation on each sample is done by each method (numerous samples are estimated).[4] This may have value where the analytic techniques are particularly laborious.

To achieve quality control in clinical chemistry, control charts may be used as an expedient to obtain simultaneously information about accuracy and precision of quantitative chemical methods. Control charts depend upon the use of the concept of the standard deviation as a measure of precision, and upon the use of chemical standards.

The procedure for their use is as follows. Daily, or with each batch of determinations, the analyst includes a specimen, usually of serum, the chemical composition of which is accurately known, but which is diluted by a factor unknown to him. When his result is obtained, and corrected by the dilution factor, it should be identical with, or close to, the known value of the standard. The permitted variation is arbitrarily taken as $\pm 3\sigma$, corresponding to limits of $100 \pm$ C.V. on a percentage basis, where $\sigma$ (or C.V.) is based upon sets of determinations with good technique and established chemical methods.

The control chart plots results of determinations of the standard as ordinates. The abscissa is time (for the date of the determination). Horizontal lines are drawn corresponding to the upper and lower permitted variations (for example, those listed by Benenson *et al.*[5] and by Varley[6]). Otherwise, they may be computed as has already been described, from the coefficient of variation for the repeated observations upon a standard, using the limits of $100 \pm 3$ C.V. Figure 2 is a control chart for a thymol turbidity test. The example illustrates how the use of a control chart can detect deterioration of reagents. In general, the permitted variations for inorganic constituents is smaller than that for organic constituents. Variations as wide as $\pm 10$ percent are permissible for certain organic substances, but variations no greater than $\pm 3$ percent are possible with many chemical methods. The variations toler-

18

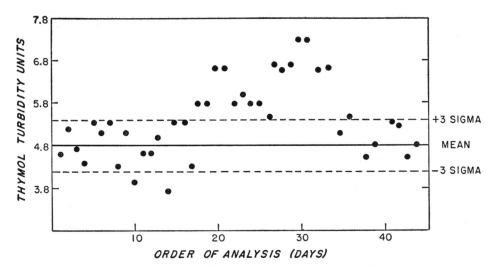

Fig. 2. A control chart showing changes due to deterioration of thymol turbidity buffer (modified from Benenson, Thompson, and Klugerman [5]).

ated by Belk and Sunderman,[7] though excessively lax, were often exceeded in their survey of clinical laboratories in 1947.

Another way of constructing a control chart uses a short-cut calculation [8] which may be made as follows. Arrange a series of $N$ results in chronologic sequence (as on the control chart), and repeat the first two results at the end of the series. The graph will be zigzag, with certain of the points at maxima or "peaks" and certain others at minima or "troughs." If the sum of all the results that occur at "trough" positions is subtracted from the sum of all the results that occur at "peak" positions, and the difference is multiplied by $16/9N$, the result is equal to $\sigma$. Lines drawn at $\pm 3\sigma$ from the known value can then be used as control lines.

Observations on a standard that falls outside the control limits are "out of control" and should be rejected as due to avoidable error. (All analyses belonging to this batch should be repeated.) Approximately 99 percent of observations should be "in control," in the absence of avoidable error.

Standard solutions for some substances are supplied by the College of American Pathologists (Prudential Plaza, Chicago

1, Illinois) and by the National Bureau of Standards (NBS Circular 552, U.S. Government Printing Office, Washington, D.C.).[9]

### THE DISTRIBUTION OF NORMAL VALUES

So far as biochemical determinations are concerned, the distribution of values among the general healthy population occupies a certain range, and the standard deviation will be larger than that due to permitted variation alone. This distribution tends to be skew, that is, the mode, or value corresponding to the peak of the distribution curve, is not central. Therefore there is difficulty in stating a normal range in terms of the mean and the standard deviation. King and Wootton [10] publish ranges of normal values within which 80 percent and 99 percent, respectively, should lie, without reference to any mean normal value.

### PRECISION IN HEMATOLOGY

For reasons that have been discussed previously, with the less accurate measurement used in hematology, a probability of 95 percent of an accurate location of the true count is regarded as satisfactory, if all reasonable efforts have been made to avoid technical error. In doubtful cases, a count can be repeated. Confidence limits locate the true value for an individual result with the stated degree of probability. In Unit 9, such confidence limits are given for the differential white-cell count and for the reticulocyte count. In white-cell and red-cell counts, the standard deviation is equal to the square root of the number of cells counted. The coefficient of variation is given by

$$\text{C.V.} = \frac{100}{\sqrt{(\text{No. of cells counted})}}.$$

This is further dealt with in Unit 4.

To demonstrate the statistical significance of a difference between two values of a differential or reticulocyte count, it is sufficient, for practical purposes, that one should be outside the confidence limits of the other. Two red- or white-cell counts are significantly different (at the 95-percent level) if

$$\frac{A - B}{\sqrt{(A + B)}} \geqslant 2,$$

where $A$ and $B$ are the numbers of cells enumerated.

## REFERENCES

1. S. S. Stevens, "Measurement and man," *Science 127,* 383 (1958).
2. M. G. Kendall, *The Advanced Theory of Statistics* (ed. 3; Hafner, New York, 1951), vol. 2, pp. 62–95.
3. F. Garwood, "Fiducial limits for the Poisson distribution," *Biometrika 28,* 437 (1936).
4. C. White, "Comparison of precision of two methods of measurement, with special reference to the measurement of hemoglobin," *Amer. J. clin. Path. 26,* 1277 (1956).
5. A. S. Benenson, H. L. Thompson, and M. R. Klugerman, "Application of laboratory controls in clinical chemistry," *Amer. J. clin. Path. 25,* 575 (1955).
6. H. Varley, *Practical Clinical Biochemistry* (Interscience, New York, 1958), p. 28.
7. W. P. Belk and F. W. Sunderman, "A survey of the accuracy of chemical analysis in the clinical laboratory," *Amer. J. clin. Path. 17,* 853 (1947).
8. B. Woolf, "Rapid estimation of standard deviations," *Nature 170,* 631 (1952).
9. B. Copeland, "The standard deviation: A practical means for the measurement and control of the precision of chemical laboratory determinations," *Amer. J. clin. Path. 27,* 551 (1958).
10. E. J. King and I. D. P. Wootton, *Microanalysis in Medical Biochemistry* (ed. 3; Grune and Stratton, New York, 1956).

## RECOMMENDED READING

11. A. B. Hill, *Principles of Medical Statistics* (ed. 6; Oxford University Press, New York, 1955).
12. D. Mainland, *The Treatment of Clinical and Laboratory Data. An Introduction to Statistical Ideas and Methods for Medical and Dental Workers* (Oliver and Boyd, London, 1938).
13. R. A. Fisher, *Statistical Methods for Research Workers* (ed. 11; Oliver and Boyd, London, 1950).
14. L. Bernstein and M. Weatherall, *Statistics for Medical and Other Biological Students* (Williams and Wilkins, Baltimore, 1952).

# Unit 3

## Collection of Blood Samples

The major components of blood and tissue are similar except that blood has no connective tissue. Since blood perfuses all tissues, crystalloid substances liberated by many different types of cells may be found in blood by appropriate methods. A sample of blood may, in fact, be regarded as a "biopsy specimen" of the most widely distributed, most representative, and most easily obtained "tissue" in the body. In addition to being a fluid that is representative of the whole body, blood exhibits many unique features not shared by other tissues. Among its unique characteristics are rapid changes in number and type of circulating cells which occur in response to a wide variety of stimuli. Many of the changes that occur in blood in response to disease are nonspecific. Nevertheless, some deviation from normal in one or more of the measurable constituents or activities of blood is detectable in most human illnesses. It is not surprising, therefore, that a majority of the currently used diagnostic laboratory procedures are "blood tests."

In obtaining blood samples for the laboratory, special requirements must be met for certain tests. Some tests require whole blood while many others are carried out on fractions of blood such as plasma, serum, or cells. For certain tests, preservatives or anticoagulants must be added at the time the samples are obtained. A few tests require arterial blood, although venous or capillary blood is satisfactory for the majority. A knowledge of these special requirements must be a part of the physician's equipment, since failure to observe the necessary precautions in obtaining blood samples is an important source of erroneous and misleading laboratory values. Many of these special requirements are summarized in the Tables of Normal Values in Unit 1. They are also discussed at greater length in subsequent units in connection with the individual tests.

*Fasting blood samples.* Only a few of the tests commonly used in clinical medicine require that blood samples be drawn with patients in the fasting state. These include *blood-glucose* and *serum-lipid* measurements, in which elevated values are obtained after meals, and *serum inorganic phosphorus* measurements, in which values are depressed after meals. Slight elevations in blood urea, creatinine, and other nitrogenous constituents of serum may also be found following meals, but, except in patients on very high-protein diets, these changes are not of sufficient magnitude to require that blood be obtained in the fasting state. None of the blood tests commonly used in clinical medicine is compromised by allowing patients to drink water. The routine deprivation of all food and water when blood is to be drawn for chemical determinations produces needless discomfort. Water deprivation is, of course, required in tests of urine-concentrating ability (Units 20 and 21).

*Promptness of examination.* When labile constituents of blood are to be meas-

21

ured, tests must be performed immediately after the sample is drawn. Examples of tests with this requirement are the prothrombin-consumption test and measurement of serum acid phosphatase. Determinations of blood gases require special handling of blood samples and must be performed soon after the samples are drawn, before significant loss by diffusion occurs. In the case of pH determinations, delay is associated with a progressive change in value due to cellular glycolysis. The erythrocyte sedimentation rate must be performed within 3 hr after the blood sample is drawn; otherwise an erroneously low value is found. For some tests, serum must be separated promptly from cells, since the substance being measured diffuses out of cells and enters the serum. Examples are measurements of potassium and uric acid concentrations in serum.

### Varieties of Blood Samples

WHOLE BLOOD. When whole blood is obtained by capillary puncture for hematologic counts, it is usually processed before it has a chance to clot. If any delay is necessary, an anticoagulant must be used. Whole blood collected with an anticoagulant is used for a variety of chemical and hematologic tests. The choice of the anticoagulant is dictated by the test for which the blood is to be used. This is discussed below. Clotted blood is often preferred for blood typing and cross-matching, since the cells keep well in their own serum, and can be teased out of the clot as needed. Either venous or capillary blood may be used for this purpose.

PLASMA. Plasma is obtained from whole blood collected with an anticoagulant. It contains all the stable components of blood except the cells.

SERUM. Serum is obtained from clotted or defibrinated blood, and contains all the stable constituents of plasma except fibrinogen. Serum may be prepared by introducing whole blood into a clean test tube containing no anticoagulant, and allowing it to clot and undergo clot retraction. If serum is needed promptly, clot retraction can be accelerated by incubating the tube at 37.5°C for 30 min. Serum and cells should always be separated as soon as possible after the clot has retracted. Serum is used for a wide variety of chemical and immunologic tests.

DEFIBRINATED BLOOD. Blood may be defibrinated by introducing it into an Erlenmeyer flask containing glass beads. The volume of the flask should be about 10 times that of the blood. One glass bead, 3 or 4 mm in diameter, should be used for each milliliter of blood. The sample is gently rotated for 10 or 15 min, until the beads are clumped in a ball of fibrin, or until they no longer "sing" during rotation. Slight hemolysis may occur from the trauma of agitation, but it is minimized by gentleness in rotation. The procedure can be carried out under sterile conditions when necessary. Defibrinated blood may be centrifuged for separation of serum from cells. To defibrinate capillary blood, a sample is collected by allowing blood to drip from the puncture site into a serologic test tube. The blood is then gently agitated with a wooden applicator until fibrin is visible on the applicator. This procedure is somewhat more traumatic than the technique described above and usually results in moderate hemolysis. Defibrinated blood is used for a variety of immunologic, bacteriologic, and chemical tests, and for blood-grouping studies. Satisfactory morphologic studies can be made on samples of defibrinated blood, but it is not satisfactory for cell counts, because some of the red cells are destroyed by mechanical agitation.

### Anticoagulants

A variety of anticoagulants are available for use in collecting blood samples.

The majority, including citrate, oxalate, and EDTA, act by binding calcium, while others, such as heparin, have more complex mechanisms of action. The special requirements of many tests dictate which anticoagulant should be used.

*Heparin* is a valuable anticoagulant in certain biologic studies but is not required in general laboratory procedures. It is expensive and prevents coagulation for only a limited period. Commercial heparin solution usually contains 1000 U.S.P. Units or approximately 10 mg of heparin per milliliter. For preservation of 10 ml of blood, 0.1 ml (or 1 mg) of this solution is necessary.

*Ethylene diamine tetraacetic acid (EDTA)*, available as Sequesterene or Versene, is a valuable anticoagulant for certain purposes.[1] This substance acts by chelating calcium and also inhibits the conversion of fibrinogen to fibrin. As an anticoagulant, it is especially useful for the separation of platelets for transfusion purposes and for concentration of the white cells for histologic or biochemical studies. The degenerative changes usually seen in the white cells when other anticoagulants are used are less striking when EDTA is used. One milligram of EDTA will keep 1 ml of blood from coagulation (0.005 to 0.01 ml of 10-percent solution for each milliliter of blood).

*Potassium oxalate* is usually used for chemical analyses of whole blood, plasma, or red blood cells. When a 20-percent solution is used, 0.01 ml is necessary for each milliliter of blood. Bottles containing the necessary amount may be prepared in quantities for convenience. If the oxalate solution in the bottle dries, it is still satisfactory. It is not advisable to use the 20-percent potassium oxalate for hematocrit determinations because potassium oxalate shrinks the cells. At a concentration of 200 mg/100 ml of whole blood, the shrinkage of the hematocrit is approximately 8 percent. Accordingly, the reading of the volume of red cells must be multiplied by the factor 1.08 to get the correct value. It is necessary to use the exact proportions of blood and anticoagulant if this correction is to be used.

*Balanced oxalate mixture.* A mixture of ammonium and potassium oxalates is commonly used as an anticoagulant for hematologic counts. Ammonium oxalate alone causes swelling, and potassium oxalate alone causes shrinkage of red cells. However, a "balanced" mixture containing 3 parts of ammonium oxalate and 2 parts of potassium oxalate causes no change in red-cell volume. Two milligrams of this mixture is used for each milliliter of blood.

Balanced oxalate mixture may be prepared as follows: 1.2 gm of crystalline ammonium oxalate and 0.8 gm of potassium oxalate are dissolved in distilled water with the aid of heat, and water is added to make a final volume of 100 ml. The solution can then be pipetted into test tubes using 0.1 ml of the 2-percent oxalate solution (2 mg of mixed oxalate) for each milliliter of blood. The test tubes are then dried in a desiccator or by gentle heating in a drying oven until all water is driven off. By using dry oxalate, dilution of the blood samples is prevented. Drying must be done at a temperature less than 180°C, since at higher temperatures ammonium oxalate is broken down.

It is common practice to prepare tubes with balanced oxalate in quantities, using 0.5 ml of oxalate solution (sufficient for 5 ml of blood) in each tube.

Because of its nitrogen content, balanced oxalate cannot be used when any chemical test involving nitrogen determination is to be done. It is also unsatisfactory when morphologic studies of blood cells are to be made. It is usually used when blood is obtained for determination of hemoglobin, hematocrit, sedimentation rate, and hematologic counts.

### Preservation of Blood Samples

Many of the constituents of blood undergo rapid deterioration as soon as they are removed from the body. Some of these labile factors, including complement, immune bodies, fibrinogen, and other coagulation factors, certain enzymes, uric acid, and other substances, can be preserved for weeks or months in plasma or serum that is promptly frozen and kept at −18°C or below. Clotted blood remains satisfactory for blood-grouping studies for several days when kept at icebox temperature (4°C). Methods of preserving blood for transfusion are not discussed here.

FLUORIDE-OXALATE MIXTURE. To prevent coagulation and arrest cellular glycolysis in samples where glucose concentration is to be determined, a mixture of sodium fluoride and potassium oxalate must be added at the time the blood is drawn. This mixture can be conveniently prepared as follows: 10 gm of potassium oxalate and 10 gm of sodium fluoride are diluted to 100 ml with distilled water. The mixture is shaken and filtered. It can then be pipetted into test tubes or bottles and dried by gentle heating. Five-tenths milliliter of the solution is sufficient for 10 ml of blood.

Various other preservative anticoagulant mixtures are available. Mixtures of sodium fluoride and thymol [2] or monochlorobenzine and fluoride [3] may be used when samples of blood for determination of glucose, urea, creatinine, and other nitrogenous constituents must be sent through the mails. They will delay bacterial breakdown for up to 3 or 4 days. A mixture of oxalate and iodoacetate must be used when lactic or pyruvic acid concentration is determined.

### Obtaining Blood Samples

VENIPUNCTURE. Good technique in venipuncture is a surgical art that causes only moderate discomfort to the patient. It is a simple procedure which can be learned rapidly, but it is too often performed in a haphazard manner. Sterile syringes and needles should be used.

With good technique and a sharp needle, the same vein may be used for scores of venipunctures without damage to the vein and without undue distress to the patient. Prolonged periods—more than 1 or 2 min—of application of the tourniquet are to be avoided since there is progressive hemoconcentration, which is roughly proportional to the time the tourniquet is applied. Vigorous pulling on the plunger of the syringe collapses the vein, may cause air to enter the syringe, and may produce hemolysis of the blood sample. Complications of venipuncture for collection of blood include syncope, continued bleeding, the formation of hematomas, and, rarely, thrombosis of the vessel. Transmission of the virus of serum jaundice may occur from the use of one syringe for multiple venipunctures. It has been demonstrated that blood from the syringe regurgitates into the vein at the time of release of the tourniquet, thus introducing any infectious material present into the patient's blood stream. Syncope is rarely encountered if the physician reassures the patient and shows no anxiety himself. Continued bleeding is usually avoided by applying a sterile pad with pressure to the venipuncture site. Thrombophlebitis from venipuncture for collection of blood rarely occurs. The formation of a hematoma does more to render a vein useless for future venipunctures than any other complication of routine venipuncture. One cause of hematoma formation is the puncture of the two sides of the vein. Another important cause is the partial (incomplete) penetration of the vein, so that blood leaks into the soft tissue by way of the bevel of the needle. This is corrected by advancing the needle further into the vein. At the first sign of uncontrolled hematoma formation, the tourniquet should be released, the needle removed immediately, and gentle pressure applied to the site with gauze. Arms covered with ecchymoses from venipuncture are usually the hallmark of poor technique and dull needles. When a patient has "poor" or "difficult" veins which are not visible or are difficult to palpate, it is of first importance to have the patient lying down and to spend the time necessary to locate the vein.

When a blood sample is transferred from the syringe into a tube, the needle should first be removed from the syringe, and the blood ejected slowly and steadily against the side of the tube to prevent foaming and mechanical hemolysis. When the blood sample is introduced into the tube under oil for blood-gas determinations, the needle should remain on the syringe while the blood is ejected.

The use of disposable vacuum containers for collection of blood samples has many advantages over the use of syringes. These containers are available with a variety of anticoagulants and preservatives for special purposes.

CAPILLARY PUNCTURE. Obtaining blood from the capillary bed by a small puncture wound through the skin is one of the oldest techniques in the collection of blood samples. In adults and children, the sample may be obtained from either the ear lobe or the tip of the finger. In infants, the heel is usually chosen as the site of the puncture.

The puncture site should be wiped off with an alcohol sponge, leaving no moisture. The puncture should be made with a quick stabbing motion, using a sharp blade which should enter the tissue to a depth of about 3 mm. It is advisable to use disposable sterile blades to avoid transmitting any viral disease from one patient to another. When the lobe of the ear is used, the puncture should be made in the dependent portion of the ear, cutting in a line with the long axis of the ear lobe. Usually the first drop is wiped off and counts and smears are taken on successive drops as needed. It is essential that free-flowing blood be used for the samples, and squeezing should be avoided since the addition of tissue juices renders the results unreliable. If the first puncture is not satisfactory, a second puncture should be made. The lobe of the ear or finger can be massaged distally from the cut to enhance the blood flow, but one should never exert undue pressure.

The puncture of the ear causes less pain than puncturing the finger. The ball of the finger or the flesh at the base of the nail may be used. If frequent finger punctures are to be made, it is best to take the fingers that are least used by the patient.

The red-cell counts and hemoglobin values in the blood from the lobe of the ear are essentially the same as those from the finger and vein, unless there is some unusual stasis due to cold or emotional disturbance. It has been found that the white-cell count from the ear lobe normally is slightly higher than that from the finger [4, 5] and that the larger white cells may be present in greater numbers. The values for the finger and vein are quite comparable. In pathologic conditions such as bacterial endocarditis, infectious mononucleosis, and leukemias, there may be a striking difference between the white-cell counts and differential counts from the ear lobe and those from finger and vein. This relative increase in the total white-cell count when drawn from the ear lobe rather than the finger or vein involves all types of white cells, but especially the large cells such as monocytes and histiocytes which are seen in increased numbers in bacterial endocarditis.[5] The relative increase of these cells may be explained largely by the greater selective filtering capacity of the vascular bed of the ear lobe as compared to that of the finger tip.

The ear lobe is a desirable source of blood for the preparation of blood films when a search for abnormal forms is to be made as in certain infections, leukemias, or leukopenias.[6] The first or second drop from the ear lobe may have more large cells than subsequent drops. After several drops have been taken, the sample is comparable to that of the finger or vein.

Capillary blood may be collected in capillary tubes and used for a variety of chemical, immunologic, and hematologic tests. Capillary tubes should be allowed to fill by capillary action, leaving 5 mm at one end unfilled. They may be sealed with heat, or with rubber caps or other devices. Capillary tubes having a uniform internal diameter are available commercially for microhematocrit determinations.

## REFERENCES

1. F. V. Sander, "The preservation of blood for chemical analysis," *J. biol. Chem.* 58, 1 (1923).
2. R. C. Lewis and G. E. Mills, "The comparative value of monochlorobenzene and thymol when used with fluoride as preservatives of blood for chemical analysis," *Amer. J. clin. Path.* 3, 17 (1933).
3. G. G. Hadley and N. L. Larson, "Use of sequestrene as an anticoagulant," *Amer. J. Path.* 23, 613 (1953).
4. G. A. Daland, *Color Atlas of Morphologic Hematology with a Guide to Clinical Interpretation* (rev. ed.; Harvard University Press, Cambridge, 1959).
5. G. A. Daland, L. Gottlieb, R. O. Wallerstein, and W. B. Castle, "Hematologic observations in bacterial endocarditis," *J. lab. clin. Med.* 48, 827 (1956).
6. H. C. Lucey, "Fortuitous factors affecting the leucocyte count in blood from the ear," *J. clin. Path.* 3, 146 (1950).

# Unit 4

# The Red-Cell and White-Cell Counts

The white-cell count is a basic laboratory examination that should be performed as part of the initial study of the new patient. The red-cell count is not considered a basic laboratory examination, since it may be normal in hypochromic anemias and thalassemia. In place of the red-cell count, determination of the hematocrit or hemoglobin should be used as a basic screening procedure to detect the presence of anemia. If anemia is present, the red-cell count is of value as one of the factors employed in the determination of the red-cell corpuscular values (Unit 7).

Knowledge of the limits of significance of the determination of the red-cell count and white-cell count is of great practical importance. For this reason, considerable emphasis will be given to defining their accuracy as related to obtaining a representative blood sample from the patient, the technique of the test, and the error of random distribution of cells in the counting chamber.

A variety of mechanical and electronic devices have been developed in recent years for the automatic counting of blood cells. A satisfactory counter has been designed by Coulter Electronics. Evaluation of this apparatus has been discussed by Brecher et al.[1]

## Equipment

PIPETTES. Pipettes for dilution of the blood samples are available from many reliable companies. A cheap pipette is not an economy. The U.S. Bureau of Standards requires that the markings on the red-cell pipettes have an accuracy of ±5 percent and white-cell pipettes, an accuracy of ±3.5 percent. The pipettes made by some companies are calibrated and the correction factor is marked on the pipette so the count can be corrected, or two pipettes may be chosen, one with a negative correction and the other with a positive correction of the same magnitude to balance the error. The divisions on the pipettes represent proportions and not absolute measurements. The pipettes for white-cell counts are marked at 0.5, 1.0, and 11. When the blood is drawn to the mark 1.0 and diluted to 11, there is one part of blood in 10 parts of diluting fluid (1/10); the dilution is 1/20 if the blood is drawn to the 0.5 mark. The solution left in the stem of the pipette is not mixed with the solution in the bulb and therefore must be discarded before the mixture is placed in the counting chamber. The marks on the red-cell pipette are 0.5, 1.0, and 101, making a dilution of 1/100 if blood is drawn to the 1.0 mark or 1/200 if drawn to the 0.5 mark, which is the usual technique. When new pipettes are purchased, they should be examined carefully to see that the marks are correct. Pipettes with broken tips should be discarded. Pipettes should be cleaned by rinsing in water, using a suction pump on the faucet. To dry the pipettes, acetone or alcohol and ether in succession may be used until the glass bead moves freely in the bulb. Dirty pipettes can be avoided if pipettes are rinsed in water immediately after use.

USE OF THE HEMOCYTOMETER. Red cells are counted in a sample of blood that has been diluted to a known volume with a fluid serving as an anticoagulant. For the white-cell count, the red cells are hemolyzed by the diluting fluid. For both the red-cell count and the white-cell count, samples of blood diluted with appropriate solutions are introduced into the two chambers of a hemocytometer. Each chamber has a depth of 0.1 mm and a

ruled area measuring 3 mm on a side. Factory standards for the manufacture of the instrument require that the error in length of any line in the ruled area does not exceed ±1 percent, and that the error in the depth of the chamber does not exceed ±2 percent. The ruled area is composed of nine large squares of equal area. Therefore, each chamber has a ruled area of 9 mm$^2$, a depth of 0.1 mm, and a volume of 0.9 mm$^3$. Each of the nine large squares is outlined by triple lines. The center line of the three is the boundary line of the square. Details of the improved Neubauer ruling for a

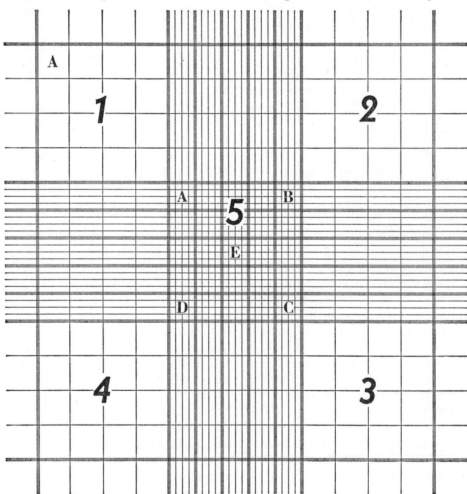

Fig. 3. Improved Neubauer ruling for one counting chamber. The white-cell count is done on the four large corner squares (1, 2, 3, 4) of each of two counting chambers (see Fig. 5). The red-cell count is done on the squares 5(*A, B, C, D, E*) of each of two counting chambers (see Fig. 4). The platelet count is done on two large corner squares (1, 3) of each of two counting chambers.

counting chamber are shown in Fig. 3 and Table 8.

The counting chamber and coverslips must be treated as precision instruments. They are cleaned immediately after each determination to prevent drying of pro-

tein on the surfaces. Both chamber and coverglass are washed with running warm tap water and with soap if necessary. Subsequent rinsing in alcohol and drying with clean gauze may be of value in eliminating grease, lint, or other par-

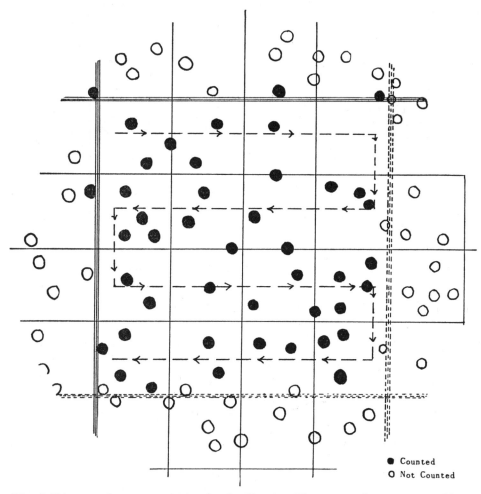

● Counted
O Not Counted

Fig. 4. Diagramatic representation of red-cell count. The square shown, comparable to square 5A in Fig. 3, is magnified 400 times using the high dry objective of the microscope. The order of counting of the small squares is indicated by the arrows. A red cell is counted only once by counting those within the small square and those touching any line at the left or top but not counting those touching any line at the right or bottom of the small square. By this procedure, all cells touching the triple lines shown as broken lines will be excluded. The count by individual small squares, showing the accumulating total, is as follows:

$$3 \rightarrow 6 \rightarrow 8 \rightarrow 9$$
$$\downarrow$$
$$21 \leftarrow 16 \leftarrow 14 \leftarrow 12$$
$$\downarrow$$
$$23 \rightarrow 25 \rightarrow 28 \rightarrow 33$$
$$\downarrow$$
$$44 \leftarrow 40 \leftarrow 38 \leftarrow 36$$

ticulate matter. Grease from the hands prevents uniform spreading of the fluid; it can be avoided by holding the chamber and coverslip by the edges.

The red cells are counted in the central large square, which is subdivided into 400 small squares. In the improved Neubauer ruling, these small squares are arranged in 25 groups of 16 each, each group being outlined by triple lines, as shown in Figs. 3 and 4. The center line of the three is the boundary line of each

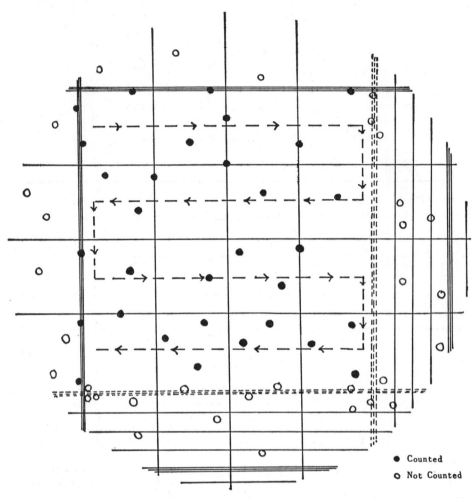

Fig. 5. Diagrammatic representation of white-cell count. The square shown, comparable to square 1 in Fig. 3, is magnified 100 times using the low-power objective of the microscope. The order of counting of the medium-sized squares is the same as that shown in Fig. 4. A white cell is counted only once by counting those within the medium-sized square and those touching any line at the left and top but not counting those touching any line at the right and bottom of the medium-sized square. By this procedure, all cells touching the triple lines shown as broken lines will be excluded. The count by individual medium-sized squares showing the accumulating total for the figure is as follows:

$$3 \to 5 \to 6 \to 8$$
$$\downarrow$$
$$14 \leftarrow 12 \leftarrow 11 \leftarrow 9$$
$$\downarrow$$
$$16 \to 17 \to 19 \to 20$$
$$\downarrow$$
$$31 \leftarrow 28 \leftarrow 25 \leftarrow 23$$

Table 8. *Dimensions of counting chamber and subdivisions.*

| Square | Length (mm) | Area (mm²) | Depth (mm) | Volume (mm³) |
|---|---|---|---|---|
| Chamber | 3 | 9 | 0.10 | 0.90 |
| 1 | 1 | 1 | .10 | .10 |
| 1A | 0.25 | 0.0625 | .10 | .00625 |
| 5A | .20 | .040 | .10 | .0040 |

group of small squares. The actual counting of erythrocytes is performed on one group of 16 small squares at a time. Five such groups, or a total of 80 small squares, are examined in the standard procedure. This represents 80/400, or 0.2, of the area of the large square.

The white cells are enumerated in a series of the large squares and the *average number* of leukocytes *per single large square* is calculated. Each of the large squares has the following measurements: area, 1 mm²; depth, 0.1 mm; volume, 0.1 mm³. Each of the four corner squares is subdivided for convenience into 16 medium-sized squares, as shown in Figs. 3 and 5. The number of white cells in the four large corner squares of each of two chambers is usually counted.

### Technique for the Red-Cell Count

Red cells may be enumerated in samples of free-flowing capillary blood or in blood containing dry oxalate mixture or other anticoagulants that do not produce significant dilution of the blood sample. They may also be counted in conjunction with measurement of hematocrit and hemoglobin on a sample of venous blood, dry oxalate mixture being used as the anticoagulant.

GOWER'S SOLUTION. This solution is made by dissolving 12.5 gm of sodium sulfate and 33.3 ml of glacial acetic acid in 200 ml of distilled water. Gower's solution is distinctly superior to Hayem's solution, since Gower's solution prevents rouleau formation. In cases of hyperglobulinemia, Hayem's solution may cause the precipitation of protein, which interferes

seriously with enumeration of erythrocytes.

SAMPLING, DILUTION, AND MIXING. If blood containing an anticoagulant is used, it is essential, as the first step, to mix the sample thoroughly by gently inverting the receptacle approximately ten times. The blood sample should *not* be shaken, since hemolysis results from trauma. Blood is then drawn into the red-cell pipette exactly to the 0.5 mark and the excess is wiped off. The pipette is always held in an almost horizontal position in filling and in adjusting the level, to facilitate control of the column of blood. If there has been a slight excess of blood drawn up, this may be removed by touching the tip of the pipette lightly with the finger. If a large excess of blood has been drawn up, the pipette should be cleaned and the procedure repeated. If capillary blood is used, the sample is drawn up promptly and exactly to the 0.5 mark and diluted immediately.

The sample is diluted with Gower's solution, the pipette being held in an almost horizontal position and agitated gently as it is filled, so that the column of concentrated blood is distributed evenly and the bead contained in the bulb of the pipette moves freely. When the bulb is almost full, the pipette is raised to the vertical position and the level of diluting fluid is drawn exactly to the 101 mark. The pipette is shaken immediately for about ½ min to facilitate the initial mixing. If the count is not performed at once, the pipette should be placed in a horizontal position to prevent leakage or entry of air bubbles. The two ends of the pipette may be closed by a rubber band or other device for transportation.

The diluted blood sample is thoroughly mixed by hand for at least 3 min or in a mechanical agitator. An arbitrary method for mixing by hand is as follows. One or two pipettes are held firmly between the thumb and fingers of one hand; the base of this hand is struck repeatedly

31

against the other hand for 3 min. The motion should be at right angles to the long axis of the pipette. The first 6 drops from the pipette are discarded to eliminate the cell-free fluid from the capillary tube. Then the well-mixed sample is introduced promptly into the counting chamber as described below. If there is a delay, or if it is desired to repeat the count, the diluted sample in the pipette must be mixed thoroughly in the same manner each time.

ENUMERATION OF ERYTHROCYTES IN THE COUNTING CHAMBER. After thorough mixing of the diluted sample and expulsion of the first 6 drops from the pipette, the fluid is introduced into the hemocytometer. The flow of the sample from the pipette may be readily controlled by pressure of the index finger on the open end or of the tongue on the mouthpiece of the tubing. The pipette being held at an angle of about 35°, the tip is rested gently at the orifice made by the coverslip and counting chamber. The chamber is filled by capillary action, the fluid being allowed to enter in a controlled manner so that it spreads slowly and evenly over the entire surface. The procedure must be repeated if either of the chambers is filled unevenly, if the moat is filled, or if air bubbles appear. A small excess remaining at the mouth of the counting chamber can be removed by touching the drop gently with the finger (not with gauze or absorbent paper).

The hemocytometer is allowed to stand for a few minutes to permit settling of the red cells. If the count is not made within a few minutes, it is advisable to prevent evaporation by covering the chamber with a Petri dish or other suitable cover containing a moistened piece of filter paper which is applied to the top inner surface.

*Red cells* are counted under the high dry magnification of the microscope. To avoid breaking the coverslip with the objective of the microscope, the ruled area should first be located under low magnification. The erythrocytes are counted in the four corner squares and the central square of the central large square of the chamber; these five squares are shown as *A, B, C, D, E* in Fig. 3. Since each of these squares contains 16 small squares, the red cells are counted in a total of 80 small squares. This represents 80/400 or 0.2 of the area of the large square. For any one group of 16 small squares, the cells are counted in each small square, including in the count those cells that touch any one of the three lines or the single line on the *left-hand* and the *top* borders of the square, but *excluding* those cells that touch any of the lines on the right-hand and bottom borders of the square. This method of counting is an arbitrary one, by which every cell is assigned to one square and no cell is counted twice. The cells are counted in each small square, first from left to right beginning with the top row of four small squares, then from right to left for the next row, and so on. A typical red-cell count is shown in Fig. 4. The number of cells for each of the 5 groups of 16 squares is recorded separately and the results are added. The erythrocytes in the second counting chamber are counted and recorded in the same manner. For reasons discussed below (p. 35), two pipettes and two chambers should be used for routine counts. In severe anemia, a larger number of squares should be counted.

CALCULATION OF THE RED-CELL COUNT. The *volume* of diluted blood contained in the chamber above the 80 small squares—5 groups of 16 each—is 0.02 $mm^3$. Hence the number of erythrocytes counted in each chamber is multiplied by 50 to convert the number found in 0.02 $mm^3$ to the number contained in 1.0 $mm^3$. Since the dilution is 1/200, the *combined conversion factor* is $50 \times 200 = 10,000$. It is standard practice to count the cells in 80 small squares in each of two separate chambers, obtain the average, and multiply this result by 10,000. Modifications of the standard method are shown in Tables 9 and 10.

Table 9. *Conversion factors for red-cell counts made in various numbers of small squares for the standard dilution of 1/200.*

| Number of groups of small squares | Total number of small squares | Volume of chamber (mm³) | Conversion factor |
|---|---|---|---|
| 5 (standard) | 80 | 0.02 | 10000 |
| 10 | 160 | .04 | 5000 |
| 15 | 240 | .06 | 3333 |
| 20 | 320 | .08 | 2500 |
| 25 (maximum) | 400 | .10 | 2000 |

*Example 1. Two pipettes, one for each of two chambers.* The counts on 5 groups of 16 small squares of one chamber are 100, 110, 115, 95, 90; total, 510. In the second chamber, the counts are 99, 102, 107, 87, 95; total, 490. The average of the two chamber counts is 500. Multiplication by the factor 10,000 gives the red-cell count of $5.00 \times 10^6/\text{mm}^3$.

In *polycythemia*, the number of cells in the counting chamber may be too large to permit accurate enumeration if the dilution is 1/200. In this case, blood is drawn up to the 0.3 division of the red-cell pipette, instead of the 0.5 mark, and the sample is diluted to the 101 mark. Enumeration is done in the same way as for a normal count, 5 groups of 16 small

squares being used in each of two chambers. The average of the two counts is multiplied by 10,000. To correct for the difference from the usual dilution, the result is multiplied by the fraction 5/3, since only 3 parts instead of 5 parts were taken.

*Example 2. Polycythemia.* Blood drawn to the 0.3 division is diluted to the 101 mark of the pipette. The total number of cells in 16 small squares is counted in each of two chambers. The average of the two chamber counts is 500. The usual conversion factor is 10,000. Since 0.3 part rather than 0.5 part of blood was used, the calculated count will be $500 \times 10,000 \times 5/3 = 8.3 \times 10^6/\text{mm}^3$.

In *anemia*, the number of red cells available for enumeration by the standard procedure may be inadequate for accurate measurement. This difficulty may be solved by two different procedures, as follows.

(1) The dilution may be decreased from 1/200 to 1/100 by drawing the blood up to the 1.0 mark of the red-cell pipette, instead of the 0.5 mark, and diluting the sample to the 101 mark. To correct for the difference from the usual dilution, the result is multiplied by 5000 ($50 \times 100$) instead of 10,000.

*Example 3. Anemia, dilution 1/100.* The average count for two chambers is 498. The

Table 10. *Coefficient of variation and normal limits of data obtained from formula of Berkson, Magath, and Hurn.*[2]

| Example No. | Total number of red cells counted in $N_c$ chambers, $N_b$ | Total number of small squares examined in each chamber | Number of chambers examined, $N_c$ | Number of separate pipettes, $N_p$ | Coefficient of variation, C.V. (percent) | 2 C.V. (percent) | True red-cell count ($10^6/\text{mm}^3$) | Normal limits of data: true count $\pm 2$ C.V. ($10^6/\text{mm}^3$) |
|---|---|---|---|---|---|---|---|---|
| *Samples with normal red-cell count* | | | | | | | | |
| A | 500 | 80 | 1 | 1 | ±7.9 | ±15.8 | 5.00 | 4.21–5.79 |
| B | 1000 | 80 | 2 | 1 | ±6.4 | ±12.8 | 5.00 | 4.36–5.64 |
| C | 1000 | 80 | 2 | 2 | ±5.5 | ±11.0 | 5.00 | 4.45–5.55 |
| *Samples with decreased red-cell count* | | | | | | | | |
| D | 500 | 80 | 2 | 2 | ±6.2 | ±12.4 | 2.50 | 2.2–2.8 |
| E | 1000 | 160 | 2 | 2 | ±5.5 | ±11.0 | 2.50 | 2.2–2.7 |
| F | 200 | 80 | 2 | 2 | ±7.9 | ±15.8 | 1.00 | 0.84–1.16 |
| G | 1000 | 400 (25 squares) | 2 | 2 | ±5.4 | ±10.8 | 1.00 | 0.89–1.11 |

result would be $498 \times 5000 = 2.49 \times 10^6/mm^3$ for the red-cell count.

(2) The dilution may be kept constant at 1/200 and the erythrocytes counted in 10 groups of 16 small squares instead of 5 in each chamber, or in a volume of 0.04 mm³ instead of 0.02 mm³.

*Example 4. Anemia, dilution 1/200.* The average count for two chambers is 500. If 160 squares are counted instead of 80, the conversion factor is $25 \times 200$, or 5000, as shown in Table 9. The result is $500 \times 5000 = 2.5 \times 10^6/mm^3$.

In severe anemia, it is more satisfactory to count the whole area (25 groups of 16 small squares), which gives the number of cells in 0.1 mm³ in each chamber.

*Example 5. Severe anemia, dilution 1/200.* The average count for two chambers is 495. Since 400 small squares are counted, the factor is $10 \times 200 = 2000$, as shown in Table 9. The result is $495 \times 2000 = 0.99 \times 10^6/mm^3$.

### Errors and Precautions in the Red-Cell Count

The error in enumeration of erythrocytes may be so great in unskilled hands as to render the data valueless. Even under excellent technical control, the inherent error in the procedure is of considerable magnitude. Three varieties of error that may influence the final result are considered below.

ERRORS RELATED TO THE PATIENT AND TO OBTAINING THE BLOOD SAMPLE. The number of erythrocytes in the circulating blood is altered following exercise. Blood samples should be taken after the patient has had a brief period of rest. Satisfactory agreement occurs with either capillary or venous blood if the blood samples are secured properly. If stasis is prolonged during venipuncture, the increase in the number of red cells resulting from hemoconcentration is progressive and significant.

TECHNICAL ERRORS. Technical errors resulting from inferior equipment or unskilled manipulations must *all* be eliminated or the error in enumerating red cells becomes excessive. In filling the pipette, precision is required to adjust the levels in the pipette exactly to the proper marks and, with capillary blood, to avoid clotting. In taking a sample of blood from the receptacle, failure properly to mix the whole sample vitiates the results. Failure to wipe off the outside of the pipette allows blood to contaminate the diluting fluid. The diluting fluid should be used in small amounts from stock and changed frequently to avoid the introduction of dirt into the chamber. In general, best results are obtained by using samples of venous blood and an anticoagulant that produces no dilution. This permits the leisurely filling of the pipette and allows for repetition of the observations in case of doubt. After dilution of the blood sample, thorough mixing in the pipette is essential. The accuracy of the count depends, also, on the exactness and uniformity of the volume of liquid contained under the coverglass of the chamber. The coverglass provided with the chamber is specially ground to uniform flatness. It is incorrect in the extreme to substitute an ordinary coverglass for that furnished with the hemocytometer. The filling of the chamber as described above must also be correctly done. The counting chamber must be chemically clean and free of detritus. Counts should be performed promptly, since drying may set up convection currents that will alter the distribution of cells in the chamber.

THE INHERENT ERROR OF DISTRIBUTION OF CELLS IN THE CHAMBER. The distribution of red cells in the counting chamber follows the law of chance,[2-4] and may be influenced by currents in the fluid within the counting chamber.[5] It must be emphasized that the chance distribution of cells in the chamber introduces an *inher-*

*ent error* into the method which cannot be controlled. The error inherent in the chance distribution of erythrocytes, when all technical factors are eliminated, has been estimated by Berkson *et al.*[2] and by Berg.[4] The coefficient of variation C.V. (percent) of an individual determination of the red-cell count, when the technical factors are controlled, is given by

$$\text{C.V.} = \sqrt{\left(\frac{8464}{N_b} + \frac{21}{N_c} + \frac{22}{N_p}\right)},$$

where $N_b$ is the total number of cells counted in $N_c$ chambers, $N_c$ is the number of chambers examined, and $N_p$ is the number of separate pipettes employed.

The examples shown in Table 10 represent the results of substituting different values in this formula. The coefficient of variation C.V. is the value for one standard deviation, expressed as a percentage of the mean (Unit 2). Sixty-seven percent of the results, based on chance distribution, are included within one standard deviation on each side of the mean. Two standard deviations, or 2 C.V., on each side of the mean include 95 percent of all results. Results falling outside the range of two standard deviations are usually due to errors in technique.

From the analysis of the red-cell count as shown in Table 10, the following conclusions can be drawn. The accuracy of the count is inadequate when only one pipette and one chamber are used (*A*). The results when one pipette and two chambers are used are more accurate (*B*). For still greater accuracy, two pipettes and two chambers (*C*) are recommended when red-cell corpuscular values (Unit 7) are to be determined. When the red-cell count is decreased, as in the anemias, the error is increased because comparatively fewer cells are present in each chamber count. There is an optimum number of cells (400–600) that should be counted in each chamber. In Table 10, in *A*, *B*, and *C*, it is shown that increasing the number of chambers and pipettes will decrease the

coefficient of variation, with C as the condition recommended.

To obtain the same degree of accuracy with lower counts ($2.5 \times 10^6/\text{mm}^3$ and $1.0 \times 10^6/\text{mm}^3$), a larger number of squares must be counted. Compare the coefficient of variation in *C*, *E*, and *G* of Table 10 to get the same degree of accuracy at red-cell count levels of 5.0, 2.5, and $1.0 \times 10^6/\text{mm}^3$ respectively. Compare the coefficient of variation in *C*, *D*, and *F* to see the comparative accuracy of different red-cell counts using the standard technique (80 small squares, 2 chambers, and 2 pipettes).

ESTIMATE OF ERROR FROM CHAMBER COUNTS. Berkson, Magath, and Hurn[2] have prepared a review of the rules recommended by several authors for maximum discrepancies to be allowed in performing red-cell counts. It is concluded that many of the rules "are meaninglessly stringent and serve only to encourage erroneous counting by requiring an attempt to live up to impossible standards." There is no simple rule by which chance distribution of erythrocytes in the chamber can be checked. Obviously, all technical error must be eliminated and the counts must be performed and recorded as accurately as possible.

It is often of value to determine whether two counts made with different pipettes, or done at different times on the same patient, differ significantly. To do this, an estimate of the chance error of the counts may be made by the following procedure.[2, 6]

Let *A* be the number of cells counted in the first chamber and *B* the number of cells counted in the second chamber. Then $(A + B)/2$ is the average of the two chamber counts. A rough approximation of the standard deviation ($\sigma$) of the difference between the two counts is given by the formula $\sigma = \sqrt{[2(A + B)/2]} = \sqrt{(A + B)}$. Two standard deviations, or $2\sigma$, is taken as the figure for comparison with the difference *C* between the two chamber counts *A* and *B*. The assumption is made in this formula that *A* and *B*, the actual number of cells counted (400–600) in each chamber, are distributed in a Poisson series.[2, 6] In calculating $\sigma$, the actual count per chamber is used, and *not* the calculated red-cell count in millions per cubic millimeter. The use of the latter value would imply that several million red cells (instead of 400–600) had been counted by the observer. The actual steps are as follows:

1. Record the number of cells observed, *A* and *B*, in each of the two chambers.

2. Obtain the numerical difference *C* between *A* and *B*.

3. Calculate $2\sigma = 2 \sqrt{(A + B)}$.

4. If *C* is less than $2\sigma$, the difference is not significant. If *C* is greater than $2\sigma$, the difference is significant.

If the comparison is made for the purpose of checking the accuracy of a given chamber count and a significant difference is found between counts in two chambers, then the count should be repeated. The *average* of the values of all four chamber counts is then taken for the calculation of the red-cell count, even though the difference between the third and fourth counts may also exceed $2\sigma$.

*Example 6. Estimate of error between two counts.* If the true red-cell count of a blood sample were $5.0 \times 10^6/\text{mm}^3$, the chamber counts observed might be as follows. First chamber: 97, 105, 100, 93, 105; total, 500. Then *A* = 500. Second chamber: 80, 95, 100, 90, 85; total, 450. Then *B* = 450. Then $C = A - B = 500 - 450 = 50$, and $2\sigma = 2\sqrt{(500 + 450)} = 2\sqrt{950} = 2 \times 31 = 62$. Since *C* (50) is less than $2\sigma$ (62), the results are considered significant by this estimate of chance error. Since the average of the two chamber counts is $(500 + 450)/2$, or 475, the red-cell count is reported as $4.75 \times 10^6/\text{mm}^3$.

### The White-Cell Count

SAMPLING, DILUTION, AND MIXING. For the white-cell count, blood is usually drawn to the 0.5 mark in the white-cell pipette and diluted to the 11 mark, thus producing a dilution of 1/20. Two-percent acetic acid is used as diluting fluid, producing hemolysis of all the nonnucleated erythrocytes. Nucleated red cells cannot be distinguished from leukocytes in the counting chamber and will be included in the white-cell count. The general procedure for the white-cell count is the same as for the red-cell count.

ENUMERATION OF LEUKOCYTES IN THE CHAMBER. Both chambers of the hemocytometer are filled and the white cells are allowed to settle. For enumeration of the leukocytes, the low-power magnification is used. The cells in all four large corner squares of each chamber are counted. Each large square is made up of 16 medium-sized squares. The cells are counted in each of the 16 medium-sized squares, including those cells that touch any of the lines on the left-hand and upper borders. The number of cells counted in each large square is recorded separately, and the numbers are added. The sum of the leukocytes found in the 8 large squares of two chambers is divided by 8 to obtain the average number per single large square. The average number of white cells per single large square is multiplied by 10 to convert the number found in 0.1 $\text{mm}^3$ to the number contained in 1.0 $\text{mm}^3$. The number in 1.0 $\text{mm}^3$ is multiplied by 20 to correct for the dilution of 1/20. The conversion factor is, therefore, $10 \times 20 = 200$.

*Example 7.* The counts on 8 large corner squares of two counting chambers are 46, 54, 58, 52, 47, 50, 55, 49; total, 411. The average number of leukocytes per single large square is $411/8 = 51.4$. Multiplication by the factor 200 gives 10,280, which is reported as a white-cell count of $10.3 \times 10^3/\text{mm}^3$.

FACTORS USED IN CALCULATION. In disease, the white-cell count may vary from 500 to 1,000,000 or more per cubic millimeter. It may be necessary, because of either insufficient cells or crowding in the chamber, to use dilutions other than

1/20. This may be accomplished with either the white-cell pipette or the red-cell pipette, acetic acid being used as diluting fluid. Any deviation from the standard procedure requires correction of the results for such changes.

In *leukopenia,* the blood is drawn to the 1.0 mark instead of the 0.5 mark and diluted to the 11 mark, thus producing a dilution of 1/10 instead of 1/20. The conversion factor is $10 \times 10 = 100$.

*Example 8. Leukopenia.* The average number of leukocytes per single large square is found to be 10. Then the result is $10 \times 100 = 1000$ white cells/mm³ or $1 \times 10^3$/mm³.

In *leukocytosis* or *leukemia,* a dilution of 1/200 may be made in the red-cell pipette, instead of 1/20 in the white-cell pipette. The conversion factor is $10 \times 200 = 2000$.

*Example 9. Leukocytosis or leukemia.* The average number of leukocytes per large square is 100 cells, when diluted 1/200 in a red-cell pipette. Then the white-cell count is $100 \times 2000 = 200,000$ white cells/mm³ or $200 \times 10^3$/mm³.

ERRORS AND PRECAUTIONS IN THE WHITE-CELL COUNT. The process of enumeration of leukocytes is subject to the same errors already discussed under the red-cell count.[1-4] Berkson, Magath, and Hurn [2] have devised a formula for analysis of the chance error of distribution of leukocytes in the counting chamber. This formula, which is similar to that for the red-cell count, will not be discussed. In general, the clinical significance of the leukocyte count does *not* require the degree of accuracy that is essential for the enumeration of red cells. It is sufficient to use one pipette to enumerate the cells in the four large corner squares of *two* counting chambers, and to obtain the average for one square as described above.

## REFERENCES

1. G. Brecher, M. Schneiderman, and G. Z. Williams, "Evaluation of the electronic red blood cell counter," *Amer. J. clin. Path. 26,* 1439 (1956).

2. J. Berkson, R. B. Magath, and M. Hurn, "The error of estimate of the blood cell count as made with the hemacytometer," *Amer. J. Physiol. 128,* 309 (1940).

3. P. Plum, "Accuracy of hematological counting methods," *Acta med. scand. 90,* 342 (1936).

4. W. Berg, "Blood cell counts. Their statistical interpretation," *Amer. Rev. Tuberc. 52,* 179 (1945).

5. M. Hynes, "The distribution of leukocytes on the counting chamber," *J. clin. Path. 1,* 25 (1947).

6. J. Worcester, personal communication.

# Unit 5

# Hemoglobinometry

**Hemoglobinometry in Clinical Medicine**

Hemoglobin has physiologic significance in the transport of oxygen from the lungs to the tissues and of carbon dioxide from the tissues to the lungs. The oxygen-combining capacity of blood is directly proportional to the concentration of hemoglobin rather than to the number of red blood cells in a standard volume of blood.

The quantitative determination of the concentration of hemoglobin in the peripheral blood is one of the most frequently performed laboratory procedures. It has importance as a screening test to yield a clue to disease that might not be suspected from the history or physical examination. In addition, serial determinations can be used to evaluate the degree of response to specific therapy. When measured with requisite precision, the concentration of hemoglobin can be used in the calculation of the mean corpuscular hemoglobin concentration (MCHC), one of the red-cell corpuscular values useful in the morphologic classification of the anemias (Unit 7).

The concentration of hemoglobin is best expressed as grams of hemoglobin per 100 ml of whole blood. In the past, it was customary to express it as a percentage of an arbitrarily selected "normal" value. However, there was no uniformity of the value selected as "normal" and equal to 100 percent. This ranged from 13.8 to 17.2 gm/100 ml, according to the method and instrument used, so that there was very poor correlation between measurements made in different laboratories.

When expressed as grams of hemoglobin per 100 ml of blood, the concentration of hemoglobin is found to vary widely in the blood of normal individuals. There are differences with age, sex, and altitude of habitation. In the case of adults residing at sea level, the normal range for males is $16 \pm 2$ gm/100 ml; that for females is $14 \pm 2$ gm/100 ml.

Because of the wide range of normal values and because of the efficiency of the body's adaptation to mild chronic anemia, it is impossible to define, either from laboratory data or from the patient's symptoms, the point at which a given patient becomes anemic. It is, however, useful to set such a limit arbitrarily, and in men and women a hemoglobin level below 12 gm/100 ml may be considered to represent anemia.

A number of methods are available for measuring the concentration of hemoglobin in blood. Since hemoglobin is not easily crystallized and weighed quantitatively, all methods for its determination are necessarily indirect. Those most frequently used measure hemoglobin by either its ability to combine with oxygen in a known stoichiometric relation, its iron content, or its color. In addition, hemoglobin concentration can be estimated grossly from the specific gravity of whole blood. Also, low concentrations can be determined by means of the reaction of hemoglobin with benzidine and hydrogen peroxide to form a colored compound.

It is important to differentiate between methods of hemoglobin determination that can be used to provide primary standards for hemoglobinometry and those which are useful clinically because of simplicity of technique and required equipment. The methods based on the oxygen-combining capacity and the iron content are technically difficult and require considerable training, so they are not useful for clinical purposes. They are, however, useful in providing primary standards for the colorimetric methods which generally have wide clinical application.

### General Principles of Methods

#### Gasometric Method

The determination of the concentration of hemoglobin in blood by measuring the oxygen-combining capacity of blood in the Van Slyke blood-gas apparatus is based on the following principles. Since the molecular weight of hemoglobin is 68,000, 1 mM weighs 68 gm. Furthermore, 1 mM of hemoglobin contains 4 mM of $Fe^{++}$ and combines with 4 mM of oxygen. Expressed in terms of volume, $1 \text{ mM O}_2 = 22.4 \text{ ml O}_2$ (under standard conditions of temperature and pressure). Hence, 1.32 ml $O_2$ is bound by and is equivalent to 1.0 gm of hemoglobin.

In principle, a sample of blood is equilibrated with oxygen under standard conditions of pressure and temperature. A measured volume of blood so equilibrated is then analyzed for its content of oxygen. An error of only ±0.5 percent can be obtained by *skilled* technicians. Accordingly, this method is used for standardization of other methods. The method requires rigid control, is technically demanding if the accuracy mentioned is to be attained, and is so time-consuming that it is not applicable to clinical use.

The reader is referred elsewhere for detailed discussions of the technique.[1,2]

Only the functional hemoglobin of the blood is measured in this way. Hemoglobin derivatives such as methemoglobin, sulfhemoglobin, and carbon monoxide hemoglobin which do not combine with oxygen are not included. Ammundsen has shown that in 40 percent of urban residents these functionally inactive pigments may represent from 2 to 10 percent of the total hemoglobin.[3]

Carbon monoxide may be substituted for oxygen with advantage and is preferred by some. Total hemoglobin may be determined by this method if the blood is first reduced completely by an active reducing agent.

#### Chemical Methods

IRON CONTENT.[4] The iron of the hemoglobin molecule can be detached by the action of sulfuric acid, and, after the proteins have been precipitated, the concentration of iron can be measured colorimetrically using a solution of known iron concentration as a standard. The iron content of hemoglobin is 0.335 gm/100 gm of hemoglobin. Although the plasma iron concentration may introduce a small error in this method, it can be disregarded since the magnitude of such error is only 0.1 to 0.2 percent in the blood of a nonanemic individual. Thus, the hemoglobin iron concentration of whole blood is about 50 mgm/100 ml, while the plasma iron concentration of whole blood (hematocrit 50 percent) is only 0.05 to 0.1 mgm/100 ml.

BENZIDINE METHOD. This method is used for the determination of micro amounts of hemoglobin. It is described in Unit 11.

#### Colorimetric Methods

These methods depend upon the production of a colored derivative of hemoglobin and, as noted above, have the advantage of clinical practicality. In general, they require minimal time, training, and equipment.

Of the many colored derivatives of hemoglobin, oxyhemoglobin, cyanmethemoglobin, and acid hematin have been most widely used for hemoglobinometry. Methods making use of each of these derivatives will be described. Beer's law, that the optical density of monochromatic light of a colored solution is proportional to the concentration of the colored material, is the basis of all colorimetric methods.

VISUAL COLORIMETRY

In visual colorimetric methods, solutions of the various hemoglobin derivatives are compared with permanent colored standards by eye. Probably the simplest procedure is to compare the color of a drop of blood applied to white filter paper with a series of lithographed color standards. Because of the variables, such as the size of the drop of blood, the degree of saturation of the hemoglobin with oxygen, the amount of spreading of the drop, and the degree of drying, this method, known as the Tallqvist method, is so unreproducible and inaccurate that it is unacceptable for clinical hemoglobinometry. The acceptable methods involve either comparison of a fixed dilution of blood with a prism of colored glass, or dilution of the hemoglobin derivative until the color of its solution matches a colored-glass standard. The accuracy of visual colorimetry varies with both the eye and the instrument. With the best of visual colorimeters and techniques, the measurement is resolved to one of matching the *brightness* of light. Differences of hue and saturation are eliminated by using proper standards and light of optimum wavelength.

There are inherent differences among persons in the ability to appreciate small changes in light intensity at different wavelengths. This appreciation can be improved somewhat by training. In general, the human eye has maximum sensitivity in the green, with rapid decrease in sensitivity in both the violet and the red. Thus, with suitable light and under the best of conditions, an experienced observer can match the brightness of two fields within ±1 percent, although in the extreme red and violet this error will increase to ±5 percent. Precision in matching light intensity is quite low with dilute solutions, which transmit most of the light, and also with concentrated solutions, which transmit little light. Fatigue of the eye may introduce an unpredictable error. Accordingly, there are inherent subjective errors which may not be easily eliminated in photometry that employs the human eye as the measuring instrument.

SAHLI METHOD. A measured quantity of blood is converted to acid hematin with dilute hydrochloric acid and is then diluted in a calibrated tube until a color match is obtained with a permanent yellow-glass standard. The color match is made using blue filtered light from an incandescent lamp. The yellow-brown color of acid hematin is easier to match visually than is the red color of oxyhemoglobin.

**Method.** The calibrated Sahli tube is filled to a mark corresponding to about 2 gm of hemoglobin with $0.1N$ HCl which is prepared by diluting 1 ml of concentrated hydrochloric acid to 100 ml with distilled water. A sample of 0.02 ml of capillary or venous blood is delivered slowly from a calibrated pipette into the hydrochloric acid with constant agitation. The pipette should be rinsed out three or four times with the acid solution in the tube. The outside tip of the pipette is rinsed with several additional drops of $0.1N$ HCl from a medicine dropper. After agitation, the mixture is allowed to stand at room temperature for at least 20 min. The concentrated acid hematin is then diluted with water until the color matches that of the glass standard. The concentration of hemoglobin in grams per 100 ml of blood is read directly from the gram scale etched on the tube, the meniscus of the hematin suspension being used as the level for reading. It is recommended that the scale showing the percent of normal hemoglobin be disregarded.

INTERPRETATIONS AND LIMITATIONS. Although there are numerous possible errors, an experienced observer using calibrated equipment can attain a reproducibility and accuracy within an error of ±5 percent. The more usual error is probably in the range of ±15–30 percent unless calibrated equipment is used. Care should be taken to wipe the outside of the pipette free of blood prior to adding the blood to the acid. The hydrochloric acid must be 0.1N since lower concentrations fail to produce acid hematin. The rate and degree of color development of acid hematin are variable. However, after 20 min, the color development is approximately 98 percent complete; it is 99 percent complete in 40 min. A standard time interval of not less than 20 min is essential.

The problem of standardization of equipment is difficult. It would be of great advantage if all manufacturers stated the correction factors for pipettes and instruments. Some manufacturers do state the correction factor for the pipettes. The reliability of these statements is not known. It is possible to purchase, at somewhat higher cost, 0.02-ml pipettes which have been certified by the U.S. Bureau of Standards as delivering volumes within a required limit of error. These pipettes bear a certification number. The variation in the uncertified pipettes is so great that they should not be used unless they have been calibrated by the user. Pipettes can be calibrated and re-marked, as described elsewhere,[5, 6, 7] but this is a tedious operation.

Many types of Sahli instruments are on the market. It is important that the tubes used should be made by the same manufacturer as that of the standards. The observer may calibrate and prepare a correction factor for a Sahli tube and color standards as follows. The hemoglobin content of a blood sample is determined within an error of ±2 percent by the oxygen-capacity method of Van Slyke.[1] A sample of 0.02 ml of the known blood is measured with a calibrated pipette and introduced into the Sahli tube. The hemoglobin concentration is determined as described above. Four separate determinations are made, and the mean of the results is recorded. The ratio of the hemoglobin concentration as determined by the Van Slyke method to the concentration determined by the Sahli apparatus may then be used as the correction factor for that particular Sahli apparatus to correct subsequent readings, provided a calibrated pipette and the same glass standards are used. The Sahli apparatus and method may also be calibrated by using a photoelectric colorimetric method to establish the "true" concentration. It is *not* recommended that one Sahli instrument be used to standardize another, since the Sahli method has a larger inherent error than that of either the Van Slyke or the photoelectric colorimetric method.

An inherent disadvantage of the Sahli method derives from the fact that the end point is reached by diluting the acid hematin suspension until a color match is reached. If the end point is inadvertently passed, the procedure must be started again from the beginning.

MEASUREMENT OF OXYHEMOGLOBIN WITH THE SPENCER HEMOGLOBINOMETER. The limitations of measuring oxyhemoglobin by direct visual matching in the red have already been mentioned. The Spencer hemoglobinometer avoids this visual difficulty by using relatively monochromatic green light for matching colors. It compares the transmission of light in an accurately prepared thin layer of hemolyzed blood (oxyhemoglobin) with that of a standardized glass wedge, the transmission of which closely approximates that of oxyhemoglobin in the green (wavelength 540 m$\mu$). Proper light is obtained by means of a green filter, so that only the *intensity* of transmitted light of uniform hue is matched in the split field. The method does *not require* quantitative measurement of the blood sample in a pipette. A constant and known thickness of the unknown sample of blood is obtained simply by filling a chamber of defined depth comparable to that of a hemacytometer. The blood is then hemolyzed by saponin.

**Method.** The blood chamber is removed from the slot on the left-hand side of the instrument and the glass containing the raised platform is slipped out from under the coverglass to expose one of the platforms completely. One drop of capillary or venous blood is placed on the exposed platform and hemolyzed by mixing with an applicator stick that carries saponin on its tip. When hemolysis is complete, as indicated by loss of turbidity of the blood sample, the platform is pushed back under the coverglass. When this is done, the chamber should be completely filled with blood, entirely free of air bubbles. A moat is provided to contain any excess blood when the capillary chamber is full. The chamber is replaced in the instrument so that the portion of the chamber filled with blood enters the instrument and is away from the metal clip. The instrument is then held to the eye with the left hand in such a manner that the left thumb rests on the button of the light switch, located on the bottom of the case. When the light is on, a split green field appears in the instrument. The slide button on the right is moved until the two fields are of equal intensity. The position of the index mark on the slider knob then indicates the hemoglobin concentration in grams per 100 ml. It is suggested that four readings be made with each sample of blood (one chamber filling) and that the mean result be reported.

INTERPRETATIONS AND LIMITATIONS. The Spencer instrument is theoretically sound. However, the wedge used in matching is short, so that accuracy is necessarily limited. The method is an ideal one for rapid screening for determination of hemoglobin, since it does not require the use of a calibrated pipette as the basis of measurement. For hemoglobin determinations on a large number of bloods, other methods, such as the photoelectric colorimeter, may be used more rapidly and with greater accuracy. However, the hemoglobin concentration can probably be measured to within $\pm$5–10 percent by most observers with the Spencer hemoglobinometer. As in all visual colorimetry, there is physiologic variation from one eye to another, so that the manufacturer's calibration is of necessity limited by the eye of the observer. It is suggested that the physician calibrate his instrument and himself by his ability to match blood samples of known hemoglobin content as determined either by the Van Slyke method or by a photoelectric colorimetric method. It is essential that all optical and glass parts be kept clean and free from dust and finger marks. Adequate light is needed for this color match; therefore the batteries must be replaced as needed or a transformer must be used.

The simplicity and reproducibility of this method and the minimal equipment required combine to make it the method of choice for determining hemoglobin concentrations when a photoelectric colorimeter is not available. It is useful for screening prospective blood donors and also can be used by the physician either in the office or at home.

PHOTOELECTRIC COLORIMETRY

The optical density of standard dilutions of the various hemoglobin derivatives at appropriate wavelengths may be measured directly and objectively by means of a photoelectric colorimeter.[8] Photoelectric colorimeters have been developed to a point where they have replaced visual instruments almost entirely. They have a marked advantage in speed and elimination of personal variations. The light-sensitive elements are now inexpensive and reliable. The photoelectric instruments measure differences in light intensity only, so that, by increasing the intensity of the light used, the range of densities that can be measured is readily increased.

The disadvantages of photoelectric colorimetry include a high initial cost and a demand for considerable technical knowledge in proper maintenance, standardization, and use of the instrument. Another disadvantage of the photoelectric cell is that it always "gives an answer" and is therefore subject to uncritical use. The galvanometer reading is a nonspecific measurement of light intensity, and may be altered by extraneous causes, such as turbidity of the solution and dirty glassware, which would preclude any comparison in a visual colorimeter. Thus, the ease of the photoelectric method introduces a real danger of false confidence in results and lack of control of the instrument and of the solution tested.

In order to calculate the hemoglobin concentration from the optical density of a solution of a hemoglobin derivative, it is necessary first to construct a calibration curve for the particular colorimeter being used. This curve relates the optical density of solutions of the same derivative of hemoglobin to the concentration of these solutions as determined by either the gasometric or the iron-content method. It has been shown that solutions of cyanmethemoglobin are stable for many years if kept in sealed amber-glass tubes, and such solutions, of known concentration, are available commercially for use as standards with which to calibrate photoelectric colorimeters.

In choosing a method to be used with a particular photoelectric colorimeter, one must consider the hemoglobin derivative to be used and also the appropriate dilution. The Coleman, Evelyn, and Klett colorimeters are among the more widely used instruments, and all are acceptable. In the Evelyn and Klett colorimeters, the "monochromatic" light source is obtained by the use of colored glass filters. In the Coleman instrument, monochromatic light of a narrower band of wavelengths is obtained by refracting light through a prism. For instructions in the use of these instruments, reference should be made to the manufacturers' instruction manuals.

Satisfactory final dilutions of blood for these instruments are as follows: Klett, 1:200; Coleman, 1:250; and Evelyn, 1:500. It is obvious that in these methods the accuracy of the pipettes and flasks used to make these final dilutions is critical in determining the accuracy and reproducibility of the results. It is customary to dilute either 0.02 ml or 0.1 ml of whole blood to the appropriate final volume. A Sahli pipette is used to measure the 0.02-ml volume and should be calibrated as noted above. A method of calibrating such pipettes is given by Crosby.[7]

The micro blood pipette for the Folin micro blood-sugar method is a precision instrument and can be used to deliver 0.1 ml with a tolerance of ±0.00025 ml. It is thus a more accurate instrument than the 0.02-ml Sahli pipette. In general, large volumes are measured with less error than small volumes. Therefore the 0.1-ml micro blood-sugar pipette is preferred for diluting blood for hemoglobinometry in all cases where the volume of blood that can be used is not severely restricted. Usually it is best to make all determinations of hemoglobin concentration on venous blood to which anticoagulant has been added. However, in some clinical situations, venous blood is difficult to obtain. Freely flowing blood may be obtained from a prick of the finger or ear lobe sufficient to obtain 0.02 ml for a Sahli pipette. The use of such a sample introduces an error beyond that of the pipette by virtue of the admixture of varying amounts of tissue juices with the blood sample.

Hemoglobin concentration is conveniently measured in a colorimeter either as cyanmethemoglobin or as oxyhemoglobin. Obviously, methods using either of these derivatives may be employed with any of the colorimeters. Only two specific methods will be given in detail: determination of total hemoglobin as cyanmethemoglobin with the Coleman Jr. Spectrophotometer using 0.02 ml of whole blood and determination of total hemoglobin as oxyhemoglobin with the Evelyn colorimeter using 0.1 ml of whole blood. These methods may be modified by appropriate change in the volumes used when colorimeters other than the two specified are supplied.

DETERMINATION OF TOTAL HEMOGLOBIN AS CYANMETHEMOGLOBIN WITH THE COLEMAN JR. SPECTROPHOTOMETER.[7] A sample of whole blood is diluted quantitatively with a solution containing potassium ferricyanide $(K_3Fe(CN)_6)$ and potassium cyanide (KCN). The former oxidizes hemoglobin to methemoglobin, which then reacts with KCN to form cyanmethemoglobin. The optical density of the solution is then determined by using light at a wavelength of 540 m$\mu$. Optical density is converted into concentration of hemoglobin by using a constant determined experimentally from the optical densities of a series of standards of known concentrations. Stable standard cyanmethemoglobin solutions of concentrations representing 1:250 dilutions of whole blood containing 5, 10, and 15 gm/100 ml of hemoglobin are available commercially and can be kept in the laboratory for original calibration of the colorimeter and also for periodic checks of the accuracy of the instrument.

**Method.** (*a*) *Preparation of the diluent* (Drabkin's solution). The amount to be

prepared should be governed by the amount of hemoglobinometry required of the laboratory. Five milliliters of solution is used for each test. To prepare 1 L of solution, 1 gm of $NaHCO_3$, 52 mg of KCN, and 198 mg of $K_3Fe(CN)_6$ are used. These are dissolved in distilled water to make 1 L of solution, which should be stored in a brown bottle because light causes a precipitate to form. Although Drabkin's solution contains little cyanide, it is regarded as a poison.

(*b*) *Precautions regarding the use of cyanide.* Salts and solutions of cyanide are poisonous and care should be taken to avoid getting them into the mouth or inhaling their fumes. Cyanide should be handled with the same caution as concentrated acids and pathogenic bacteria. The minimum lethal dose of anhydrous cyanic acid for humans is 36 mg.[9] In 1 L of Drabkin's solution there are 115 mg of cyanide as CN. The smallest dose of potassium cyanide that has been known to kill a human is 300 mg.[9] This amount of potassium cyanide is equivalent to that present in 6 L of Drabkin's solution.

The following specific precautionary measures are recommended: pipettes should be filled with a suction bulb; blood should be mixed with the cyanide solution by swirling; if small amounts of cyanide compounds are accidentally spilled on the laboratory bench or on the floor during the weighing procedure, the dry powder should be wiped up with a damp cloth and discarded in a suitable container; cyanide salts should be stored in a locked cupboard.

(*c*) *Calibrating the Coleman Jr. Spectrophotometer for the cyanmethemoglobin method.* To span the light beam of the Coleman Jr. Spectrophotometer, there must be at least 6 ml of solution in the 19-mm cuvette. The use of a 6-ml sample is cumbersome because transfer pipettes are not available in that size and serologic pipettes are inaccurate. Therefore it is recommended that the instrument be slightly modified to permit accurate readings with a smaller volume of solution. A 5-mm slice should be cut from the top of a No. 1 rubber stopper and dropped into the cuvette adapter so that it lies flat on the bottom. This elevates the cuvette sufficiently that 5 ml of solution spans the light beam.

The tubes containing the hemoglobin standards, after removal from the refrigerator, should be wiped free of condensed moisture before they are used. When they are placed in the well of the spectrophotometer, the arrow on the side of the tube should face squarely toward the source of light.

The spectrophotometer must be warmed up. The blank tube is placed in the well, and the galvanometer beam is adjusted to 100-percent light transmittance (at the right of the black scale) with the wavelength scale set at 540.

A tube containing the standard solution representing an original whole-blood concentration of 5 gm/100 ml of hemoglobin is next placed in the well. The reading on the black scale (the percentage of light transmittance) is recorded. The blank is checked and the percentage of light transmittance is recorded for the standard solutions representing whole-blood concentration of hemoglobin of 10 and 15 gm/100 ml.

The readings are transcribed onto semilogarithmic graph paper. The abscissa represents grams per 100 ml of hemoglobin, and the ordinate the percentage of light transmittance. A line is drawn through the three points and a table is prepared from this graph to show what each reading of the percentage of light transmittance corresponds to in grams of hemoglobin per 100 ml of blood. The table can be mounted between sheets of plastic or clear x-ray film. Each spectrophotometer must be standardized individually against the cyanmethemoglobin solutions and should be rechecked at weekly intervals thereafter. The standards should be kept in a refrigerator.

(d) *Procedure for hemoglobin deter-* *mination as cyanmethemoglobin.* Exactly 5 ml of Drabkin's solution is measured into each of two matched Coleman Jr. spectrophotometer tubes. To one tube, 0.02 ml of whole blood is delivered with a Sahli pipette which is rinsed repeatedly so that all of the blood is delivered. Blood and solution are mixed by swirling and allowed to stand for 10 min. The other tube serves as a blank.

The cuvette adapter is altered as described above.

The blank tube is placed in the well of the warmed-up spectrophotometer and the wavelength scale is set at 540. By means of coarse- and fine-adjustment knobs, the galvanometer light beam is adjusted to coincide with 100-percent light transmittance. The tube containing the hemoglobin solution is substituted for the blank tube and the percentage of light transmittance is read on the black scale. The result is translated into grams per 100 ml of hemoglobin by use of the calibration curve or table.

Where a large number of hemoglobin determinations are to be made sequentially, the same 0.02-ml pipette can be used for each. Two small beakers, one containing water, the other acetone, should be available. The pipette is attached to a length of latex tubing about 20 in. long with an ordinary plastic mouthpiece at one end. After the first specimen of blood has been measured, the pipette is rinsed first with water and then three times with acetone, the outside is wiped, and air is sucked through the pipette until the inside is dry. The whole procedure requires about 10 sec. It reduces the number of calibrated pipettes needed for a large laboratory service and it simplifies the use of the correction factor of the pipette. Pipettes should be cleaned with concentrated nitric acid at least once a week.

INTERPRETATIONS AND LIMITATIONS. Photoelectric methods are rapid, potentially accurate, and reproducible in good hands. With clean glassware, calibrated pipettes, and a standardized instrument, an accuracy of ±2–3 percent in routine determinations is usual. It must be emphasized that the photoelectric cell measures differences in light intensities only, so that large, variable errors occur unless clean glassware and nonturbid solutions are used. Careful attention to the manufacturer's instructions for operation is essential for reproducibility from day to day.

Since precision 0.02-ml pipettes are not available, it is necessary either to use certified pipettes or to calibrate the pipettes and apply the appropriate correction.

Pellets containing the ingredients of Drabkin's solution are available commercially. The diluent for the cyanmethemoglobin method is conveniently prepared from such pellets by dissolving them in the specified volume of distilled water. It has been found that Drabkin's solution prepared from such pellets deteriorates rapidly, so that falsely low values for hemoglobin concentration are obtained after several days. When the commercially available pellets are used, the diluting fluid should therefore be prepared fresh each day it is to be used. Drabkin's solution prepared from reagent-grade chemicals has been found to be stable for at least one week.

DETERMINATION OF TOTAL HEMOGLOBIN AS OXYHEMOGLOBIN WITH THE EVELYN PHOTOELECTRIC COLORIMETER. A sample of whole blood is hemolyzed in distilled water or a dilute solution of ammonium hydroxide (0.007N, pH 10). Active hemoglobin is converted immediately to oxyhemoglobin, whereas methemoglobin, carboxyhemoglobin, and sulfhemoglobin are not altered. A stronger alkali tends to produce variable proportions of alkaline hematin. The optical density of the hemoglobin solution is determined in the Evelyn photometer, using a light filter whose maximum transmission is at a wavelength of 540 m$\mu$. At this wavelength and pH, the absorption is so nearly the same for the various forms of hemoglobin mentioned above that the total content of hemoglobin is determined as oxyhemoglobin. Optical density is converted into grams of hemoglobin by multiplying by an experimentally determined constant.

**Method.** Dilute 0.007N ammonium hydroxide is prepared by diluting 0.04 ml of concentrated ammonium hydroxide (specific gravity 0.88) to 100 ml with distilled water. Approximately 25 ml of 0.007N ammonium hydroxide is added to a 50-ml volumetric flask. A sample of venous blood is measured, using a calibrated pipette; the pipette is wiped off to remove blood from the outside, and the sample is introduced into the solution. The pipette is rinsed three or four times with the solution. The sample is then mixed, made to the volume of 50.0 ml with 0.007N ammonium hydroxide, and mixed thoroughly. The solution should always be bright red and clear.

Evelyn tubes are selected that give galvanometer readings which agree within ¼ scale division when the tubes are filled with samples of the same dilute solution of hemoglobin. Each tube is marked with a vertical line so that it can always be centered to correspond with the vertical line on a tube holder of the instrument. One tube from the selected series serves as a blank, being filled with 10 ml of 0.007N ammonium hydroxide that contains no blood. To a second tube is added at least 10 ml of the unknown hemoglobin solution, diluted as described above. The tube should be handled only by the top to avoid fingerprints on the lower portion through which the beam of light passes. The tube holder of the instrument is adjusted to the 10 mark and the tube is inserted and centered. The 540 filter is inserted in the filter slot and the instrument is turned on. The light intensity is adjusted by varying the rheostats, marked fine and coarse, so that transmittance of light, as read on the galvanometer, is 100. With no change in this adjustment, the blank tube is removed and the tube containing the diluted unknown is introduced. The galvanometer reading is recorded to the nearest ¼ division. There is a correction for the galvanometer itself, which is obtained from the chart supplied with it by the manufacturer.

*Calculation.* The corrected galvanometer reading $G$ may be converted to optical or photometric density $L$ from a table supplied with the instrument, or from the equation $L = 2 - \log G$. From Beer's law it is known that the concentration $C$ of a colored solute is directly proportional to its optical density, so that

$$C \text{ (gm Hb/100 ml)} = \frac{100L}{K},$$

where $K$ is an experimentally determined constant, which is 2.58 for oxyhemoglobin measured in the Evelyn photometer as calibrated by the manufacturer. This constant should be checked by the laboratory using the instrument. Only small variations are found from one Evelyn colorimeter to another, but each instrument should be calibrated and any necessary changes made in the value for $K$.

INTERPRETATIONS AND LIMITATIONS. The comments noted under the cyanmethemoglobin method apply here also.

PHYSICAL METHOD: MEASUREMENT OF
HEMOGLOBIN BY COPPER SULFATE
METHOD

The hemoglobin concentration of whole blood can be determined from the specific gravities of whole blood and of plasma measured with solutions of copper sulfate (Unit 16). The hemoglobin is read from the line chart in Fig. 6.[10, 11]

The method is as described in Unit 16. In addition, specific gravity is also determined on a sample of well-mixed whole blood containing dry oxalate mixture,

200 mg/100 ml. A separate set of 40 copper sulfate solutions is required (for whole blood) with specific gravities from 1.035 to 1.075, at intervals of 0.001. For rougher work, sixteen solutions at intervals of 0.004 suffice to cover the entire range of plasma and whole blood (1.015–1.075).

*Example.* A sample of 5 ml of venous blood is taken with dry oxalate mixture, 200 mg/100 ml, the sample is mixed, and a drop of whole blood is introduced into each of a series of copper sulfate solutions until the specific gravity is estimated (Unit 16). A sample of 2 ml of whole blood is centrifuged, the plasma is removed, and its specific gravity is determined. Both results are corrected for the effect of anticoagulant by subtracting 0.0008. If the specific gravity of whole blood is read as 1.061, then 1.061 − 0.0008 = 1.0602. If the specific gravity of the plasma is 1.027, then 1.027 − 0.0008 = 1.0262, corresponding to a protein concentration of 7.25 gm/100 ml. A straight line connecting the values of specific gravity for plasma and whole blood on the line chart (Fig. 6) intersects the scale for hemoglobin at 16.2 gm/100 ml.

The results were found, in the original investigation, to be within ±2 percent of the mean hemoglobin value determination by the oxygen-capacity method of Van Slyke. Accordingly, this method, which requires no absolute measurements of volumes of blood, is a most practical and rapid procedure for determining both plasma protein and hemoglobin concentration with considerable accuracy. However, the Spencer hemoglobinometer as described above is perhaps less complicated to use and more reliable.

## Identification and Quantitative Determination of Methemoglobin and Sulfhemoglobin

Methemoglobin is a derivative of hemoglobin in which the ferrous ion has been oxidized to the ferric form. This change is reversible and, in itself, is not necessarily accompanied by any red-cell damage or destruction. Methemoglobin

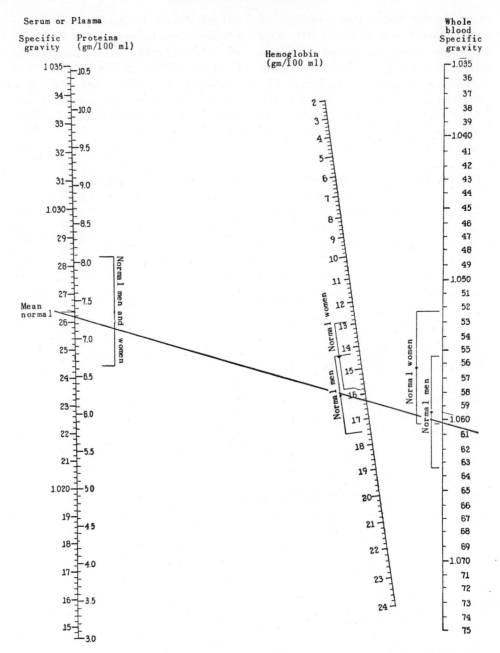

Fig. 6. Line chart for obtaining protein content of serum or plasma and hemoglobin content of corresponding sample of whole blood. The hematocrit scale has been deleted from the original publication.[10]

is inert in that it does not transport oxygen and does not combine reversibly with oxygen. About 1 to 2 percent of the total hemoglobin is in the form of methemoglobin in the normal individual and normal red cells have an active enzymatic glycolytic system which operates to reduce methemoglobin back into hemoglobin. Sulfhemoglobin is an abnormal pigment, not found at all in the body under ordinary circumstances. The exact nature of sulfhemoglobin is not known, and it has not been prepared in pure form. It is considered to be a derivative of hemoglobin formed by the action of certain drugs and chemicals such as sulfanilimide and trinitrotoluene. It is inactive with respect to oxygen transport.

Methemoglobinemia occurs as a congenital anomaly with polycythemia.[12] Also, transient methemoglobinemia and, occasionally, sulfhemoglobinemia occur following the ingestion of certain drugs such as sulfonamides, acetanilid, primaquinine, and certain oxidant compounds.[12] Rarely, hemolytic anemia occurs following intoxication from these compounds and may be severe, with hemoglobinemia and hemoglobinuria. Such hemolytic reactions are often associated with a deficiency of an intraerythrocytic enzyme, glucose-6-phosphate dehydrogenase, which appears to be required to maintain adequate levels of reduced glutathione within red cells (see Unit 11). Methemoglobin and sulfhemoglobin, which are in the red cells, may be identified by spectroscopic analysis.[12] In addition, they are readily detected and quantitated by the method of Evelyn and Malloy.[13]

IDENTIFICATION BY SPECTROSCOPIC ANALYSIS. The hand spectroscope or the Hartridge reversion spectroscope may be used to identify these pigments. Advantage is taken of the fact that the dark band of methemoglobin at a wavelength of 635 m$\mu$ disappears after the addition of cyanide ions to a solution of methemoglobin to form cyanmethemoglobin. The dark band of sulfhemoglobin at 620 m$\mu$ is not affected by cyanide ion but is dispersed by hydrogen peroxide [14] and shifts its position when the blood is equilibrated with carbon monoxide.[13] The spectroscopic methods probably cannot detect these pigments unless they represent at least 5 to 10 percent of the total hemoglobin and hence are not useful for detecting subtle changes in the blood.

QUANTITATION BY METHOD OF EVELYN AND MALLOY.[13] *Methemoglobin.* When sodi-um cyanide is added to a solution of methemoglobin, the characteristic absorption band at 635 m$\mu$ is almost completely abolished by the conversion of methemoglobin into cyanmethemoglobin. The resulting change in optical density is directly proportional to the concentration of methemoglobin. This change in optical density may be measured on the photoelectric colorimeter with a color filter that transmits a narrow spectral band in the vicinity of 635 m$\mu$.

*Sulfhemoglobin.* The depth of the 620-m$\mu$ absorption band of sulfhemoglobin is unchanged by the addition of cyanide, hence the concentration of sulfhemoglobin in a solution containing oxyhemoglobin can be determined after methemoglobin has been converted into cyanmethemoglobin by addition of cyanide. This measurement can be made by means of the photoelectric colorimeter, with a suitable filter, on the same solution used for the methemoglobin determination. A correction must of course be made for the small, though not negligible, absorption of oxyhemoglobin and methemoglobin at 620 m$\mu$.

*Oxyhemoglobin.* The concentration of oxyhemoglobin is obtained by subtracting the values for methemoglobin and sulfhemoglobin from the concentration of total hemoglobin determined by the cyanmethemoglobin method. The various forms of hemoglobin are converted into cyanmethemoglobin and the concentration of this pigment is determined by measuring the optical density of the solution in the photoelectric colorimeter, with a filter that transmits a spectral band in the vicinity of the cyanmethemoglobin absorption maximum at 540 m$\mu$.

**Method.** (*a*) *Reagents:* (1) M/15 phosphate buffer of pH 6.6; (2) M/60 phosphate buffer of pH 6.6 prepared from the above by dilution as required; (3) 20-percent aqueous potassium ferricyanide; (4) 10-percent aqueous sodium cyanide; (5) a neutralized solution of sodium cyanide prepared within 1 hr of the time of use by mixing equal parts of 10-percent sodium cyanide and 12-percent acetic acid; (6) concentrated ammonium hydroxide. Reagents (3) to (6) should be kept in dropper bottles that deliver approximately 25 drops/ml.

(*b*) *Procedure.* One-tenth milliliter of fresh whole blood (finger blood or venous blood to which not more than 2 mg/ml of potassium oxalate has been added) is delivered into 10 ml of M/60 phosphate buffer of pH 6.6 in a colorimeter tube. The solution is allowed to stand for 5 min, and a reading is made with light at a wavelength of 635 m$\mu$, after the galvanometer is first adjusted to 100 with a blank tube containing water only. The optical density is recorded as $L_1$. One drop of the neutralized sodium cyanide is then added to the solution to convert any methemoglobin into cyanmethemoglobin, and after 2 min a second reading $L_2$ is made with the same filter and blank tube. The difference ($L_1 - L_2$) is proportional to the concentration of methemoglobin. The solution, which up to this time will have been very slightly turbid, is now cleared for the sulfhemoglobin determination by addition of 1 drop of concentrated ammonium hydroxide, and a reading $L_3$ is made with light at a wavelength of 620 m$\mu$ and a blank tube containing water only. Finally, 2 ml of the solution is pipetted into a second colorimeter tube containing 8 ml of M/15 phosphate buffer of pH 6.6 and 1 drop of 20-percent potassium ferricyanide. The tube is allowed to stand for 2 min in order that all the oxyhemoglobin may be converted into methemoglobin; then 1 drop of 10-percent sodium cyanide is added to convert the methemoglobin into cyanmethemoglobin for the total-hemoglobin determination. At the end of 2 min a reading is made with light at a wavelength of 540 m$\mu$ and a blank tube containing 10 ml of water and 1 drop each of

20-percent potassium ferricyanide and 10-percent sodium cyanide.

*Calculations.* The concentrations of the various hemoglobin derivatives are calculated from the following equations, in which *T*, *M*, and *S* represent grams per 100 ml of blood of total hemoglobin, methemoglobin, and sulfhemoglobin respectively:

$$T = \frac{100L_4}{2.38}, \tag{1}$$

$$M = \frac{100(L_1 - L_2)}{2.77}, \tag{2}$$

$$S = \frac{1000L_3 - (8.5M + 4.4T)}{100}, \tag{3}$$

$$\text{Percent MHb} = \frac{M}{T}\,100. \tag{4}$$

The value for *T* obtained from Eq. (1) is not strictly accurate when the blood contains sulfhemoglobin, because it is not possible to convert sulfhemoglobin into cyanmethemoglobin with the reagents used. Fortunately, this error is not very serious, because the absorption (at 540 m$\mu$) of the compound formed from sulfhemoglobin by the action of ferricyanide is almost as great (78 percent) as that of a corresponding amount of cyanmethemoglobin. Since the error introduced in the total-hemoglobin determination is directly proportional to the concentration of sulfhemoglobin, the true value of *T* may be calculated from the formula

$$T_{\text{corr}} = T + 0.22S. \tag{5}$$

The concentration of oxyhemoglobin is obtained from the equation

$$\text{HbO}_2 = T_{\text{corr}} - (M + S). \tag{6}$$

The numerical values of the calibration constants that appear in the foregoing equations apply only to the Evelyn photoelectric colorimeter, but the form of the equations will be the same for all photoelectric colorimeters, and no difficulty should be encountered in adapting the method to other instruments.

INTERPRETATIONS AND LIMITATIONS. The comments noted above in connection

50

with the photoelectric determinations of hemoglobin concentrations apply here too.

The determination of methemoglobin is subject to an error of not more than 0.2 gm/100 ml and this also represents the smallest amount that can be detected with certainty. This method is, therefore, much more sensitive than the spec-

troscopic methods in detecting methemoglobin.

As little as 0.1 gm of sulfhemoglobin per 100 ml of blood can be detected, but the absolute accuracy of the measurement is somewhat less than that of the methemoglobin determination, since it is not possible to prepare pure sulfhemoglobin for a standard.

## REFERENCES

1. J. P. Peters and D. D. Van Slyke, *Quantitative Clinical Chemistry, Vol. II, Methods* (Williams and Wilkins, Baltimore, 1932).
2. C. F. Consolazio, R. E. Johnson, and E. Marek, *Metabolic Methods* (Mosby, St. Louis, 1951), p. 261.
3. E. Ammundsen, "Studies on the presence of non-carbon-monoxide-combining (inactive) hemoglobin in the blood of normal persons," *J. biol. Chem. 138,* 563 (1941).
4. S. Y. Wong, "Colorimetric determination of iron and hemoglobin in blood," *J. biol. Chem. 77,* 409 (1928).
5. M. A. Andersch and M. S. Sachs, "The hemoglobin pipette as a source of error in photoelectric hemoglobinometry," *Amer. J. clin. Path. 15,* 105 (1945).
6. E. C. Peffer, "Device for testing hemocytometers and other pipettes of small capacity," *J. Research Nat. Bur. Standards 19,* 177 (1937).
7. W. H. Crosby, J. I. Munn, and F. W. Furth, "Standardizing a method for clinical hemoglobinometry," *U.S. armed Forces med. J. 5,* 693 (1954).
8. D. L. Drabkin, in O. Glasser, ed., *Photometry and Spectrophotometry in Medical Physics* (Yearbook Publishers, Chicago, 1944), vol. 1.
9. J. J. P. Glaister, *Medical Jurisprudence and Toxicology* (ed. 8; Livingstone, Edinburgh, 1945), p. 558 quoted by Crosby *et al.*
10. R. A. Phillips, D. D. Van Slyke, V. P. Dole, K. Emerson, Jr., P. B. Hamilton, and R. M. Archibald, "Copper sulfate method for measuring specific gravities of whole blood and plasma, with line charts for calculating plasma proteins, hemoglobin, and hematocrit from plasma and whole blood gravities" (United States Navy Research Unit at the Hospital of the Rockefeller Institute for Medical Research, 1943–44, republished by Josiah Macy Foundation, New York, 1945).
11. P. B. Hawk, B. L. Oser, and W. H. Summerson, *Practical Physiological Chemistry* (ed. 12; Blakiston, Philadelphia, 1947), pp. 546–556.
12. C. A. Finch, "Methemoglobinemia and sulfhemoglobinemia," *New Engl. J. Med. 239,* 470 (1948).
13. K. A. Evelyn and H. T. Malloy, "Microdetermination of oxyhemoglobin, methemoglobin, and sulfhemoglobin, and in a single sample of blood," *J. biol. Chem. 126,* 655 (1938).
14. H. O. Michel and J. S. Harris, "Blood pigments: properties and quantitative determination with special reference to spectrophotometric methods," *J. lab. clin. Med. 25,* 445 (1939).

## Unit 6

# Determination of Hematocrit: Macroscopic Examination of Centrifuged Blood

The hematocrit may be defined as the percentage of the volume of a blood sample contributed by the red cells contained in it. If adequate technical methods are used for its determination, the hematocrit is a measurement of considerable accuracy. It finds particular application as a screening test for blood dyscrasias, and it provides necessary data for the computation of the mean corpuscular volume and the mean corpuscular hemoglobin concentration. Inspection of the plasma and buffy coat after centrifugation will sometimes yield valuable diagnostic information.

### Factors Involved in Hematocrit Determination

#### EFFICIENCY OF COMPONENT SEPARATION

If accurate and reproducible determinations of the hematocrit are to be made, the blood must be separated as completely as possible into its three main components. If blood is allowed to stand in a tube on the bench, some degree of separation by sedimentation will eventually occur. However, the forces resisting separation, namely plasma viscosity and convection currents, are large in relation to the forces producing separation; thus complete separation of cells and plasma, although approached, is never realized. When blood is subjected to a power-

ful centrifugal field, the components rapidly separate into layers determined by their respective specific gravities, since the forces tending to retard separation now become vanishingly small in relation to the forces producing it.

The efficiency with which this separation may be achieved depends upon three major factors: the magnitude of the centrifugal force; the duration of application of the force; the packed-cell volume of the blood. These three factors interact in a complex manner (each is an independent exponential variable), but it is relatively simple to define a set of limiting conditions that will meet the ordinary demands of hematocrit determination in clinical practice. The minimum magnitude and duration of the centrifugal field required to pack red cells so that further centrifugation produces no further change of packed-cell volume are given in Table 11 for a blood of 75-percent packed-cell volume. Lower values of packed-cell volume would not

Table 11. *Magnitude and duration of centrifugal field required to produce complete packing of blood having 75 percent packed-cell volume.*

| Centrifugal field ($Cg$) | Duration (min) |
|---|---|
| 10,000$g$ | 4 |
| 5,500$g$ | 10 |
| 2,500$g$ | 30 |

52

require the application of such high centrifugal fields to produce equivalent packing. Blood with a hematocrit higher than 75 percent might not be efficiently packed by these fields. Although the term "relative centrifugal force" is widely used, what is meant is actually centrifugal acceleration. The centrifugal field at the tip of the centrifuge tube, in units of $g$, the acceleration due to gravity ($980$ cm/sec$^2$), is calculated from the formula

$$C_g = (1.118 \times 10^{-5})n^2 r,$$

where $C$ is the numerical measure of the field, $n$ (rev/min) is the speed of rotation of the centrifuge, and $r$ (cm) is the radius of rotation measured to the tip of the centrifuge cup.

Even after centrifugation, about 20 percent of the white cells and platelets may remain trapped in the upper part of the red-cell layer and contribute to the apparent red-cell volume. This is not, normally, an important source of error, but in cases where the red cells have low specific gravity (that is, in severe hypochromic anemia) the edge of the red-cell layer may be blurred beyond definition. Another contribution to inefficient component separation is the fact that the curvature of the surfaces of red cells does not permit them to pack together without some interstitial spaces remaining. This results in an entrainment of plasma in the red-cell layer which is quantitatively dependent on the packed-cell volume and qualitatively dependent on the size, shape, and deformability of the cells. Estimates have been made of the volume of plasma trapped in the red-cell layer in hematocrit determinations. Ebaugh *et al.*[1] give the range of 0–2 percent of the observed cell volume for cells of normal morphology in the hematocrit range 33 to 68 percent. The difficulty of making satisfactory corrections for the error due to trapped plasma has resulted in its being ignored for routine clinical observations.

The application of hematocrit techniques to research problems, particularly those concerned with blood-volume measurements in blood diseases, should involve consideration of whether a correction for trapped plasma is necessary to the interpretation of the results.

REPRESENTATIVE SAMPLING

The blood plasma is in a state of dynamic equilibrium with the extravascular spaces. In the capillaries, shifts of fluid across the vessel wall may occur with extraordinary rapidity, influencing the hematocrit of blood within these vessels. Fluid shifts occur mainly in response to local changes in hydrostatic and osmotic pressure. Pronounced changes in hydrostatic pressure can be produced within the capillaries by unduly prolonged venous obstruction, such as might occur during venipuncture. Thus, in the collection of venous-blood samples for hematocrit determination the tourniquet should be applied for the minimum time necessary for insertion of the needle.

For the collection of specimens for microhematocrit measurements similar precautions are necessary. It is customary to speak of such specimens as being of "capillary" blood. The blood obtained by puncture of the finger tip emanates mainly from metarterioles and venules, with very little contribution from capillaries. A correctly performed stab of the finger pulp with a sharp scalpel blade should result in a free flow of blood without any necessity for congestion or squeezing of the finger. Representative blood samples, adequate for most clinical and experimental purposes, can be obtained in this way.

The question frequently arises whether stab specimens and venous specimens are truly representative of the "total body hematocrit." This is a field of esoteric debate best ignored by the clinical worker. Total body hematocrit is a physiologic concept rather than a directly mensurable parameter, and blood specimens collected from peripheral vessels can be taken as being sufficiently representative for practical purposes. Account should be taken, however, of the possible unreliability of hematocrit measurements made immediately following moderate hemorrhage (including enthusiastic blood-specimen collection in infants!) or shortly after the infusion of whole blood, plasma, or packed red cells. It would also be considered unwise to attempt to compute blood indices from red-cell count and hemoglobin based on "capillary" blood and hematocrit based on venous blood.

### THE RED CELL AS AN OSMOMETER

Because of the sharp structural differentiation between its membrane and its contents, the red cell responds, by changes in size and shape, to alterations in the osmotic pressure of its environment. Minor increase of the plasma osmotic pressure results in loss of water from the cell, with consequent shrinkage. Reduction of plasma osmotic pressure causes swelling of the cell owing to imbibition of water.

The membrane of the red cell cannot, however, be regarded as a simple semipermeable membrane. Because of the relatively high osmotic pressures within the cell, there is a continual tendency for water to enter. In the normal, freshly collected cell, resistance to entry of water (and hence change of cell volume) is high, but after storage in certain media the cell begins to "leak" potassium. Potassium leakage is known to be associated with loss of integrity of the membrane and is rapidly followed by loss of the ability of the cell to resist the entry of water. The cell consequently swells, assumes a spheroidal shape, and eventually bursts.

From these basic facts it can be seen that it is necessary to pay careful attention to factors influencing the environment of the red cell. Serious errors may be introduced into hematocrit measurements if cell shrinkage or swelling is permitted to occur.

### THE CHOICE AND USE OF ANTICOAGULANTS

The most probable source of osmotic errors lies in the use of unsatisfactory anticoagulants (or in the incorrect use of satisfactory ones). The ideal anticoagulant remains to be discovered, but of those at present available balanced oxalate and heparin have been shown, by experience, to produce sufficiently small distortion of the red cells to permit accurate hematocrit measurements.

Both these reagents are used in the dry state, since dilution of the plasma by anticoagulant solutions would cause falsely low readings of packed-cell volume. *Balanced oxalate* is suitable for use in circumstances where it is possible to collect quantities in excess of 1 ml of venous blood. This anticoagulant has the advantage that the red cells of blood collected into it do not suffer significant disturbance of their size or shape by osmotic forces. This advantage is fully achieved only when the proper volume of blood is added to the dried anticoagulant (see Unit 3). Because of measuring difficulties, it is not feasible to collect capillary blood into balanced oxalate without special precautions: venous samples of less than 1 ml cannot be easily or accurately mixed with this reagent. For these reasons the use of balanced oxalate is confined to samples (generally 5 ml in volume) intended for testing by the Wintrobe technique. Considerable shrinkage of leukocytes occurs after contact with oxalate for several hours at room temperature, and the finer aspects of nuclear structure (such as chromatin patterns and nucleoli) are rapidly lost. If critical examination of the buffy coat is indicated, a further specimen should be collected into the dried sodium salt of EDTA (see Unit 3). Salts of EDTA are not recommended for hematocrit measurements. Experience with their use is not sufficient at the present time. They probably cause some degree of cell shrinkage.

For microhematocrit methods, the dried sodium salt of *heparin* is the anticoagulant of choice. While heparin is not a "permanent" anticoagulant, it delays clotting for many hours or days when used in slight excess. In useful concentrations it does not cause any appreciable shrinkage of red cells. When heparin is used, distortion of the leukocytes is not as severe as with oxalated blood, but if examination is delayed for several hours marked clumping and disintegration of white cells may occur.

## Procedure for Inspection of Hematocrit Tube

The importance of the macroscopic examination of blood as an essential part of hematocrit determination is stressed by Wintrobe.[2] In determining hematocrits it is important to note and record the following observations.

### RAPID SEDIMENTATION OF RED CELLS

Even when measurement of the erythrocyte sedimentation rate is not made, or is made separately, observation of the filled hematocrit tube immediately prior to centrifugation may reveal the presence of a high rate of red-cell sedimentation. For such an observation to be valid, the tube must have been kept as near to vertical as possible from the time of filling, and the approximate period of standing should be known. A striking degree of settling (20 percent or more of the plasma cleared of cells) in 5 to 10 min may indicate the presence of rouleaux or of agglutinins.

### EXAMINATION OF THE PLASMA

Attention should be directed particularly to color and opacity. The presence of excessive bilirubin is easily recognized. Acute intravascular hemolysis may produce the characteristic reddish color-ation of hemoglobinemia, but caution should be exercised in interpreting the clinical significance of apparent free hemoglobin in the plasma, since the commonest cause of the appearance of this pigment in a blood specimen is poor collection technique or shaking the specimen. True hemoglobinemia almost always occurs in association with some degree of bilirubinemia and methemalbuminemia.

A cloudy appearance of the plasma may usually be taken to indicate abnormally high plasma lipid levels, such as may be found in nephrosis. However, specimens collected from normal persons within 1 or 2 hr after a fatty meal may show striking lipemia. A rare cause of clouding of plasma is a hyperglobulinemic state such as myeloma.

### EXAMINATION OF THE BUFFY COAT

The buffy coat (packed white cells and platelets) normally appears as a sharply demarcated gray zone occupying 0.5–1 percent of the blood-specimen volume, separating red cells from plasma. Leukemia or acute infections associated with high white-cell counts cause an obvious extension of the buffy coat, while leukopenic states cause its reduction. Loss of the sharp dividing line between red cells and buffy coat indicates the presence of abnormal red cells (usually hypochromic) with specific gravities close to that of leukocytes. The hematocrit tube provides a convenient source for the microscopic examination of buffy-coat material.

## Methods of Determining the Hematocrit

Two methods are now widely used for hematocrit measurement. The Wintrobe, or macro, method has for many years been regarded as the standard by which other techniques must be judged. Almost every laboratory possesses a centrifuge suitable for this method. The microhematocrit method, developed from a procedure described by Guest,[3] offers **many** advantages in economy of time, labor, and blood and is as accurate as Wintrobe's technique.[4]

WINTROBE METHOD

EQUIPMENT. *Hematocrit tubes.* The Wintrobe hematocrit tube is a thick-walled glass tube with a uniform internal bore. The bottom of the tube is flattened and the wall is marked with millimeter graduations from zero to 105 mm. The tube should be provided with a suitable rubber cap to prevent evaporation of the contents during centrifugation.

*Filling pipette.* This is a long-stemmed capillary pipette, of which various commercial patterns are available. The most satisfactory type has a metal stem which is either fused to a glass chamber or fitted to it by a ground joint. A 2-ml syringe provided with a long aspirating needle makes a satisfactory filling pipette. Whatever the design, the delivery tip of the pipette must be capable of reaching the bottom of the hematocrit tube.

*Centrifuge.* Many of the standard laboratory centrifuges will be satisfactory but it should be established that the model used is capable of generating a centrifugal field of at least 2500g at the bottom of the cup. Angle heads, preferably of not more than 45° inclination, have proved to yield satisfactory results and, on account of better streamlining, have the advantage of higher speed of rotation than the swing-out head.

**Procedure.** *Mixing the sample.* The sample will usually be taken from a bottle or tube containing 5 ml of blood mixed with balanced oxalate. Before attempting to fill the hematocrit tube, check that the level of blood in the bottle is such as to indicate that the correct volume of blood has been placed in it. The importance of representative sampling has been stressed. This is best achieved by mixing cells and plasma by a minimum of 30 slow and complete inversions of the bottle. On no account should the bottle be shaken. Rolling or

swirling the bottle contents does not give adequate redistribution of the cells if sedimentation has occurred. The most reliable means of mixing the specimen is the mechanical system described by Dacie.[5] After mixing, the hematocrit tube should be filled without delay.

*Filling the tube.* The hematocrit tube is filled by means of the filling pipette previously described. Sufficient blood should be drawn into the pipette to enable the tube to be filled in one operation and filling should commence from the *bottom* of the tube, the pipette being raised as filling proceeds but with the delivery tip always under the surface of the blood in the tube. Bubbles must be avoided. With skill the tube can be filled to the 100-mm mark with fair precision; however, there is no advantage in attempting to adjust the level exactly to this point. It is better to fill near to the 100-mm mark and then to derive the percentage packed-cell volume after centrifugation by simple computation.

Hematocrit tubes should be capped after filling in order to prevent evaporation of their contents during centrifugation. If caps are not available, the filling level of the tube should be noted before centrifugation. If the tubes are capped, the reading of the filling level may be taken after centrifugation.

*Centrifugation.* In accordance with the principles already discussed, the filled tube should be centrifuged for 30 min at 2500g. If a lower centrifugal force is applied, some reservation is necessary in interpreting the results of hematocrits over 70 percent.

*Mensuration.* Tubes should be removed from the centrifuge with the minimum disturbance and observed in the upright position in a good light against a neutral gray or green background. The thick wall of the tube tends to introduce parallax errors in reading, and care should be taken to avoid this error. The filling level (approximately 100 mm) is read against the lowest point of the plasma meniscus, as in reading a burette or pipette. The red-cell level is read at the lower margin of the buffy coat. At this point the red-cell layer frequently shows a well-defined dark band.

*Computation of results.* The following formula is used:

$$\text{Hematocrit (percent)} = 100L_1/L_2,$$

where $L_1$ (mm) is the height of the red-cell column and $L_2$ (mm) is the total height of the red cells plus plasma (the filling level).

*Recovery of buffy coat.* A drop of a highly concentrated suspension of white cells and platelets may be obtained by careful aspiration with a fine-pointed capillary pipette at the grayish interface of plasma and red cells. When smears made from this material are examined, allowance should be made for alterations in appearance and staining properties of cells that have been in contact with balanced oxalate.

### MICROHEMATOCRIT METHOD

EQUIPMENT. *Hematocrit tubes.* Considerable latitude of choice is possible in the selection of tubes. The essential requirements are that they should be capable of fitting comfortably in the radial grooves of the microhematocrit centrifuge head and that they should be of uniform bore throughout their whole length. Drawn glass tubing tends to have a taper but this is usually so slight as to contribute no significant error to the result. The most widely used type of tube is the so-called "melting-point" capillary tube with a bore of about 1 mm and a length of about 7 cm. The walls of this tubing are thin and it is easily sealed by the heat of a very small flame.

Before they can be used, a suitable amount of dried heparin must be introduced into the tubes. This is best accomplished by diluting commercial heparin solution with distilled water to yield a reagent with a heparin concentration of 0.1 mg/ml. The tubes are filled with the diluted solution by capillary action and then placed in a 56°C drying oven or 37°C incubator until all moisture is driven off. The tubes may then be stored in tightly stoppered containers until required for use.

*The centrifuge.* Microhematocrit tubes may, of course, be used in any of the centrifuges suitable for the macro method. If this is done, the centrifuging time will be at least 30 min and, because of the risk of breakage, the thin-walled tubes must be supported in the axis of the centrifuge cup by placing them in other, larger tubes.

Full use is made of the advantages of the micro method only when centrifuging is carried out in one of the specially designed high-speed units that are commercially available. Several satisfactory types are on the market and most are capable of producing centrifugal fields of the order of 10,000g. This high value of centrifugal field permits shortening of the centrifuging time to 4 or 5 min, while at the same time giving greater assurance of complete packing of high-hematocrit bloods than can be gained at lower values. Recently a microhematocrit head has been made available for the International Equipment Company "Clinical" centrifuge that permits speeds up to 7500 rev/min and centrifugal fields up to 5500g. Centrifuging time with this head should be 10 min.

*Reading device.* Since the microhematocrit tube is ungraduated, some means must be provided for measuring the lengths of the columns of packed red cells and plasma. Several semiautomatic measuring devices are commercially available, each operating on a different principle, but reasonably accurate measurements may be made by using a clearly graduated millimeter rule and a low-power magnifying lens. If large numbers of specimens are to be tested, errors in measurement due to fatigue will be reduced by using a commercial reading device that expresses the percentage of packed red cells directly on a scale without the necessity for computation by the operator.

**Procedure.** *Sampling.* Occasionally the microhematocrit tube may be filled from a venous specimen. If this is the case, proper care should be taken in mixing the blood before sampling. Usually the tube will be filled with blood obtained from skin puncture. The stab wound should be deep enough to insure a free and generous flow of blood. The first two or three drops should be wiped away and the tube filled by capillary action from the next drop as it forms. Blood should not fill the tube from end to end, but at least 1 cm of the tube should be left empty. The skin of the finger should be perfectly dry at the time of puncture; no alcohol or other antiseptic should be permitted to dilute or hemolyze the blood. The skin should be warm to the touch but not hyperemic. It should never be necessary to apply congestion to make the blood flow. If specimens are collected outside the laboratory, the microhematocrit head with its numbered radial slots makes a convenient carrier.

*Sealing the tube.* Once the tube has been charged with blood, the empty end should be sealed by passing the tip through a small flame or plugging it with modeling clay (Plasticene). A micro burner is conveniently made by connecting a 24-gauge needle to a suitable gas outlet by rubber tubing on which is an adjustable clamp. Larger flames may cook the blood.

*Centrifuging.* After the tubes have been sealed, they are placed in the centrifuge head with the closed end outermost. At this time there will be an air gap between the seal and the blood but this air will be later displaced by the centrifugal force. Tubes that have been plugged with modeling clay may show a tendency to leak during centrifugation unless the hematocrit head is fitted with a rubber gasket at its periphery to act as a cushion for the ends of the tubes to

bear against. The very rapid acceleration of high-speed microhematocrit centrifuges can lead to breakage of the tubes if there is even a slight gap between the end of the tube and the periphery of the head. It is good practice to spin the centrifuge head by hand before switching on the motor in order to force the tubes into firm contact with the peripheral retaining shoulder. Refer to Table 11 for centrifuging time.

*Mensuration.* After a suitable time of centrifuging has elapsed, the tubes may be removed from the head for reading. If an automatic reading device is used, the manufacturer's instructions must be followed exactly for best results. Otherwise, the lengths of the packed-cell and plasma columns should be carefully measured with a millimeter rule and the same method of computing the packed-cell volume should be used as is described for the macro method.

*Buffy-coat recovery.* If it is desired to recover the buffy coat for microscopic examination, a very small piece of modeling clay should be inserted in the open end of the tube and a diamond scratch made on the tube just *below* the buffy coat. The tube may then be snapped easily into two pieces, with the buffy coat in the section containing the plasma. The broken end of the tube is held over a coverglass or microscope slide and a larger piece of modeling clay is forced into the upper end of the tube to act as a piston which will drive a drop of material from the lower end. A smear may then be made in the usual way.

### Interpretation of Results

In addition to the information that may be obtained from qualitative examination of the hematocrit tube, the percentage packed-cell volume is one of the most important and precise measurements that can be made on a blood sample in the evaluation of anemia and polycythemia. It is more accurate and less laborious to make than the red-cell count. Wintrobe gives the mean value of packed-cell volume for normal males as $(47.0 \pm 7.0)$ percent and for normal females as $(42.0 \pm 5)$ percent. The packed-cell volume is used to derive values for mean corpuscular volume (MCV) and mean corpuscular hemoglobin concentration (MCHC) (Unit 7).

It is important to appreciate that the hematocrit does not give information as to total red-cell mass of a patient. A normal or near-normal total red-cell mass may exist in the face of wide varia-tions of hematocrit. Examples of this are to be found in cases of hemodilution such as the physiologic hydremia of pregnancy where a falling hematocrit may not necessarily indicate anemia in the sense of a reduction of the total number of circulating red cells. On the other hand, the hemoconcentration of shock may produce an apparently normal, or a raised, hematocrit even though a considerable proportion of the total red-cell mass has been lost through hemorrhage.

## REFERENCES

1. F. G. Ebaugh, Pearl Levine, and C. P. Emerson, "The amount of trapped plasma in the red cell mass of the hematocrit tube," *J. lab. clin. Med.* 46, 409–415 (1955).

2. M. M. Wintrobe, *Clinical Hematology* (ed. 3; Lea and Febiger, Philadelphia, 1951).

3. G. M. Guest and V. E. Siler, "A centrifuge method for the determination of the volume of cells in blood," *J. lab. clin. Med.* 19, 757 (1934).

4. J. J. McGovern, A. R. Jones, and A. G. Steinberg, "The hematocrit of capillary blood," *New Engl. J. Med.* 253, 308 (1955).

5. J. V. Dacie, *Practical Hematology* (Chemical Publishing Co., Brooklyn, 1951), p. 30.

# Unit 7

# Red-Cell Corpuscular Values

The anemias may be classified in terms of morphologic characteristics of the red cells, such as size, shape, and hemoglobin content. Measurement of these features is often helpful in arriving at an etiologic diagnosis.

### SIZE

AVERAGE SIZE. The average size of red cells, compared to the normal, can be estimated by inspection and comparison (see Unit 9), by direct measurement of the diameters of cells on the stained blood smear, or by determination of the mean corpuscular volume (MCV).[1] The red cell is then described as macrocytic, normocytic, or microcytic in size.

VARIATION IN SIZE. The degree of variation in size of red cells can be estimated by inspection or by measurement of the diameters of red cells on the smear [2] (see Fig. 7), but not by measurement of mean red-cell corpuscular values. Red cells are then reported as showing normal, moderate, marked, or extreme variation in size (anisocytosis). The variation in size may be more quantitatively expressed as the standard deviation of the diameters or as the coefficient of variation of the diameters in percent.

### SHAPE

AVERAGE SHAPE. The shape of the average red cell is estimated by inspection of the smear. It is usually round. Rarely, the congenital anomaly of ovalocytosis is observed.[3]

VARIATION IN SHAPE. The degree of variation in shape of the red-cell population is estimated from inspection of the smear, and is reported as normal, moderate, marked, or extreme. The shapes of individual abnormal forms are reported as oval, spheroidal, sickled, oat-shaped, pencil-formed, pear-shaped, tailed, or fragmented. The term poikilocyte (literally, varied cell, that is, of various shapes) is used generically to indicate red cells of abnormal shapes. It is preferable that a description be recorded of the actual shape.

### HEMOGLOBIN CONTENT

The average concentration of hemoglobin per red cell and the degree of variation in hemoglobin content can be estimated from inspection of the smear. The red cells are described as normochromic, hypochromic, or hyperchromic. The average hemoglobin content of the red cells may be calculated and expressed as the mean corpuscular hemoglobin (MCH) and as the mean corpuscular hemoglobin concentration (MCHC).

### IMMATURE AND ABNORMAL FORMS

Immature red cells are detected by the presence of polychromatophilia and nucleated forms. Stippling of cells, and cells

60

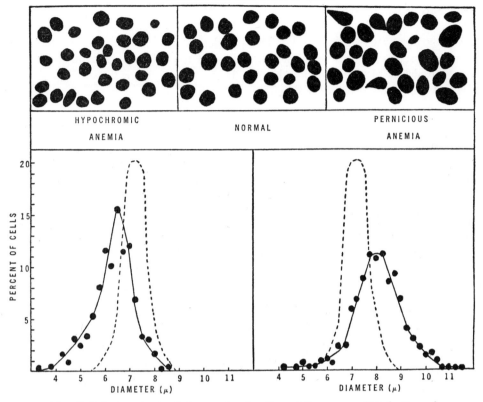

Fig. 7. Relative size and shape of red cells and frequency distribution of diameters of red cells.

|  | Hypochromic anemia | Normal | Pernicious anemia |
|---|---|---|---|
| Red-cell count $(10^6/mm^3)$ | 4.3 | 5.2 | 1.16 |
| Hemoglobin (gm/100 ml) | 4.8 | 15 | 4.2 |
| MCV [mean corpuscular volume $(\mu^3)$] | 52 | 90 | 125 |
| MCD [mean cell diameter $(\mu)$] | 6.3 | 7.2 | 8.1 |
| $\sigma$(MCD)$(\mu)$[a] | 0.83 | 0.50 | 1.01 |
| C.V.(MCD)(percent)[a] | 13 | 7.1 | 12.5 |

[a] $\sigma$ is one standard deviation and C.V. is one coefficient of variation of the diameters of 500 red cells measured in each case.

containing nuclear remnants such as Cabot rings and Howell-Jolly bodies, may be noted.

### Determination of Average Size and Hemoglobin Content of Red Cells

#### METHOD OF CALCULATION

The average size and hemoglobin content of red cells can be calculated by the method of Wintrobe from a knowledge of the red-cell count in millions per cubic millimeter, the hemoglobin content in grams per 100 ml, and the hematocrit in percent. The determinations of red-cell count, hemoglobin content, and hematocrit are described in Units 4, 5, and 6 respectively. Venous blood is used, containing as anticoagulant either heparin or a mixture of dry ammonium and potassium oxalates, as described in Unit 3. Each of these determinations must be accurate within ±5 percent (2 coefficients of variation).

MEAN CORPUSCULAR VOLUME (MCV). The mean corpuscular volume expresses the average volume of the individual red cells and is calculated from the equation

$$MCV = \frac{\text{Hematocrit (percent)} \times 10}{\text{Red-cell count } (10^6/\text{mm}^3)}.$$

The result is expressed in cubic microns ($\mu^3$) per cell.

*Examples.* In a normal subject, the red cells are normocytic, as indicated by a normal MCV: hematocrit, 45 percent; red-cell count, $5.0 \times 10^6/\text{mm}^3$; MCV = 45 $\times$ 10/5 = 90 $\mu^3$. In severe pernicious anemia, the macrocytosis is indicated by the increased MCV: hematocrit, 14 percent; red-cell count, $1.0 \times 10^6/\text{mm}^3$; MCV = 14 $\times$ 10/1.0 = 140 $\mu^3$. In severe hypochromic anemia, the microcytosis is indicated by the low MCV: hematocrit, 14 percent; red-cell count, $2.5 \times 10^6/\text{mm}^3$; MCV = 14 $\times$ 10/2.5 = 56 $\mu^3$.

MEAN CORPUSCULAR HEMOGLOBIN (MCH). The mean corpuscular hemoglobin expresses the average content of hemoglobin of the individual red cell in absolute terms; it is calculated from the equation

$$MCH = \frac{\text{Hemoglobin concentration (gm/100 ml)} \times 10}{\text{Red-cell count } (10^6/\text{mm}^3)}.$$

The result is expressed in micromicrograms ($\mu\mu$g or $10^{-12}$ gm) per cell.

*Examples.* In a normal subject, the hemoglobin concentration per red cell is calculated: hemoglobin, 15 gm/100 ml; red-cell count, $5.0 \times 10^6/\text{mm}^3$; MCH, 15 $\times$ 10/5.0 = 30 $\mu\mu$g. In severe pernicious anemia, the absolute amount of hemoglobin in each cell is greater than normal because the average volume of the red cells (MCV) is larger than normal: hemoglobin, 5 gm/100 ml; red-cell count, $1.0 \times 10^6/\text{mm}^3$; MCH, 5 $\times$ 10/1.0 = 50 $\mu\mu$g. In severe hypochromic anemia, the absolute amount of hemoglobin in each cell is reduced, for two reasons: the average volume of the red cells (MCV) is markedly reduced and the red cells themselves contain less than the average amount of hemoglobin. Therefore, the MCH is greatly reduced: hemoglobin, 4 gm/100 ml; red-cell count, 2.5 $\times$ $10^6/\text{mm}^3$; MCH = 4 $\times$ 10/2.5 = 16 $\mu\mu$g.

In most types of anemia, the MCH and MCV vary in a corresponding manner. The MCH is measured in absolute terms and is a measure of two variables: the size of the cell and its hemoglobin content.

MEAN CORPUSCULAR HEMOGLOBIN CONCENTRATION (MCHC). The mean corpuscular hemoglobin concentration expresses the average hemoglobin concentration per unit volume (per 100 ml) of packed red cells and is calculated from the equation

$$MCHC = \frac{\text{Hemoglobin concentration (gm/100 ml)} \times 100}{\text{Hematocrit (percent)}}.$$

The result is expressed in grams per 100 ml of *red cells.*

*Examples.* In a normal subject: hemoglobin, 15 gm/100 ml; hematocrit, 45 percent; MCHC = 15 $\times$ 100/45 = 33 gm/100 ml. In severe pernicious anemia, in spite of a large cell (increased MCV) and an increased absolute amount of hemoglobin in each cell (increased MCH), the average concentration of hemoglobin per unit volume of packed red cells is normal: hemoglobin, 5 gm/100 ml; hematocrit, 14 percent; MCHC = 5 $\times$ 100/14 = 36 gm/100 ml. In severe hypochromic anemia, the concentration of hemoglobin per unit volume of packed red cells is reduced: hemoglobin, 4 gm/100 ml; hematocrit, 15 percent; MCHC = 4 $\times$ 100/15 = 27 gm/100 ml.

The MCHC does not exceed the normal value except in spherocytosis. A decrease in the MCHC indicates that a unit volume of packed red cells contains less hemoglobin than normal or that stroma is present in cells in the place of hemoglobin.

ACCURACY

Determinations of the MCV, MCH, and MCHC require an accuracy of at least ±5 percent (2 coefficients of variation) in observations of the red-cell count, hemoglobin, and hematocrit. It is essential to use accurate data to calculate these corpuscular values. It is useful to check the appearance of the red cells on the stained film against the cal-

Table 12. *Normal values for red cells at various ages.*[3]

| Age | Red-cell count $(10^6/mm^3)$ | Hemoglobin (gm/100 ml) | Hematocrit (percent) | Corpuscular values [a] | | | |
|---|---|---|---|---|---|---|---|
| | | | | MCV $(\mu^3)$ | MCH $(\mu\mu g)$ | MCHC (gm/100 ml) | MCD $(\mu)$ |
| First day | 5.1 ± 1.0 | 19.5 ± 5.0 | 54.0 ± 10.0 | 106 | 38 | 36 | 8.6 |
| 2–3 days | 5.1 | 19.0 | 53.5 | 105 | 37 | 35 | |
| 4–8 days | 5.1 | 18.3 ± 4.0 | 52.5 | 103 | 36 | 35 | |
| 9–13 days | 5.0 | 16.5 | 49.0 | 98 | 33 | 34 | |
| 14–60 days | 4.7 ± 0.9 | 14.0 ± 3.3 | 42.0 ± 7.0 | 90 | 30 | 33 | 8.1 |
| 3–5 months | 4.5 ± 0.7 | 12.2 ± 2.3 | 36.0 | 80 | 27 | 34 | 7.7 |
| 6–11 months | 4.6 | 11.8 | 35.5 ± 5.0 | 77 | 26 | 33 | 7.4 |
| 1 year | 4.5 | 11.2 | 35.0 | 78 | 25 | 32 | 7.3 |
| 2 years | 4.6 | 11.5 | 35.5 | 77 | 25 | 32 | |
| 3 years | 4.5 | 12.5 | 36.0 | 80 | 27 | 35 | 7.4 |
| 4 years | 4.6 ± 0.6 | 12.6 | 37.0 | 80 | 27 | 34 | |
| 5 years | 4.6 | 12.6 | 37.0 | 80 | 27 | 34 | |
| 6–10 years | 4.7 | 12.9 | 37.5 | 80 | 27 | 34 | 7.4 |
| 11–15 years | 4.8 | 13.4 | 39.0 | 82 | 28 | 34 | |
| *Adults* | | | | | | | |
| Females | 4.8 ± 0.6 | 14.0 ± 2.0 | 42.0 ± 5.0 | 87 ± 5 | 29 ± 2 | 34 ± 2 | 7.5 ± 0.3 |
| Males | 5.4 ± 0.8 | 16.0 ± 2.0 | 47.0 ± 7.0 | 87 ± 5 | 29 ± 2 | 34 ± 2 | 7.5 ± 0.3 |

[a] MCV, mean corpuscular volume;
MCH, mean corpuscular hemoglobin;
MCHC, mean corpuscular hemoglobin concentration;
MCD, mean corpuscular diameter.

culated values. The values may also be cross-checked against each other. Thus extremely low values for MCH are not consistent with macrocytosis. Replicate observations of corpuscular values should check within ±5 percent.

### CORPUSCULAR VALUES IN DISEASE

The normal red-cell corpuscular values for children and adults are shown in Table 12. The approximate ranges observed in normal adults and in anemias are given in Table 13 and discussed in Unit 11.

### Measurement and Estimation of Variation in Size and Shape of Red Cells

The variation in size of erythrocytes can be measured by the method of Price-Jones,[2] in which the diameters of a large number of cells are measured from a stained film or a wet preparation of blood. The procedure is too laborious for routine clinical use. It is informative, however, to recognize the variation in diameters, as shown in Fig. 7 [4, 5] for the

Table 13. *Ranges of red-cell corpuscular values.*

| Condition | MCV $(\mu^3)$ | MCH $(\mu\mu g)$ | MCHC (gm/100 ml) |
|---|---|---|---|
| Normal | 82–92 | 27–31 | 32–36 |
| Normocytic anemia | 82–92 | 25–30 | 32–36 |
| Macrocytic anemia | 95–150 | 30–50 | 32–36 |
| Microcytic anemia | 50–80 | 12–25 | 25–30 |

normal blood and for a microcytic and a macrocytic anemia. For clinical purposes, the inspection of the stained blood smear and comparison with a smear of normal blood will permit an estimate and description of variation in size and shape of the individual red cells (Unit 9). Examination of a wet preparation (Unit 9) will also permit assessment of the size and shape of red cells.

### Other Methods of Measuring Red Cells

Certain methods are available for the measurement of red cells other than those described above. The color index is calculated by dividing the hemoglobin concentration in "percent of normal" by the red-cell count. This is based on the erroneous assumption that a single normal value for hemoglobin concentration can be selected. The color index has been largely replaced by calculation of the corpuscular values of Wintrobe. The measurement of the average diameter of red cells by their diffraction of light (halometer) has been used.[3] The osmotic-fragility test as a measure of the geometric form of red cells is discussed in Unit 11.

## REFERENCES

1. M. M. Wintrobe, "The direct calculation of the volume and hemoglobin content of the erythrocyte," *J. lab. clin. Med. 17*, 899 (1932).
2. C. Price-Jones, *Red Blood Cell Diameters* (Oxford Medical Publications, London, 1933).
3. M. M. Wintrobe, *Clinical Hematology* (Lea and Febiger, Philadelphia, ed. 4, 1956).
4. G. A. Daland, C. W. Heath, and G. R. Minot, "Differentiation of pernicious anemia and certain other macrocytic anemias by the distribution of red blood diameters," *Blood 1*, 67 (1946).
5. M. M. Wintrobe, "Classification and treatment on the basis of differences in the average volume and high content of the red corpuscles," *Arch. intern. Med. 51*, 256 (1934).

# Unit 8

## The Platelet Count

The blood platelet, or thrombocyte, one of the three formed elements of the blood, has an important role in hemostasis. It maintains the resistance of the blood-vessel wall against mechanical and possibly other types of trauma; it participates in the coagulation mechanism (see Unit 14) and is required for the normal retraction of the clot. The platelet also serves as a carrier for 5-hydroxy-tryptamine (serotonin) and possibly for other amines.

The platelet is a colorless irregularly rounded body with a diameter of 1–5 $\mu$. It can undergo ameboid movement and is capable of extending filamentous pseudopods, the length of which may considerably exceed that of the body of the platelet. By electron microscopy, the platelet is found to have a thin membrane, a central dense area (granulomere), and a peripheral band of less dense material (hyalomere). The central dense area has a diameter which is about ⅓ to ½ that of the whole platelet and is tightly packed with granules (0.03–0.06 $\mu$ in diameter). The hyalomere has a finely fibrillar appearance. The platelet does not contain nuclear material and is all but free of desoxyribonucleo-protein. This is consistent with the currently available data on the origin of platelets, which indicate that they arise from the cytoplasm of the megakaryocytes.

The number of platelets in the blood represents the balance between their production on the one hand, and their utilization, loss, or destruction on the other hand. The level of circulating platelets, although not an absolute measure of the number of available platelets, frequently serves as a good indicator of a deficiency of platelets (thrombocytopenia) or of the rare excess of platelets (thrombocytosis or thrombocythemia).

The normal number of platelets, depending in part on the method used for their enumeration, varies from 130,000 to 700,000/mm³ of blood, with averages of 250,000–300,000/mm³. Disturbances involving platelets may also be qualitative, involving a defect in one or more of the normal functions of platelets.

A decrease in the count to below 100,000 platelets/mm³ may be associated with a generalized bleeding tendency together with a prolonged bleeding time, with or without petechiae or ecchymoses. Thrombocytopenia may further be associated with inadequate retraction of the clot and a diminished prothrombin consumption. The severity of these manifestations increases as the platelet count decreases.

An excess of platelets, as indicated by a platelet count of 700,000/mm³ or more, may be associated with a tendency toward thrombosis. Rarely, an exceedingly high platelet count (above 3,000,000/mm³) may be associated with a bleeding tendency.

The number of circulating platelets may be increased following hemorrhage, trauma, a number of infectious diseases, or splenectomy, and in polycythemia, idiopathic thrombocythemia, and megakaryocytic or myelogenous leukemia.

The quality of the platelets may be altered in regard to one or more of their activities (thrombopathia or thrombasthenia). Qualitative changes occur in the presence of a normal number of circulating platelets and may be attended by a hemorrhagic state. Qualitative defects may be reflected by large and bizarrely formed platelets. One or more of the following disturbances may be encountered: reduced clot retraction; inadequate plasma thromboplastin generation; increased vascular fragility; prolonged bleeding time. Qualitative defects in platelets are frequently inherited and may occur in the absence of other disturbances.

The number and morphology of the platelets should be examined as an integral part of the inspection of the blood film stained with Wright's stain as described in Unit 9. When abnormality of the platelet number or of their morphology is suspected, the number of circulating platelets should be determined and appropriate studies of platelet functions should be carried out (see Unit 14).

A large number of methods for the determination of the platelet count have been described,[1] as reviewed by Wintrobe[2] and by Tocantins.[3] Two types of method are used commonly, namely, direct[1] and indirect.[3] In the direct methods, the platelets are counted in a hemocytometer, as described below.[4] In indirect methods, the number of platelets per 1000 red cells is determined, the red-cell count is determined separately, and the platelet count is converted to the number of platelets per cubic millimeter on the basis of the red-cell count. Four methods are described below: two indirect methods for the semiquantitative estimation of the number of platelets from the stained film of blood, and two direct methods for counting platelets by ordinary microscopy[4] and by phase microscopy.[5]

### Semiquantitative Estimation of the Number of Platelets from the Blood Film Stained with Wright's Stain

A film of blood stained with Wright's stain should always be inspected for the morphology of the platelets and to obtain a semiquantitative estimate of the number of platelets present in relation to the number of red cells. Since clumping of platelets usually occurs in various degrees on the blood film made from capillary or venous blood, accurate counts of platelets from this type of smear are not possible. The examiner can inspect the blood film and estimate by comparison with the normal blood smear whether the number of platelets is increased, normal, or decreased. These semiquantitative designations will serve for screening in diagnosis and to indicate whether or not direct methods should be employed for counting of platelets.

#### INDIRECT PLATELET COUNT IN STAINED BLOOD FILM

When Wright's stain is used, the platelets appear as formed elements usually measuring 1–5 $\mu$ in diameter. They contain granules which appear purple or purplish-red in a background of pale blue cytoplasm. In some platelets, the number of granules is so great that the cytoplasm is indistinct. At other times, there may be relatively few granules and a larger amount of pale blue cytoplasm. The platelet does not have a nucleus. In disease, the size of the platelets may vary from very small structures containing only a few granules to masses of cytoplasm larger than that of the red blood cell. If the blood film has been stained with brilliant cresyl blue, as in the reticulocyte method, and then with Wright's stain, the cytoplasm of the platelets will have a more intense blue color. Platelets are best observed in the thin parts of the blood film.

**Method.** A blood film is prepared as described in Unit 9. The accuracy of the indirect test may be increased by placing a large drop of a 14-percent magnesium sulfate solution on the clean, dry skin and puncturing the skin through the liquid.[6]

The ratio of platelets to erythrocytes should be established from at least 1000 red cells. The number of platelets is calculated from this ratio on the basis of a red-cell count carried out on a specimen of blood obtained at the same time. The mean count by that method in 30 male adults was found to be 234,000 platelets/mm³, ranging from 140,000 to 350,000.

*Example.* Ratio of RBC:platelets = 1000:50 = 20. If RBC count = 5,000,-000/mm³, then platelet count = 5,000,-000/20 = 250,000/mm³.

INDIRECT PLATELET COUNT USING WET PREPARATION AND BRILLIANT CRESYL BLUE [7]

**Method.** A clean glass slide is coated with a thin layer of a saturated alcoholic solution of brilliant cresyl blue. A coverslip containing a small amount of capillary blood is inverted on a stained slide. The blood is allowed to spread by itself at first and then, by gently pressing down the coverslip, the red blood cells are spread into a unicellular layer. The smear can be examined directly, but examination can be delayed for about 1 hr if drying is prevented by sealing the edges of the coverslip with molten paraffin. Platelets are estimated by counting in different areas a total of 1000 red cells and simultaneously counting the number of platelets. The actual red-cell count in the same drop of capillary blood need not be determined, since for routine purposes it is sufficiently accurate to estimate the red-cell count from the known hemoglobin content or hematocrit value.

The *normal range* is 500,000 to 1,000,-000 platelets/mm³.

*Example.* If the hemoglobin content is known to be 10 gm/100 ml, the estimated red-cell count is 3,000,000/mm³. If 100 platelets are found per 1000 red blood cells, the platelet count is 3000 × 100 = 300,000/mm³.

## Direct Method of Counting Platelets with the Ordinary Light Microscope

PRINCIPLE. Capillary blood or venous blood (containing an anticoagulant) is drawn up in a red-cell pipette and diluted with a special fluid.[6] The diluting fluid contains an anticoagulant, a fixing agent, and brilliant cresyl blue, which gives the platelets a faint bluish stain. After proper mixing, the diluted blood sample is introduced into the two chambers of the hemocytometer and the platelets are counted directly as described below.

DILUTING FLUID FOR COUNTING PLATELETS. The diluting fluid employed is a modification[6] of that originally described by Rees and Ecker.[5] The solution is made by dissolving 8 gm of cane sugar and 2 gm of sodium citrate in approximately 75 ml of distilled water. The solution is then filtered. Brilliant cresyl blue dye, 0.04 gm, is ground in a mortar with three or four separate samples of 5 ml each of distilled water. The solution is then filtered and mixed with the solution of sodium citrate and sucrose. The mixture is made up to 100 ml with distilled water and allowed to stand 4 to 6 hr with occasional shaking. The final solution is filtered and then centrifuged at 1000g (2500 rev/min in a clinical centrifuge) for 30 min to remove particulate matter. The preparation is stored in the icebox in glass-stoppered bottles. Whenever the diluting fluid is used, a small amount of the stock solution is filtered immediately before use and the unused diluting fluid is discarded to prevent contamination of the stock solution.

**Method.** Capillary or venous blood is drawn to the 0.5 mark of a red-cell pipette, the excess blood is wiped off, and the pipette is filled immediately with platelet diluting fluid to the 101 mark. This makes a dilution of 1/200. The pipette is then shaken for from 3 to 5 min. Both the pipette and the counting chamber must be completely free of grease and particulate matter. After the pipettes are shaken, the two counting chambers of the hemocytometer are filled and the platelets are allowed to settle for 15 min. To prevent drying, the hemocytometer must be covered with a receptacle (a Petri dish) containing filter paper moistened with water. Since the platelets have the lowest specific gravity of the formed elements of the blood, the period of 15 min for settling is necessary in order that platelets may be visible at the lower level of the counting chamber.

APPEARANCE OF THE PLATELETS IN THE COUNTING CHAMBER. In the counting chamber, the platelets appear as highly refractile forms that may be round, oval, or comma-shaped, varying in dimensions from 1 to 5 $\mu$. For adequate visualization, a magnification of 400× is required. The amount of light and the position of the condenser should be so adjusted that, with continual focusing with the fine adjustment, the platelet will appear as a highly refractile object. The platelet must be distinguished especially from yeasts that are similar in appearance and also from debris, such as precipitated stain. Since the red cells are present in the preparation, any hemolysis may introduce artifacts from the stroma of destroyed cells. Occasional clumps of platelets may be seen containing two or three platelets that can be readily counted. If large aggregates occur, the count is vitiated.

**Method of counting.** The total number of platelets is counted in two large corner squares in each of two separate counting chambers (that is, in a total of four squares). The average number of platelets per large square (0.1 mm³) is obtained and multiplied by 10 to convert it to the number present in 1.0 mm³ and by 200 to correct for the dilution (that is, by a factor of 2000). The count is reported to three significant figures, as the number of platelets per cubic millimeter of blood. The correction factor for the red-cell pipette may be disregarded.

*Example.* The platelet counts in 16 medium-sized squares in each of 4 larger corner squares are 128, 120, 140, 120; total, 508. Then the average number of platelets per square is 127 and the total platelet count is $127 \times 2000 = 254,000$ platelets/mm³ or $254 \times 10^3$/mm³.

ERRORS AND PRECAUTIONS IN COUNTING PLATELETS. The counting of platelets has the same limitations of distribution and is susceptible to the same technical errors as obtain for the red-cell count and the white-cell count. The accuracy of the platelet count in experienced hands is of the same order as that of the erythrocyte count. Therefore, when determinations are made infrequently, it is recommended that a platelet count be performed on a normal subject as a control observation on the method.

A source of error may be contamination of the diluting fluid or of the counting chamber with particulate matter which may easily be confused with platelets. As a precaution, a control observation may be made on the diluting fluid alone, when introduced into the counting chamber, to observe the number of particles present in the system. If this so-called "blank count" exceeds 5000 platelet-like bodies per cubic millimeter, a platelet count should not be attempted until the diluting fluid has been centrifuged and filtered free of contaminants and the hemocytometer has been thoroughly cleaned.

The largest error may occur with low platelet counts of the order of 10,000/mm³, since the blank count may be of the order of 5000 particles/mm³ of the diluting fluid. When a low platelet number is obtained, the platelets in a larger area of the hemocytometer are counted and the correction factor is altered correspondingly. Alternatively, the count may be repeated with twice the amount of blood used in the procedure described above, the appropriate factor (namely, 100 instead of 200) being applied. The procedure may also be repeated with a white-cell counting pipette and the dilution factor appropriately adjusted.

Since platelets agglutinate when mixed with tissue fluid, it is essential to use free-flowing capillary blood or to use venous blood that has been collected in chemically clean glassware, even though loss of platelets by their removal on glassware may be encountered. For these reasons, a number of laboratories employ siliconed glassware and needles coated with a hemo-repellent agent for all procedures in which the integrity of the formed blood elements has to be preserved.

INTERPRETATION. In the study of 40 normal male subjects, Tocantins [6] found that the average number of platelets per cubic millimeter in samples of blood from the arm was: capillary blood, 250,000 (standard deviation, ±59,999); venous blood, 310,000 (standard deviation, ±110,000); arterial blood, 350,000 (standard deviation, ±128,000).

### Direct Method of Counting Platelets with the Phase Microscope

This method [7] has largely supplanted older methods in investigative work. The better resolution afforded by phase microscopy permits morphologic identification of the platelet on the basis of its structure rather than on the basis of its size and shape alone, to which ordinary light microscopy is limited. Thus platelets can be differentiated from cellular debris and other round particles of approximately the same size. Phase microscopy, therefore, facilitates accurate counting of platelets and is particularly

useful for observers with limited experience.

The optical properties of the phase system are such that materials with different densities appear to differ from each other in the intensity and the shade of the light transmitted through them. The need for staining is therefore eliminated. Thus biologic material may be examined by phase microscopy without the modifications induced by stains.

The principle of platelet counting is the same as described above under the direct method. A 1-percent solution of ammonium oxalate is used as the diluting fluid. This fluid hemolyzes the red cells, while the platelets and white cells remain intact.

The platelets appear highly refractile by phase microscopy, and fibrillar processes may be seen. White cells and foreign particles can easily be distinguished. The absence of the red cells also makes counting easier than in the method employed for the ordinary light microscope. The presence of platelet clumps indicates that dilution of the specimen has been delayed too long and a new sample must be taken. Because of the relatively small working distance (between specimen and objective of the microscope), it is essential to have a counting chamber designed for use with a phase optical system.[7] The error in a single count by this method is 11 percent when 50–150 platelets per chamber are actually counted. This error can be reduced to 4 percent if eight pipettes and chambers are counted on a single sample. Normal values range from 150,000 to 450,000 platelets/mm³ with a mean of 250,000 platelets/mm³.[8]

GENERAL COMMENTS. Pohle [4] has reported that the capillary blood from the ear showed, on the average, 15 percent fewer platelets than were obtained on samples of venous blood from the arm. There is a fluctuation of about 6 percent at different times during the day and from day to day in the same individual.[3] In normal women, there is a slow progressive decrease in number of platelets during 14 days prior to menstruation and a rapid return to normal soon after the onset of the menses.[4]

In thrombocytopenia of 100,000 platelets/mm³ or less, there is a decrease in the retraction of the blood clot that is roughly proportional to the degree of thrombocytopenia, as discussed in Unit 14. Accordingly, there are two methods of screening for an apparent decrease in the number of platelets, namely, inspection of the film of blood stained with Wright's stain and observation of the reaction of the clot

## REFERENCES

1. L. M. Tocantins, "Technical methods for the study of blood platelets," *Arch. Path.* (*Chicago*) *23,* 850 (1937).
2. M. M. Wintrobe, *Clinical hematology* (ed. 4; Lea and Febiger, Philadelphia, 1956).
3. L. M. Tocantins, "The mammalian blood platelet in health and disease," *Medicine 17,* 155 (1938).
4. F. S. Pohle, "The blood platelet count in relation to the menstrual cycle in women," *Amer. J. med. Sci. 197,* 40 (1939).
5. H. M. Rees and E. E. Ecker, "An improved method for counting platelets," *J. Amer. med. Ass. 80,* 621 (1923).
6. L. M. Tocantins, "Counting platelets in the blood," in L. M. Tocantins, ed., *The Coagulation of Blood* (Grune and Stratton, New York, 1955), p. 33.
7. B. M. Jacobson and W. D. Sohier, "Effects of ACTH and cortisone on the platelets in idiopathic thrombopenic purpura," *New Engl. J. Med. 246,* 247 (1952).
8. G. Brecher, M. Schneiderman, and E. P. Cronkite, "The reproducibility and constancy of the platelet count," *Amer. J. clin. Path. 23,* 15 (1953).

# Unit 9

# Methods for the Study of the Morphology of Blood

In a wide variety of diseases and other forms of physiologic stress, characteristic changes occur in the number and proportions of the cells that comprise the peripheral blood. These changes in most instances reflect alterations in the rate of formation of the various cells in the blood-forming organs. Knowledge of the nature and intensity of the hematologic response to disease is of great importance in diagnosis and in following the response to therapy. The examination of stained films of peripheral blood is an integral part of the initial examination of patients in all branches of medicine. This examination includes a differential count of the white cells, a description of the red cells, and an estimation of the number of platelets. Further information concerning the nature of cells can be obtained by the use of special stains and techniques. Examination of bone-marrow samples gives additional information concerning the processes of development and maturation of the various cells. Bone-marrow aspiration is especially useful when a marked excess or deficiency of any cell is evident in the circulating blood, or when abnormal or immature forms appear in the peripheral blood.

All morphologic examinations of blood and bone marrow depend on the ability of the examiner to recognize and discriminate among the various cell types that are encountered in health and disease. This knowledge must be acquired through training and practice, using representative stained blood films and hematologic atlases as guides.[1-5]

## Methods of Preparing and Staining Blood Films

### MATERIALS AND REAGENTS

WRIGHT'S STAIN. A compound dye composed of methylene blue and eosin was probably first used by Ehrlich in 1879 and subsequently modified by Romanovski, Wright, and others. Wright's stain is one of many dyes that have been employed successfully in staining blood. To prepare Wright's stain, methylene blue solution containing sodium bicarbonate is heated, and then eosin is added. Eosin enters into chemical combination with the basic dyes present, forming an insoluble precipitate. This precipitate dissolved in methyl alcohol is Wright's stain.[6, 7]

Since reliable solutions made from certified Wright's stain may be purchased, detailed instructions for preparation of the stain are omitted here. If a previously prepared solution is not available, Wright's stain may be purchased in the powdered form that has been certified by the Commission on Staining.[8] The solution is then prepared by dissolving 0.1 gm of powder per 60 ml of chemically pure absolute methyl alcohol. The dye is filtered at the time it is made and whenever samples are taken from the stock solution. Care should be taken to avoid

71

contamination with water of the reagents or glassware containing Wright's stain. The reagent bottles *must be kept stoppered,* since methyl alcohol rapidly takes up water vapor which spoils the stain. Exposure of the stain to acid fumes or ammonium hydroxide should be avoided.

Wright's stain is classified as a polychrome stain because of the variety of colors it produces. The fixed material in the blood cells that is acid in reaction is stained by a basic dye (methylene blue) and is termed basophilic; neutral material is stained violet in color and is termed neutrophilic; basic material is stained by an acid dye (eosin) and is termed eosinophilic. The reader is referred elsewhere for information on other Romanovski stains and dyes.[4-9]

*Buffer for use with Wright's stain.* For dilution of Wright's stain in the process of staining blood films, control of pH is desirable. This may be done by the use of Sorensen's phosphate buffer at pH 6.7 and $M/15$; this solution is prepared by mixing 43.5 ml of $M/15$ $Na_2HPO_4$ (anhydrous, 9.47 gm/L) and 56.5 ml of $M/15$ $KH_2PO_4$ (9.08 gm/L).

COVERGLASSES. Coverglasses must be of the proper thinness for the examination of blood films under the oil-immersion objective of the microscope. Either No. 0 or No. 1 coverglasses ⅞ in. square are satisfactory. No. 2 coverglasses are too thick to allow focusing with the oil-immersion objective. To prepare satisfactory blood films, it is essential to use clean, grease-free coverslips. They may be cleaned as needed by washing the surfaces of each coverslip, held between the thumb and forefinger, using soap and water, rinsing under running tap water, and polishing with a clean, lint-free cloth or gauze. Pairs of coverslips may be placed cornerwise in slits made in a cardboard box or in a holder made by folding a piece of paper into a small envelope. To protect the surfaces from grease, coverglasses are handled by their edges only. Larger numbers of coverglasses may be prepared in advance by washing them as described above and storing them in alcohol. Each coverglass should be washed separately and dropped into a beaker containing tap water. All traces of soap should be removed by multiple rinses. The wet coverglasses may then be drained and stored in a clean covered dish containing 95-percent ethyl alcohol. They may be removed from the alcohol as needed and polished with a cloth. Dry coverslips may also be stored satisfactorily in a clean dry Petri dish or other covered container.

Large numbers of coverglasses may also be cleaned in advance with acid cleaning solution. Potassium dichromate–sulfuric acid cleaning solution is prepared as follows: dissolve, with the aid of heat, 25 gm of powdered potassium dichromate in 25 ml of water; allow this solution to cool and add cautiously 1 L of technical grade sulfuric acid to the dichromate solution, using Pyrex glassware because of the intense heat evolved. Coverglasses are separated, dropped individually into the acid cleaning solution, and allowed to stand 4 to 24 hr. The acid cleaning solution is decanted and the coverslips are washed with multiple changes of tap water. Heating may hasten the removal of the acid. The last wash water should be tested for the presence of acid with litmus paper. The water is drained off and the coverslips are stored as described above.

GLASS SLIDES. Glass slides, measuring $1 \times 3$ in., are standard for hematologic studies. They may be washed and stored by one of the methods described above. For ordinary use, "previously cleaned" slides may now be purchased.

## PREPARATION OF FILMS OF PERIPHERAL BLOOD

COVERGLASS METHOD. The differential count of white cells should be made from a stained film of blood prepared on coverglasses. In such films, the blood spreads by capillary action and the dispersion of the leukocytes is that of chance distribution. A thin film of capillary blood may be prepared rapidly and simply between coverglasses by the following procedure. A capillary puncture is made and wiped clean with a dry piece of gauze. When a small drop of blood has appeared, the operator touches it with the center of a clean coverglass, without touching the skin. A drop of blood 2 to 3 mm in diameter is thus taken on the coverslip. This coverglass, with its drop of blood, is now placed crosswise over a second coverglass, so that the corners appear as an eight-pointed star. The blood should spread evenly and quickly by capillary action between the two surfaces. The operator waits briefly until the spreading is nearly complete and then separates the two coverglasses by sliding them apart quickly in the same plane in which they are lying. They should never be separated by lifting. The blood films may then be placed back to back and supported by one corner in a cardboard box.

A blood film may be prepared from venous blood by touching the tip of the hypodermic needle gently to a coverglass, delivering a drop 1 to 2 mm in diameter. A second coverglass is placed over the drop of blood and the procedure completed as described above. Blood films made from samples of venous blood containing oxalate as an anticoagulant are unsatisfactory for the study of white cells because the presence of the oxalate produces changes in their morphology and staining characteristics. Vacuoles and phagocytized crystals of oxalate are apparent and the nuclei of lymphocytes and monocytes may appear divided or in clover-leaf forms. Some degenerative changes are seen when other anticoagulants are used, or in defibrinated blood whenever there is a delay before the blood films are made.

GLASS-SLIDE METHOD. Distribution of leukocytes is *not* uniform in blood films that are prepared by spreading a drop on a glass slide and using the edge of another glass slide as a spreader. However, use of the slide technique is reliable and valuable for the examination of the red cells and for detecting malarial parasites. For the preparation of a blood film by this method, the slides must be chemically clean and free from grease. A drop of blood 3 to 4 mm in diameter is placed on one slide approximately one-quarter of the distance from one end. The slide is placed on a flat surface and held down firmly by the opposite end. The narrow side of a second slide is used as a spreader. The spreader slide is held at an angle of approximately 30° from the horizontal. The edge of the spreader slide is moved toward the drop of blood until contact is made within the acute angle formed by the two slides. By capillary action, the drop of blood spreads promptly along the edge of the spreader slide. The thin film is then made by moving the spreader slide slowly in the reverse direction so that the blood flows *behind* the edge of the spreader slide. The thickness of the blood film may be varied by changing the size of the drop of blood, the angle at which the spreader slide is held, and the speed of spreading. A good blood film should have a smooth, even appearance, free from ridges, waves, or holes. The film should not extend to the edges or to the ends of the slide. The use of a narrower slide as a spreader prevents the blood from running over the edge of the slide on which the preparation is made.

### STAINING OF BLOOD FILMS WITH WRIGHT'S STAIN

**Method.** The coverglass or glass slide bearing the air-dried blood film is placed on a flat support, such as a cork stopper, with the blood film uppermost. The coverglass or glass slide is covered with a thick layer of stain and the stain is allowed to remain for 3 min. More stain must be added if evaporation occurs during this period. Conditions favoring excessively rapid evaporation should be avoided. The stain is then diluted with an equal volume of buffer. (In many parts of the country, fresh tap water is equally satisfactory.) The mixture of stain and buffer should *not* run off the glass surface. Three minutes after dilution, the stain is floated off the glass surface by holding the coverslip in a horizontal plane under gently running tap water. This prevents contamination of the preparation by precipitate. The film is washed under running water for a brief period. If the color is somewhat too dark, some of the excess blue color will be removed by further washing. The preparation is then dried thoroughly either by evaporation or by blotting gently with filter paper. When dry, the stain on the *back* of the preparation is removed by rubbing with gauze moistened with alcohol.

Coverglass blood films may be quickly mounted by placing them blood side down on a glass slide on which a drop of immersion oil has been placed. Films mounted in this way rapidly become dirty and must be discarded after examination. Permanent mounts may be made by using 1 drop of isobutyl methacrylate dissolved in xylol or toluol. The mounting fluid should be at approximately neutral pH. Enough mounting fluid must be used to spread completely under the coverslip so as to avoid air pockets. The slide should be properly labeled.

COMPLICATIONS IN STAINING. The foregoing directions for staining serve only as a guide. Different lots of stain may require different periods for staining and dilution. Well-stained preparations have a lavender color. If the film is excessively blue, the cause may be excessive thickness of the blood film, overstaining, inadequate washing, or excess alkalinity of the stain or diluent. In some parts of the country, tap water is too alkaline for use in the washing of Wright's-stained preparations. In these areas, the buffer at pH 6.7 should be used for both dilution and washing. If the film is excessively pink, the cause may be insufficient staining, prolonged washing, mounting the coverslips before they are dry, or increased acidity of the stain or diluting fluid. Precipitate on the film may be due to drying during the period of staining or of dilution, to contamination with precipitated stain that is not floated off in the washing, or to sediment in the stain itself, which should have been removed by filtration. Staining in proximity to fumes from strong acids or alkalis should be avoided.

EXAMINATION OF THE QUALITY OF THE STAINED BLOOD FILM. Initially, the stained film of blood should be inspected for its quality under the low-power magnification of the microscope. In most fields examined, the red cells and white cells should be clearly separated and should show no artifacts such as vacuoles in the red cells. There should not be significant amounts of precipitate. The color of the stained film should be uniform without areas of paleness or dark greenish color resulting from thick areas of blood that are densely stained. If the stained blood film is not satisfactory, results will be unreliable and may be seriously misleading. Another blood film should be prepared.

### Examination of Red Cells on Wright's-Stained Films of Peripheral Blood

Methods for quantitative measurements of the average volume (MCV), average hemoglobin concentration (MCHC), and average diameter [10] of red cells are described in Unit 7.

Information of clinical importance can be derived quickly and with considerable reliability by semiquantitative evaluation of the red cells on a film of

Wright's-stained blood. Variations from the normal in size, shape, and hemoglobin content of the red cell, as well as abnormal forms, may be observed. The morphologic characteristics of red cells are listed in Table 14.

Table 14. *Morphologic characteristics of red cells that may be evaluated semiquantitatively by inspection of blood films.*

| Morphologic characteristics | Descriptive term |
| --- | --- |
| Size (diameter) | Normal: normocytic<br>Abnormal: macrocytic, microcytic |
| Shape | Normal: round<br>Abnormal forms: oval, sickled, oat-shaped, pencil, tailed, spheroidal, fragmented |
| Hemoglobin content | Normal: normochromic<br>Abnormal: hypochromic, hyperchromic |
| Immature and abnormal forms | Polychromatophilic<br>Nucleated red cells<br>Inclusion bodies, stippling, Cabot rings, Howell-Jolly bodies, refractile granules, siderocytes, malarial parasites |

Variations from the normal in size, shape, and hemoglobin content can be reported as slight, moderate, marked, or extreme. Variations in shape from the normal are frequently described by the term *poikilocytosis.* Since this term is not definitive, it is preferable that abnormal shapes be *described* and that the degree of variation in shape be expressed by the terms that are indicated. Variations in size (diameter) are frequently reported by the general term *anisocytosis,* but may be described semiquantitatively by the terms indicated.

### ESTIMATION OF RED-CELL SIZE

While marked macrocytosis or microcytosis can be recognized easily by an experienced observer, moderate or slight variations from the normal in the diameter of red cells are difficult to detect without some standard for reference. Three simple methods for the evaluation of red-cell diameter are described below.

INDIRECT COMPARISON WITH FILM OF NORMAL BLOOD. Comparison can be made by alternately examining the patient's blood

film and a normal control under the same microscope. A normal film should always be kept for this purpose.

DIRECT COMPARISON WITH SUPERIMPOSED FILM OF NORMAL BLOOD. A satisfactory coverglass preparation of the patient's blood, stained with Wright's stain, is mounted on a glass slide, stained side *up.* A coverglass film of normal blood, stained with Wright's stain, is then mounted with immersion oil, stained side *down,* so that the two blood films are face to face. The films are placed in this arrangement to permit focusing on the lower film. The normal blood film may be slipped off and used repeatedly.

Since the two films are face to face, the unknown and the normal red cells can be compared for diameter, shape, and hemoglobin content by focusing on them alternately.

DIRECT MEASUREMENT WITH MICROMETER DISK. The diameter of a red cell can be measured directly by means of a scale etched on a micrometer disk which is placed in one ocular of the microscope. A good area of the blood film is located and the diameters of a number of cells are measured as the slide is moved about. Since the magnification differs from one microscope to another, the scale on the disk must be calibrated for the instrument in use. This can be done by comparison with the calibrated scale of a commercially available stage micrometer or with the ruled area of a hemocytometer. For example, since the smallest square in the center of the hemocytometer measures 50 $\mu$, the divisions on the micrometer disk may be compared with this known measurement and the absolute value in microns of each division on the disk calculated. Blood films from a few normal subjects should be measured first to make sure that the method is giving reliable results.

A more accurate method of measuring the diameters of red cells is described by

Price-Jones,[10] but the technique is laborious and demanding.

### VARIATIONS IN SIZE AND SHAPE OF RED CELLS

Variations in size may be evaluated by the direct and indirect methods of comparison described above. The degree of variation in size and the morphologic characteristics of the large and small cells are very important. A careful description of this variation means much more than the term "anisocytosis." Abnormal shapes, such as pencil, tailed, spheroidal, or oval forms, can be identified easily on the blood film. A careful description of these forms is of greater value than the term "poikilocytosis."

### ESTIMATION OF HEMOGLOBIN CONTENT OF RED CELLS

The variation in intensity of staining is a manifestation of the hemoglobin content of the cells. It is relatively easy to recognize hypochromic cells in a film if the hypochromia is extreme or if some normal (or transfused) cells are present in the patient's blood for comparison. It is more difficult to judge hypochromia if the hemoglobin content of *all* of the cells is slightly decreased, except by comparison of the patient's blood film with a normal control or by the direct method of comparison described above. Sharply defined holes appearing in red cells usually are artifacts, especially if seen in thick smears.

Macrocytes that carry a large amount of hemoglobin often appear hyperchromic. The absolute increase in the amount of hemoglobin per cell is due to the increase in the diameter and thickness of the cells. The mean corpuscular hemoglobin concentration (MCHC) is normal.

The spherocyte is a small deeply staining cell without the central pallor of the normal biconcave red cell. Although the volume of the cell is approximately normal, the diameter is decreased and the thickness increased.[11, 12] The spherocytes appear hyperchromic not only because of this increased thickness but also because of their increased corpuscular hemoglobin concentration. The increased thickness of the spherocyte may be seen in wet preparations.

## Examinations of Platelets on Stained Films of Peripheral Blood

It is important to estimate the number of platelets in the Wright's-stained films of peripheral blood. This is done by surveying several oil-immersion fields and estimating whether the number of platelets is normal, increased, or decreased as compared with those on a film of normal blood (Unit 8). The number of platelets is considered in relation to the number of red cells on the blood film. If severe anemia is present, the number of platelets may appear to be normal, relative to the number of red cells, but actually the absolute number of platelets per unit volume of whole blood may be reduced.

*Example.* If the red-cell count is $5.0 \times 10^6/mm^3$ and the platelet count is normal, namely 200 to $400 \times 10^3/mm^3$, then the number of platelets will be 4 to 8 percent of the number of red cells. However, if the same percentages of platelets are observed at a red-cell count of $1.0 \times 10^6/mm^3$, the platelet count is only 40 to $80 \times 10^3/mm^3$— a definite thrombocytopenia.

If the platelets appear significantly decreased in number or absent, this important observation should be checked by performing a platelet count (see Unit 7). Morphologically, the platelets may be abnormal in size and shape.

## Differential Count of White Cells on Stained Films of Peripheral Blood

### METHOD OF PERFORMING THE DIFFERENTIAL COUNT

The differential count of white cells should be performed on samples of capillary or venous blood containing no anticoagulants and using blood films made on coverglasses, rather than spread on glass slides, for reasons discussed elsewhere. The oil-immersion objective of the microscope is used, since lower magnification does not permit sufficient delineation of structure to assure accurate classification. A mechanical stage is used and the film is moved progressively so that each cell is counted only once. Beginning at the upper left-hand corner, the cells are counted from left to right. The film is then moved up for a distance of one or two microscopic fields and across in the reverse direction. This process is continued, *all nucleated cells,* including nucleated red cells, being counted and classified. Since the differential count concerns only the leukocytic series, the number of white cells is recorded separately from other nucleated forms. In recording results, the number of each class of white cells is expressed as a percentage of the total number of white cells enumerated. Abnormal white cells should be classified or described in detail and are also recorded as a percentage of the total number of leukocytes. Cells that are ruptured, fragmented, or degenerated ("basket" cells or "smudges") usually cannot be identified and are not included in the differential count. They may be noted separately and reported as the number seen per 100 white cells. Differential counts are performed in multiples of 100 cells, preferably using the two "matched"

coverglass blood films from the same drop of blood. At least 200 cells should always be counted (p. 81).

### NUCLEATED RED CELLS

When immature forms of the erythrocytic series are present in small numbers, they should be reported as the number seen while counting 100 white cells, but they are *not* included in the differential count of leukocytes. If there are large numbers of nucleated red cells, the types encountered should be noted and an actual count made of the number of nucleated red cells per 1000 red cells and the percentage determined. From this figure, the absolute number of nucleated red cells per cubic millimeter is calculated. Since the nucleated red cells are not hemolyzed by acetic acid, they are included in the total white-cell count. This is corrected by subtracting the number of nucleated red cells per cubic millimeter.

*Example.* The following data might be obtained in hemolytic anemia, such as sickle-cell disease or thalassemia: red-cell count, $2.5 \times 10^6/\text{mm}^3$; apparent white-cell count, $70 \times 10^3/\text{mm}^3$. Inspection of the blood film reveals 20 nucleated red cells per 1000 red cells, or 2 percent. Taking this fraction of the red-cell count, there are $50 \times 10^3$ nucleated red cells per cubic millimeter. Therefore, the corrected white-cell count is the difference, or $(70 \times 10^3) - (50 \times 10^3) = 20 \times 10^3/\text{mm}^3$.

Table 15. *Mean values of white-cell counts and differential white-cell counts in 20 apparently healthy young adults in blood taken from the antecubital vein.*[1]

| Cells | Mean (percent) | Standard deviation (percent) | Observed range (percent) | Mean (cells/mm³) | Observed range (cells/mm³) |
|---|---|---|---|---|---|
| White-cell count (cells/mm³) | 6700 | 1400 | 4400–9500 | 6700 | 4400–9500 |
| Differential white-cell count | | | | | |
| Neutrophils, adult | 47.9 | ±7.3 | 36.5–61.5 | 3210 | 2100–5350 |
| Neutrophils, band | 12.5 | ±5.6 | 4.5–22.5 | 837 | 220–1240 |
| Eosinophils | 2.6 | ±1.6 | 0.5– 6.5 | 174 | 34–475 |
| Basophils | 0.4 | ±1.6 | 0.0– 1.5 | 27 | 0–80 |
| Lymphocytes, small | 23.8 | ±6.3 | 15.5–33.0 | 1604 | 750–2900 |
| Lymphocytes, large | 4.0 | ±1.5 | 1.0–10.0 | 270 | 58–840 |
| Lymphocytes, atypical and young | 1.3 | — | 0.0– 7.0 | 87 | 0–480 |
| Monocytes | 7.1 | ±3.3 | 2.0–17.0 | 475 | 168–1140 |
| Histiocytes | 0.4 | — | 0.0– 0.5 | 27 | 0–114 |

Table 16. Normal values for white blood cells at different ages.[13]

| Age | White cells | | Neutrophils | | | | Eosinophils | | Basophils | | Lymphocytes | | Monocytes | |
|---|---|---|---|---|---|---|---|---|---|---|---|---|---|---|
| | | | Adult | | Band | | | | | | | | | |
| | No./mm³ | 95% range | % | No./mm³ | % | No./mm³ | % | No./mm³ | % | No./mm³ | % | No./mm³ | % | No./mm³ |
| Birth | 18,240 | 9,000–30,000 | 52 | 9,400 | 9.1 | 1,650 | 2.2 | 400 | 0.6 | 100 | 31 | 5,500 | 5.8 | 1,050 |
| 12 hours | 22,781 | 13,000–38,000 | 58 | 13,200 | 10.2 | 2,330 | 2.0 | 450 | 0.4 | 100 | 24 | 5,500 | 5.3 | 1,200 |
| 24 | 19,045 | 9,400–34,000 | 52 | 9,800 | 9.2 | 1,750 | 2.4 | 450 | 0.5 | 100 | 31 | 5,800 | 5.8 | 1,100 |
| 1 week | 12,279 | 5,000–21,000 | 39 | 4,700 | 6.8 | 830 | 4.1 | 500 | 0.4 | 50 | 41 | 5,000 | 9.1 | 1,100 |
| 2 | 11,400 | 5,000–20,000 | 34 | 3,900 | 5.5 | 630 | 3.1 | 350 | 0.4 | 50 | 48 | 5,500 | 8.8 | 1,000 |
| 4 | 10,800 | 5,000–19,500 | 30 | 3,300 | 4.5 | 490 | 2.8 | 300 | 0.5 | 50 | 56 | 6,000 | 6.5 | 700 |
| 2 months | 11,000 | 5,500–18,000 | 30 | 3,300 | 4.4 | 490 | 2.7 | 300 | 0.5 | 50 | 57 | 6,300 | 5.9 | 650 |
| 4 | 11,500 | 6,000–17,500 | 29 | 3,300 | 3.9 | 450 | 2.6 | 300 | 0.4 | 50 | 59 | 6,800 | 5.2 | 600 |
| 6 | 11,900 | 6,000–17,500 | 28 | 3,300 | 3.8 | 450 | 2.5 | 300 | 0.4 | 50 | 61 | 7,300 | 4.8 | 580 |
| 8 | 12,200 | 6,000–17,500 | 27 | 3,300 | 3.3 | 410 | 2.5 | 300 | 0.4 | 50 | 62 | 7,600 | 4.7 | 580 |
| 10 | 12,000 | 6,000–17,500 | 27 | 3,200 | 3.3 | 400 | 2.5 | 300 | 0.4 | 50 | 63 | 7,500 | 4.6 | 550 |
| 12 | 11,450 | 6,000–17,500 | 28 | 3,200 | 3.1 | 350 | 2.6 | 300 | 0.4 | 50 | 61 | 7,000 | 4.8 | 550 |
| 2 years | 10,680 | 6,000–17,000 | 30 | 3,200 | 3.0 | 320 | 2.6 | 280 | 0.5 | 50 | 59 | 6,300 | 5.0 | 530 |
| 4 | 9,100 | 5,500–15,500 | 39 | 3,500 | 3.0 | 270 | 2.8 | 250 | 0.6 | 50 | 50 | 4,500 | 5.0 | 450 |
| 6 | 8,500 | 5,000–14,500 | 48 | 4,000 | 3.0 | 250 | 2.7 | 230 | 0.6 | 50 | 42 | 3,500 | 4.7 | 400 |
| 8 | 8,300 | 4,500–13,500 | 50 | 4,100 | 3.0 | 250 | 2.4 | 200 | 0.6 | 50 | 39 | 3,300 | 4.2 | 350 |
| 10 | 8,100 | 4,500–13,500 | 51 | 4,200 | 3.0 | 240 | 2.4 | 200 | 0.5 | 40 | 38 | 3,100 | 4.3 | 350 |
| 12 | 8,000 | 4,500–13,500 | 52 | 4,200 | 3.0 | 240 | 2.5 | 200 | 0.5 | 40 | 38 | 3,000 | 4.4 | 350 |
| 14 | 7,900 | 4,500–13,000 | 53 | 4,200 | 3.0 | 240 | 2.5 | 200 | 0.5 | 40 | 37 | 2,900 | 4.7 | 380 |
| 16 | 7,800 | 4,500–13,000 | 54 | 4,200 | 3.0 | 230 | 2.6 | 200 | 0.5 | 40 | 35 | 2,800 | 5.1 | 400 |
| 18 | 7,700 | 4,500–12,500 | 54 | 4,200 | 3.0 | 230 | 2.6 | 200 | 0.5 | 40 | 35 | 2,700 | 5.2 | 400 |
| 20 | 7,500 | 4,500–11,500 | 56 | 4,200 | 3.0 | 230 | 2.7 | 200 | 0.5 | 40 | 33 | 2,500 | 5.0 | 380 |
| 21 | 7,400 | 4,500–11,000 | 56 | 4,200 | 3.0 | 220 | 2.7 | 200 | 0.5 | 40 | 34 | 2,500 | 4.0 | 300 |

## NORMAL RANGE FOR TOTAL WHITE-CELL COUNT AND DIFFERENTIAL COUNT

ADULTS. Relative and absolute values for leukocyte counts for the normal adult [1] are shown in Table 15. The proportions of the differential count of leukocytes that appear in the adult are probably reached about puberty.[2] No significant difference has been found between the differential counts observed in the young adult and in the aged. Variations in the white cells in disease are discussed in Unit 12.

INFANTS AND CHILDREN. Average normal values for infants and children are shown in Table 16, from Albritton.[13] From the age of 3 weeks to 4 years, the granulocytes are much lower in both relative and absolute total numbers than the lymphocytes.[13] There is a slight monocytosis in the neonatal period, lasting the first 2 weeks. Thereafter, the absolute number of monocytes falls to a level more or less constantly maintained throughout childhood. After the fifth year, the lymphocytes steadily decrease until the fifteenth year, when their number is approximately half that of the granulocytes.

## QUALITATIVE CHANGES IN WHITE-CELL MORPHOLOGY

IMPORTANCE OF TECHNIQUE IN THE PREPARATION OF BLOOD FILMS AS RELATED TO THE RESULTS OF DIFFERENTIAL COUNT. To identify and classify leukocytes, it is necessary that the cells be separated one from another in the spreading of the film and that they be well stained. If the leukocytes are crowded by red cells, their staining characteristics are changed and the cytoplasm cannot be well seen. If the staining is too light, nuclei may fail entirely to stain and the characteristic granules of cells may not stain or may not show their usual color reaction with Wright's stain. If the film is too thick or the staining too dark, there may be no differentiation of the structure of the nucleus and cytoplasm. Unless these technical factors are controlled, the results of the differential count may be worthless.

QUALITATIVE CHANGES IN LEUKOCYTES. The detection and identification of abnormal leukocytes is of major importance in diagnosis (see Unit 12), since the presence of immature or atypical white cells in the peripheral blood frequently denotes an abnormality of the bone marrow or the presence of a specific infectious disease such as infectious mononucleosis. If an abnormal form cannot be identified, a sketch or description should be recorded. Statistical considerations are relatively unimportant when considering qualitative changes in leukocytes, as compared with the importance of statistical analyses of quantitative changes in the differential count. Nucleated red cells must be distinguished from cells of the leukocytic series. The presence of small numbers of nucleated red cells in the peripheral blood indicates unusual erythropoietic activity, which may be a normal physiologic response or may represent disease of the bone marrow (see Units 11 and 12).

## RESULTS OBTAINED FROM COVERGLASS PREPARATIONS COMPARED WITH GLASS-SLIDE PREPARATIONS

It has been demonstrated that the distribution of leukocytes on glass-slide films is not uniform, and is characterized by a predominance of neutrophils and monocytes along the edges and at the "tail" of the film.[14, 15] On the other hand, as shown by Barnett,[16] the dispersion of leukocytes in coverglass preparations is that of chance alone. Because of this important fact, differential counts of leukocytes should always be made on coverslip preparations. The statistical evaluation of the differential count is discussed below.

In summary, the results of counting 200 white cells in the differential count are adequate for ordinary clinical use.

STATISTICAL EVALUATION OF THE ERROR
OF CHANCE DISTRIBUTION IN THE
DIFFERENTIAL COUNT OF WHITE CELLS

ERRORS IN SAMPLING. In his excellent analysis of the differential count of white cells, Barnett [16] eloquently states the problem of sampling: "An error due entirely to chance occurs whenever in dealing with a universe composed of a very large number of individual units our estimate of the distribution of different types of units must be based upon the study of an extremely small proportion of them. Thus in differential counting we study a few hundred cells in order to determine the proportion of the various types in the entire blood stream, which, if we assume a white count of 10,000 cells per cubic millimeter, and a blood volume of 5 liters, will contain 50,000,-000,000 cells. It is obvious that when from such a tremendous total number of cells, samples as small as 100 are taken, each will differ slightly from another, and no single count will give a true picture of the actual distribution. This error is completely independent of technique or interpretation and is entirely unavoidable. It can be decreased by increasing the number of cells studied in the total count, but it cannot be eliminated, and when small numbers of cells are counted, it leads to a large variation."

There is no definite information available that indicates the degree of reproducibility of differential counts of white cells made from coverglass preparations that are *made serially* and at the same time from free-flowing capillary blood. For example, 100 films might be taken serially from a capillary puncture of the ear or finger from each of several normal subjects and from patients with disease (such as leukocytosis or leukemia) to determine the reproducibility of sampling, using the statistical methods of Barnett. From such data, if large numbers of cells are counted and the statistical error is thus minimized, it would be possible to state the *error of sampling* of capillary blood as opposed to the *error of chance distribution* of white cells on the coverglass.

ERROR OF CHANCE DISTRIBUTION. Barnett [16] has made a classic report in which he confirmed empirically that the error of the differential white-cell count conforms to the value of the theoretical statistical error, when technical errors are minimized.

Confidence limits for the differential white-cell count are based, except for very small percentages, on the binomial distribution and are calculated using the formula [17] for the standard deviation:

$$\sigma = \sqrt{(Npq)},$$

where $\sigma$ is the standard deviation, $N$ is the number of cells counted, $p$ is the fraction of cells of a certain type, and $q$ is the fraction of all other types of cells $(q = 1 - p)$.

*Examples.* (*a*) *100 cells:* If 100 white cells are counted and 25 percent are lymphocytes, then $N = 100$, $p = 0.25$, $q = 0.75$, and $\sigma = \pm\sqrt{(100 \times 0.25 \times 0.75)} = \pm 4.3$ percent.

(*b*) *200 cells:* If 200 white cells are counted, $\sigma = \pm\sqrt{(200 \times 0.25 \times 0.75)}$. Therefore the standard deviation per 100 white cells is $2\sigma/2 = \pm\frac{1}{2}\sqrt{(200 \times 0.25 \times 75)} = \pm 3.05$ percent.

(*c*) *400 cells:* If 400 white cells are counted, $\sigma = \pm\sqrt{(400 \times 0.25 \times 0.75)}$. The standard deviation per 100 white cells is $2\sigma/4 = \pm\frac{1}{4}\sqrt{(400 \times 0.25 \times 0.75)} = \pm 2.15$ percent.

Thus it will be seen that the standard deviation of a differential count, expressed per 100 cells, is inversely proportional to the square root of the number of cells counted, so that to double the accuracy one must quadruple the number of cells counted.

The question often arises whether two differential counts in a series are really different. This can be settled by calculating the standard deviation of the difference by the formula

$$\sigma = \sqrt{(\sigma_1{}^2 + \sigma_2{}^2)}.$$

If the difference is equal to or greater than $2\sigma$ it is significant. More simply, the following rule of thumb can be applied: for practical purposes, if the range for one count, represented by the count $\pm\sigma_1$, does not overlap that for the other, represented by that count $\pm\sigma_2$, then they are significantly different. If tables of confidence limits are available which can be applied, and one number lies outside the confidence limits of the other, then the difference can be regarded as statistically significant. Where one count is just within the confidence limits of the other, the count should be repeated.

Goldner and Mann,[18] in their account of the statistical error of the differential white-cell count, express their results in terms of confidence limits. Table 17

Table 17. *Confidence limits for differential white-cell count.*[16, 17]

| Percentage of given type of cell | For 100 cells, $\pm 2\sigma$ | For 200 cells, $\pm \dfrac{2\sigma}{2}$ | For 400 cells, $\pm \dfrac{2\sigma}{4}$ |
|---|---|---|---|
| 10 | 4.0–16.0 | 5.8–14.2 | 7.0–13.0 |
| 15 | 7.9–22.9 | 10.0–20.0 | 11.5–18.5 |
| 20 | 12.0–28.0 | 14.3–25.7 | 16.0–24.0 |
| 25 | 16.4–33.6 | 18.9–31.1 | 20.7–29.3 |
| 30 | 20.8–39.2 | 23.5–36.5 | 25.4–34.6 |
| 35 | 25.6–44.4 | 28.3–41.7 | 30.3–39.7 |
| 40 | 30.2–49.8 | 33.1–46.9 | 35.2–44.8 |
| 45 | 35.1–54.9 | 38.0–52.0 | 40.1–49.9 |
| 50 | 40.0–60.0 | 42.9–57.1 | 45.0–55.0 |
| 55 | 45.1–64.9 | 48.0–62.0 | 50.1–59.9 |
| 60 | 50.2–69.8 | 53.1–66.9 | 55.2–64.8 |
| 65 | 55.6–74.4 | 58.3–71.7 | 60.3–69.7 |
| 70 | 60.8–79.2 | 63.5–76.5 | 65.4–74.6 |
| 75 | 66.4–83.6 | 68.9–81.1 | 70.7–79.3 |
| 80 | 72.0–88.0 | 74.3–85.7 | 76.0–84.0 |
| 85 | 77.9–92.1 | 80.0–90.0 | 81.5–88.5 |
| 90 | 84.0–96.0 | 85.8–94.2 | 87.0–93.0 |

shows how such limits are affected by basing the differential white-cell count on the enumeration of 100, 200, and 400 white blood cells. In the left-hand column, the percentages of a particular type of white cell and the upper and lower confidence limits are given and each value of $2\sigma$ can be obtained in the proper rank and column. For very small percentages, the appropriate confidence limits

are derived from the Poisson distribution and not from a consideration of the ordinary binomial distribution.[19] Table 18

Table 18. *Confidence limits for differential white-cell counts, for small percentages.*[a, 19]

| Percentage of given type of cell | For 100 cells | For 200 cells | For 400 cells |
|---|---|---|---|
| 0 | 0.00– 3.00 | 0.00–1.50 | 0.00–0.75 |
| 1 | 0.51– 4.74 | 0.18–3.15 | 0.34–2.29 |
| 2 | 0.36– 6.30 | 0.68–4.57 | 0.99–3.61 |
| 3 | 0.82– 7.75 | 1.30–5.92 | 1.73–4.86 |
| 4 | 1.37– 9.15 | 1.99–7.22 | 2.51–6.07 |
| 5 | 1.97–10.51 | 2.72–8.48 | 3.31–7.27 |

[a] The true value may be expected to lie between the limits in only 90 percent of instances, but it should lie either below an upper limit or above a lower limit in 95 percent of instances.

gives confidence limits for small percentages in the differential white-cell count.

As mentioned in Unit 2, confidence limits are used not to control and eliminate erroneous estimates, but to interpret the results of isolated counts, by providing limits within which the true value probably lies. The range given by $\pm 2\sigma$ is preferred, because it more precisely locates the true value, although at a lower level of probability. It will be seen from Table 17 that even these limits include a rather wide range, especially for counts based on 100 cells. For this reason, we regard the differential white-cell count as adequate only when it is based on 200 cells or more.

## Methods of Staining and Counting Reticulocytes

The enumeration of the number of immature erythrocytes provides data that are essential in classifying the physiologic activity of the bone marrow in diagnosis and in determining the response to treatment (see Unit 11).

It is important to realize that the immature erythrocyte, the polychromatophilic cell, and the reticulocyte are the *same* cell. When stained with Wright's stain, the basophilic material in the immature erythrocyte gives a diffuse and homogeneous blue color. This may be removed by ribonuclease and is therefore a ribonucleoprotein.[20, 21] The hemoglobin stains red. Combinations of varying amounts of basophilic material and of hemoglobin result in a variation in color from gray-blue to gray-red, called polychromatophilia or polychromasia.

When the young cells are stained with brilliant cresyl blue or other "vital" dyes which enter the living cell before fixation, the ribonucleoprotein is precipitated, appearing as a blue network or reticulum in the cell. The cell stained in this way is termed a reticulocyte. Polychromatophilic cells containing only small amounts of basophilic substance are difficult to recognize as young cells with Wright's stain. However, they are readily identified when stained with brilliant cresyl blue or new methylene blue. The examination of the reticulocytes may be made in a wet preparation or in a dry preparation that is counterstained with Wright's stain and preserved. Either coverglass or glass-slide preparations may be used. The variety of methods available allows a choice based on the equipment and needs of a particular laboratory.

### REAGENTS

ALCOHOL SOLUTION OF BRILLIANT CRESYL BLUE. An alcohol solution is made by dissolving 0.4 gm of powdered brilliant cresyl blue dye in 100 ml of 95-percent ethyl alcohol. This dye solution is stable but should be filtered to remove sediment when it is made up and at frequent intervals thereafter.

SALINE SOLUTION OF BRILLIANT CRESYL BLUE. A saline solution is made by dissolving 1 gm of brilliant cresyl blue dye in 100 ml of solution containing 0.85 gm of sodium chloride and 0.4 gm of sodium citrate per 100 ml of distilled water.

NEW METHYLENE BLUE.[22] A solution containing both an anticoagulant and a dye

is made by dissolving 0.5 gm of new methylene blue (color index 927) and 1.6 gm of potassium oxalate in 100 ml of distilled water.

### METHODS OF STAINING RETICULOCYTES

WET PREPARATION—SALINE BRILLIANT CRESYL BLUE. As recommended by Wintrobe,[2] one drop of capillary or venous blood is placed on a glass slide and approximately twice as much saline solution of brilliant cresyl blue is added and mixed with the corner of a coverglass. The mixture is then covered with a coverglass and gentle pressure is exerted with a piece of filter paper to make a thin preparation which may then be sealed around the edges with isobutyl methacrylate, vaseline, or melted paraffin. The preparation may be examined after it has stood for a few minutes and will keep for at least a day, but is not permanent. This procedure requires no specially prepared glassware and permits critical examination of the formal elements in a wet preparation.

WET PREPARATION—ALCOHOL BRILLIANT CRESYL BLUE. A drop of alcohol brilliant cresyl blue is allowed to dry on a clean glass slide. A drop of blood is added and mixed; a coverglass is then placed over the mixture, pressed to make a thin preparation, and sealed.

DRY PREPARATION USING GLASS SLIDES AND ALCOHOL. Two drops of alcohol solution of brilliant cresyl blue is allowed to dry near the end of a clean glass slide. One drop of blood is placed near the area of the stain and mixed with the dye. During the brief period when the preparation is wet, the dye enters the red cells. The blood-and-dye mixture, now stained blue, is spread promptly, by means of a second spreader slide, and allowed to dry before being counterstained with Wright's stain.

DRY PREPARATION USING COVERGLASSES. This method is more technically demanding than the slide method, since it may be difficult to prepare coverglasses that are evenly covered with dye unless the glassware is entirely free from grease. Clean, dry coverglasses are placed on a flat surface and enough (1 or 2 drops) alcohol solution of brilliant cresyl blue is added just to cover the surface of each coverglass. The coverglasses are then covered with a beaker or other glass vessel to reduce the rate of evaporation of the alcohol. When dry, the surface appears gray. It is polished to a purple color by rubbing it on smooth paper. This should result in a smooth, uniformly purple-stained preparation. Such preparations can be made and stored in a clean dry receptacle until needed. Films of blood are made with two stained coverglasses, as described above (p. 72). When dry, they are counterstained with Wright's stain.

TEST-TUBE METHOD—DRY PREPARATION OR WET PREPARATION FROM SALINE BRILLIANT CRESYL BLUE. One convenient method is available that utilizes prolonged contact of red cells with the dye and also allows for examinations as a wet preparation or as a dry preparation. The procedure is as follows. Two drops of saline solution of brilliant cresyl blue is placed in a small test tube (8 × 75 mm) and an equal amount of venous or capillary blood is added. The mixture may stand for a convenient period, such as ½ to 1 hr, before being examined. The mixture can then be handled in either of two ways: (1) a drop can be set up in a wet preparation as in method 1; (2) a drop can be added to a glass slide or to a coverglass and a film spread, dried, and counterstained with Wright's stain as in method 3. Prolonged or multiple contacts of red cells with glass surfaces increase the tendency to formation of crenated red cells.

NEW METHYLENE BLUE METHOD. Mix approximately equal parts of this staining solution and blood and allow to stand 10 min either on a slide, in a pipette, or in a test tube. A wet preparation can be made by placing a drop of this mixture on a slide, covering with a coverglass, and sealing, or a dry preparation can be made by spreading a drop on either a slide or a coverglass. The dry preparations are more satisfactory if counterstained with Wright's stain. The reticulum stains blue and is sharply defined. Counts may be a little higher than in the other methods because the cells are in contact with the methylene blue for a longer period than in the usual methods using brilliant cresyl blue.

### COUNTING RETICULOCYTES

In a dry or a wet preparation, the number of reticulocytes is determined in the counting of 1000 red cells. All red cells, including nucleated forms, that contain reticulum are counted as reticulocytes. The results are usually expressed as a percentage of the red cells. The absolute number of reticulocytes per unit volume may be calculated from the red-cell count. Because of the large number of cells in an oil-immersion field, it is helpful to cut down the area by inserting in one ocular of the microscope a mask that has a central hole about 3 to 4 mm in diameter. This can be improvised or a fiber washer from a plumber's supply company may be used. One standard washer is ¾ in. in diameter with a central hole $\frac{3}{16}$ in. in diameter. Different areas throughout the blood film should be selected for counting where the film is thin and the cells are separated, well stained, and easily identified.

DRY METHOD. Counterstaining the vitally stained preparation with Wright's stain gives sharp contrast between the blue of the reticulum and the red of the cell. No polychromatophilic cells should be present if the film is sufficiently stained with the brilliant cresyl blue. A film that is poorly stained should be discarded. Precipitated stain is often confused with reticulum but may be recognized because it also appears between the cells. This confusion may be avoided by thorough washing after staining and by frequent filtering of the cresyl blue and Wright's stain. Platelets, superimposed on red cells, may also be confused with reticulum. However, platelets stain purple and not the blue color of reticulum.

WET PREPARATIONS. In wet preparations the film of blood must be thin enough to permit inspection of individual red cells without excessive movement of the cells when focusing with the oil-immersion objective of the microscope. The reticulum of the red cells, the nuclei of white cells, and the platelets are stained blue. Crenation of the red cells, with formation of "thorn-apple" forms, may cause confusion. However, the spinelike projections on the red blood cells are refractile but *do not* stain. Crenation is caused, not by faulty technique, but by the removal by glass of the antisphering factor (crystalbumin).[23]

### LIMITATIONS AND SIGNIFICANCE

The normal values for reticulocytes vary slightly with the method employed but are usually in the range of 0.5–1.5 percent. Compared with the use of alcoholic solutions of dye, methods employing saline solutions of brilliant cresyl blue may give slightly higher values for reticulocytes because of the prolonged contact with the red cells in a wet preparation. For comparative studies, in following the course of a patient, the same method should be used throughout. The confidence limits for reticulocyte counts based on the counting of 1000 red cells are shown in Table 19.

One crude check on the results of the reticulocyte count is obtained from inspection of the Wright's-stained film in which the number of polychromatophilic cells should correspond to the number of reticulocytes observed on preparations stained with brilliant cresyl blue. If

Table 19. *Confidence limits for reticulocyte counts, based on 1000 red cells.*

| Percentage of reticulocytes | Limits | Percentage of reticulocytes | Limits |
|---|---|---|---|
| 0 | 0 –0.30 | 4.0 | 3.02– 5.21 |
| 0.1 | 0.01–0.47 | 4.5 | 3.46– 5.77 |
| 0.2 | 0.04–0.63 | 5.0 | 3.90– 6.33 |
| 0.3 | 0.08–0.78 | 6 | 4.50– 7.50 |
| 0.4 | 0.14–0.91 | 7 | 5.39– 8.61 |
| 0.5 | 0.20–1.05 | 8 | 6.28– 9.72 |
| 0.6 | 0.26–1.18 | 9 | 7.19–10.8 |
| 0.7 | 0.33–1.32 | 10 | 8.10–11.9 |
| 0.8 | 0.40–1.44 | 11 | 9.02–13.0 |
| 0.9 | 0.47–1.57 | 12 | 9.95–14.1 |
| 1.0 | 0.54–1.70 | 13 | 10.9 –15.1 |
| 1.1 | 0.62–1.82 | 14 | 11.8 –16.2 |
| 1.2 | 0.69–1.94 | 15 | 12.7 –17.3 |
| 1.3 | 0.77–2.07 | 16 | 13.7 –18.3 |
| 1.4 | 0.85–2.19 | 17 | 14.6 –19.4 |
| 1.5 | 0.92–2.31 | 18 | 15.6 –20.4 |
| 1.6 | 1.00–2.43 | 19 | 16.5 –21.5 |
| 1.7 | 1.08–2.55 | 20 | 17.5 –22.5 |
| 1.8 | 1.16–2.67 | 25 | 22.3 –27.7 |
| 1.9 | 1.24–2.79 | 30 | 27.1 –32.9 |
| 2.0 | 1.33–2.91 | 35 | 32.0 –38.0 |
| 2.5 | 1.74–3.49 | 40 | 36.9 –43.1 |
| 3.0 | 2.16–4.07 | 45 | 41.9 –48.1 |
| 3.5 | 2.59–4.64 | 50 | 46.8 –53.2 |

Above 5 percent, the true reticulocyte count should lie within the limits in 95 percent of instances; limits are calculated from the formula for the standard deviation of a binomial distribution.[18] For 5 percent and less, the limits are based on the confidence limits of the Poisson distribution.[19] In this case, the true value may be expected to lie within the limits in only 90 percent of instances, but it should lie either below an upper limit or above a lower limit in 95 percent of instances.

the dry methods are used, the preparation can be kept for future reference.

In wet preparations, the platelets may also be counted (Unit 8). Also, the three-dimensional configuration of the red cells can be observed. Wet films cannot be preserved and must be counted within the day of preparation.

### Examination of Blood in Wet Preparations

Much can be learned by careful observation of the cells in a drop of blood, previously preserved with an anticoagulant, mounted on a glass slide, and covered with a coverglass. To obtain a very thin film, slight pressure with a filter paper may be exerted to absorb excess fluid. To study motility of the white cells, a small drop of blood just sufficient to cover the film should be used and no pressure should be exerted. For prolonged observation, the preparation should be sealed around the edge with methacrylate or paraffin.

In wet preparations, the shape of the cells can be observed in three dimensions. Spherocytes are readily identified and the identification of rouleaux and of agglutinated red or white cells is facilitated. Wet preparations are also useful in detecting the presence of Heinz bodies [24] (see Unit 11) or the presence of the crystals that may be seen in Hemoglobin C disease.[25]

## Preparation of Buffy Coat

In certain cases of leukopenia, leukemia, or carcinoma, the white cells may be concentrated and examined for abnormal or unusual forms. This is done by making blood films from the buffy coat after centrifugation. Good preparations are obtained by taking the blood sample in EDTA and centrifuging immediately for 10 min at 1500 rev/min. The immediate centrifugation and preparation of the films will avoid some of the morphologic changes in the white cells that take place if the blood is allowed to stand. Various modifications of this method are used to study tumor cells or leukemic cells, especially when leukopenia is present. The "LE Test" is discussed in Unit 13.

## Free Iron in Red Cells—Siderocytes

It has been shown [26] that in the blood of normal human embryos and in hemolytic anemia there occur cells that, in addition to hemoglobin, contain "free" or easily detachable iron, possibly belonging to a hemoglobin precursor. The free iron can be stained by the Prussian blue reaction and appears in the form of small, single or multiple, bluish-green particles in the red cell. The particles have been termed *siderotic granules,* and red cells

containing them have been termed *siderocytes*. Siderocytes may also be seen in films stained with Wright's stain. They appear as blue-purple granules (Pappenheimer bodies).[27] They are easily confused with stipple cells, and often appear in groups. The Prussian blue stain is necessary for identification.

PRUSSIAN BLUE REACTION—GRUNEBERG METHOD.[26] A dried film of blood is fixed in methyl alcohol for 10 min and dried. It is then immersed for approximately 10 min in a freshly prepared mixture of equal parts of aqueous potassium ferrocyanide (2 gm/100 ml) and aqueous hydrochloric acid (1 percent by volume). The slide is washed, dried, and counterstained for 1 min (no more) in aqueous Biebrich scarlet dye, 1 gm/100 ml. The finished preparation is washed, mounted, and examined under the oil-immersion objective.

INTERPRETATION AND LIMITATIONS. Siderotic granules are found in small numbers in normal nucleated red cells but are not found in the normal mature erythrocyte.[28] The role of siderocytes has been reviewed by Mills and Lucia,[29] who have also classified inclusion bodies of red cells. The physiologic significance of siderocytes is not known. In disease and in anemias, the number of siderocytes may vary from 0 to 35 percent or more.[28] Increased concentrations are seen in some instances of hemolytic anemia and especially after splenectomy.

## Peroxidase Stain

Staining with benzidine and hydrogen peroxide is of occasional value in distinguishing various species of leukocytes. Peroxidase-positive granules are found in neutrophils, eosinophils, monocytes, and myelocytes. Lymphocytes, plasma cells, and all forms of blasts are peroxidase-negative. Histiocytes are also peroxidase-negative but may contain phagocytosed material which is peroxidase-positive.

**Method of Washburn as Modified by Osgood and Ashworth.**[30] *Solution 1.* Benzidine base, 0.3 gm, is dissolved in 99 ml of ethyl alcohol and to this is added 1 ml of a saturated aqueous solution of sodium nitroprusside. This staining solution will remain active for 8 to 10 months. *Solution 2.* A dilute solution of hydrogen peroxide is made just before use by adding 0.3 ml of fresh 3-percent hydrogen peroxide to 25 ml of distilled water. Films of blood, dried in the air, are stained preferably within 3 to 4 hr or at least within 12 hr of the time when the blood was collected. Ten drops of Solution 1 is placed on the slide and allowed to remain for 1 to 1½ min; 5 drops of Solution 2 is added directly and allowed to stand 3 to 4 min. The slide is then washed thoroughly in tap water for 3 to 4 min and counterstained with Wright's stain as already described.

INTERPRETATION. The granules in neutrophils are large, blue-black, and abundant. In myelocytes, the granules are small and blue-green in color. Fewer granules appear in the younger myelocytes. The granules of monocytes are small and blue-green in color like those of the myelocytes, but fewer in number and more widely separated. The characteristic shape of the monocyte nuclei aids in differentiating them from the myelocytes. Eosinophils have large bronze-colored granules. The granules of basophils may appear partially "empty" when counterstained with Wright's stain.

## Histochemical Methods of Staining

Histochemical methods for staining films of blood in hemopoietic tissues have been reviewed by Wislocki and Dempsey.[31] Supravital stains such as Janus green and neutral red may be used for staining cells in the living state and have been used for studying motility and other characteristics of leukocytes. However, they are seldom of practical aid in clinical diagnosis. At present, the most useful histochemical technique is the alkaline phosphatase stain. An even better method is the determination of alkaline phosphatase in a white-cell suspension. Both tests are useful in distinguishing between leukemic and normal cells, and are especially valuable in identifying normal cells in leukemoid reactions (see Unit 12).

HISTOCHEMICAL TECHNIQUE FOR ALKALINE PHOSPHATASE [32]

REAGENTS. 1. *Fixative solution:* Formalin (36–39 percent formaldehyde, 10 ml; absolute methanol, 90 ml). Should be stored in frozen state when not in use.

2. *Substrate mixture* (prepare immediately before use): sodium alpha naphthyl acid phosphate, 35 mg; fast Blue RR (diazonium salt of 4–benzoyl-2:5–methoxy-aniline), 35 mg; working 0.05$M$ propanediol buffer, pH 9.75, 35 ml. Filter directly onto slides or into Coplin jars and use at once. The pH of the mixture is 9.5–9.6.

INTERPRETATION. The alkaline phosphatase stains cytoplasmic granules within the cell brown or black. The results are expressed as a "score" per 100 mature neutrophils. Cells with no cytoplasmic staining are scored 0; those with diffuse brown staining, 1; those with distinct brown-black granules, 2; those with uniform distribution of granules throughout the entire cytoplasm, 3; and those with heavy black staining of cytoplasm, 4. A control group of 14 healthy adults gave a score range of 16 to 53, with an average of 30.

Histochemical staining demonstrates alkaline phosphatase activity only in mature and band-form granulocytes and is absent in immature granulocytes, lymphocytes, and monocytes. From a practical standpoint, the histochemical technique is satisfactory and useful but the biochemical determination is more accurate and quantitative.

QUANTITATIVE DETERMINATION
OF LEUKOCYTE ALKALINE
PHOSPHATASE [33]

REAGENTS. 1. Fibrinogen solution freshly prepared by mixing 200–250 mg of bovine fibrinogen (3.5 ml of the dry powder) with 0.9-percent sodium chloride solution to make a final volume of 13.0–13.5 ml.

2. 0.026$M$ sodium beta-glycerophosphate solution buffered to pH 9.9 with NaOH and sodium diethyl barbiturate.

3. 2-percent saponin in 0.9-percent sodium chloride solution

4. 0.050$M$ $MgCl_2$ solution

5. 30-percent trichloracetic acid

**Method.** *Preparation of Leukocyte Suspension.* (1) Mix 20–25 ml of unclotted venous blood with the freshly prepared fibrinogen solution. The citrate content of commercial fibrinogen acts as an anticoagulant. Remove the foam from the top of the mixture with a spatula and let the mixture sediment at room temperature for 20–30 min.

(2) Remove the supernatant plasma without contaminating it with red blood cells, and centrifuge this fraction for 5 min at approximately 600$g$.

(3) Remove and discard the supernatant fluid and resuspend the cell mass in 50 ml of 0.9-percent sodium chloride solution.

(4) Centrifuge the suspension for 5 min at approximately 600$g$.

(5) Resuspend the cells in 1.5–2.0 ml of sodium chloride solution and perform two white-cell counts on the suspension. The cell count (average of two counts) should be between 40,000 and 80,000/ mm$^3$. Even higher counts are desirable when the test is performed on patients suspected of having leukemia.

*Determination of Alkaline Phosphatase.* (1) Prepare four incubation mixtures, by mixing, in each of four tubes, 9.0 ml of the buffered glycerophosphate solution, 0.5 ml of saponin solution, and 0.2 ml of $MgCl_2$ solution (total volume of each mixture: 9.7 ml). Number the

tubes and warm them to 37°C in an incubator.

(2) To tubes 1 and 2, add 0.3 ml of the leukocyte suspension, and incubate them at 37°C for 60 min. At the end of the incubation period, add 2.0 ml of 30-percent trichloracetic acid to each tube.

(3) While tubes 1 and 2 are incubating, add 2.0 ml of 30-percent trichloracetic acid to tube 3 and then add 0.3 ml of the leukocyte suspension.

(4) To tube 4, add 2 ml of 30-percent trichloracetic acid and 0.3 ml of 0.9-percent sodium chloride solution.

(5) Filter the mixtures in the four tubes through No. 42 Whatman filter paper into clean centrifuge tubes.

(6) Determine inorganic phosphorus concentration of the filtrates by the method of Fiske and SubbaRow.[34] A modification of this method, using 0.5 ml of *p*-methylamino phenol made up in 3-percent sodium bisulfite, in place of the less stable amino naphthol sulfonic acid reagent, is recommended. The filtrate from tube 4 is used as a blank in the determination.

*Calculation of Results.* The difference between the phosphorus content of tube 3 and the mean value of tubes 1 and 2 represents the phosphate liberated by alkaline phosphatase. The alkaline phosphatase activity is expressed in units, where one unit is equal to 1 mg of phosphorus liberated by $10^{10}$ white cells in 1 hr.

INTERPRETATION. Normal values are 15 to 40 units. In patients with leukemia, alkaline phosphatase is almost always below 10 units. Patients with myeloid metaplasia and polycythemia usually have alkaline phosphatase above 40 units. Polycythemia vera or myeloid metaplasia turning into leukemia has not been studied by this method.

The low level of alkaline phosphatase in lymphocytic and monocytic leukemia is probably due to a relative decrease in granulocytes. Alkaline phosphatase also is low in infectious mononucleosis and other conditions associated with a decrease in granulocytes. At present it is not known whether the low level of alkaline phosphatase in leukemia is due to a decrease in the number of mature forms of granulocytes or a true enzymatic defect produced by the leukemia. In polycythemia vera, the alkaline phosphatase is usually elevated, whereas in secondary polycythemia, the alkaline phosphatase is normal.

## REFERENCES

1. G. A. Daland, *Color Atlas of Morphologic Hematology with a Guide to Clinical Interpretation* (rev. ed.; Harvard University Press, Cambridge, 1959).
2. M. M. Wintrobe, *Clinical Hematology* (ed. 4; Lea and Febiger, Philadelphia, 1956).
3. L. W. Diggs, D. Sturm, and A. Bell, *The Morphology of Human Blood Cells* (Saunders, Philadelphia, 1956).
4. J. B. Miale, *Laboratory Medicine—Hematology* (Mosby, St. Louis, 1958).
5. H. Downey, *Handbook of Hematology* (Hoeber, New York, 1938).
6. H. J. Conn, *Biological Stains. A Handbook on the Nature and Uses of the Dyes Employed in the Biological Laboratory* (ed. 6; Williams and Wilkins, Baltimore, 1953).
7. J. H. Wright, "A rapid method for the differential staining of blood films and malaria parasites," *J. med. Res. 7,* 138 (1902).
8. H. J. Conn and M. A. Darrow, *Staining Procedures Used by the Biological Stain Commission* (Biotech Publications, Geneva, N. Y., 1943–1944).
9. R. D. Lillie, "Factors influencing the Romanovsky staining of blood films and the role of methylene violet," *J. lab. clin. Med. 29,* 1181 (1944).
10. C. Price-Jones, *Red Blood Cell Diameters* (Oxford Medical Publications, London, 1933).
11. R. L. Haden, "The mechanism of the increased fragility of the erythrocytes in congenital hemolytic jaundice," *Amer. J. med. Sci. 188,* 441 (1934).
12. W. B. Castle and G. A. Daland, "Susceptibility of mammalian erythrocytes to hemolysis with hypotonic solutions; a function of differences between discoidal volume and volume of a sphere of equal surface," *Arch. intern. Med. 60,* 949 (1937).
13. Abridged from Errett C. Albritton, ed., *Standard Values in Blood* (Saunders, Philadelphia, 1952); see also Miale, ref. 4.
14. C. C. Sturgis and F. H. Bethell, "Quantitative and qualitative variations in normal leukocytes," *Physiol. Rev. 23,* 279 (1943).
15. R. G. S. MacGregor, W. Richards, and G. L. Loh, "The differential leukocyte count," *J. Path. Bact. 51,* 337 (1940).
16. C. W. Barnett, "Unavoidable error in differential count of leukocytes of blood," *J. clin. Invest. 12,* 77 (1933).
17. G. U. Yule and M. G. Kendall, *An Introduction to the Theory of Statistics* (ed. 14; Griffin, London, 1950).
18. F. M. Goldner and W. N. Mann, "The statistical error of the differential white count," *Guy's Hosp. Rep. 88,* 54 (1938).
19. F. Garwood, "Fiducial limits for the Poisson distribution," *Biometrika 28,* 437 (1936).
20. N. S. Burt, R. G. E. Nurray, and R. J. Rossiter, "Nucleic acids of rabbit reticulocytes," *Blood 6,* 906 (1951).

21. B. W. Holloway and S. H. Ripley, "Nucleic acid content of reticulocytes and its relation to uptake of radioactive leucine in vitro," *J. biol. Chem. 196*, 695 (1952).

22. G. Brecher, "New methylene blue as a reticulocyte stain," *Amer. J. clin. Path. 19*, 895 (1949).

23. R. F. Furchgott and E. Pond, "Disksphere transformation in mammalian red cells. II. The nature of the anti-sphering factor," *J. Exper. Biol. 18*, 117 (1940).

24. M. H. Fertman and M. B. Fertman, "Toxic anemias and Heinz bodies," *Medicine 34*, 131 (1955).

25. L. W. Diggs, A. P. Kraus, D. B. Morrison, and R. P. T. Rudnicki, "Intro-erythrocytic crystals in a white patient with hemoglobin C in the absence of other types of hemoglobin," *Blood 9*, 1172 (1954).

26. H. Grüneberg, "The anemia of flexed-tail mice. II. Siderocytes," *J. Genet. 44*, 246 (1942).

27. A. M. Pappenheimer, W. P. Thompson, D. D. Parker, and K. E. Smith, "Anemia associated with unidentified erythrocytic inclusions after splenectomy," *Quart. J. Med. 14*, 75 (1945).

28. J. V. Dacie, *The Haemolytic Anaemias, Congenital and Acquired* (Grune and Stratton, New York, 1954).

29. H. Mills and S. P. Lucia, "Familial hypochromic anemia associated with postsplenectomy erythrocytic inclusion bodies," *Blood 4*, 891 (1949).

30. E. E. Osgood and C. M. Ashworth, *Atlas of Hematology* (Stacey, San Francisco, 1937), p. 206.

31. G. B. Wislocki and E. W. Dempsey, "Observations on the chemical cytology of normal blood and hemopoietic tissues," *Anat. Rec. 96*, 249 (1946).

32. L. S. Kaplow, "Histochemical procedure for localizing and evaluating leukocyte alkaline phosphatase activity in smears of blood and marrow," *Blood 10*, 1023 (1955).

33. W. N. Valentine and W. S. Beck, "Biochemical studies on leukocytes. I. Phosphatase activity in health, leukocytosis, and myelocytic leukemia," *J. lab. clin. Med. 38*, 39 (1951).

34. C. H. Fiske and Y. SubbaRow, "The colorimetric determination of phosphorus," *J. biol. Chem. 66*, 375 (1925).

## Unit 10

# Methods for the Study of the Morphology of Bone Marrow

The morphologic study of bone marrow is an important aid in the diagnosis of a variety of diseases, as listed in Table 20. Certain of the methods used in the study of bone marrow are outlined below. For more details the reader is referred to the textbooks, monographs, and original reports that are available on this subject, and especially to the critical article by Dacie and White [2] concerning erythropoiesis.

### Aspiration of the Bone Marrow by Needle Puncture

Bone-marrow aspiration by needle puncture is a minor procedure of great diagnostic value. The samples of bone marrow may be studied by a variety of methods. The morphology of formed elements may be examined on direct films stained with Wright's stain or a supravital stain. The morphology may also be examined in aspirated material that is fixed and cut in sections, employing the standard methods of pathology. Hemosiderin may be demonstrated on the direct smear, or the formed elements, plasma, and fat may be separated by centrifugation and the volumes determined as in the hematocrit method.

#### SITES FOR NEEDLE PUNCTURE OF BONE MARROW

In adults any of three sites is satisfactory for aspiration of the bone marrow: (a) the body of the sternum at the level of the second interspace, (b) the spinous processes of the vertebrae, and (c) the iliac crest. The first of these has been used most commonly for years; the others give samples comparable to those obtained from the sternum. In the premature and newborn infant, iliac crest, tibia, and femur may be used. In the child from 1 to 4 years of age, the medial aspect of the tibia can be punctured and satisfactory samples obtained. The spinous process and iliac crest may also be used in the child. The availability of multiple sites for puncture permits the comparison of results from more than one area of bone marrow and allows the examiner to choose the site that is least distressing to the patient. Frequently it is less strain psychologically and less painful to puncture a spinous process than the sternum.

#### NEEDLES FOR PUNCTURE OF BONE MARROW

A variety of needles have been found satisfactory for puncture of the marrow cavity. In general, the needle must be short and rigid to prevent bending or breaking. Some types are provided with a guard to prevent excessive penetration. The lumen should be 1–2 mm in diameter and should have a tight-fitting stylet. The bevel should be short, and the point sharp.

90

Table 20. *Comparison of needle aspiration and surgical biopsy of the bone marrow* (*see also* Units 11 and 12).

| Diagnosis, physiologic mechanism, or anatomic change | Problem presented by examination of peripheral blood | Bone-marrow aspiration (differential count on direct film—Wright's stain) | Surgical-trephine biopsy (examination of stained sections of tissue) |
|---|---|---|---|
| 1. *Anemias:* In the anemias, examination of the bone marrow may confirm the diagnosis, may give data that are consistent with other observations, or may be of no diagnostic aid (see Unit 11) [1-9] | | | |
| Deficiency of vitamin $B_{12}$, folic acid, and related substances | Macrocytic anemia with low reticulocyte numbers | Abnormal forms of the erythrocytic series, including megaloblasts, are demonstrable in bone marrow and are presumptive evidence for deficiency of vitamin $B_{12}$, folic acid, and related substances | |
| Deficiency of iron | Hypochromic, microcytic anemia with low reticulocyte numbers | Hemosiderin is *absent* from marrow. Morphologically, the marrow is normoblastic. Normoblasts with deficient amount of cytoplasm are often seen. The data are confirmatory rather than diagnostic | |
| Hypoplasia of the marrow | Variable degrees of anemia, low reticulocyte numbers, leukopenia, neutropenia, thrombocytopenia, or pancytopenia | Bone-marrow aspiration will usually be indeterminate, giving a "dry tap" or a small number of marrow cells. If found repeatedly, this result is suggestive but not diagnostic | Biopsy is diagnostic since the hypoplasia is evident from the anatomic sections. In fibrosis or osteosclerosis, the sections are also diagnostic |
| Fibrosis or osteosclerosis of marrow | Immature cells of granulocyte and red-cell series with or without thrombocytopenia | | |
| Myelophthisic anemia (infiltration or replacement of bone marrow by leukemia, neoplasm, lymphoma, or granuloma) | (1) Variable degrees of anemia with variable numbers of reticulocytes and nucleated red cells; (2) white cells varying from leukopenia to leukocytosis to leukemia; (3) variable thrombocytopenia | Bone-marrow aspiration may give definite evidence for leukemia, metastatic tumor, or granuloma. Biopsy may be necessary to demonstrate these abnormalities, especially in granulomata, such as miliary tuberculosis, sarcoidosis, eosinophilic granuloma, and Hodgkin's disease | |
| Anemia in chronic infection, azotemia, liver disease | In infection, the chronic anemia is usually normocytic; in azotemia and liver disease, it is slightly macrocytic. The numbers of reticulocytes are usually low in infection but may be moderately elevated in the anemia of azotemia and liver disease | Examination of the bone marrow may exclude other diseases, but is not diagnostic of the cause or mechanism for the anemia. The iron content may be elevated in infection | |
| Hemolytic anemias, acute and chronic | The anemia is characterized by *reticulocytosis* and evidence of increased destruction of red cells (see Unit 11) | Examination of bone marrow usually shows increased normal erythropoiesis with immature forms. The immaturity of the nucleated red cells indicates the activity of the hemolytic process. The adult red cells in the background may give diagnostic information if sickled cells, polychromatophylic macrocytes, spherocytes, or fragmented forms are present | |
| Acute and subacute blood loss without deficiency of iron | The anemia is normocytic or slightly macrocytic (young red cells) with moderate reticulocytosis. In acute blood loss there may be marked leukocytosis, leukemoid reaction, nucleated red cells, and reticulocytosis | The bone marrow shows a normal physiologic response with increased erythropoiesis. In acute hemorrhage, there is increased erythropoiesis and myelopoiesis. These data are confirmatory but not diagnostic | |

Table 20. *Comparison of needle aspiration and surgical biopsy of the bone marrow* (*continued*).

| Diagnosis, physiologic mechanism, or anatomic change | Problem presented by examination of peripheral blood | Bone-marrow aspiration (differential count on direct film— Wright's stain) | Surgical-trephine biopsy (examination of stained sections of tissue) |
|---|---|---|---|
| **2.** *Polycythemia:* A critical differentiation between polycythemia vera and secondary polycythemia cannot usually be made on the basis of bone-marrow examination [4, 5, 10] | | | |
| Polycythemia of arterial anoxia, polycythemia vera, polycythemia associated with early leukemia, certain tumors, or myeloid metaplasia (osteosclerosis of marrow) | In polycythemia of arterial anoxia, the white cells and platelets are normal. However, in polycythemia vera there is usually leukocytosis and increased platelets. In early leukemia, leukemic cells may or may not be found. In myeloid metaplasia, there may be a leukemoid reaction of granulocytic elements | Examination of the bone marrow is of particular value to *exclude* fibrosis, leukemia, or early metastatic tumor. In polycythemia of arterial anoxia, there is hyperplasia of all elements. In polycythemia vera, myelopoiesis may be increased as well as erythropoiesis, and there is often an increased number of megakaryocytes | |
| **3.** *Malignant diseases:* Leukemia, lymphoma, and metastatic carcinoma [11–18] | | | |
| Manifest leukemia | There is marked increase in white-cell count with an increase of immature forms of leukocytes. There may be a myelophthisic or hemolytic anemia and thrombocytopenia | The marrow should always be examined for confirmation of the diagnosis of leukemia. In leukemoid reactions, examination of the bone marrow may exclude leukemia | |
| Leukemia with normal or low white-cell counts | The white cell count may be normal or low, without *marked* evidence of leukemic cells in the peripheral blood. The abnormal cells may be overlooked because of their scarcity. There may be variable degrees of anemia and thrombocytopenia | In "aleukemic" leukemia, the bone marrow will frequently give evidence of leukemic involvement before abnormal cells are evident in the peripheral blood. Repeated aspirations may be necessary to demonstrate bone-marrow involvement | |
| Hodgkin's disease, reticulum-cell sarcoma, plasmacytoma, multiple myeloma, and lymphomas | Usually there are no characteristic changes in the white cells of the peripheral blood. The presence of a few abnormal cells may be of great importance (histiocytes, plasma cells) | Bone-marrow aspirations may show evidence of infiltration. A biopsy may be necessary to allow anatomic study of infiltrating lesions | |
| Carcinoma with metastatic lesions in the bone marrow | Rarely, tumor cells may be seen in the blood, but are not easily identifiable. Anemia with nucleated red cells and myelocytes is usually present | Aspiration may reveal tumor cells in the bone marrow. Although single cells may be present, clumps of cells with amorphous masses of cytoplasm are necessary for diagnosis | |

Table 20. *Comparison of needle aspiration and surgical biopsy of the bone marrow (continued).*

| Diagnosis, physiologic mechanism, or anatomic change | Problem presented by examination of peripheral blood | Bone-marrow aspiration (differential count on direct film— Wright's stain) | Surgical-trephine biopsy (examination of stained sections of tissue) |
|---|---|---|---|
| **4** *Nonneoplastic diseases involving white cells:* Study of bone marrow is of value largely to exclude other diseases or to confirm a diagnosis [19-21] | | | |
| Agranulocytosis due to drugs and chemicals | Agranulocytosis without anemia or thrombocytopenia. There is a relative increase in lymphocytes and monocytes. Plasma cells may be increased | Examination of the bone marrow may not be necessary to make the diagnosis. Usually, mature granulocytes are absent from the bone marrow. The number and immaturity of the granulocytes vary with the severity of the disease process. Plasma cells, young lymphocytes, and reticulum cells are often increased | |
| | Leukopenia, neutropenia, lymphocytosis, atypical lymphocytosis, infectious mononucleosis, leukemoid reactions, eosinophilia. These changes may occur without anemia or thrombocytopenia | The bone marrow may be examined to exclude such diseases as leukemia. It may or may not show variations comparable to those of the peripheral blood | |
| **5.** *Thrombocytopenia:* Bone-marrow examination often shows characteristic changes of idiopathic or of secondary thrombocytopenia [22-27] | | | |
| Idiopathic thrombocytopenic purpura | Thrombocytopenia occurs as the only abnormality unless anemia is present due to hemorrhage | Bone-marrow aspiration reveals normal marrow with a normal or increased number of megakaryocytes which show diminished or absent budding of platelets | |
| Secondary thrombocytopenia purpura | Thrombocytopenia may occur without other abnormalities or with the changes of the primary disease such as leukemia (myelophthisic anemia) | There may be no demonstrable abnormality of the marrow or its megakaryocytes. There may be the changes of hypoplastic or invaded marrow with decreased numbers of megakaryocytes | |
| **6.** *Histiocytosis X and lipid-storage diseases:* [28-30] | | | |
| Histiocytosis X  Letterer-Siwe's disease  Eosinophilic granuloma  Hand-Schüller-Christian's disease  Nieman-Pick's disease  Gaucher's disease | Abnormal cells are rarely seen in peripheral blood taken from finger or vein. They may be more evident in blood taken from the ear lobe. The degree of anemia is variable | Aspiration may be helpful in demonstrating the abnormal cells. Usually trephine biopsy is necessary. When the spleen is enlarged, splenic aspiration may be necessary | |
| **7.** *Granulomata:* Granulomata of the bone marrow may be associated with the variable changes of a myelophthisic or hemolytic anemia. Granulomata are best observed with *surgical biopsy* in such conditions as miliary tuberculosis, syphilis, brucellosis, actinomycosis, leprosy, sarcoidosis, coccidiomycosis, histoplasmosis, and visceral leishmaniasis [20, 31, 33] | | | |
| **8.** *Hemochromatosis and hemosiderosis:* Aspiration or surgical marrow biopsy may show large deposits of hemosiderin in the bone marrow [33-35] | | | |

A lumbar-puncture needle (18-gauge) with stylet may be cut down to a length of 4 to 5 cm and the point ground to a short bevel. A 14-gauge needle has also been used. The needle described by Turkel and Bethell [47] may be used where bone samples are desired. This consists of an outer 14-gauge cutting needle and stylet 2 cm in length, and a 17-gauge inner needle, 6 cm in length, equipped with a serrated cutting tip for trephining the bone. The Turkel-Bethell needle may also be used for parenteral administration of fluids by way of the bone marrow.

Tocantins, O'Neill, and Jones [46] have described a needle for the parenteral infusion of bone marrow that may be used for aspiration of marrow samples. This is available in three different lengths for use in infants, children, and adults. The outer needle is fitted with an adjustable guard.

The Klima and Rosegger needle [39, 45] is 5.5 cm in length and has an adjustable guard (screw-thread adjustment) on which pressure may be exerted. It has been modified by Leitner.

A Vim-Silverman needle has been found satisfactory when aspiration has been unsatisfactory. With this needle, sufficient material may be obtained for histologic study as well as for cover-glass preparations.

### PERFORMANCE OF NEEDLE PUNCTURE OF BONE MARROW

STERNAL PUNCTURE. For puncture of the sternum, a point in the center of the body of the sternum and halfway between the second and third ribs is cleaned with iodine and alcohol and a local anesthetic is introduced into the skin, subcutaneous tissue, and periosteum. The patient usually lies flat in bed. A puncture needle with stylet is held at a 45° angle from the chest wall, with the butt of the needle toward the patient's feet. For an adult, the guard may be set at 1 cm. With firm pressure the needle is introduced through the skin, soft tissue, and cortex of the sternum into the spongy marrow. Rotation aids the penetration. A sudden "give" in resistance usually occurs when the needle enters the marrow cavity. Otherwise, the needle is advanced to a 1-cm depth or until blood is obtained. Suction is then applied to obtain a sample from the marrow. Excessive suction causes pain.

TREPHINE-NEEDLE BIOPSY. If the Turkel-Bethell needle is used for biopsy, the outer needle with fitting stylet is introduced until the point is embedded firmly in the outer lamella of the sternum. The stylet is then removed and the cutting needle is introduced and rotated back and forth until the trephine tip enters and cuts a sample from the bone marrow. The cutting needle is removed and the section of bone and marrow is forced out by a stylet into fixative solution.

PUNCTURE OF SPINOUS PROCESS. Puncture of a spinous process is done with the patient either in the prone position or on one side. A lower thoracic or lumbar vertebra is selected and the skin is cleaned. Local anesthetic is infiltrated down to the periosteum of the spinous process. The needle is then introduced vertically or at a slight angle to prevent slipping.

PUNCTURE OF ILIAC CREST. For puncture of the iliac crest, an area about 2.5 cm below the anterior superior spine is selected on the side of the ilium. Preparation and marrow aspiration are performed as described above.

### PREPARATION OF DIRECT FILMS OF MATERIAL ASPIRATED FROM BONE MARROW

Several satisfactory methods are available for the preparation of films from the material aspirated by needle puncture from the bone marrow. From 0.25 to 4 ml (usually 1 ml) of material may be aspirated by suction on the barrel of the syringe. A small drop of aspirated material may be placed directly on each of a series of clean coverslips and films prepared in the manner described for making films of peripheral blood (see Unit 9). The marrow fragments can be concentrated by placing a series of drops from the syringe on glass slides and allowing the blood to run off. The marrow particles adhere to the glass. Another method of concentrating the marrow particles is to obtain 4 ml of material from the marrow and introduce it into a watch glass containing 4-percent sodium citrate. The gray marrow particles are then picked up with a capillary pipette and transferred to a coverslip and a film is prepared. Concentrated preparations may also be fixed in formalin and examined by standard histologic methods.

STAINING OF DIRECT FILMS OF MATERIAL ASPIRATED FROM THE BONE MARROW

WRIGHT'S STAIN. The films are thoroughly dried in the air and then stained with Wright's stain for morphologic study and differential count of the nucleated formed elements. Because of the high concentration of nucleated cells, somewhat longer staining is usually necessary than for films of peripheral blood.

SUPRAVITAL STAINING. Fresh preparations of bone marrow may be stained without fixation, using vital dyes for identification of cells, as described by Epstein and Tompkins.[38]

PRUSSIAN BLUE STAIN—HEMOSIDERIN. Films of material from the bone marrow may be mounted unstained or may be stained by Prussian blue reaction for hemosiderin by the method of Rath and Finch [51] as a test for the amount of iron stored in tissues. Prussian blue stain is prepared by dissolving 4 gm of potassium ferrocyanide in 20 ml of distilled water. Concentrated hydrochloric acid is added until a white precipitate is formed. This mixture is then filtered. The film made from concentrated marrow material is covered with the filtrate for 30 min.

INTERPRETATIONS AND LIMITATIONS. In unstained films, the hemosiderin appears as golden-yellow granules under reduced illumination. When stained with Prussian blue, the hemosiderin granules appear blue. The amount of hemosiderin is graded on an arbitrary scale from none to very heavy. Structures other than hemosiderin may be stained occasionally. The iron in ferritin and hemoglobin is not stained. Clinically, the following variations have been found. In iron deficiency, there is no hemosiderin. In hemochromatosis and hemosiderosis, the deposits are very heavy. In pernicious anemia and infection, there is a greater deposit of hemosiderin than normal. The hemosiderin is increased following multiple transfusions. In general, the deposits of iron in the morphologic form of hemosiderin in the bone marrow correlate well with stores of iron elsewhere in the body.

QUANTITATIVE DETERMINATION OF BONE-MARROW ELEMENTS IN SAMPLES OBTAINED BY NEEDLE PUNCTURE

Aspirated samples from the bone marrow contain an unpredictable and uncontrollable admixture of whole blood together with particles and cells from the bone-marrow cavity. As shown by Weisberger and Heinle and others, the determination of the number or volume of nucleated cells or the volume of red cells or fat may not correlate with morphologic appearance of fixed sections of bone marrow.[42, 48, 49, 50] Statistically, the correlation of mean values may be satisfactory, but for the individual case the variation in the number of nucleated cells is too great to serve as a reliable diagnostic aid.

### Surgical Trephine Biopsy of Bone Marrow

Biopsy of bone marrow, usually of the sternum, is a minor surgical procedure. A small incision is made over the body of the sternum at the level of the second interspace, the periosteum is incised and elevated, and a trephine with a saw-toothed crown, 5 mm in diameter and 5 mm in depth, is used to remove a section of cortical and medullary bone. From the sample of bone marrow, imprints can be made directly on coverslips for staining with Wright's stain and the specimen of marrow may be put into tissue fixative and decalcified for the preparation of microscopic sections which are examined for anatomic relations and cellular structure. Differential counts of nucleated forms are made on tissue sections of bone marrow, and tissue sections are examined for cells which are identified and estimated quantitatively in relation to the structures of the marrow, such as connective tissue, blood vessels, bone, and fat.

### Interpretations and Limitations of Examinations of Bone Marrow

NORMAL RANGE. The normal range for the differential count of formed elements in direct films of material obtained by bone marrow puncture and stained by Wright's stain is shown in Table 21. When the differential count is made for clinical purposes, at least 200 cells should be examined. For investigative

Table 21. *Relative number of nucleated cells in normal bone marrow, based on 20 normal individuals.*

| Formed elements | Mean (per- cent) | Standard deviation (percent) | Range (percent) |
|---|---|---|---|
| Granulocytes: | | | |
| Neutrophils | 16.5 | 4.9 | 11.6–21.4 |
| Eosinophils | 0.7 | 0.7 | 0– 1.3 |
| Basophils | 0.1 | 0.3 | 0– 3.7 |
| Granulocytes, young (bands): | | | |
| Neutrophils | 25.6 | 8.1 | 17.5–33.7 |
| Eosinophils | 0.4 | 0.7 | 0– 1.1 |
| Basophils | 0.0 | 0.1 | 0– 0.2 |
| Metamyelocytes: | | | |
| Neutrophils | 9.2 | 3.5 | 5.7–12.7 |
| Eosinophils | 0.4 | 0.6 | 0– 1.0 |
| Basophils | 0.0 | 0.1 | 0– 0.1 |
| Myelocytes: | | | |
| Neutrophils | 10.2 | 4.4 | 5.9–14.6 |
| Eosinophils | 1.0 | 1.2 | 0– 2.2 |
| Basophils | 0.1 | 0.2 | 0– 0.3 |
| Myelocyte A | 0.4 | 0.5 | 0– 0.9 |
| Myeloblast | 0.7 | 0.5 | 0.2– 1.2 |
| Lymphocytes | 14.7 | 6.0 | 8.7–20.7 |
| Plasma cells | 0.9 | 0.8 | 0.1– 1.7 |
| Monocytes | 3.0 | 1.3 | 1.6– 4.3 |
| Reticulum cells or histiocytes | 0.5 | 0.1 | 0– 1.3 |
| Megakaryocytes | 0.1 | 0.1 | 0– 0.2 |
| Normoblasts | 11.1 | 4.6 | 6.5–15.6 |
| Late erythroblasts | 3.6 | 1.5 | 2.1– 5.1 |
| Early erythroblasts | 0.5 | 0.7 | 0– 1.2 |
| Proerythroblasts | 0.2 | 0.3 | 0– 0.4 |

work, 1000 cells should be counted. Since the published normal values vary considerably,[42, 48] the ranges given in Table 21 must be regarded as approximate only. The errors of performing a differential count of nucleated cells from puncture of the marrow have been discussed for different methods by Epstein and Tompkins.[38] It is evident that the errors will be similar in kind to those of the differential count of leukocytes of peripheral blood. In addition, the puncture of bone marrow is an attempt to sample a fixed tissue that is mixed with blood. Therefore, the reproducibility of sampling of bone marrow is considerably more limited than that of capillary blood.

The morphologic study of material obtained by bone-marrow aspiration is valuable in establishing many diagnoses that formerly required more demanding procedures of the patient and laboratory. Some of the indications together with the significance and limitations of results are outlined in Table 20.

LIMITATIONS OF DIRECT FILMS MADE FROM BONE MARROW. The positive identification of normal and abnormal cells in the bone marrow requires well-stained preparations and adequate training and skill of the observer. Accordingly, the reliability of differential counts will depend in part directly on the ability of the examiner. In general, any procedure that attempts to sample an organ as extensive as the bone marrow of an adult may miss a lesion that is not uniformly distributed. Furthermore, bone marrow is not a homogeneous structure, being composed of formed elements, fat, connective tissue, and a framework of bony trabeculae. There is therefore an inevitable sampling error in any one small specimen of marrow. In many diseases of blood, such as refractory anemias, aleukemic leukemia, myelophthisic anemia, neutropenia, and thrombocytopenia, there may be a lack of correlation between the morphologic findings in the bone marrow and those observed in the peripheral blood stream. In many instances, abnormality of the marrow may be demonstrable in the peripheral blood at a later stage of the development of the disease. A specific limitation of bone-marrow aspiration results from the procedure of spreading marrow tissue which frequently obliterates the anatomic relations of the cells. From the film, it is impossible to evaluate quantitatively the amount of fibrosis and replacement by fat, or to judge accurately the degree of cellularity per unit volume of tissue. Accordingly, the diagnosis of fibrosis of marrow or of hypoplasia cannot be made in a definitive manner. It may only be inferred from a "dry" tap or from low cellularity of the sample. Such an inference may be in error. Aspiration of bone marrow may fail to obtain certain cells that can be demonstrated by trephine biopsy. Thus, in granulomas, carcinoma, and leukemia (particularly of primitive cell types), aspirated marrow samples may show very few cells.[49, 50]

FIXED TISSUE SECTIONS. As has been described, anatomic sections can be made of material aspirated from the marrow,[13] or from trephined material.[12] Both of these procedures have the advantage of providing a small anatomic unit of marrow which may be examined for such changes as fibrosis, hypoplasia, and sheets of abnormal cells. However, the amount of tissue obtained by these methods may be insufficient for diagnosis.

Surgical trephine biopsy of bone marrow provides a specimen of tissue of sufficient size to be reliable as a representative sample of marrow. It also allows anatomic relations to be studied in a variety of sections. As indicated in Table 20, trephine biopsy is particularly helpful in identifying and evaluating fibrosis, hypoplasia, or aplasia of marrow, aleukemic leukemia, neoplasm, or granulomatous disease of the marrow. In hemorrhagic disorders, the danger of bleeding is greater with this procedure than with bone-marrow aspiration.

# REFERENCES

1. W. B. Castle, in W. A. Sodeman, ed., *Pathologic Physiology and Mechanisms of Disease* (ed. 2; Saunders, Philadelphia, 1956), chap. 28, "Diseases of the blood."
2. J. V. Dacie and J. D. White, "Erythropoiesis with particular reference to its study by biopsy of human bone marrow: a review," *J. clin. Path. 2*, 1 (1949).
3. J. L. Scott, "Acquired aplastic anemia: An analysis of 35 cases and review of the pertinent literature," *Medicine 38*, 2 (1959).
4. D. R. Korst, D. V. Clatanoff, and R. F. Schilling, "On myelofibrosis," *Arch. intern. Med. 97*, 169 (1956).
5. M. Block and L. O. Jacobson, "Myeloid metaplasia," *J. Amer. med. Ass. 143*, 1390 (1950).
6. C. H. Jaimet and H. E. Amy, "Cancer diagnosis by bone marrow smears," *Ann. intern. Med. 44*, 617 (1956).
7. A. S. Weisberger and R. W. Heinle, "Study of fixed tissue sections of sternal bone marrow obtained by needle aspiration. III. Metastatic carcinoma in sternal bone marrow," *Amer. J. med. Sci. 217*, 263 (1949).
8. J. H. Jandl, "The anemia of liver disease: observations on its mechanism," *J. clin. Invest. 34*, 390 (1955).
9. J. H. Jandl and M. S. Greenberg, "Bone marrow failure due to relative nutritional deficiency in Cooley's hemolytic anemia," *New Engl. J. Med. 260*, 461 (1959).

10. I. H. Manning, "The diagnostic value of the sternal bone marrow puncture in polycythemia vera," *Amer. J. med. Sci. 214,* 469 (1947).
11. C. H. Jaimet and H. E. Amy, "Cancer diagnosis by bone marrow smears," *Ann. intern. Med. 44,* 617 (1956).
12. W. Dameshek, "Biopsy of the sternal bone marrow. Its value in the study of diseases of blood-forming organs." *Amer. J. med. Sci. 190,* 617 (1935).
13. W. Dameshek, H. H. Henstell, and E. H. Valentine, "The comparative value and the limitations of the trephine and puncture methods for biopsy of the sternal bone marrow," *Ann. intern. Med. 16,* 801 (1937).
14. I. Snapper, L. B. Turner, and H. L. Moscovitz, *Multiple Myeloma* (Grune and Stratton, New York, 1953).
15. B. A. Bouroncle, B. K. Wiseman, and C. A. Doan, "Leukemic reticulo-endotheliosis," *Blood 13,* 609 (1958).
16. I. J. Wolman and B. Dickstein, "Clinical applications of bone marrow examinations in childhood," *Amer. J. med. Sci. 214,* 676 (1947).
17. E. D. Bayrd, "The bone marrow on sternal aspiration in multiple myeloma," *Blood 3,* 987 (1948).
18. T. Cooper and C. H. Watkins, "An evaluation of sternal aspiration as an aid in diagnosis of the malignant lymphomata," *Blood 4,* 534 (1949).
19. R. M. Jones, "Human sternal marrow in hyperthyroid and myxedematous states," *Amer. J. med. Sci. 200,* 211 (1940).
20. R. F. Houde and R. D. Sundberg, "Granulomatous lesions in the bone marrow in infectious mononucleosis. A comparison of the changes in the bone marrow in infectious mononucleosis with those in brucellosis, tuberculosis, sarcoidosis, and lymphatic leukemia," *Blood 5,* 209 (1950).
21. F. Kolouch, R. A. Good, and B. Campbell, "The reticulo-endothelial origin of the bone marrow plasma cells in hypersensitive states," *J. lab. clin. Med. 32,* 759 (1955).
22. W. Dameshek and E. B. Miller, "The megakaryocytes in idiopathic thrombocytopenic purpura, a form of hypersplenism," *Blood 1,* 27 (1946).
23. L. W. Diggs and J. S. Hewlett, "A study of the bone marrow from thirty-six patients with idiopathic hemorrhagic (thrombopenic) purpura," *Blood 3,* 1090 (1948).
24. D. A. Nickerson and D. A. Sunderland, "The histopathology of idiopathic thrombocytopenic purpura hemorrhagica," *Amer. J. Path. 13,* 463 (1937).
25. S. O. Schwartz, "The prognostic value of marrow eosinophils in thrombocytopenic purpura," *Amer. J. med. Sci. 209,* 579 (1945).
26. E. H. Valentine, "Idiopathic thrombocytopenic purpura. A study of three cases with special reference to changes in the megakaryocytes," *Amer. J. med. Sci. 214,* 260 (1947).
27. L. Whitby, "The significance of megakaryocytes in the peripheral circulation," *Blood 3,* 934 (1948).
28. L. Lichtenstein, "Histiocytosis X: Integration of eosinophilic granuloma of bone," *Arch. Path. 56,* 84 (1953).
29. J. Groen, "The hereditary mechanism of Gaucher's disease," *Blood 3,* 1238 (1948).
30. T. Cooper and C. H. Watkins, "An evaluation of sternal aspiration as an aid in diagnosis of the malignant lymphomata," *Blood 4,* 534 (1949).
31. J. W. Rebuck, "The structure of the giant cells in the blood-forming organs," *J. lab. clin. Med. 32,* 660 (1947).

32. D. R. Sundberg and W. W. Spink, "The histopathology of lesions in bone marrow of patients having active brucellosis," *Morphological Hematology* (*Blood*, special issue No. 1; Grune and Stratton, New York, 1947).

33. E. E. Muirhead, G. Crass, F. Jones, and J. M. Hill, "Iron overload (hemosiderosis) aggravated by blood transfusions," *Arch. intern. Med. 83*, 477 (1949).

34. C. E. Rath and C. A. Finch, "Sternal marrow hemosiderin. A method for determination of available iron stores in man," *J. lab. clin. Med. 33*, 81 (1948).

35. S. O. Schwartz and S. A. Blumenthal, "Exogenous hemochromatosis resulting from blood transfusions," *Blood 3*, 617 (1948).

36. I. Snapper, *Bone Diseases in Medical Practice* (Grune and Stratton, New York, 1957).

37. J. B. Miale, *Laboratory Medicine Hematology* (Mosby, St. Louis, 1958).

38. R. D. Epstein and E. H. Tompkins, "A comparison of technics for the differential counting of bone marrow cells," *Amer. J. med. Sci. 206*, 249 (1943).

39. R. Klima and H. Rosegger, "Zur Methodik der diagnostischen Sternalpunktion," *Klin. Wchnschr. 14*, 541 (1935).

40. L. R. Limarzi, "Evaluation of bone marrow concentration techniques," *J. lab. clin. Med. 32*, 732 (1947).

41. J. P. Loge, "Spinous process puncture. A simple clinical approach for obtaining bone marrow," *Blood 3*, 198 (1948).

42. E. E. Osgood and A. J. Seaman, "The cellular composition of normal bone marrow as obtained by sternal puncture," *Physiol. Rev. 24*, 46 (1944).

43. P. Pizzolato and J. Stasney, "Quantitative cytological study of multiple sternal marrow samples taken simultaneously," *J. lab. clin. Med. 32*, 741 (1947).

44. J. J. Rheingold, L. Weisfuse, and W. Dameshek, "Multiple sites for bone marrow puncture with particular reference to children," *New Engl. J. Med. 240*, 54 (1949).

45. E. M. Schleicher and E. A. Sharp, "Rapid methods for preparing and staining bone marrow," *J. lab. clin. Med. 22*, 949 (1937).

46. L. M. Tocantins, J. F. O'Neill, and H. W. Jones, "Infusions of blood and other fluids via the bone marrow," *J. Amer. med. Ass. 117*, 1229 (1941).

47. H. Turkel and F. H. Bethell, "Biopsy of bone marrow performed by a new and simple instrument," *J. lab. clin. Med. 28*, 1246 (1942).

48. A. S. Weisberger and R. W. Heinle, "Study of fixed tissue sections of sternal bone marrow obtained by needle aspiration. I. Method and the morphology in various conditions," *Amer. J. med. Sci. 215*, 170 (1948).

49. J. V. Dacie and J. D. White, "Erythropoiesis with particular reference to its study by biopsy of human bone marrow: a review," *J. clin. Path. 2*, 1 (1949).

50. A. S. Weisberger and R. W. Heinle, "Study of fixed tissue sections of sternal bone marrow obtained by needle aspiration. II. Comparison of nucleated cell count and volumetric pattern with histological appearance," *Amer. J. med. Sci. 215*, 170 (1948).

51. C. E. Rath and C. A. Finch, "Sternal marrow hemosiderin. A method for determination of available iron stores in man," *J. lab. clin. Med. 33*, 81 (1948).

# Unit 11

# Anemia and Polycythemia

Anemias are generally defined as conditions in which the hemoglobin concentration of blood is decreased below normal. Polycythemias, despite the term, are similarly defined as conditions in which the blood hemoglobin concentration is increased above normal.[1,2]

These definitions express the important physiologic fact that anemias are characterized by a decreased, and polycythemias by an increased, ability of the circulating blood to carry oxygen from the lungs to the tissues. It has been suggested that anemias and polycythemias should be expressed in terms of total red-cell mass. However, oxygen transport to the tissues depends on the concentration of oxygenated hemoglobin and on cardiac output but is not directly related to total red-cell mass.

Anemias and polycythemias are caused by changes in the rate of production or destruction of red blood cells. In either case, the normal homeostatic mechanisms, which balance the demand for oxygen in the tissues with the supply, will influence the pathophysiologic picture.

## PHYSIOLOGY OF THE RED CELL

### PRODUCTION AND DESTRUCTION OF CIRCULATING RED BLOOD CELLS

The red blood cells are designed primarily for the purpose of synthesizing, carrying, and protecting hemoglobin molecules. The synthesis of hemoglobin begins as soon as multipotential stem cells in the bone marrow differentiate into the most immature of the nucleated red cells, the proerythroblasts.[3] In the presence of an adequate supply of enzymes and metabolic substrates, porphyrin rings and globin molecules are formed and bonded together with iron atoms. Finished hemoglobin molecules can be recognized spectrophotometrically in the early erythroblasts [4] and visually in the late erythroblasts. During this period of hemoglobin synthesis and concomitant decrease in the cytoplasmic content of ribonucleic acid, the nucleated red cells go through a series of mitotic divisions and their number increases geometrically (Fig. 8).[5-9] The number of divisions and the exact duration of the period of cellular multiplication are not known, but it has been estimated that 1 to 2 days after the initial differentiation the cells reach the normoblastic stage in which the nucleus is condensed and incapable of further divisions. Approximately 1 day later, the nucleus is extruded and the cells take on the appearance of reticulocytes. The hemoglobin synthesis and the uptake of iron into the cells continue until the ribonucleic acid is exhausted and the cells have matured into adult red blood cells. At some point

100

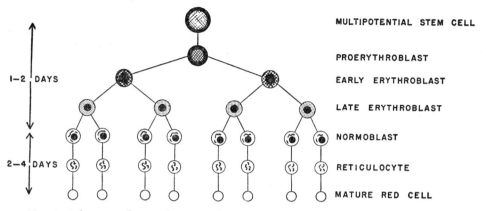

MULTIPOTENTIAL STEM CELL

PROERYTHROBLAST

1–2 DAYS

EARLY ERYTHROBLAST

LATE ERYTHROBLAST

NORMOBLAST

2–4 DAYS

RETICULOCYTE

MATURE RED CELL

Fig. 8. Scheme outlining the normal maturation and multiplication of nucleated red blood cells.

during the maturation of reticulocytes, the cells leave the bone marrow and the remaining maturation, lasting a few days, takes place in the circulating blood.

The mature red cells circulate through the vascular system for about 120 days, during which period they slowly grow old, lose their enzymatic vigor, and finally are destroyed, their component parts being either reutilized or excreted.[10] The destruction of 1 ml of red cells will result in the release of approximately 1 mg of iron and 10 mg of bilirubin into the circulation.

### STRUCTURE AND FUNCTION OF CIRCULATING RED BLOOD CELLS

The mature red cell structurally consists of a lipoprotein framework enclosing and supporting 200 to 300 million hemoglobin molecules. It is an actively metabolizing structure, deriving its energy from anaerobic glycolysis.[11, 12] It contains a number of enzymatic systems necessary for this glycolysis, for the preservation of its structural integrity, and for the maintenance of hemoglobin in its biologically active state. In addition, it contains the enzyme carbonic anhydrase, which assists in the transport of carbon dioxide.

The principal functions of the circulating red cells are to provide transportation for oxygen by means of hemoglobin, and to facilitate transportation of carbon dioxide by means of carbonic anhydrase.

### HEMOGLOBIN

The transport of large amounts of oxygen in the circulating blood is made possible by hemoglobin molecules, which are packed in high concentration in the red cells. Each molecule of hemoglobin consists of four porphyrin rings bonded to a protein matrix by means of iron atoms in the ferrous state (Fig. 9). The ferrous atoms have six co-ordination bonds. Four of these are attached to the pyrrole nitrogens of the porphyrin radical, the fifth is attached to the imidazole nitrogen of a histidine radical in a polypeptide chain of globin, and the physiologically all-important sixth is held reversibly by an oxygen molecule. When reduced hemoglobin is exposed to oxygen at increasing pressures, more and more oxygen will be taken up until each hemoglobin molecule has bound four molecules of oxygen and fully saturated oxyhemoglobin has been formed containing 1.34 ml of oxygen per gram of hemoglobin. Owing to intramolecular interactions between the heme groups, the oxygen binding and oxygen dissociation can be related graphically to the oxygen pressure by means of a sigmoid curve, the oxygen dissociation curve (Fig. 10).[13, 14] The shape of the oxygen

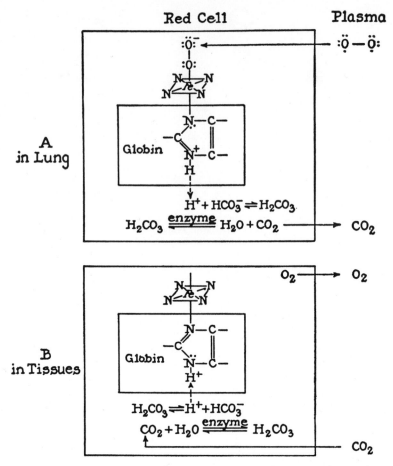

Fig. 9. Scheme outlining the heme binding and dissociation of oxygen and its effect on $CO_2$. [By permission from S. Granick, "The chemistry and functioning of the mammalian erythrocyte," *Blood 4,* 404 (1949).]

dissociation curve permits a stable and efficient transport of oxygen from the lungs to the tissues. The flat upper part of the curve signifies that the hemoglobin molecules in the lungs will be saturated with oxygen not only at the normal alveolar oxygen pressure, $P(O_2)$, of 100 mm Hg, but at considerably lower pressures as well. This provides a stable oxygen uptake, despite moderate changes in the pulmonary function or in the partial pressure of oxygen in atmospheric air. The steep middle portion of the curve signifies that a smaller or larger number of oxygen molecules can be released to the tissues at almost identical pressures. Under situations of increased or decreased cellular demand for oxygen,

these demands can then be fulfilled without materially changing the oxygen pressure that propels the molecules through the tissues from the capillaries to the cells.

The oxygen dissociation curve is influenced by the hydrogen-ion concentration (Bohr effect) with a shift to the left at a more alkaline pH and a shift to the right at a more acid pH. In other words, at a constant oxygen pressure more oxygen is released to tissues with a high metabolic activity and a high hydrogen-ion concentration than to dormant tissues with a low concentration of acid metabolic by-products.

The changes in red-cell pH are kept within the physiologic range primarily

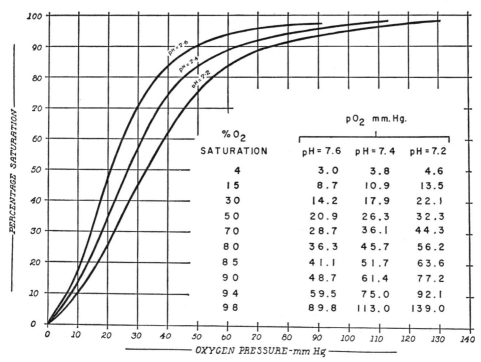

| % $O_2$ SATURATION | $pO_2$ mm. Hg. | | |
|---|---|---|---|
| | pH = 7.6 | pH = 7.4 | pH = 7.2 |
| 4 | 3.0 | 3.8 | 4.6 |
| 15 | 8.7 | 10.9 | 13.5 |
| 30 | 14.2 | 17.9 | 22.1 |
| 50 | 20.9 | 26.3 | 32.3 |
| 70 | 28.7 | 36.1 | 44.3 |
| 80 | 36.3 | 45.7 | 56.2 |
| 85 | 41.1 | 51.7 | 63.6 |
| 90 | 48.7 | 61.4 | 77.2 |
| 94 | 59.5 | 75.0 | 92.1 |
| 98 | 89.8 | 113.0 | 139.0 |

Fig. 10. Oxygen dissociation curves for human blood.[15]

by means of the buffering capacity of the hemoglobin molecules. When oxygen molecules are bonded to the heme radicals of reduced hemoglobin, an intramolecular rearrangement of electric forces takes place and hydrogen ions are liberated. Oxyhemoglobin, consequently, behaves as a stronger acid than reduced hemoglobin (Fig. 9). This change in the acidity of hemoglobin results in free hydrogen ions being formed in the pulmonary capillaries and hydrogen ions being neutralized in the tissue capillaries. It neatly counterbalances changes in the hydrogen-ion concentration caused by the transport of $CO_2$ from the tissues to the lungs, and it is partly responsible for the small difference between arterial and venous pH.

### CARBONIC ANHYDRASE

The transport of carbon dioxide from the tissues to the lungs is greatly facilitated by an enzyme, carbonic anhydrase, present in the red cells. Some carbon dioxide is absorbed physically in the blood, but the main bulk is carried as bicarbonate. The process that transforms carbon dioxide into bicarbonate in the tissue capillaries and releases carbon dioxide from bicarbonate in the pulmonary capillaries is catalyzed by this intracellular enzyme. Figure 11 outlines the biochemical pathway of carbon dioxide from tissues to the lungs and shows its important relation with carbonic anhydrase, hemoglobin, and chloride anions.

### PHYSIOLOGIC REGULATION OF RED-CELL PRODUCTION

Under physiologic conditions, the red blood cell count and hemoglobin concentration in circulating blood are determined by the rate of red-cell production. Normally, the rate of red-cell destruction does not appear to vary and the bone marrow alone must be responsible for maintaining a level of red cells in blood that is optimal for the fulfillment of its functional objectives. It seems likely that the red-cell production is controlled primarily, if not exclusively, by the effects

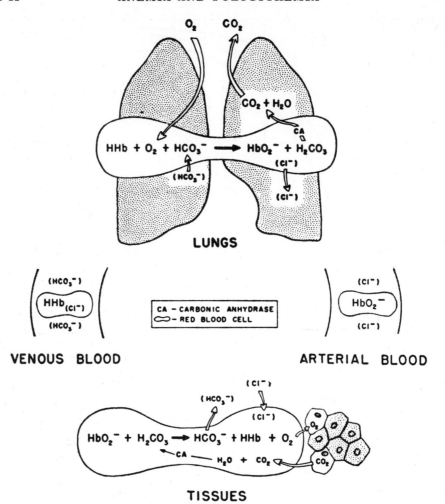

Fig. 11. Outline of the $CO_2$ transport and its dependence on hemoglobin and carbonic anhydrase.[16] (By permission of *Surgery, Gynecology and Obstetrics.*)

of oxygen transport on the tissues, or more specifically on the oxidative tissue metabolism, and almost all clinical and experimental observations have so far been compatible with this hypothesis.[17] Impaired transport of oxygen to the tissues, as in anemia, at high altitudes, or in pulmonary and cardiovascular disorders, results in accelerated production of red cells. Increased transport of oxygen, as in transfusion polycythemia, or during exposure to high atmospheric oxygen pressure, leads to a less rapid production of red cells. These changes in the rate of red-cell production are probably accomplished by changes in the rate at which multipotential stem cells are differen-

tiated into nucleated red cells or proerythroblasts (Fig. 7). When the nutritional and hormonal environment is adequate, subsequent multiplication and hemoglobin synthesis appear to proceed at a fixed rate, which has no relation to demands for accelerated or reduced red-cell production.[18]

The mechanism by which the oxidative tissue metabolism regulates the rate of stem-cell differentiation is not thoroughly understood. Recently it has been demonstrated that plasma from anemic animals is erythropoietically active and will stimulate red-cell production when infused into a normal animal.[19] Similar erythropoietic activity is displayed by plasma from animals exposed to low oxygen pressure and by plasma and urine from some anemic and polycythemic patients.[20, 21, 22] The existence of erythropoietic activity in plasma suggests that red-cell formation may be controlled through the production or release of variable amounts of an erythropoietic factor.

### PHYSIOLOGY OF OXYGEN TRANSPORT

The production of red cells in the bone marrow is influenced by the functional activity of the lungs, the heart, and the vascular system. The integrated action of these four organ systems is responsible for the transfer of oxygen from the atmospheric air to the tissues. Furthermore, they are responsible for making oxygen available in the tissues, both in amounts adequate for aerobic cellular metabolism and at pressures sufficient to permit oxygen to diffuse from the capillaries to the cytochrome system of even the most remote cell.[23] Whenever the tissue demand for oxygen exceeds the supply, compensatory changes in the rate of red-cell production, the pulmonary vital capacity, the cardiac output, and the distribution of blood among the tissues take place until the tissue demand has been fulfilled. As is the case with red-cell production, it seems most likely that the oxidative tissue metabolism in some way is responsible for the mobilization of these compensatory changes. Consequently, the oxidative tissue metabolism may provide a servomechanism as a pivot for feedback mechanisms which influence the bone marrow, the heart, the lungs, and the blood vessels.

Under normal conditions, the steady state for this integrated oxygen-transport mechanism is reached when the rate of red-cell production is sufficient to maintain a hemoglobin concentration of about 15 gm/100 ml. Adequate amounts of oxygen can be delivered to the tissues at considerably lower levels of hemoglobin with only slight changes in vascular distribution of blood or in the cardiac output. However, most mammals stabilize their level of hemoglobin between 12 and 15 gm/100 ml, a level that must be considered advantageous in the body economy. Many factors are probably at work in the selection of this level as "normal." One of these factors is undoubtedly the fact that an increase in the number of oxygen-carrying red blood cells is associated with increased viscos-

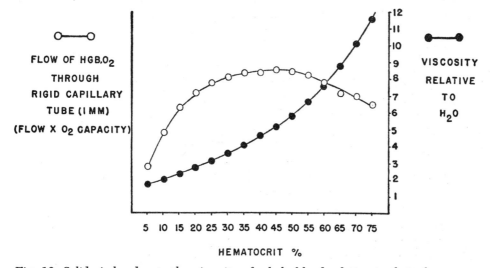

FLOW OF HGB.O₂ THROUGH RIGID CAPILLARY TUBE (I MM) (FLOW X O₂ CAPACITY)

VISCOSITY RELATIVE TO H₂O

HEMATOCRIT %

Fig. 12. Solid circles denote the viscosity of whole blood relative to that of water at various hematocrits measured in an Ostwald viscosimeter. The open circles denote the flow of oxyhemoglobin through the viscosimeter in arbitrary units at various blood hematocrits.[25]

ity of blood and consequently a slower flow. If the oxygen transport is expressed as the product of hematocrit and flow (Fig. 12), it can be calculated that the oxygen transport through a narrow, rigid tube reaches optimal values at hematocrits between 30 and 60 percent, or hemoglobin concentrations between 10 and 20 gm/100 ml.

A decreased supply of oxygen to cells will result in tissue anoxia and an increased supply in tissue hyperoxia. On pathogenetic grounds, Barcroft[24] has subdivided the anoxic conditions into "anoxic anoxia," "anemic anoxia," and "stagnant anoxia." "Histotoxic anoxia" is a term used when the cellular supply of oxygen is adequate but the cells are unable to metabolize oxygen. Of these conditions, "anoxic anoxia" and "anemic anoxia" are of clinical importance, while "stagnant anoxia," "histotoxic anoxia," and "hyperoxia" are of more theoretic interest.

### ANOXIC ANOXIA

Anoxic anoxia is met at high altitudes, in pulmonary diseases, and in cardiac and vascular abnormalities where venous unsaturated blood is being shunted directly into the arterial circulation. The arterial oxygen pressure is less than is necessary for complete saturation of the hemoglobin with oxygen and less oxygen is delivered to the tissues. If the extraction of oxygen in the tissues remains the same, this oxygen must be delivered at lower mean capillary pressure and the cells most distant from the capillaries will suffer.[23] To overcome the resulting cellular anoxia, respiratory activity is increased, red-cell production is accelerated, and cardiac output is increased.[26, 27]

In terms of oxygen transport, an increase in red-cell production resulting in polycythemia is not a very effective compensating device, but it can be maintained indefinitely with little expenditure of energy and without exhausting any bone-marrow reserve. There is, however, a limit to the number of red cells that can be accommodated by the blood. At hematocrit levels above 60 percent the viscosity of blood increases sharply, thus impeding the flow through vascular channels (Fig. 12). Under conditions of continued tissue anoxia and continued stimulation of the bone marrow, the blood volume will eventually increase in order to prevent the bone marrow from clogging the vessels with viscous blood.[28] This increase in blood volume will result in a slower circulation, but it might facilitate the oxygen diffusion in the tissues by keeping more capillary channels open. The increased viscosity and increased blood volume seem to be tolerated very well by mountain dwellers, in whom visual disturbances, nosebleed, and vascular thrombosis, so common in patients with polycythemia vera, are quite rare.

Increased cardiac output results in a rapid circulation, with oxygen being made available to the tissues in greater amounts per unit time and at greater mean capillary pressures. This compensatory device is very effective in increasing the oxygen delivery to the tissues, but it appears to be a mechanism that is saved primarily for conditions in which there is an acute demand for more oxygen. In persons well acclimatized to their anoxic anoxia, cardiac output at rest is almost normal[29] and compensation for low atmospheric oxygen is achieved by the lungs and the bone marrow alone.

### ANEMIC ANOXIA

The compensatory devices utilized in anemic anoxia are, as in anoxic anoxia, designed to provide the tissues with an adequate amount of oxygen at an adequate pressure. This is accomplished by an accelerated rate of red-cell production, by an increase in cardiac output, and by a redistribution of blood among the tissues. An increase in pulmonary ventilation is of little help in anemic anoxias since the blood already is saturated with oxygen and hyperventilation would cause only a slight additional increase in physically absorbed oxygen. Actually, it is unusual to observe an increase in respiratory activity except in severe anemias. One suggested explanation is that the metabolism in the carotid and aortic bodies that influences pulmonary ventilation is dependent on the arterial oxygen pressure rather than on the oxygen-carrying capacity of blood.[30]

Anemic anoxia will stimulate the erythropoietic tissues, but the effectiveness of this stimulation in counteracting the anemic anoxia depends upon the pathogenesis of the anemia. In blood-loss anemias and in hemolytic anemias, the anoxic stimulus will increase the output of red blood cells from the bone marrow from a normal daily output of 20 ml of packed cells to as high as 120–140 ml.[31] In nutritional anemias, the bone marrow becomes hyperplastic and is packed with nucleated red cells, but the output of mature red cells is decreased owing to faulty red-cell maturation. In anemias caused by toxic inhibition of the bone marrow, and in aplastic anemias, there is no bone-marrow evidence to indicate the existence of an effective anoxic stimulus of red-cell production. However, it has been reported that plasma from patients with aplastic anemia is erythropoietically active,[32] which suggests the presence of an anoxic erythropoietic stimulus but the lack of an erythropoietic bone-marrow response to this stimulus.

In anemias, the fall in total red-cell mass is usually balanced by an increase in plasma volume, leaving the blood volume within normal limits. In severe anemia, there may be a decrease in blood volume, presumably in an attempt to keep the hemoglobin concentration from falling below values compatible with life.[33]

The oxygen dissociation curve in chronic anemias is shifted slightly to the right, thereby increasing the amount of oxygen delivered to the tissues at a certain oxygen pressure.[34] This shift is not caused by a change in the hemoglobin molecule, since the dissociation curve of hemolysates is normal, but must be caused by a change in the intracellular environment of the red cell.

A compensatory increase in cardiac output takes place in acute anemias associated with a sudden decrease in blood volume and in chronic anemias when the hemoglobin concentration is below a level of approximately 7 gm/100 ml.[35] In chronic anemias with a hemoglobin concentration above 7 gm/100 ml, the cardiac output is normal at rest, and tissue anoxia in vital organs is prevented solely by a redistribution of blood. The donor areas in this redistribution are organs with a blood supply greater than that dictated by their oxygen needs, like the skin and the kidneys, and the recipient areas are oxygen-sensitive tissues like the brain, or tissues with a large oxygen consumption like the heart and the muscles.[36]

### STAGNANT ANOXIA

Increased circulation time as observed in congestive heart failure results in an increased extraction of oxygen from the sluggishly moving blood in the capillaries and a decrease in mean capillary oxygen pressure. This stagnation must lead to a certain degree of anoxia in cells situated at a distance from the capillaries and should theoretically result in an anoxic stimulation of red-cell production. Owing to the concomitant pulmonary and cardiovascular changes in congestive heart failure it has been difficult to demonstrate this stimulation, but the total red-cell mass is frequently increased, suggesting an accelerated rate of red-cell production.[37]

### HISTOTOXIC ANOXIA

A toxic inhibition of the oxidative cellular metabolism leads to metabolic changes that may be similar to the changes observed under conditions of oxygen deprivation. It has been suggested that the increase in red-cell production observed after cobalt administration is a compensatory response to such a toxic inhibition of tissue respiration.[38] This suggestion has received some support from the observation that cobalt induces the formation of reversible complexes of oxygen with histidine.[39] Furthermore, oxygen in subcutaneous gas pockets is not utilized in a normal manner in cobalt-treated mice.[40] In addition, recent studies have demonstrated that rats respond to cobalt administration with an increase in the erythropoietic activity of plasma in the same manner as rats exposed to anemic or anoxic anoxia.[41]

TISSUE HYPEROXIA

Under artificial conditions, it is possible to make oxygen available in the tissues at an abnormally high mean capillary pressure. In transfusion polycythemia, the tissues can extract the needed oxygen with only a small decrease in oxygen saturation of hemoglobin and the mean capillary oxygen pressure will approach arterial pressure.[42] Exposure to high atmospheric oxygen pressures will increase the amount of physically absorbed oxygen in blood, and will increase the pressure at which oxygen is delivered in the tissues.[43] It has been shown that a decrease in the rate of red-cell production occurs under these conditions, which supports the hypothesis that the rate of red-cell production is regulated by the degree of tissue oxygenation.

## THE ANEMIAS

Anemia exists when the hemoglobin concentration is decreased below the lower limit of normal, or below approximately 12 gm/100 ml. The anemias can be divided into two main groups: those caused by impaired red-cell production (Table 22) and those caused by red-cell loss or increased destruction (Table 23).

### Anemias Associated with Defective Red-Cell or Hemoglobin Production

Anemia caused by diminished release of red cells from the bone marrow into the circulation may or may not be accompanied by diminution in marrow cellularity, in the rates of plasma iron turnover or utilization, or in the excretion of bile pigments, depending upon the mechanism of the disorder. The most reliable general indication of this category of anemias is the presence of a low percentage of circulating reticulocytes despite continued anemia. These anemias are classified on an etiologic basis in Table 22 and on a functional basis in Table 24 and in the following text.

### Hypochromic Anemias

These anemias are caused by impaired hemoglobin synthesis, most commonly from a lack of iron.

#### IRON-DEFICIENCY ANEMIA

##### PATHOLOGIC PHYSIOLOGY

The absorption of iron from the diet is limited to a few milligrams daily, even during iron deficiency. Absorbed iron is transferred to the sites of utilization by the serum iron-binding protein, "transferrin." Normally, over 60 percent of the body's store of iron is present in the hemoglobin of circulating red cells, which contain about 1 mg of iron/ml of cells, a small portion (3 or 4 percent) of which exists in heme enzymes and myoglobin and the rest in storage sites in the form of hemosiderin and ferritin. Since very little iron is excreted from the body, the body stores of iron are almost quantitatively reutilized. Thus dietary deficiency or intestinal malabsorption of iron will cause iron deficiency only when combined with increased requirements, as

Table 22. *Etiologic classification of anemias caused by impaired red-cell production.*

==========================================

### I. *Nutritional deficiency*

A. Deficiency of vitamin $B_{12}$
   1. Dietary deficiency
   2. Defective absorption
      a. Intrinsic-factor deficiency
         i. Pernicious anemia
         ii. Gastrectomy
      b. Intestinal disease
         i. Intestinal malabsorption (sprue, operative removal, short-circuit, etc.)
         ii. Fish-tapeworm infestation
         iii. "Blind-loop syndrome"
B. Deficiency of folic acid
   1. Dietary deficiency
   2. Defective absorption
      a. Intestinal malabsorption (as above)
      b. "Blind-loop syndrome"
   3. Metabolic derangement
      a. Folic acid antagonists
      b. ? Pernicious anemia of pregnancy
      c. ? Administration of anticonvulsants (rarely)
      d. ? Cirrhosis (rarely)
      e. Ascorbic acid deficiency (rarely)
C. Deficiency of iron
   1. Insufficient neonatal iron stores
   2. Dietary deficiency
   3. Defective absorption
   4. Chronic blood loss

### II. *Endocrine deficiency*

A. Hypothyroidism
B. Hypopituitarism
C. Hypoadrenocorticism

### III. *Toxic inhibition*

A. Internal: Chronic infection and inflammation, renal disease, tumors
B. External:
   1. Chemical (benzol, nitrogen mustards, chloromycetin, etc.)
   2. Irradiation

### IV. *Replacement of bone marrow by nonerythroid tissue*

A. Myelophthisis: Myelofibrosis, carcinomatosis, leukemia, etc.

### V. *Idiopathic "aplasia" or "hypoplasia"*

A. Congenital
B. Acquired

### VI. *Erythremic myelosis (DiGuglielmo's disease)*

==========================================

during phases of rapid growth, during pregnancy, or as a result of blood loss, as from menstrual or intestinal bleeding.

### SCREENING TESTS

The peripheral blood in iron deficiency is hypochromic and microcytic, and an-

isocytosis becomes pronounced only when severe anemia develops. Unlike Cooley's anemia, iron deficiency does not involve extreme anisocytosis, abnormal

Table 23. *Etiologic classification of anemias caused by red-cell loss or increased destruction.*

==========================================

A. Acute blood loss
   1. Hemorrhage, external
   2. Hemorrhage, internal (trauma, purpura, scurvy, etc.)
B. Hemolytic anemias
   1. Intrinsic defects of red cells
      a. Hereditary
         i. Hereditary spherocytosis
         ii. Hemoglobinopathies: sickle-cell anemia, hemoglobin C disease, etc.
         iii. Hereditary microcytosis: Cooley's anemia, "hemoglobin H disease," etc.
         iv. Hereditary ovalocytosis
      b. Acquired
         i. Paroxysmal nocturnal hemoglobinuria
   2. Extrinsic defects of red cells
      a. Immune mechanisms
         i. Isoimmune
            (a) Natural: transfusion of ABO-incompatible plasma
            (b) Acquired: sensitization to Rh factor
         ii. "Autoimmunity": acquired hemolytic anemia
            (a) Primary (idiopathic)
            (b) Secondary to lymphatic leukemia, lymphoma, sensitization to certain drugs and pollens, syphilis (P.C.H.), virus pneumonia, disseminated lupus erythematosus, etc.
      b. Drugs and chemicals
         i. "Oxidant" compounds that cause methemoglobinemia and Heinz-body formation
            (a) Usually not requiring hypersusceptible red cells: phenylhydrazine, $\alpha$-naphthol, naphthalene, acetanilide and other aniline derivatives, etc.
            (b) Usually requiring hypersusceptible red cells: sulfonamides, naphthoquinone, primaquine, pamaquin, etc.
         ii. Other chemicals: arsine, lead, etc.
      c. Infections
         i. Bacterial hemolysins: Welch bacillus, hemolytic streptococcus
         ii. Red-cell parasitization: malaria, *Bartonella*, etc.
      d. Heat: extensive third-degree burns
      e. Miscellaneous: terminal renal disease and carcinomatosis
   3. Defects of red-cell environment
      a. Splenic hyperfiltration: splenomegaly caused by portal hypertension, cellular infiltration, infection, etc.

==========================================

Table 24. *Functional classification of anemias caused by impaired red-cell production.*

| Functional defect in erythropoiesis | | Blood changes | Marrow changes | Causes |
|---|---|---|---|---|
| Late: | Failure of hemoglobin synthesis | Microcytic, hypochromic | Hyperplastic, deficient hemo-globinization | Iron deficiency, pyridoxine deficiency, chronic lead poisoning |
| Middle: | Failure of nucleoprotein synthesis | Macrocytic, normochromic | Hyperplastic, maturation arrest (megaloblastic) | $B_{12}$ deficiency, folic acid deficiency |
| Early: | Failure of stem-cell differentiation | Normocytic, normochromic | Hypoplastic, normal cytology | Endocrine, toxic, physiologic, idiopathic |

nuclear remnants (Howell-Jolly bodies and Cabot rings), and basophilic stippling. In iron deficiency, hypochromia and microcytosis usually go hand in hand, whereas in Cooley's anemia (thalassemia) or Cooley's trait microcytosis is striking while the MCHC is normal or only mildly reduced (Fig. 13). Characteristically, in iron deficiency the nucleated red cells of the bone marrow are small and contain scanty blue cytoplasm that is visibly deficient in hemoglobin.

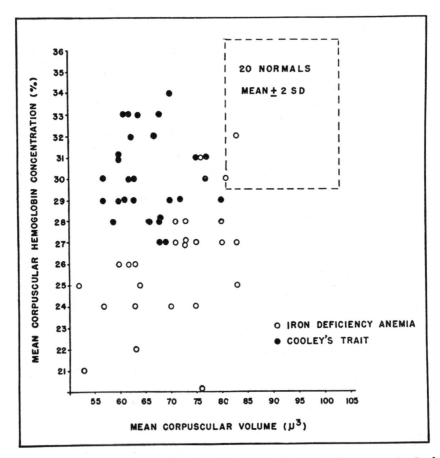

Fig. 13. Comparison of red-cell corpuscular values in "microcytic" anemias. In Cooley's trait, microcytosis is usually accompanied by little or no hypochromia. In iron-deficiency anemia, hypochromia is more striking and is roughly proportional in severity to the degree of microcytosis. (By permission of Geneva A. Daland.)

SPECIAL TESTS

(*a*) A therapeutic trial of oral or parenteral iron may aid in establishing the diagnosis, although morphologic criteria generally suffice. The specific reticulocyte response to iron at a given hemoglobin level is less striking than the response to vitamin $B_{12}$ or to folic acid when deficiency of these substances is present (Fig. 14).

(*b*) The bone-marrow aspirate may be examined for the presence of iron as hemosiderin, either directly [44] or by staining by the Prussian blue reaction (Unit 10). The direct examination is preferable in that it is simpler and not as subject to false positives as is the staining method. In either case, it is important that observations be made on a good cellular marrow specimen containing reticuloendothelial elements.

(*c*) Several methods are available for the measurement of serum iron levels.[45, 46] In general, normal serum iron levels range from about 80 to 180 μg/

100 ml. Although levels below this are found in iron deficiency, hypoferremia is also encountered in many diseases, especially in infection or in some chronic disease states. Determination of the total iron-binding capacity of serum [47, 48] helps differentiate these causes of hypoferremia, since this capacity tends to increase in iron deficiency and is usually diminished during infection or chronic disease.

OTHER HYPOCHROMIC ANEMIAS

Pyridoxine deficiency leads to a hypochromic microcytic anemia morphologically resembling that of iron deficiency, but associated with high serum iron levels, increased tissue hemosiderin, and the urinary excretion of abnormal derivatives of tryptophan.[50] The pathogenesis of the deficiency is unclear.

Hypochromia is often a feature of the anemia of chronic lead poisoning (see below) since the heme-synthesizing mechanism is particularly susceptible to lead poisoning.

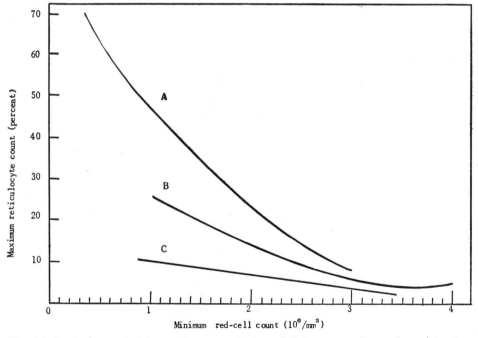

Fig. 14. Reticulocytosis in pernicious anemia, iron-deficiency anemia, and anemia after hemorrhage: [49] (*A*) maximum response in pernicious anemia treated with liver extract; (*B*) response in iron-deficiency (hypochromic) anemia; (*C*) response after acute hemorrhage in patients who did not receive iron.

### Nutritional Macrocytic (Megaloblastic) Anemias

These anemias are caused by defects in nuclear development, as the result of deficiencies in substances necessary for desoxyribonucleic acid synthesis.

#### DEFICIENCY OF VITAMIN $B_{12}$

PATHOLOGIC PHYSIOLOGY. Vitamin $B_{12}$ (cyanocobalamin) is synthesized almost exclusively by bacteria and is available in diets containing the flesh (particularly the livers) of animals having access to bacterial products. The absorption of dietary vitamin $B_{12}$ requires its interaction with the so-called gastric intrinsic factor, which is released by the fundus of the stomach and which has a strong binding affinity for vitamin $B_{12}$. The site of absorption of vitamin $B_{12}$ bound to intrinsic factor is the small intestine, particularly the lower portion. Excess vitamin $B_{12}$ is stored in the liver, which in normal adults contains 1–2 $\mu$g/gm of liver. Accordingly, a dietary inadequacy may not lead to deficiency of vitamin $B_{12}$ in persons on a diet free of animal or bacterial products for several years and such a dietary deficiency is rare in temperate climates except among extreme vegetarians. The great majority of cases of vitamin $B_{12}$ deficiency are due to a lack of intrinsic factor.[51] This lack may arise from a spontaneous degeneration of the fundic glands of the stomach, pernicious anemia, or total gastrectomy. Even in the presence of adequate intrinsic factor, however, vitamin $B_{12}$ absorption may be curtailed by any of a variety of conditions causing intestinal malabsorption (for example, sprue, regional enteritis, surgical removal of small-bowel segments, and so forth). Indeed, competitive utilization of intraluminal vitamin $B_{12}$ by the fish tapeworm, *Diphyllobothrium latum,* occasionally results in clinical vitamin $B_{12}$ deficiency.[52] The existence of intestinal anomalies that predispose toward blind intestinal loops in some cases impairs the absorption of vitamin $B_{12}$. This impairment may reflect competition for vitamin $B_{12}$ by the entrapped bacteria, for it may be reversed by the oral administration of antibiotics.[53]

#### SCREENING-TEST FINDINGS

(*a*) Regardless of the mechanism of induction of vitamin $B_{12}$ deficiency, changes in the blood and bone-marrow morphology are identical. As in all nutritional macrocytic anemias, there is evident a macrocytic normochromic anemia, associated with oval macrocytes, large multilobed polymorphonuclear granulocytes, and a hyperplastic marrow containing abnormal erythroid and myeloid elements of various stages of maturity. Similar cytologic changes are visible in cells removed from the buccal, esophageal, gastric, and vaginal epithelium.[54]

(*b*) In pernicious anemia, aspiration of the gastric contents reveals a paucity of gastric juice even after stimulation by histamine or its analogues. That which is obtained has a pH greater than 3.5 and thus fails to turn red upon the addition of Topfer's reagent, dimethylaminoazobenzene (see Unit 23). In "juvenile pernicious anemia," [55] in which there often exists a strong hereditary tendency toward pernicious anemia,[55, 56] and possibly in rare cases of classical pernicious anemia, "free gastric hydrochloric acid" (that is, a red color upon the addition of Topfer's reagent) may exist. Despite these rare exceptions, the finding of free hydrochloric acid in the gastric juice almost excludes the diagnosis of pernicious anemia.

#### SPECIAL TESTS

(*a*) The most generally applicable specific test for vitamin $B_{12}$ deficiency is the therapeutic trial.[57] Ideally, the subject is observed for a week or ten days on a reasonably constant diet low in animal products, and then is given either daily small injections (1–5 $\mu$g) or a single large (30 $\mu$g) injection of vitamin $B_{12}$. If there are no important hematologic changes during the initial control period, and if there is a sharp rise in reticulocyte levels from 2 to 8 days after the start of therapy, associated with general hematologic improvement, one may conclude that vitamin $B_{12}$ deficiency existed (Fig. 15). The height of the reticulocyte response is proportional to the severity of the anemia (Fig. 13). If there is an insufficient initial control period, a "false positive" may arise from dietary sources of folic acid and, in some instances, of vitamin $B_{12}$. A failure of reticulocyte response ("false negative") may occur if, at the time of therapy, the patient's marrow is depressed by infection or inflammation.

(*b*) Determination of the serum vitamin $B_{12}$ level [58] is extremely helpful in diagnosing vitamin $B_{12}$ deficiency, particularly when a therapeutic trial cannot be conducted. However, the microbiologic assay of this vitamin, which usually involves measurement of the growth response of *Euglena gracilis* or of *Lactobacillus leishmannii,* is a specialized procedure not carried out in most laboratories and therefore it will not be described here.

(*c*) Determination of the intestinal absorption of $Co^{60}$-labeled vitamin $B_{12}$ is a useful method for differentiating intrinsic-factor deficiency (pernicious anemia) from intestinal malabsorption, particularly in patients in therapeutic remission who cannot be subjected to a therapeutic trial. In the method, small quantities (usually 0.5–2.0 μg) of $Co^{60}$-labeled vitamin $B_{12}$ are administered orally and the

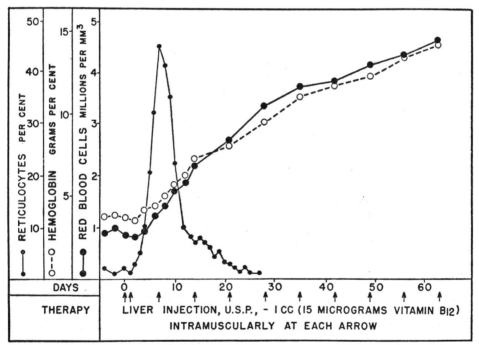

Fig. 15. Reticulocyte response to specific therapy. This is a characteristic maximal response to the parenteral administration of vitamin $B_{12}$ by a severely anemic patient with pernicious anemia. Note that (1) there is the usual 2-day delay between the first injection and the first significant rise in reticulocyte levels; (2) the maximum reticulocyte level is attained on about the 7th day of therapy; (3) as in patients with folic acid deficiency, there is a striking reticulocytosis (a reticulocyte "peak") early in the response, because of the release from the marrow of reticulocytes derived from a large population of megaloblasts in the marrow which had accumulated during the deficiency, and (4) since the defect being corrected was one of cell formation, and not of hemoglobin formation, the rise in red count is disproportional to the rise in hemoglobin.

absorption with or without the addition of an intrinsic-factor preparation is determined by the measurement of (i) the fecal excretion of $Co^{60}$;[59] (ii) the urinary excretion of $Co^{60}$, often involving the injection of a large "flushing" dose of non-radioactive vitamin $B_{12}$ to facilitate the excretion of radioactive vitamin (the "Schilling test"),[60] or (iii) the hepatic radioactivity, as determined by body-surface counting.[61] The finding by any of these methods of subnormal absorption of vitamin $B_{12}$ that can be corrected by the simultaneous administration of vitamin $B_{12}$ and an intrinsic-factor preparation is good evidence for pernicious anemia. Once again, however, these techniques are usually not essential to clinical diagnosis and management and are beyond the scope of this Syllabus.

## DEFICIENCY OF FOLIC ACID

### PATHOLOGIC PHYSIOLOGY

Folic acid (pteroylglutamic acid) is synthesized by the higher plants, as well as by bacteria, and is plentiful in diets containing fresh vegetables or liver. Approximately 90 percent of dietary folic acid is conjugated with glutamic acid, most commonly as the heptoglutamate, which must be deconjugated for intestinal absorption to occur. Although free folic acid normally is very readily absorbed, only about one-third of the 500–1500 $\mu$g of conjugated folic acid in the average daily diet is absorbed. Of this, only 4–5 $\mu$g is normally excreted in the urine. Although the metabolic fate of the remainder is not well known, there appears to be little storage of the vitamin as compared with vitamin $B_{12}$.

In the temperate zone, dietary deficiency of folic acid is more common than that of vitamin $B_{12}$, and is found particularly among chronic alcoholics and elderly people who subsist on diets deficient in meats and vegetables. As with vitamin $B_{12}$, diseases causing intestinal malabsorption or involving intestinal

blind loops[62] are commonly complicated by a deficiency of folic acid. A derangement in the metabolism of folic acid is known to attend the administration of aminopterin and other "folic acid antagonists." Similarly, derangements in folic acid metabolism are suspected, but as yet unproved, in patients with the "pernicious anemia of pregnancy," and in occasional patients receiving anticonvulsant drugs[63] or having alcoholic cirrhosis.[64] The active, physiologic metabolite of folic acid in the body is believed to be $N^{10}$ formyltetrahydrofolic acid.

### SCREENING-TEST FINDINGS

Changes in blood and bone-marrow morphology occur which closely resemble those seen in vitamin $B_{12}$ deficiency, although the abnormalities in myeloid elements usually appear more severe in folic acid deficiency.

### SPECIAL TESTS

(a) As with vitamin $B_{12}$ deficiency, the therapeutic trial is the most widely applicable clinical test for folic acid deficiency. The use of small (0.5–2.0 mg) daily doses of the medication, after a suitable control period, is advisable. It is well established that large (10–100 mg) doses of folic acid will cause partial therapeutic responses in patients with known vitamin $B_{12}$ deficiency, thus provoking, possibly by a mass-action effect, "false positive" responses. It is probable, but less well established, that, conversely, large doses of vitamin $B_{12}$ may elicit a partial response in patients with folic acid deficiency.

(b) Special bioassay methods are available for measuring urinary and serum levels of folic acid.[65] Similarly, the presence in the urine of abnormal quantities of formiminoglutamic acid, a metabolite of histidine that accumulates during folic acid deficiency, can be determined microbiologically[66] or enzymatically.[67] These procedures are only carried out in specialized laboratories.

## Normocytic Normochromic Anemias

In general, these anemias arise from disturbances of red-cell formation, probably at the "stem-cell" or erythroid-precursor level. Many acute or chronic illnesses are associated with some depression of erythroid activity in the marrow, frequently causing anemias that are normocytic and normochromic, or only slightly macrocytic or hypochromic. These anemias especially may accompany endocrine deficiencies, chronic inflammation, chronic renal disease, and carcinomatosis. They usually lack peculiar diagnostic features and respond to improvement in the underlying disease. Isolated injury to bone-marrow function, causing "aplastic or hypoplastic anemias," may arise from chemical or radiologic injury or may be idiopathic. Although uneven or diminished marrow cellularity, and bizarre nucleated forms which often resemble megaloblasts, may be found in these conditions, there are no specific diagnostic tests. On the other hand, "myelophthisis," meaning displacement of the marrow by nonerythroid tissue (such as fibrous tissue, leukemia, carcinoma, and so forth), is often morphologically distinctive. In these anemias, extreme anisocytosis and aberrations of cell form characteristically appear and nucleated red cells often enter the peripheral blood anomalously, that is, in the absence of extreme anoxia and unassociated with marked reticulocytosis. Erythremic myelosis (DiGuglielmo's disease) is an incompletely defined rare disease of immature red cells, characterized by their pathologic, possibly neoplastic, proliferation with failure to mature. Thus, functionally, there is erythroid marrow hypoplasia with bizarre megaloblastoid cells, diminished release of red cells by the marrow, erythroblastemia, and systemic tissue infiltration by erythroblasts. In some instances, this syndrome may accompany a stage of myelogenous leukemia. Chronic "anerythroblastic" forms are included in this syndrome by some authors. However, the criteria for separating such forms from the "aplastic" anemias are indistinct.

## Anemias Caused by Red-Cell Loss or Increased Destruction: General Considerations

These are anemias (classified etiologically in Table 23) in which the primary event is the loss or increased destruction of red cells. Usually, a secondary, compensatory increase in red-cell production is thereby stimulated, thus increasing the rate of red-cell turnover, although in some diseases the compensatory response of the marrow may be deficient. Diseases such as pernicious anemia, in which red-cell survival is somewhat diminished but in which the predominant defect is a failure of the bone marrow to release red cells, have already been discussed. In some diseases, such as chronic renal disease in which anemia is most commonly caused by bone-marrow failure, instances may occur, often terminally or during acute azotemia, in which a hemolytic state clearly supervenes.

### ACUTE BLOOD LOSS

#### PATHOLOGIC PHYSIOLOGY

External loss of blood sufficient to produce anemia is readily observed except when the loss is into the gastrointestinal tract, where an extensive hemorrhage may be overlooked. Serious internal hemorrhage when secondary to such conditions as thrombocytopenic purpura or scurvy is generally attended by visible hemorrhagic manifestations. However, bleeding into the abdominal cavity or into major muscle groups, as during trauma or in hemophilia, may at times go unrecognized. Acute blood loss is followed by a rapidly progressing anemia as the plasma volume is restored, and within 2 to 4 days reticulocyte levels increase and remain elevated until the red-cell mass is restored. If blood loss is external, depletion of the bodily iron stores by recurrent or chronic bleeding eventually will impair the bone-marrow response and produce a hypochromic, iron-deficient anemia, whereas in sustained internal blood loss, as in scurvy, the hemoglobin iron is reutilized.

### SCREENING-TEST FINDINGS

These are largely circumstantial. The finding of an acute anemia without morphologic abnormalities and without icterus and followed by a reticulocytosis should stimulate a search for a site of blood loss. Especially valuable in this regard are the stool guaiac examination (Unit 22) and the screening tests for a hemostatic defect (Unit 14).

### HEMOLYTIC ANEMIAS

The destruction of red cells in most hemolytic anemias involves three main steps. First, the red cell possesses or develops an abnormality, and this can often be recognized in vitro microscopically or by certain laboratory tests. Second, the cell is destroyed or is filtered from the circulation, so that the red-cell survival is diminished. This survival may be measured on autogenous red cells by use of the $Cr^{51}$-labeling method [68] or on homologous cells by the Ashby method of differential agglutination.[69] Third, the destroyed red cells release hemoglobin which is catabolized to various pigments, including bilirubin and urobilinogen (Unit 24).

### TESTS RELATED TO HEMOGLOBIN CATABOLISM

Since in most hemolytic anemias hemoglobin is metabolized readily to bilirubin at the sites of red-cell destruction such as the spleen and liver (that is, "extravascularly"), hemoglobin levels in the plasma rise little. When the rate of hemolysis is rapid, or when it occurs intravascularly, however, free hemoglobin appears in the plasma (hemoglobinemia). Initially, during hemolysis, plasma hemoglobin is bound to a specific hemoglobin-binding globulin, haptoglobin, and the hemoglobin-haptoglobin complex is removed and catabolized by the reticuloendothelial system.[70] When plasma hemoglobin levels exceed 100–130 mg/100 ml, however, or when the plasma haptoglobin has been exhausted, the unbound hemoglobin in the plasma is excreted in the urine (hemoglobinuria). Some of the hemoglobin is catabolized while passing through the renal tubules and the derived iron is excreted and identifiable as hemosiderin, while the remaining hemoglobin may be partially oxidized in the urine to the brown methemoglobin. Normally, the plasma contains only 2 or 3 mg/100 ml of hemoglobin (that is, about 0.02 percent of the whole blood hemoglobin). Plasma containing 5 to 10 mg/100 ml of hemoglobin shows a yellow to orange discoloration, and at somewhat higher levels a distinct pink color is visible. Most methods for quantitative measurement of these low concentrations of hemoglobin are based upon the peroxidative activity of heme, as in the modification of the quantitative benzidine method of Bing and Baker [71] described below.

### HAM MODIFICATION OF THE BENZIDINE METHOD FOR MEASURING PLASMA HEMOGLOBIN

Nine parts of blood, collected gently in a syringe, rinsed with 0.9-percent sodium chloride solution, are added to 1 part of 3-percent sodium citrate or 1-percent EDTA. The sample is mixed by gentle inversion and centrifuged without delay at about 800–1000g. To minimize turbidity, all plasma specimens are diluted with an equal volume of saline before sampling. If pink or red, the plasma is diluted with a known amount of saline until the color is faintly pink. If a colorimeter is unavailable, the color can be measured visually by comparison with a solution of hemoglobin derived from blood measured by standard blood hemoglobinometry and treated as described for the unknown.

REAGENTS. (1) *Benzidine reagent:* Dissolve 1 gm of purified benzidine dihydrochloride in 20 ml of glacial acetic acid; add 30 ml of distilled water; add 50 ml of 95-percent ethyl alcohol. A slight yellow color may be disregarded. If purified benzidine is not available, ordinary benzidine may be purified and dissolved in the same manner as described by Bing and Baker.[71] It is advisable to make up this reagent fresh each day.

(2) *Acetic acid:* 20-percent glacial acetic acid is diluted 1 part to 4 parts of distilled water.

(3) *Hydrogen peroxide solution:* 0.6 percent. The usual 3-percent solution of hydrogen peroxide is diluted with distilled water to give a 0.6-percent solution. (If possible, it is better to use superoxol diluted 1 to 50.) All solutions should be stored in dark bottles at icebox temperature.

**Method.** To 2 ml of benzidine solution prepared as described add 1 ml of hemoglobin solution or plasma, then 1 ml of 0.6-percent hydrogen peroxide solution. A blank is prepared by using 1 ml of distilled water or physiologic saline in place of the solution to be tested. Allow the samples to stand for 60–100 min at room temperature (preferably in the dark). Then add 21 ml of 20-percent acetic acid to each tube.

Read the tubes in the Evelyn colorimeter with filter No. 620, using the blank tube to set the galvanometer scale at 100.

It is essential that all glassware be very clean, for gross errors may result from contamination with small amounts of hemoglobin.

*Calculation.* $C = L/K$, where $C$ is the chromogen (mg/100 ml of hemoglobin), $L$ is the $L$ value of the colorimeter reading, and $K$ is the constant calculated from determinations on standard solutions of known hemoglobin concentration.

CROSBY AND FURTH MODIFICATION OF THE
BENZIDINE METHOD FOR MEASURING
PLASMA HEMOGLOBIN

In this method,[72] the colorimetric interference by turbid plasmas is reduced by using "micro" volumes of plasma.

REAGENTS. (1) *Benzidine reagent:* Dissolve 1 gm of benzidine base in 90 ml of glacial acetic acid and make up to 100 ml with distilled water. Store in refrigerator.

(2) *Hydrogen peroxide:* 1.0 percent. Prepare freshly from concentrated stock solutions free of sulfate.

(3) *Standard hemoglobin solution:* This can most simply be prepared and measured by using a 1/500 dilution of normal whole blood in water. The hemoglobin concentration of this solution will be 1/500 of the standard hemoglobin reading, or normally about 30 mg/100 ml.

(4) *Diluent:* 10-percent (v/v) glacial acetic acid in distilled water.

**Method.** Using calibrated Sahli pipettes, add 0.02 ml of the unknown plasma, of the hemoglobin standard, and of a water "blank" respectively to three 15-ml test tubes containing 1 ml of benzidine reagent. Add 1 ml of hydrogen peroxide to each tube and mix immediately. When the color change is completed (approximately 20 min) add 10 ml of the diluent, mix, and allow to stand for 10 min. Transfer the solutions to cuvettes and read in the spectrophotometer at 515 m$\mu$.

The optical density $D$ of the hemoglobin standard represents a hemoglobin concentration of approximately 30 mg/100 ml, as determined above, whereas the $D$ value of the water blank is 0. On ordinary graph paper, a line connecting the two points will provide corresponding values in milligrams of hemoglobin per 100 ml of blood for the $D$ readings of the unknown plasmas.

The avoidance of hemolysis by the act of blood collection is crucial to these determinations. Plasma hemoglobin levels exceeding 5 mg/100 ml are significant. Atlhough levels up to 25 or 30 mg/100 ml are encountered in many hemolytic states, higher levels are usually indicative of intravascular processes such as hemolysinic transfusion reactions, paroxysmal nocturnal hemoglobinuria, and paroxysmal cold hemoglobinuria. The benzidine method does not differentiate hemoglobin from methemoglobin, sulfhemoglobin, or methemalbumin. Fairley [73] has shown that the golden-brown pigment methemalbumin is formed by the combination of hematin (ferriheme) with plasma albumin and may persist in the plasma for several days. Thus, following intravascular hemolysis, the plasma may acquire a brown rather than a pink color and, in chronic hemolytic anemias, such as paroxysmal nocturnal hemoglobinuria, methemalbuminemia may be continuously present.

THE SHUMM TEST FOR METHEMALBUMIN

Nine volumes of plasma (or serum) are covered with a layer of ether, and then one volume of a saturated solution of ammonium sulfide is run in with a pipette and mixed with the plasma. A positive reaction is indicated by the appearance of a hemochromagen with a sharply defined absorption band at 558 m$\mu$, when the plasma is viewed with a hand spectroscope.

INTERPRETATION

The finding of methemalbuminemia is subject to the same interpretation as is hemoglobinemia.

For most clinical purposes, the direct visual examination of plasma, obtained as described above, for the presence of hemoglobin or its immediate derivatives is sufficient and reliable. Quantitation of the level of hemoglobin and the detection of methemalbumin should be re-

served for special or problematic situations.

TESTS FOR HEMOGLOBIN IN THE URINE

See Unit 19.

## Hemolytic Anemias Caused by Intrinsic Defects of Red Cells

These anemias are caused by intrinsic, usually hereditary, abnormalities of red cells which impair their survival in the circulation.

HEREDITARY SPHEROCYTOSIS (CONGENITAL HEMOLYTIC ANEMIA OR JAUNDICE)

PATHOLOGIC PHYSIOLOGY

Hereditary spherocytosis is a familial disease, transmitted as a Mendelian dominant gene that expresses itself quite variably. Thus the disease ranges from a mild or "trait" form to a hemolytic process of great severity. The fundamental defect in this disease apparently exists in the red-cell membrane, which is deficient in area and manifests certain metabolic abnormalities.[74] As a result, the red cells are more nearly spherical than normal (despite normal or subnormal cell volumes), they are mechanically fragile, the MCHC is high, and, on standing, the cells take in water and sodium, lose potassium, and undergo autohemolysis to abnormal extents. From the pathogenetic standpoint, the most significant feature is that the spheroidal shape of the red cells renders them susceptible to filtration by the vascular filter bed of the normal spleen.[75] Thus in hereditary spherocytosis red cells are trapped while perfusing the spleen, and, while so sequestered from metabolic substrates, they slowly undergo autohemolysis. Meanwhile, the spleen, which is chronically congested with red cells and other debris, undergoes progressive enlargement. Apparently the spleen alone possesses sufficiently refined filter beds to trap these red cells, for splenectomy invariably corrects the

118

hemolytic process, although the red-cell defect persists.

### SCREENING-TEST FINDINGS

In addition to the general findings of a chronic hemolytic process (reticulocytosis, acholuric jaundice, elevated levels of fecal urobilinogen), the presence of spherocytes on the blood smear is characteristic. However, spherocytosis is also found in various unrelated hemolytic diseases; the differentiation of hereditary spherocytosis from these is based upon (i) its chronic, congenital course, (ii) the absence of other red-cell alterations, (iii) the family history, and (iv) the characteristics of the spherocytes as determined quantitatively by the osmotic-fra-

gility technique. It should be borne in mind that the spherocytes in hereditary spherocytosis are usually relatively small cells with high values of MCHC, whereas the spherocytes of acquired hemolytic anemia are usually relatively large and tend to have low MCHC (Fig. 16).

### DETERMINATION OF RED-CELL OSMOTIC FRAGILITY

When red cells are introduced into hypotonic solutions of plasma, serum, or sodium chloride, they imbibe water and swell until the spheroidal or critical volume is reached at which rupture occurs. The spherical shape contains the maximum volume for the surface area of the cell, and any further increase in volume

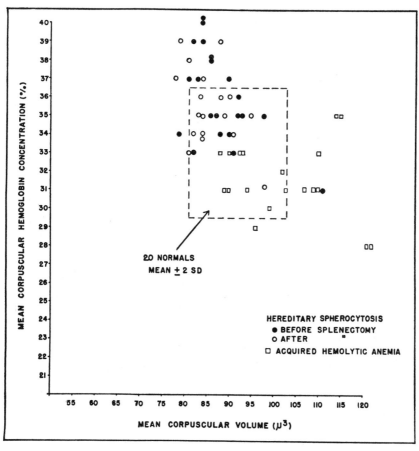

Fig. 16. Comparison of red-cell corpuscular values in "spherocytic" anemias. The spherocytic red cells of patients with hereditary spherocytosis tend to be microcytic and hyperchromic, whereas those of patients with acquired hemolytic anemia tend to be macrocytic and hypochromic. (By permission of Geneva A. Daland.)

119

would require increase of the area of the membrane. The flat or thin cell, as seen in hypochromic anemias, has a decreased osmotic fragility (or an increased resistance) in hypotonic solutions because it can swell to a large extent in solutions of low tonicity before it reaches a spheroidal form and ruptures. However, a cell that is already spheroidal, as in congenital spherocytosis, has an increased osmotic fragility (or a decreased resistance) in hypotonic solutions because it can swell to only a small extent before it reaches a spheroidal form and ruptures. If the osmotic fragility is determined quantitatively, the resultant summation curve indicates the distribution of cells of a different geometric configuration,

that is, the percentage of cells that have reached a spheroidal form and ruptured at different levels of hypotonicity. Representative curves are shown in Fig. 17.

### SCREENING TEST FOR INCREASED OSMOTIC FRAGILITY

A crude screening test for the detection of an increase in the osmotic fragility may be performed with only two concentrations of sodium chloride, namely, 0.85 and 0.50 gm/100 ml. Samples of 0.1 ml of venous blood are added to 1.0 ml of the above saline solutions, mixed, and centrifuged. If a pink color occurs in the sodium chloride solution of 0.50 gm/100 ml and not in physiologic saline, the osmotic fragility of the red cells is proba-

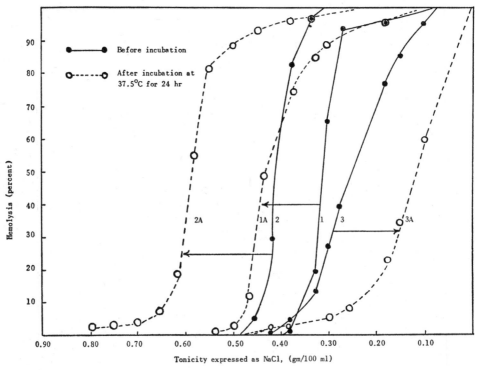

Fig. 17. The effect of sterile incubation on the osmotic fragility of defibrinated whole blood. *Curves 1 and 1A:* Normal subject. There is a moderate "symmetric" increase in osmotic fragility on incubation. *Curves 2 and 2A:* The "trait" of hereditary spherocytosis in a patient who showed no anemia or jaundice but a chronic reticulocytosis of 4–7 percent. Note that the osmotic fragility of the unincubated sample is only slightly increased above the normal range, a result that is indeterminate. The incubated sample, however, shows the striking symmetric increase in osmotic fragility that is characteristic of this disease. *Curves 3 and 3A:* Cooley's anemia. The osmotic fragility of the unincubated blood sample is decreased and, after incubation, is decreased further. The significance of this change on incubation has not been defined.

bly increased and may be studied more quantitatively, as by the methods described below.

## A SEMIQUANTITATIVE METHOD FOR MEASURING OSMOTIC FRAGILITY

In this method,[76] 0.1-ml samples of washed red cells adjusted to a concentration of 20 percent in a 0.9-percent sodium chloride solution are added to tubes containing 1.0 ml of the various concentrations of hypotonic salt solutions. These stock salt solutions can be made in large quantity once a year and kept stoppered at room temperature. They will remain uncontaminated if subsamples are poured from the stock solutions as needed, the excess being discarded. After centrifugation, the hemolysis of a patient's blood is compared with that of a normal sample by visual inspection of the amount of hemolysis in the supernatant fluid and the remaining unhemolyzed red cells.

## QUANTITATIVE METHOD FOR OSMOTIC FRAGILITY

A quantitative test [77] for osmotic fragility may be performed on freshly drawn venous blood containing dry oxalate mixture as an anticoagulant. This can be done at a pH of 7.35 to 7.5, by accurately measuring 0.1-ml samples of blood into a series of tubes each containing 1.0 ml of the following aqueous solutions of sodium chloride: hypertonic sodium chloride, 1.0 gm/100 ml; isotonic sodium chloride, 0.85 gm/100 ml; hypotonic sodium chloride, 0.80 to 0.10 gm/100 ml, each tube differing by 0.04 gm/100 ml; and distilled water. The samples are mixed and centrifuged, and 0.5-ml samples of the supernatant solutions are diluted to 10 ml with distilled water, in Evelyn colorimeter tubes. One drop of concentrated ammonium hydroxide is added to each tube, the sample is mixed, and the hemoglobin is determined in an Evelyn colorimeter using filter No. 540. The pH of 5 ml of blood, transferred to a bottle of 8-ml capacity containing dry oxalate mixture, will usually vary from pH 7.35 to 7.5 during the procedure of setting up the fragility test. Small amounts of carbon dioxide are lost. A decrease in pH produces progressive swelling of the red cell, and the osmotic fragility increases by an increment of sodium chloride of 0.01 gm/100 ml for each 0.1 decrease in pH.

*Example.* If 1 percent of red cells are hemolyzed at pH 7.5 in aqueous sodium chloride, 0.44 gm/100 ml, then a change in pH to 7.3 will be accompanied by an increase in osmotic fragility such that 1 percent hemolysis will occur in aqueous sodium chloride, 0.46 gm/100 ml.

More precise correction for the increase of pH caused by the escape of $CO_2$ from blood manipulated in vitro can be made by referring to the tables of Emerson and his associates.[78]

The colorimetric values observed in the hypertonic salt solution are used as the blank and subtracted from each value observed in the hypotonic range to give a corrected figure for hemolysis. The percentage hemolysis at each salt concentration is then calculated by dividing the corrected figure for hemolysis by the similarly corrected figure for complete hemolysis produced in distilled water. The curve of the osmotic fragility is then plotted, with the hemolysis, in percent, as the ordinate and the corrected tonicity of the hypotonic mixture as the abscissa. Since the mixtures contain 0.1 ml of whole blood and 1.0 ml of salt solutions of known but different tonicities, the blood sample alters the final tonicity. Accordingly, the final tonicity of the hypotonic mixture may be corrected by assuming arbitrarily that the amount of blood added is equivalent to a solution of aqueous sodium chloride, 0.85 gm/100 ml. In addition, the pH of blood in vitro varies, depending upon the loss of carbon dioxide. Since a decrease in pH produces a significant swelling of red cells, it is important that the pH of the blood

Table 25. *Corrected tonicity Tc (gm NaCl/100 ml) at pH 7.4 for red cells suspended in saline.*[a, 78]

| Tu (NaCl, gm/100 ml) | pH 6.6 | 6.8 | 7.0 | 7.1 | 7.2 | 7.3 | 7.4 | 7.5 | 7.6 | 7.7 | 7.8 | 7.9 | 8.0 | 8.1 | 8.2 | Tu |
|---|---|---|---|---|---|---|---|---|---|---|---|---|---|---|---|---|
| 1.00 | 0.825 | 0.860 | 0.900 | 0.920 | 0.940 | 0.965 | 0.990 | 1.010 | 1.040 | 1.065 | 1.095 | 1.125 | 1.155 | 1.190 | 1.225 | 1.00 |
| 0.90 | 0.750 | 0.780 | 0.815 | 0.835 | 0.855 | 0.875 | 0.895 | 0.920 | 0.940 | 0.965 | 0.990 | 1.020 | 1.050 | 1.080 | 1.115 | 0.90 |
| 0.88 | 0.735 | 0.765 | 0.800 | 0.820 | 0.840 | 0.855 | 0.880 | 0.900 | 0.925 | 0.945 | 0.970 | 1.000 | 1.025 | 1.055 | 1.090 | 0.88 |
| 0.86 | 0.720 | 0.750 | 0.785 | 0.800 | 0.820 | 0.840 | 0.860 | 0.880 | 0.905 | 0.925 | 0.955 | 0.980 | 1.005 | 1.035 | 1.065 | 0.86 |
| 0.84 | 0.700 | 0.735 | 0.765 | 0.785 | 0.805 | 0.820 | 0.840 | 0.860 | 0.885 | 0.905 | 0.930 | 0.960 | 0.985 | 1.015 | 1.045 | 0.84 |
| 0.82 | 0.690 | 0.720 | 0.750 | 0.765 | 0.785 | 0.805 | 0.825 | 0.845 | 0.865 | 0.890 | 0.910 | 0.935 | 0.965 | 0.990 | 1.020 | 0.82 |
| 0.80 | 0.670 | 0.700 | 0.735 | 0.750 | 0.770 | 0.785 | 0.805 | 0.825 | 0.845 | 0.870 | 0.890 | 0.915 | 0.940 | 0.970 | 1.000 | 0.80 |
| 0.78 | 0.655 | 0.685 | 0.715 | 0.735 | 0.750 | 0.770 | 0.785 | 0.805 | 0.830 | 0.850 | 0.870 | 0.895 | 0.920 | 0.950 | 0.980 | 0.78 |
| 0.76 | 0.640 | 0.670 | 0.700 | 0.715 | 0.735 | 0.750 | 0.770 | 0.785 | 0.810 | 0.830 | 0.850 | 0.875 | 0.900 | 0.925 | 0.955 | 0.76 |
| 0.74 | 0.625 | 0.655 | 0.685 | 0.700 | 0.715 | 0.735 | 0.750 | 0.770 | 0.790 | 0.810 | 0.830 | 0.855 | 0.880 | 0.905 | 0.930 | 0.74 |
| 0.72 | 0.610 | 0.640 | 0.665 | 0.685 | 0.700 | 0.715 | 0.730 | 0.750 | 0.770 | 0.790 | 0.810 | 0.835 | 0.855 | 0.880 | 0.910 | 0.72 |
| 0.70 | 0.595 | 0.625 | 0.650 | 0.665 | 0.680 | 0.695 | 0.715 | 0.730 | 0.750 | 0.770 | 0.790 | 0.810 | 0.835 | 0.860 | 0.885 | 0.70 |
| 0.68 | 0.580 | 0.605 | 0.635 | 0.650 | 0.665 | 0.680 | 0.695 | 0.715 | 0.730 | 0.750 | 0.770 | 0.790 | 0.815 | 0.840 | 0.865 | 0.68 |
| 0.66 | 0.565 | 0.590 | 0.620 | 0.630 | 0.645 | 0.660 | 0.680 | 0.695 | 0.715 | 0.730 | 0.750 | 0.770 | 0.795 | 0.815 | 0.840 | 0.66 |
| 0.64 | 0.550 | 0.575 | 0.600 | 0.615 | 0.630 | 0.645 | 0.660 | 0.675 | 0.695 | 0.710 | 0.730 | 0.750 | 0.770 | 0.795 | 0.820 | 0.64 |
| 0.62 | 0.535 | 0.560 | 0.585 | 0.600 | 0.615 | 0.625 | 0.640 | 0.660 | 0.675 | 0.690 | 0.710 | 0.730 | 0.750 | 0.770 | 0.795 | 0.62 |
| 0.60 | 0.520 | 0.545 | 0.570 | 0.580 | 0.595 | 0.610 | 0.625 | 0.640 | 0.655 | 0.670 | 0.690 | 0.710 | 0.730 | 0.750 | 0.775 | 0.60 |
| 0.58 | 0.505 | 0.530 | 0.550 | 0.565 | 0.575 | 0.590 | 0.605 | 0.620 | 0.635 | 0.650 | 0.670 | 0.690 | 0.710 | 0.730 | 0.750 | 0.58 |
| 0.56 | 0.490 | 0.510 | 0.535 | 0.550 | 0.560 | 0.570 | 0.590 | 0.600 | 0.615 | 0.635 | 0.650 | 0.670 | 0.685 | 0.705 | 0.725 | 0.56 |
| 0.54 | 0.475 | 0.495 | 0.520 | 0.530 | 0.540 | 0.555 | 0.560 | 0.585 | 0.600 | 0.615 | 0.630 | 0.650 | 0.665 | 0.685 | 0.705 | 0.54 |
| 0.52 | 0.460 | 0.480 | 0.500 | 0.515 | 0.525 | 0.535 | 0.550 | 0.565 | 0.580 | 0.595 | 0.610 | 0.625 | 0.645 | 0.665 | 0.685 | 0.52 |
| 0.50 | 0.445 | 0.465 | 0.485 | 0.495 | 0.510 | 0.520 | 0.530 | 0.545 | 0.560 | 0.575 | 0.590 | 0.605 | 0.625 | 0.640 | 0.660 | 0.50 |
| 0.48 | 0.430 | 0.450 | 0.470 | 0.480 | 0.490 | 0.500 | 0.515 | 0.530 | 0.540 | 0.555 | 0.570 | 0.585 | 0.600 | 0.620 | 0.640 | 0.48 |
| 0.46 | 0.415 | 0.430 | 0.450 | 0.460 | 0.475 | 0.485 | 0.495 | 0.510 | 0.520 | 0.535 | 0.550 | 0.565 | 0.580 | 0.595 | 0.615 | 0.46 |
| 0.44 | 0.400 | 0.415 | 0.435 | 0.445 | 0.455 | 0.465 | 0.480 | 0.490 | 0.500 | 0.515 | 0.530 | 0.545 | 0.560 | 0.575 | 0.595 | 0.44 |
| 0.42 | 0.385 | 0.400 | 0.420 | 0.430 | 0.440 | 0.450 | 0.460 | 0.470 | 0.485 | 0.495 | 0.510 | 0.520 | 0.540 | 0.555 | 0.570 | 0.42 |
| 0.40 | 0.370 | 0.385 | 0.400 | 0.410 | 0.420 | 0.430 | 0.440 | 0.450 | 0.465 | 0.475 | 0.490 | 0.500 | 0.515 | 0.530 | 0.550 | 0.40 |
| 0.38 | 0.355 | 0.370 | 0.385 | 0.395 | 0.405 | 0.415 | 0.425 | 0.435 | 0.445 | 0.455 | 0.470 | 0.480 | 0.495 | 0.510 | 0.525 | 0.38 |
| 0.36 | 0.340 | 0.355 | 0.370 | 0.380 | 0.385 | 0.395 | 0.405 | 0.415 | 0.425 | 0.435 | 0.450 | 0.460 | 0.475 | 0.490 | 0.500 | 0.36 |
| 0.34 | 0.325 | 0.340 | 0.355 | 0.360 | 0.370 | 0.375 | 0.385 | 0.395 | 0.405 | 0.415 | 0.430 | 0.440 | 0.455 | 0.465 | 0.480 | 0.34 |
| 0.32 | 0.310 | 0.320 | 0.335 | 0.345 | 0.350 | 0.360 | 0.370 | 0.380 | 0.385 | 0.400 | 0.410 | 0.420 | 0.430 | 0.445 | 0.460 | 0.32 |
| 0.30 | 0.295 | 0.305 | 0.320 | 0.325 | 0.335 | 0.340 | 0.350 | 0.360 | 0.370 | 0.380 | 0.390 | 0.400 | 0.410 | 0.420 | 0.435 | 0.30 |
| 0.28 | 0.275 | 0.290 | 0.305 | 0.310 | 0.315 | 0.325 | 0.330 | 0.340 | 0.350 | 0.360 | 0.370 | 0.380 | 0.390 | 0.400 | 0.415 | 0.28 |
| 0.26 | 0.260 | 0.275 | 0.285 | 0.295 | 0.300 | 0.305 | 0.315 | 0.320 | 0.330 | 0.340 | 0.350 | 0.355 | 0.370 | 0.380 | 0.390 | 0.26 |
| 0.24 | 0.245 | 0.260 | 0.270 | 0.275 | 0.280 | 0.290 | 0.295 | 0.305 | 0.310 | 0.320 | 0.330 | 0.335 | 0.345 | 0.355 | 0.365 | 0.24 |
| 0.22 | 0.230 | 0.240 | 0.255 | 0.260 | 0.265 | 0.270 | 0.280 | 0.285 | 0.290 | 0.300 | 0.310 | 0.315 | 0.325 | 0.335 | 0.345 | 0.22 |
| 0.20 | 0.215 | 0.225 | 0.235 | 0.240 | 0.245 | 0.255 | 0.260 | 0.265 | 0.275 | 0.280 | 0.285 | 0.295 | 0.305 | 0.315 | 0.320 | 0.20 |
| 0.18 | 0.200 | 0.210 | 0.220 | 0.225 | 0.230 | 0.240 | 0.240 | 0.245 | 0.255 | 0.260 | 0.265 | 0.275 | 0.280 | 0.290 | 0.300 | 0.18 |
| 0.15 | 0.180 | 0.185 | 0.195 | 0.200 | 0.205 | 0.210 | 0.215 | 0.220 | 0.225 | 0.230 | 0.235 | 0.245 | 0.250 | 0.260 | 0.265 | 0.15 |
| 0.10 | 0.140 | 0.145 | 0.155 | 0.155 | 0.160 | 0.165 | 0.170 | 0.170 | 0.175 | 0.180 | 0.185 | 0.190 | 0.195 | 0.205 | 0.210 | 0.10 |
| 0.05 | 0.105 | 0.105 | 0.110 | 0.115 | 0.115 | 0.120 | 0.125 | 0.125 | 0.130 | 0.130 | 0.135 | 0.140 | 0.145 | 0.150 | 0.155 | 0.05 |
| | 6.6 | 6.8 | 7.0 | 7.1 | 7.2 | 7.3 | 7.4 | 7.5 | 7.6 | 7.7 | 7.8 | 7.9 | 8.0 | 8.1 | 8.2 | |

[a] The uncorrected tonicity (Tu) of each mixture of saline and blood is corrected (Tc) for the added blood (dilution 1:11) and to a pH of 7.4. The equation for the correction is:

$$\text{Tonicity at pH 7.5 (Tc)} = (10\,Tu + 0.85) \times 0.373/(11.5 - pH),$$

where Tc (gm NaCl/100 ml) is the corrected tonicity for the blood-saline mixture, Tu is the tonicity of the saline before addition of the blood sample, and pH is the pH of the blood sample measured just before mixing.

specimen be determined and that the osmotic-fragility data be corrected to a pH of 7.4. Corrections for both the tonicity and the pH of blood are presented in Table 25, compiled by Emerson and his associates.[78] The values for the percentage of hemolysis are then plotted against the corrected tonicity values for the saline solutions.

### INTERPRETATION

In the screening test for increased osmotic fragility, there is normally a tinge of yellow in the tube containing 0.5-percent saline as compared to the 0.85-percent tube. A pink or red color in the 0.5-percent tube, with a clear 0.85-percent tube, indicates spherocytosis involving at least 1 percent of the red cells. Smaller numbers of spherocytes may be recognized in the blood smear without being discernible by osmotic-fragility tests. Table 26 shows the quantitative osmotic-fragility values for 31 normal subjects.[78]

Table 26. *Osmotic fragility of red cells from peripheral blood before and after incubation at 37.5°C for 24 hr of samples from patients with hereditary spherocytosis and from normal subjects.*[78]

| Hemolysis (percent) | Corrected tonicity (gm NaCl/100 ml), mean ± σ | | |
|---|---|---|---|
| | Normal persons (31 subjects) | Hereditary spherocytosis | |
| | | Spleen not removed (22 cases) | Spleen removed (13 cases) |
| | *Unincubated* | | |
| 1 | 0.47±0.027 | 0.60±0.080 | 0.58±0.06 |
| 2 | .46± .027 | .56± .07 | .56± .06 |
| 5 | .44± .025 | .52± .06 | .53± .06 |
| 10 | .43± .026 | .49± .06 | .52± .06 |
| 25 | .42± .024 | .47± .05 | .49± .05 |
| 50 | .40± .022 | .44± .04 | .47± .04 |
| 75 | .38± .020 | .42± .04 | .44± .04 |
| 90 | .36± .025 | .37± .05 | .40± .04 |
| | *Incubated* | | |
| 1 | 0.59±0.030 | 0.80±0.07 | 0.82±0.04 |
| 2 | .57± .029 | .77± .08 | .80± .04 |
| 5 | .55± .028 | .74± .09 | .78± .04 |
| 10 | .54± .025 | .71± .10 | .75± .04 |
| 25 | .51± .027 | .65± .09 | .69± .05 |
| 50 | .49± .028 | .59± .08 | .62± .05 |
| 75 | .46± .028 | .53± .08 | .56± .05 |
| 90 | .32± .035 | .42± .09 | .50± .06 |

It should be noted that the osmotic-fragility test is a measure neither of osmotic pressure nor of cellular fragility. It is simply an accurate means of determining how nearly spherical red cells are. Thus, the finding *increased osmotic fragility* is indicative of spherocytosis, which, as discussed above, is a nonspecific sign of in vivo hemolysis. *Diminished osmotic fragility,* on the other hand, indicates excessive red-cell flatness, and is encountered in the hypochromic anemias of iron deficiency and of thalassemia, and in conditions associated with target-cell formation and red-cell flattening of unknown mechanism (hemoglobinopathies, obstructive jaundice, hepatitis, and so forth).

*The effect on the osmotic fragility of sterile incubation* in vitro at 37°C is useful in the diagnosis of hereditary spherocytosis. When samples of blood (defibrinated or with sterile anticoagulant) from patients with hereditary spherocytosis are incubated at 37°C for 24 hr under sterile conditions, there is a marked and uniform increase in osmotic fragility that is greater than normal (Table 26, Fig. 16), even though the osmotic fragility of the unincubated blood may be fairly normal. The diagnosis of hereditary spherocytosis cannot be excluded without this procedure. The spheroidal red cells often seen in acquired hemolytic anemias are usually altered somewhat differently by sterile incubation. Thus the most osmotically fragile (spheroidal) cells become more fragile and the least osmotically fragile (discoidal) cells became less fragile, producing an abnormal "flattened" osmotic-fragility curve. It is important to avoid bacterial contamination during the incubation, since spherocytosis and hemolysis are caused by the growth of many bacteria.

### DETERMINATION OF RED-CELL MECHANICAL FRAGILITY

The susceptibility of red blood cells to destruction by mechanical trauma is always increased when there is an increase in the osmotic fragility. However, in certain clinical conditions, the mechanical fragility may be increased although the osmotic fragility is normal.

**Method.** An empirical method [79] for the measurement of the mechanical fragility consists in the rotation of a small amount of blood in a 50-ml Erlenmeyer flask containing 10 glass beads of a uniform diameter of 4 mm. The flask is clamped in a horizontal position at right angles to the circumference of a vertical wooden wheel (Fig. 18). The center of

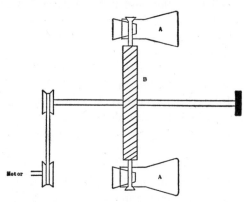

Fig. 18. Diagram of apparatus for determination of mechanical fragility of red cells: (A) 50-ml Erlenmeyer flask containing 0.5 ml of blood and 10 4-mm glass beads; (B) distance from axis to the center of the flask = 15 cm. Speed of rotation, 30 rev/min.

the flask is located approximately 15 cm from the axis of the wheel. The wheel is rotated at 30 rev/min. The beads and blood are rotated around the maximum internal circumference of the flask. The rotating device may be placed in a thermostatically controlled box that is set at 37.5°C, but this is not necessary with ordinary room temperature.

Defibrinated blood or blood containing dry oxalate mixture may be used for the test. The hematocrit of 1.0 ml of blood is adjusted to approximately 35 percent, since the percentage of cells destroyed varies directly with the concentration (hematocrit) of red cells in suspension, and 0.5 ml is introduced into a flask containing beads. The flask is stoppered and rotated for 90 min. The remainder is kept as the unrotated control sample, and 0.1-ml samples are introduced into test tubes containing 1 ml of aqueous sodium chloride, 1.25 gm/100 ml (no osmotic hemolysis), and 1 ml of distilled water (complete osmotic hemolysis). Duplicate amounts of 0.1 ml from the rotated sample are introduced into duplicate tubes containing 1.0 ml of aqueous sodium chloride, 1.25 gm/100 ml. The samples are mixed and centrifuged at 1000 rev/min for 5 min and 0.5 ml of the supernatant fluid is diluted with 9.5 ml of distilled water. The hemoglobin is determined with the Evelyn photoelectric-cell colorimeter.

The percentage of hemolysis due to trauma, that is, the mechanical fragility, is calculated as follows. Let $A$ represent the hemoglobin content of the supernatant fluid of the unrotated control sample in aqueous sodium chloride, 1.25 gm/100 ml; let $B$ represent the hemoglobin content of the sample in 1 ml of distilled water; and let $C$ represent the average hemoglobin content of the supernatant fluid of the rotated samples (duplicates) in 1 ml of aqueous sodium chloride, 1.25 gm/100 ml; then the percentage of hemolysis or mechanical fragility is $100(C - A)/(B - A)$. It is recommended that the mechanical fragility of a sample of normal blood be run for comparison with an unknown sample until the normal range is determined for the particular apparatus.

### INTERPRETATIONS AND LIMITATIONS

The normal values for human blood are between 1 and 5 percent hemolysis with this empirical system. The mechanical fragility is increased in congenital hemolytic jaundice (7–12 percent) in patients with the trait (no anemia) or with manifest anemia, and in many instances of acquired hemolytic jaundice, whether the osmotic fragility is normal or increased. The mechanical fragility is markedly increased in cells that are firmly agglutinated or sickled. When red cells are injured by heat, there is a corresponding increase in both the osmotic and the mechanical fragilities. The basis of an increase in mechanical fragility may be related to a decrease in the strength of the red-cell membrane, to increase in spheroidicity of the cell, or to firm agglutination of the cells. Biologically, an increase in mechanical fragility indicates an abnormality of the red-cell membrane and may be related to increased destruction of red cells during their circulation in vivo. However, the relation to clinical hemolysis of increased mechanical fragility is less constant than is that of increased osmotic fragility, its relation to the mechanism of red-cell destruction is less clear, and the methodology is less exact. Consequently, the determination of red-cell mechanical fragility is not a routine procedure and can be regarded chiefly as a supportive test in the study of hemolytic diseases.

### The Hemoglobinopathies

The hemoglobinopathies comprise a group of genetically determined diseases of varying degrees of severity. In some of these diseases, the abnormality of the hemoglobin leads to an increased rate of red-cell destruction. The presence of target cells in the peripheral blood is characteristic of most of the hemoglobinopathies, although it is not specific for them.

The fact that the abnormal hemoglobins can usually be distinguished by electrophoresis [80] and the availability of relatively simple methods for filter-paper electrophoresis have led to the discovery of a number of other abnormal hemoglobins. These hemoglobins have been designated alphabetically in the order of their discovery, with the exception that the hemoglobin present in the red cells of patients with sickle-cell anemia is called hemoglobin S. Normal adult hemoglobin is designated hemoglobin A and the alkali-resistant hemoglobin present in the red cells of the normal human fetus and newborn is called hemoglobin F. To date, the following other hemoglobins have been described: C, D, E, G, H, I, J, K, L, M, N, and O. The characteristics of each of the known hemoglobins are presented in Table 27.

The genetic aspects of all the abnormal hemoglobins are the same with the possible exceptions of hemoglobins G and H.[81, 82] The hemoglobins are inherited as though they were determined by allelomorphic genes occupying a single chromosomal site. Thus a pair of genes determines the hemoglobin pattern of

Table 27. *Some physical and chemical characteristics of the human hemoglobins.*

| Hemoglobin | Relative electrophoretic mobility, barbital buffer at pH 8.6 (1 = fastest) | Solubility of reduced forms | Denaturation by alkali | Racial predominance |
|---|---|---|---|---|
| A | 4 | High | Rapid | — |
| F | 5 | High | Slow | — |
| S | 7 | Low | Rapid | Negro |
| C | 10 | High | Rapid | Negro |
| D | 7 | High | Rapid | East Indian, Negro, Caucasian |
| E | 9 | High | Rapid | Southeast Asian |
| G | 5 | High | Rapid | Negro |
| H | 1 | Low | Rapid | East Asian |
| I | 1 | High | Rapid | Negro |
| J | 2 | High | Rapid | Negro |
| K | 3 | High | Rapid | East Indian, Negro |
| L | 6 | High | Rapid | East Indian |
| M | ? | ? | ? | Caucasian |
| O | 8 | ? | Rapid | Indonesian |

the individual. Each gene manifests it-self in the hemoglobin phenotype. Two identical genes result in homozygosity, while two different ones yield heterozy-gosity. The most frequently observed he-moglobin pattern is that of the normal adult, which consists of hemoglobin A alone. The next most common pattern is that found in persons with sickle-cell trait, where there is a mixture of hemo-globin A and hemoglobin S. In sickle-cell anemia, hemoglobin S is usually present alone, though in some persons there may be hemoglobin F as well. That the he-moglobin pattern is influenced by other genetic factors is certain. Thus, for ex-ample, in sickle-cell trait less than half (22–46 percent) of the hemoglobin is hemoglobin S.[83] The simultaneous inher-itance of the thalassemia trait influences the hemoglobin pattern, and in persons who inherit both this and sickle-cell trait hemoglobin S is present in greater con-centration than hemoglobin A. In gen-eral, the thalassemia trait seems to favor the production of the abnormal hemo-globin at the expense of hemoglobin A. When hemoglobins S and C occur to-gether, they are usually present in equal amounts. The number of possible combi-nations of the various hemoglobins is great, and not all have yet been found clinically.

### LABORATORY PROCEDURES USED IN THE IDENTIFICATION OF THE ABNORMAL HEMOGLOBINS

#### FILTER-PAPER ELECTROPHORESIS OF HEMOLYSATES

PRINCIPLES. Proteins can be characterized by their rate of migration in an electric field when in solution in a buffer of fixed pH (Unit 16). The rate of migration de-pends principally upon the net electric charge per molecule, the molecular weight and spatial configuration, and the magnitude of the electric field. The net electric charge of a protein molecule is a function of the isoelectric point of the protein and the pH of the solution. The isoelectric point of a protein is the pH at which the net charge per molecule of that protein is zero. At this pH, the pro-tein migrates toward neither the posi-tive nor the negative pole when an elec-tric field is imposed upon the solution. However, if the pH of the protein in so-lution is greater than the isoelectric point of the protein, the protein has a net nega-tive charge per molecule and will move toward the positive pole of an electric field. It is necessary to buffer the pH in order to keep it relatively constant. The use of filter paper as the suspending me-dium diminishes the degree of diffusion by convection of the proteins being stud-ied.

In the case of the human hemoglobins, electrophoretic separation has been found to be best accomplished at a pH greater than the isoelectric points. It is customary to use a pH of 8.6 buffered by a mixture of sodium diethylbarbiturate and diethylbarbituric acid. The magni-tude of the electric field depends upon the nature of the apparatus actually used. The use of the siliconized glass-plate apparatus as described by Smith and Conley[84] is a satisfactory way of separating hemoglobins.

MATERIALS. *Electrophoresis apparatus.* Siliconized glass plates are suspended between two buffer chambers made of lucite. Each buffer chamber is divided by a partition with a baffle. Carbon or platinum electrodes are placed in the outer sections and the paper dips into the inner ones. A source of direct current can be provided in various ways. A pow-er unit capable of supplying up to 400–500 volts output with a current of up to 200 milliamperes is satisfactory. A suit-able unit, available in kit form for as-sembly by the user, has been widely used and referred to in the literature (Heath Kit).

*Barbital buffer,* pH 8.6, ionic strength 0.05 M, may be prepared by dissolving

10.3 gm of sodium diethylbarbiturate and 1.84 gm of diethylbarbituric acid in 1 L of distilled water.

*Hemoglobin solution* of concentration 8 to 10 gm/100 ml is prepared by washing the red cells from 5 ml of unclotted blood (any anticoagulant may be used) three times with isotonic saline. To 1 volume of packed washed red cells are then added 1 volume of distilled water and 0.5 volume of toluene. This mixture is shaken vigorously for several minutes and then centrifuged at 3000 rev/min for 15 to 20 min. The upper clear layer (of toluene) and the middle layer (of sediment) are aspirated and discarded. The clear bottom layer of hemoglobin solution is filtered and used without further manipulation. The concentration of the hemoglobin solution is not critical, but best results are obtained at concentrations of 8 to 12 gm/100 ml.

**Procedure.** A pencil line is lightly drawn across the center of the piece of filter paper to be used. For the glass plates described, the filter paper should be 20 in. in length by 8 in. in width. Whatman No. 3 filter paper gives good results, but almost any thickness of filter paper may be used. The filter paper is placed on one of the siliconized glass plates so that each end of the paper hangs over an end of the glass and dips into the buffer solution in one of the buffer chambers. Buffer solution is applied to the filter paper with a capillary pipette so that the paper is wetted evenly with the buffer solution everywhere but for a strip about 1 in. wide along the penciled center line. Then 0.01 to 0.02 ml of each of the hemoglobin solutions are applied to the filter paper along the center line. It is important to leave about an inch free between hemoglobin spots so that there will be no interaction between them. The center dry strip on the filter paper is next wetted evenly with buffer solution up to the hemoglobin spots themselves. The second siliconized glass plate is then placed on top of the

filter paper. The space between the edges of the glass plates is sealed with cellophane tape to prevent evaporation and the glass plates are held evenly and firmly together by six evenly spaced Hargraves No. 2 steel spring clamps. The electrodes are attached and a voltage of 300–500 volts is placed across them. Sufficient migration of the hemoglobins to separate hemoglobin S from hemoglobin A will have occurred in 6 to 8 hr under these conditions. It is sometimes convenient to accomplish the electrophoretic separation overnight and a good separation will occur if the voltage is set at 150–200 volts for 16 to 18 hr. The optimal voltage and timing will depend upon the apparatus used, the width of the filter paper, and the room temperature, and these variables are discussed in the references cited.[85, 86] Theoretically, there is some advantage to running the electrophoresis in a cold room. However, under the conditions described above, adequate separation of the more common hemoglobins is easily accomplished at room temperatures of 15–25°C. The hemoglobin spots are red, and easily seen without staining. Electrophoresis may be discontinued when adequate separation is observed. The filter paper is allowed to dry in a horizontal position without resting on any surface. It is convenient to drop the edges of the paper over the sides of an open refrigerator dish. When the paper is dry, the amount of hemoglobin present in each component may be measured either by use of a photoelectric densitometer or by elution of the hemoglobin from the paper. When the hemoglobin spot is very faint, it may be necessary to stain the hemoglobin with a dye such as bromphenol blue. A satisfactory method, applicable to serum proteins as well as hemoglobin, is to immerse the dried filter paper in a saturated solution of mercuric chloride in absolute ethanol containing 0.1 gm bromphenol blue for 20 min. The paper is then washed in running tap water for 4 min and allowed to dry in a horizontal position.

*Results.* A diagrammatic representation of the filter-paper electrophoretic migration, under the conditions described above, of the various human hemoglobins is given in Fig. 19. It is to be noted that some of the hemoglobins are not separated from each other under these conditions. For example, hemoglobins I and H are not separated. However, they both are separated from hemoglobin A under these conditions and may be separated from each other in a different buffer at a lower pH.

ALKALI-DENATURATION TECHNIQUE
FOR HEMOGLOBIN F

Hemoglobin F is more resistant to denaturation in alkaline solution than are the other human hemoglobins, and this difference may be used in the identification and quantitation of hemoglobin F. A description of this procedure is given below in the section on thalassemia.

SOLUBILITY DETERMINATIONS TO IDENTIFY
HEMOGLOBIN D

Differences in solubility in aqueous solutions of inorganic salts such as ammo-

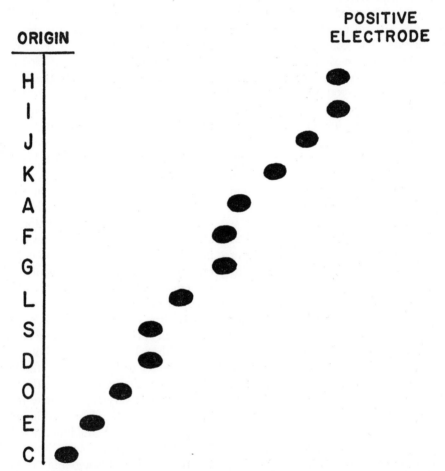

Fig. 19. Relative migrations of the human hemoglobins after electrophoresis on filter paper in 0.05 M barbital buffer at pH 8.6. Hemoglobins H and I may be separated by filter-paper electrophoresis at pH 6.5 (phosphate buffer). Hemoglobins S and D may be differentiated by virtue of their different solubilities in phosphate buffer under standard conditions. Hemoglobins F and G may be differentiated from each other by the resistance of the former to denaturation by alkali.

nium sulfate or potassium phosphate have been useful in distinguishing proteins from each other. The concentration of the salt, pH, and temperature must be controlled. This technique has been applied to the human hemoglobins and a standard solubility test in 2.24 M phosphate has been devised. Although oxyhemoglobins A and S do not differ in solubility, the corresponding reduced hemoglobins differ markedly. Reduced hemoglobin S appears to differ from all the other reduced human hemoglobins in that it has the lowest solubility. This fact is useful in the identification of hemoglobin D which is indistinguishable from hemoglobin S in its electrophoretic characteristics. Reduced hemoglobin D differs from reduced hemoglobin S in having a solubility close to that of reduced hemoglobin A and in not causing the sickling of red cells in which it is present. Since the method of determining the solubility of the hemoglobins is beyond the scope of the usual clinical laboratory, the reader is referred to the original literature.[87]

### PAPER AND ION-EXCHANGE RESIN CHROMATOGRAPHY

Chromatography also provides a means of differentiating some of the human hemoglobins from each other.[88] Immunologic studies have shown differences between hemoglobin F and hemoglobin A. In addition, antigenic differences between hemoglobins A and S have been found. However, immunologic methods have not been used clinically in the diagnosis of hemoglobinopathies.

### CLINICAL SYNDROMES ASSOCIATED WITH THE ABNORMAL HEMOGLOBINS

The known hemoglobinopathies and some of their laboratory and clinical manifestations are summarized in Table 28. Some of the more common hemoglobinopathies will be described in greater detail as well.

## SICKLE-CELL ANEMIA AND ITS VARIANTS

### PATHOLOGIC PHYSIOLOGY

Sickle-cell anemia is characterized by two main clinical features: (i) chronic hemolytic anemia and (ii) episodic painful crises. The defect underlying these features is the presence of the abnormal hemoglobin (hemoglobin S) in the red blood cells of patients with this disease. Although it is freely soluble when oxygenated, hemoglobin S upon deoxygenation forms irregular elongated molecular masses called tactoids (Fig. 20) which give to the red cells the distorted shape from which the disease derives its name.[89] Thus the red cells of patients with this disease are morphologically normal when oxygenated, but are distorted into sickle shapes when deoxygenated or chemically reduced (Fig. 20b). This change in shape of the red blood cells is associated with increased viscosity of the blood and a greater mechanical fragility of the red cells.

The chronic hemolytic anemia has been explained on the basis of the increased mechanical fragility that accompanies the sickled state, and the painful crises have been related to the increased viscosity of the blood which is proportional to the degree of sickling. Factors that impede the flow of blood, thereby causing anoxia, increase the likelihood of sickling in vivo; this in turn increases the viscosity of the blood and consequently further decreases blood flow. Thus is instituted a vicious circle leading to localized ischemia and ultimately to infarction.

The severity of these clinical manifestations is related to the amount of hemoglobin S present in the red blood cells. This may be expressed as the mean corpuscular hemoglobin S concentration (MCSHC), which is the MCHC multiplied by the percentage of the total hemoglobin that is hemoglobin S. When the MCSHC is below 15 gm/100 ml of red cells, as occurs in persons with sickle-

Table 28. *Clinical and laboratory manifestations of some of the known hemoglobinopathies.*

| "Disease" | Hemoglobin present | Spleno-megaly | Hemo-lytic anemia | Pain-ful crises | Bone lesions | Sickling phenom-enon | Oat cells (perma-nently sickled forms) | Target cells | Micro-cytosis | Hypo-chromia |
|---|---|---|---|---|---|---|---|---|---|---|
| Normal newborn | A, F | 0 | 0 | 0 | 0 | 0 | 0 | 0 | 0 | 0 |
| Normal adult | A | 0 | 0 | 0 | 0 | 0 | 0 | 0 | 0 | 0 |
| Sickle-cell trait | A, S | 0 | 0 | 0 | 0 | + | 0 | 0 | 0 | 0 |
| Sickle-cell anemia | S, (F) | +, 0 | + | + | + | + | + | + | 0 | 0 |
| Sickle-cell–Hgb. C disease | S, C | + | + | + | + | + | 0 | + | 0 | 0 |
| Sickle-cell–Hgb. D disease | D, S | 0 | + | + | ? | + | + | + | 0 | 0 |
| Sickle-cell–Hgb. G disease | G, S | 0 | 0 | 0 | ? | + | 0 | 0 | 0 | 0 |
| Sickle-cell–thalassemia | S, (A), F | + | + | + | + | + | + | + | + | + |
| Sickle-cell–Hgb. G thalassemia | S, G | + | + | + | ? | + | + | + | 0 | 0 |
| Hemoglobin C trait | A, C | 0 | 0 | 0 | 0 | 0 | 0 | + | 0 | 0 |
| Hemoglobin C disease | C | + | + | 0 | 0 | 0 | 0 | + | 0 | 0 |
| Hemoglobin C–thalassemia | C, A | + | + | 0 | 0 | 0 | 0 | + | + | + |
| Hemoglobin D trait | A, D | 0 | 0 | 0 | 0 | 0 | 0 | 0 | 0 | 0 |
| Hemoglobin D disease | D | 0 | + | 0 | 0 | 0 | 0 | + | + | 0 |
| Hemoglobin E trait | A, E | 0 | 0 | 0 | 0 | 0 | 0 | 0 | 0 | 0 |
| Hemoglobin E disease | E | ± | + | 0 | 0 | 0 | 0 | + | + | 0 |
| Hemoglobin E–thalassemia | E, F | + | + | 0 | 0 | 0 | 0 | + | + | + |
| Hemoglobin G trait | A, G | ? | 0 | 0 | 0 | 0 | 0 | 0 | 0 | 0 |
| Hemoglobin G disease | G | ? | 0 | 0 | 0 | 0 | 0 | 0 | 0 | 0 |
| Hemoglobin G–thalassemia | G | 0 | 0 | 0 | 0 | 0 | 0 | + | + | + |
| Hemoglobin H trait | A, H | + | + | 0 | 0 | 0 | 0 | + | + | + |
| Hemoglobin H–thalassemia | A, H |  |  |  |  | 0 |  |  | + | + |
| Hemoglobin I trait | A, I | 0 | 0 | 0 | 0 | 0 | 0 | 0 | 0 | 0 |
| Hemoglobin J trait | A, J | 0 | 0 | 0 | 0 | 0 | 0 | 0 | 0 | 0 |
| Hemoglobin J–Hemoglobin D disease | J, D |  |  |  |  |  |  |  |  |  |
| Hemoglobin K trait | A, K | ? | 0 | 0 | 0 | 0 | 0 | 0 | 0 | 0 |
| Hemoglobin L trait | A, L | ? | 0 | 0 | 0 | 0 | 0 | 0 | 0 | 0 |
| Hemoglobin M trait | A, M[a] | ? | 0 | 0 | 0 | ? | 0 | 0 | 0 | 0 |
| Hemoglobin O trait | A, O | ? | 0 | 0 | 0 | 0 | 0 | 0 | 0 | 0 |

[a] Methemoglobin M is also present in the red cells; this has chemical and spectral properties that differ from those of methemoglobin A.

cell trait, sickling does not take place at normal oxygen pressures and the individual is asymptomatic. When the MCSHC is above 25 gm/100 ml of red cells, as it is in persons with the homozygous condition, sickle-cell anemia, sickling occurs readily at physiologic oxygen pressures and pH and the clinical manifestations are maximal. When the MCSHC is between 15 and 25 gm/100 ml of red cells, as it may be in persons with sickle-cell–hemoglobin C disease and sickle-cell–thalassemia disease, sickling occurs less readily under physiologic conditions and the clinical manifestations are intermediate.[90]

### SCREENING-TEST FINDINGS

Examination of the Wright's-stained smear of the peripheral blood may reveal "irreversibly sickled cells," which are densely stained oat-shaped red cells with sharply pointed ends (Fig. 20). These are not found in the blood of persons with sickle-cell trait and their presence indicates that sickling occurs in vivo. Target cells (Fig. 20) are present in the blood smears of patients with many of the hemoglobinopathies. The finding of numerous target cells in the blood of a Negro strongly suggests the presence of hemoglobin C.

### DEMONSTRATION OF THE SICKLING PHENOMENON

The sickling phenomenon may be demonstrated by the removal of sufficient oxygen to permit sickling to take place. This may be accomplished in vitro by allowing cellular metabolism to use up the oxygen in a sealed preparation of whole blood, by gas evacuation, or by displacement of oxygen with hydrogen, nitrous oxide, carbon dioxide, or nitrogen. Displacement of oxygen is enhanced by lowering the pH with carbon dioxide. A number of reducing substances have been used to produce sickling: sodium hydrosulfite, hydrogen sulfide, cysteine, 2,3-dimercaptopropanol (BAL), sodium metabisulfite, vitamin C, sodium bisulfite, and buffered sodium dithionite. Three methods are given below.

### SEALED WHOLE-BLOOD METHOD FOR DEMONSTRATING SICKLING

Oxygen is removed by the metabolism of the white cells and contaminating bacteria in a drop of whole blood. This method is described because it requires a minimum of supplies.

**Method.** A drop of whole blood obtained either by finger prick or by venipuncture is placed upon a clean glass slide. A glass coverslip is put over the drop so that the blood spreads out between the coverslip and the slide. The edges of the coverslip are sealed with vaseline and the preparation is incubated at room temperature. It is examined for sickling at hourly intervals for several hours and after 24 hr. It is helpful to apply a tourniquet to the arm or finger for 5 min before drawing the blood, care being taken to expose the blood to room air as little as possible. Oxalate and heparin do not interfere with this test.

### INTERPRETATION AND LIMITATIONS

In wet preparations, red cells that undergo sickling show a variety of changes. Characteristically, there are elongated forms with sharp projections suggesting holly leaves, and crescent forms with long filamentous projections (Fig. 20). The former are considered by some to be associated with sickle-cell trait and the latter with sickle-cell anemia. Similarly, the rapidity with which sickling occurs is also used to differentiate between these states. However, there is considerable overlapping owing to the many uncontrolled conditions of the test so that differentiation between sickle-cell trait and sickle-cell anemia on the basis of such criteria is very unreliable. If 10 percent or more of the cells are sickled, the result is positive for the demonstration of the sickling phenomenon. A negative preparation is unreliable because the red cells

131

may lose their ability to sickle before sufficient oxygen has been used up by cellular metabolism.

Hemoglobin is rapidly converted to reduced hemoglobin by this chemical reducing agent and the test is therefore independent of the rate of metabolism of the leukocytes present in the preparation.

**Method.** Aqueous sodium metabisulfite ($Na_2S_2O_5$), 2 gm/100 ml, is made up fresh before use. For convenience, a 200-mg capsule has been prepared and is available commercially (Aloe), so that a fresh solution can be made each time by adding the contents of one capsule to 10 ml of water. One or two drops of this 2-percent aqueous sodium metabisulfite are added to one drop of capillary or venous blood on a glass slide. After this is mixed, a coverglass is dropped onto the preparation and the excess blood is expressed by gently pressing the coverglass with a piece of filter paper. This produces a wet preparation which is thin enough to permit examination of individual cells. It is not necessary to seal the preparation. A control preparation containing a drop of isotonic saline in place of the reducing agent should be set up simultaneously. Observations should be made immediately and 15 and 30 min after preparation.

### INTERPRETATION AND LIMITATIONS

This method gives rapid and reproducible results. Ten to 100 per cent of the red cells assume the sickled form within 15 to 30 min when the test is positive. Sickle-cell anemia cannot be distinguished from sickle-cell trait or the other hemoglobin S syndromes by this test. The presence of hemoglobin S in red cells being tested may not be revealed if the concentration of hemoglobin S is too low for sickling to occur. It can be shown that if the concentration of hemoglobin S in the red cells (MCSHC) is less than 7 gm/100 ml sickling does not occur

even in the complete absence of oxygen. The greatest source of difficulty with this test is the instability of the reducing agent. A negative sickling test must therefore be repeated with fresh reagent before being accepted. A positive test is completely reliable. The saline control is useful in differentiating ovalocytosis and extreme anisocytosis, such as occurs in thalassemia major, from the sickling phenomenon. Sickled forms are easily distinguished from crenated cells, which are round and have short spinelike projections.

### DIFFERENTIATION OF SICKLE-CELL ANEMIA FROM SICKLE-CELL TRAIT BY EQUILIBRATION WITH GAS MIXTURES

The physiologically significant difference between the blood of a patient with sickle-cell anemia and that of one with sickle-cell trait is that the former undergoes sickling at higher oxygen pressures than the latter. It has been found that if samples of each type of blood are equilibrated at 37°C with a mixture containing 90 percent of nitrogen and 10 percent of carbon dioxide, both bloods will undergo sickling. Generally, 90 percent of the red cells in sickle-cell anemia will be in the sickled form under these conditions, while 50 percent or less of those of sickle-cell trait will be so altered. If samples of each type of blood are equilibrated at 37°C with a gas mixture containing 4 percent of oxygen, 86 percent of nitrogen, and 10 percent of carbon dioxide, 90 percent or more of the red cells of sickle-cell anemia will be in the sickled form, whereas there will usually be no sickled forms at all in the blood of sickle-cell trait under these conditions. However, the sickled forms produced in this way revert promptly to the normal form if a film of blood is made and allowed to dry in air, a step that permits reoxygenation. The sickled form can be fixed by formalin and the blood examined in a wet preparation.

132

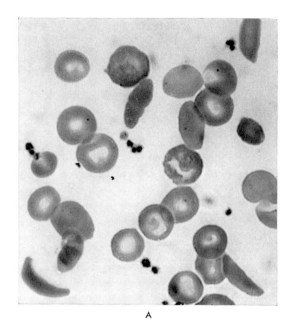

A

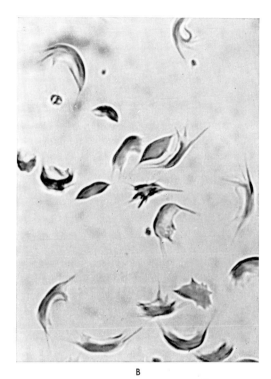

B

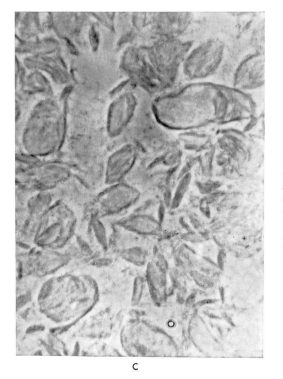

C

Fig. 20. The sickling phenomenon. (*a*) Peripheral venous blood smear from a patient with sickle-cell anemia. "Permanently" sickled red cells (that is, cells that remain sickled despite oxygenation) are evident and target cells are plentiful. Sickled red cells are not found in blood smears of patients with sickle-cell trait. (*b*) Sickling produced by chemical reduction (with sodium metabisulfite) of the red cells of a patient with sickle-cell anemia. Sickling produced in this way is usually more extreme than is encountered in vivo and the red cells may be markedly deformed and develop filaments as shown. Sickle-cell anemia and trait cannot be reliably differentiated by the extent of sickling in this technique. (*c*) Hemoglobin S tactoids. The physical basis of sickling was shown by Harris[89] to depend upon the aggregation and alignment of reduced hemoglobin S molecules into elongated, relatively insoluble molecular masses called tactoids. The photograph, taken with a phase-contrast microscope, is of a solution of hemoglobin S under nitrogen.

**Method.** Samples of 2 to 4 ml of whole blood are placed in each of two small glass vessels having a capacity of 15 to 25 ml. The glass vessels, which may be large test tubes, small bottles, or Erlenmeyer flasks, are closed with stoppers containing rubber diaphragms. Each aliquot of blood is then equilibrated with one of the gas mixtures described above. The gases are hydrated by bubbling them through water. Equilibration with a gas mixture is accomplished by allowing it to flow through the glass containers for three 3-min periods. During these periods, the containers are gently agitated. After each of these periods, including the last one, the blood is shaken gently for 15 min at 37°C. The apparatus for measuring mechanical fragility of red blood cells (Fig. 18) may be used for this purpose also, the blood being rotated at 30 rev/min for 15 min each time. After equilibration, 0.1 ml to 0.5 ml of the blood is transferred without exposure to room air into 2 to 3 ml of a solution containing 1 part of formalin (37 percent of formaldehyde in water) and 9 parts of aqueous sodium chloride, 0.85 gm/100 ml. The red cells are thereby irreversibly fixed and may then be examined in a wet preparation under a coverslip.

### INTERPRETATION AND LIMITATIONS

The presence of sickled forms in the blood at zero oxygen pressure (equilibrated with the gas mixture containing no oxygen) indicates the presence of hemoglobin S in the red cells. In sickle-cell anemia (homozygous state), 90 percent or more of the cells will be in the sickled form. Generally, less than 50 percent of the cells will be in the sickled form in sickle-cell trait (heterozygous state). When the sample of blood at an oxygen pressure of 30 mm-of-mercury (equilibrated with the gas mixture containing 4 percent of oxygen) is examined, blood from a patient with sickle-cell trait will show less than 10 percent of sickled forms (usually no sickling at all is present under the conditions described), whereas the degree of sickling present in blood from a person with sickle-cell anemia will be about the same as that which occurs at zero oxygen pressure. This makes possible differentiation between sickle-cell anemia and sickle-cell trait even in persons who have had recent transfusion with normal blood. Normal red cells do not undergo sickling, and therefore the blood of a patient with the sickling phenomenon who has been transfused recently will not show complete sickling even at zero oxygen pressure. At an oxygen pressure of 30 mm-of-mercury, however, no sickling will occur in the blood of persons with sickle-cell trait, while in the blood of those with sickle-cell anemia sickling occurs to the same extent as at zero oxygen pressure. This differentiation between sickle-cell anemia and sickle-cell trait in persons who have had recent transfusion cannot be made by electrophoretic analysis of hemolysates of red cells, since the normal hemoglobin of the normal red cells causes the electrophoretic pattern to resemble that of blood from persons with sickle-cell trait. The bloods of persons with sickle-cell–hemoglobin C disease and sickle-cell–thalassemia disease give intermediate degrees of sickling in this test.

### HEMOGLOBIN ANALYSIS BY MEANS OF PAPER ELECTROPHORESIS AND ALKALI DENATURATION

The hemoglobin phenotype can be determined by these procedures in patients who have not had transfusions within 4 months. Paper electrophoresis is easily done and requires relatively simple equipment. Comparison of the mobility of an unknown sample with those of known hemoglobins is usually sufficient to identify hemoglobin S and the more common hemoglobins with which it has been found. The method is not reliable for detecting a hemoglobin that comprises less than 10 percent of the total.

This is especially true of mixtures of hemoglobins S and A. Hemoglobin C is easily separated from hemoglobin S.

The alkali-denaturation test quantitates the amount of hemoglobin F present. When more than 10 percent of the hemoglobin is hemoglobin F (resistant to denaturation by alkali) thalassemia is suggested. The pattern of hemoglobin S plus hemoglobin A plus hemoglobin F is characteristic of sickle-cell–thalassemia disease. In sickle-cell anemia, the amount of hemoglobin F may vary from normal to 10 percent of the total hemoglobin, although even higher values have been reported. The cases having the greater amounts of hemoglobin F are probably cases of sickle-cell–thalassemia disease in which no hemoglobin A at all is present.[92]

### Hemoglobin C Disease and Trait

Hemoglobin C trait, which occurs in about 2 percent of American Negroes, is an asymptomatic condition without hematologic abnormalities, save for the appearance of increased numbers of target cells in smears of the peripheral blood. Sickling of red cells does not occur. Hemoglobin analysis reveals the presence of hemoglobins A and C in a ratio of about 2:1. Hemoglobin F is present in normal amounts.

Hemoglobin C disease, the homozygous condition, has an incidence of 1:6000 in American Negroes. It is a relatively benign condition, compatible with a normal life span, the most common symptom being vague intermittent arthralgia. Splenomegaly is usually present. Hematologic examination reveals mild normochromic anemia, slight elevation of reticulocytes, and large numbers of target cells in blood smears. The survival time of the red blood cells has been shown to be mildly decreased. Sickling of red cells does not occur. There is moderate erythroid hyperplasia of the bone marrow. Hemoglobin analysis by paper electrophoresis shows only hemoglobin

C. Hemoglobin F is usually present in normal amounts.

### Hereditary Microcytosis (Thalassemia)

This designation includes a complex of hereditary disorders, prevalent in people of Mediterranean, African, and Asian ancestry, which are characterized by microcytosis, anisocytosis, increased red-cell destruction, and frequent association with increased concentrations of normal "trace" hemoglobins or with abnormal hemoglobins. Although this complex is still not fully defined, the following disease entities are recognized.

#### cooley's anemia (homozygous thalassemia, thalassemia major)

This is usually a severe hemolytic anemia commencing in early life and classically associated with marked microcytosis, mild or moderate hypochromia, erythroblastosis, and striking deformities of the red cells, including bizarre cell shapes, basophilic stippling, siderocytosis, and the persistence of nuclear remnants (Howell-Jolly bodies, Cabot rings). The concentration of fetal hemoglobin is usually moderately or markedly increased, and the level of the normal "trace" hemoglobin fraction A2 is often elevated.[93, 94]

#### cooley's trait (heterozygous thalassemia, thalassemia minor, thalassemia minima)

The heterozygous form of Cooley's anemia, this condition is associated with little or no reduction in the blood hemoglobin concentration, with microcytosis, and with mild or moderate red-cell deformities. There is a characteristic elevation in the level of hemoglobin A2. Intermediate forms of thalassemia may occur in families with familial microcytosis in which it is difficult to determine whether the condition is a mild form of Cooley's anemia or a severe form of Cooley's trait.

### HEMOGLOBIN H DISEASE

A hereditary entity has been described recently in which hereditary microcytosis, clinically and morphologically similar to classical thalassemia of moderate severity, is associated with the abnormal hemoglobin H.[82] Hemoglobin H disease apparently is the result of the interaction between a "silent" recessive gene for hemoglobin H and a gene for thalassemia.

### COMBINATIONS OF THE TRAITS FOR THALASSEMIA AND OTHER HEMOGLOBINOPATHIES (DOUBLE HETEROZYGOSITY)

Most important is the heterozygous combination of Cooley's trait and sickle-cell trait, causing a disease (S-thalassemia) clinically resembling sickle-cell anemia of moderate severity but with the blood morphology of Cooley's anemia. Other combinations have been described, usually having less clinical severity. These include C-thalassemia, E-thalassemia, and the combination of thalassemia and so-called Lapore trait.

As a result of an inherited defect in red-cell formation, probably involving an impairment in hemoglobin synthesis, small hypochromic red cells are produced in large numbers. Many of these red cells are so abnormal that, as in pernicious anemia, they never escape the marrow; those that are released into the blood stream are destroyed with abnormal rapidity, probably by their filtration by the spleen and liver.

### SCREENING-TEST FINDINGS

The morphologic changes in the red cells are distinctive and striking on the blood smear, particularly in Cooley's anemia, and are described above. Characteristically, as determined by red-cell corpuscular values, microcytosis is relatively marked and hypochromia relatively mild, whereas in iron deficiency the MCV and MCHC tend to diminish pro-portionately (Fig. 13). Examination of the blood of other members of the patient's family is valuable in distinguishing these disease entities.

### SPECIAL TESTS

There are no specific tests apart from blood morphology for the categorical diagnosis of hereditary microcytoses. The associated changes in various trace hemoglobins, or the appearance of certain abnormal hemoglobin fractions (see above), may aid in identifying or distinguishing these syndromes. Filter-paper electrophoresis, as described previously, will reveal the presence of a significant proportion (greater than 10 percent) of hemoglobin S, C, H, E, and so forth. For the detection of small amounts of these pathologic hemoglobins, starch-block electrophoresis has been utilized. By this method it is possible to identify the characteristic increase in hemoglobin fraction A2 that is found in Cooley's trait and in patients not having a preponderance of fetal hemoglobin in Cooley's anemia. Fetal hemoglobin (hemoglobin F) tends to persist in abnormally high amounts in the familial microcytoses, particularly in Cooley's anemia, where it may constitute as much as 90 percent of the patient's hemoglobin. Fetal hemoglobin may be measured by electrophoretic, chromatographic, or immunologic means. However, it is most readily and usually determined by the alkali-denaturation technique,[95] which utilizes the fact that fetal hemoglobin is less readily denatured and precipitated by alkali than is normal adult hemoglobin.

### ALKALI DENATURATION TEST FOR HEMOGLOBIN F

A measured quantity of hemoglobin solution is made alkaline for a short period of time, whereupon the solution is neutralized, nonhemoglobin "chromogens" are precipitated, and the hemoglobin remaining in solution (which therefore is alkali-resistant) is measured and its amount expressed as a percentage of the initial amount of hemoglobin.

REAGENTS (1) Alkali solution: N/12 KOH or NaOH, kept in paraffin-lined or plastic bottles in the refrigerator.

(2) Precipitating solution: 1000 ml of 50-percent saturated $(NH_4)_2SO_4$ plus 2.5 ml of concentrated HCl.

**Method.** Prepare a hemolysate from fresh whole blood as follows: wash 5 or 10 ml of blood once with physiologic saline; to the packed cells, add 1.5 volumes of distilled water and 0.4 volume of toluene (C.P.), shake the mixture vigorously for 5 min, and spin at 3000 rev/min in a clinical centrifuge for 10 min. Discard the upper two layers, remove and filter the clear red solution, and adjust its concentration of hemoglobin to about 10 percent with distilled water before determining its exact concentration $(H_1)$. To 1.6 ml of the alkaline reagent, adjusted to room temperature, add 0.1 ml of the hemoglobin solution, rinsing the pipette 5 or 6 times and gently agitating the tube. Exactly 1 min after the hemoglobin has been pipetted, add 3.4 ml of the precipitating reagent, invert the test tube 3 or 4 times, and immediately filter. The hemoglobin concentration of the filtrate $(H_2)$ is determined, using 1/50th the dilution used to measure $H_1$, and the percentage $(H_2/H_1) \times 100$ of alkaline-resistant hemoglobin can be calculated.

### INTERPRETATION

With hemoglobin from normal adults, the filtrate is almost colorless (less than 2 percent of the initial hemoglobin is in the filtrate, and presumed to be fetal hemoglobin), whereas the filtrate of blood with increased concentrations of fetal hemoglobin (> 2 percent) is faintly brown to red. Slight to moderate elevations of fetal hemoglobin (2 − 10 percent) are encountered in some patients with Cooley's trait, hemoglobin H disease, or sickle-cell anemia, and occasionally in patients with hereditary spherocytosis. Marked elevations are chiefly encountered in normal newborn infants, in Cooley's anemia, in cases of sickle-cell–thalassemia combination, and rarely as a hereditary peculiarity in otherwise normal subjects.

### PAROXYSMAL NOCTURNAL HEMOGLOBINURIA (MARCHIAFAVA-MICHELI SYNDROME)

#### PATHOLOGIC PHYSIOLOGY

Paroxysmal nocturnal hemoglobinuria (PNH) is an acquired chronic hemolytic anemia, usually severe, of unknown cause. It is associated with continuing intravascular hemolysis, as evidenced by hemoglobinemia, methemalbuminemia, hemoglobinuria, and hemosiderinuria. The rate of hemolysis characteristically increases during sleep, resulting in the presence of hemoglobin in urine passed on awakening.

The fundamental abnormality resides in the red-cell membranes. This renders them hypersusceptible to hemolysis by certain agents that are inactive against, or only potentially hemolytic for, normal red cells. Thus a complex system of heat-labile lytic factors of normal serum, which are optimally active at a slightly acid pH, hemolyzes PNH red cells but not normal cells. This lytic system involves complement, properdin, and $Mg^{++}$ and is most active at a pH between 6.5 and 7.1 (Fig. 21). It is presumed to cause the destruction of PNH red cells in vivo and is the basis of the acid-serum (Ham) test,[96] described below. PNH red cells are often hemolyzed by antibodies that agglutinate or "coat," but do not hemolyze, normal red cells. Antibodies active in this respect include isoantibodies, certain "autoantibodies," and heterophile antibodies. This activity of the last reportedly accounts for the efficacy of commercial thrombin prepara-

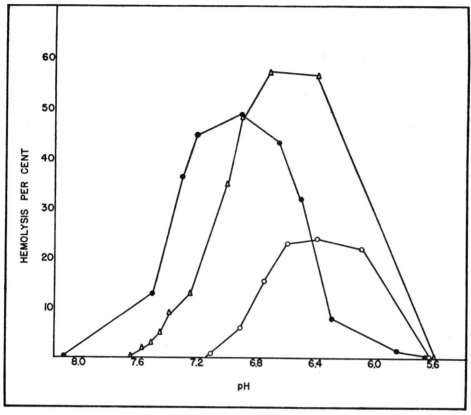

Fig. 21. The influence of pH on the hemolysis by serum of the red cells of three patients with paroxysmal nocturnal hemoglobinuria. The factors in normal serum that hemolyze these red cells are maximally effective at a pH of from 6.5 to 7.0.

tions in hemolyzing PNH red cells, for such preparations are rich in heterophile antibodies. The behavior of PNH red cells exposed to nonhemolytic antibodies resembles that of trypsinized red cells, and both types of cells are often employed for the detection of occult antibodies.[97]

### SCREENING-TEST FINDINGS

Routine morphologic studies of the blood reveal the general findings of hemolytic anemia, usually associated with granulocytopenia and often with thrombocytopenia, but no distinctive changes are evident. There is usually moderate to severe hemoglobinemia, methemalbuminemia, hemoglobinuria, hemosiderinuria, and an elevated indirect-reacting serum bilirubin. These findings, with or without

a clear history of dark urine on awakening, should suggest the possible diagnosis of paroxysmal nocturnal hemoglobinuria.

### TESTS DEPENDING ON REACTIONS IN ACID SERUM

It is remarkable that an acid pH of approximately 6.5 to 6.8 has been found necessary or optimum in four different serum-red-cell reactions that are directly related to hemolytic anemias. These are as follows.

HEMOLYSIS OF PATIENT'S RED CELLS IN PAROXYSMAL NOCTURNAL HEMOGLOBINURIA. The abnormal red cells are hemolyzed at an acid pH in normal serum.

Three different, but probably related, reactions either require or are optimum at an acid pH of the serum from patients with acquired hemolytic jaundice.

(i) PANAGGLUTINATION AT ACID PH. In some instances, the serum of these patients agglutinates all normal red cells at an acid pH but not at an alkaline pH of 8.0.[98]

(ii) INDIRECT COOMBS TEST AT ACID PH. In some instances, the indirect Coombs test is positive at an acid pH, while it is negative at pH 8.0.[98]

(iii) HEMOLYSIS AT ACID PH. Hemolysins occur (chiefly in association with high concentrations of cold agglutinins) that are active at pH 6.8 in producing hemolysis and sensitization of red cells but are not active at pH 8.0.[97]

### SCREENING TEST FOR ACID-SERUM HEMOLYSIS

A simplified screening test may be used for the detection or exclusion of these reactions based on the use of the patient's fresh serum which is acidified to approximately pH 6.5 and incubated for 1 hr at 37.5°C. If *no* abnormalities are detected, no more refined tests may be necessary. If abnormalities are found, the system involved is investigated in detail, as described in subsequent sections.

**Method.** Approximately 5 ml of the patient's venous blood is defibrinated with glass beads. Plasma *cannot* be used because anticoagulants antagonize complement. Approximately 4.5 ml of blood is centrifuged at 1000 rev/min for 10 min to obtain 2.0 ml of serum. A sample of 0.1 ml of 1/3 normal hydrochloric acid is first placed in a small test tube; then 1.8 ml of serum is added and these reagents are mixed thoroughly. To make a suspension of approximately 2 percent of red cells, 0.1 ml of the whole defibrinated blood is added and mixed. The pH of the final mixture will be approximately 6.5 to 6.8. Ideally, the pH is tested and adjusted to this range. The sample is then divided; 1 ml is centrifuged immediately as a control for color of the serum and 1 ml is incubated in a water bath at 37.5°C for 1 hr. The incubated sample is first examined for agglutination. It is then centrifuged, and the supernatant fluid is inspected for hemolysis. A sample of normal blood is treated in the same manner as a control. If hemolysis occurs in the incubated sample, it may be produced either by the PNH red-cell defect or by the presence of acid hemolysins. No hemolysis should occur in the normal control.

### PRESUMPTIVE ACID-SERUM TEST FOR PAROXYSMAL NOCTURNAL HEMOGLOBINURIA

This test distinguishes between acid hemolysis by an abnormal serum factor (an acid hemolysin) and that due to an abnormal red-cell susceptibility to a lowered serum pH, as occurs in PNH.

**Method.** (1) Separate the serum from 10–12 ml of defibrinated blood from the patient and from a normal compatible subject. Prepare a 50-percent red-cell suspension in saline.

(2) Prepare acid sera by adding to 1.8 ml each of patient and normal serum 0.1 ml of $N/3$ HCl.

(3) In a series of test tubes, make the following combinations of 1.0-ml volumes of serum and 0.1-ml volumes of 50-percent red cells:

| Tube | 1 | 2 | 3 | 4 | 5 | 6 | 7 | 8 |
|---|---|---|---|---|---|---|---|---|
| Patient serum | x | | | | x | | | |
| Patient acid serum | | x | | | | x | | |
| Normal serum | | | x | | | | x | |
| Normal acid serum | | | | x | | | | x |
| Patient cells | x | x | x | x | | | | |
| Normal cells | | | | | x | x | x | x |

(4) Incubate at 37°C for 30–60 min, centrifuge, and read for hemolysis.

### INTERPRETATION

The finding of hemolysis in tubes 2 and 4 only is presumptive evidence of paroxysmal nocturnal hemoglobinuria. A false positive may appear when the patient's red cells are spherocytic, as in hereditary spherocytosis or in certain cases of acquired hemolytic anemia. This phenomenon may be ruled out in three ways. (i) If there are no sperocytes microscopically visible, and if the osmotic fragility is normal, as is usually the case in PNH, spherocyte swelling is not responsible for the hemolysis. (ii) Heating the patient's serum at 56°C for 30 min before acidification prevents hemolysis by acid serum of PNH cells but not of spherocytes. (iii) Hemolysis of PNH red cells is maximal at only a slightly acid pH (Fig. 20), whereas spherocytes are hemolyzed in direct proportion to the degree of acidity. Provided one of these three conditions is met, the diagnosis of paroxysmal nocturnal hemoglobinuria may be regarded as established by the above test.

### COMPLETE TEST FOR PAROXYSMAL NOCTURNAL HEMOGLOBINURIA (HAM TEST)

This more exhaustive test demonstrates that, in addition to those features elicited by the presumptive test above, the human-serum factor responsible for lysis of PNH red cells is thermolabile and that the addition of fresh guinea pig serum does not restore this activity, that is, the factors destroyed by heat include substances other than complement.

REAGENTS. (1) Patient's serum, derived from defibrinated venous blood.

(2) Patient's red cells, washed three times with an equal volume of aqueous sodium chloride, 0.85 gm/100 ml, and made to a 5-percent suspension in physiologic saline.

(3) Normal serum, derived from defibrinated venous blood of the same blood group as the patient.

(4) Normal red cells, prepared in a 5-percent suspension as above.

(5) Hydrochloric acid, $N/3$, in distilled water.

(6) Fresh serum from a guinea pig, serum undiluted.

(7) Acidified serum: 1.9-ml samples of serum from the patient and the normal subject are measured into separate tubes and 0.1 ml of $N/3$ hydrochloric acid is added to each and mixed thoroughly.

(8) Heat-inactivated acidified serum: 1.9-ml samples of both serums are heated for 5 min at 56°C to inactivate complement and, after cooling, 0.1 ml of $N/3$ hydrochloric acid is added to each and mixed thoroughly.

(9) Heat-inactivated acidified serum with added guinea pig serum: 1.5-ml samples of both serums are heated as above, and 0.1 ml of $N/3$ hydrochloric acid is added to each. Then 0.4 ml of undiluted guinea pig serum is added as a source of complement.

**Method.** Samples of 0.5 ml of the suspensions of red cells are introduced into small test tubes (11 × 100 mm) as indicated in Table 29 and centrifuged, and the supernatant saline is removed with a micropipette. The saline must be removed since this hemolytic reaction is greatly decreased by dilution. Then 0.5-ml amounts of the reagents are introduced as indicated in Table 29, mixed thoroughly, incubated in a water bath at 37.5°C for 1 hr, and centrifuged, and the hemolysis is observed in the supernatant sera.

### INTERPRETATION

(1) *Paroxysmal nocturnal hemoglobinuria.* The hemolytic reaction that is specific for paroxysmal nocturnal hemoglobinuria is shown in Table 29 and establishes the features outlined at the beginning of this section.

(2) *Paroxysmal cold hemoglobinuria.* Rarely, red cells are sensitized by a cold hemolysin at room temperature. This would produce hemolysis whenever the patient's active serum was used, irrespective of the red cells (tubes 1, 3, 9, and 11 in Table 29). Hemolysis would be inhibited by heating (tubes 5 and 13). In

Table 29. *Hemolysis test with acidified serum.*

| Tube number | Packed red cells from 0.5 ml of suspension [a] (5 percent) | Unaltered serum, 0.5 ml | Acidified serum, 0.5 ml | Heated acidified serum, 0.5 ml | Heated serum plus guinea pig serum, 0.5 ml | Hemolysis in paroxysmal nocturnal hemoglobinuria (percent) |
|---|---|---|---|---|---|---|
| 1 | P [b] | P | | | | 0–10 |
| 2 | P | C | | | | 0–10 |
| 3 | P | | P | | | 2–30 |
| 4 | P | | C | | | 2–30 |
| 5 | P | | | P | | 0 |
| 6 | P | | | C | | 0 |
| 7 | P | | | | P | 0 |
| 8 | P | | | | C | 0 |
| 9 | C | P | | | | 0 |
| 10 | C | C | | | | 0 |
| 11 | C | | P | | | 0 |
| 12 | C | | C | | | 0 |
| 13 | C | | | P | | 0 |
| 14 | C | | | C | | 0 |
| 15 | C | | | | P | 0 |
| 16 | C | | | | C | 0 |

[a] All saline is removed by centrifugation before serum is added, to prevent dilution of the serum.
[b] P = Patient; C = Control.

some instances, the cold hemolysin is thermostable and hemolysis would be restored by guinea pig serum (tubes 7 and 15). An acid pH of 6.5 to 6.8 does not inhibit hemolysis by the cold hemolysin.

(3) *Hemolysin effective at acid pH.* With a hemolysin effective at acid pH, the hemolysis would occur whenever the patient's active and acidified serum was used (tubes 3 and 11). There might be no hemolysis or a slight amount in un-acidified patient's serum (tubes 1 and 9). Heating would inhibit hemolysis (tubes 5 and 13). Guinea pig serum might restore hemolysis (tubes 7 and 15) if the hemolysin is thermostable. For most purposes, the "presumptive" test described above suffices, particularly when the presence of spherocytes has been excluded.

### Hemolytic Anemias Caused by Extrinsic Defects of Red Cells

These anemias are caused by factors external to the red cell which alter the cell and thereby, directly or indirectly, promote its destruction. Although in most instances the red cells involved have no intrinsic abnormality, in some instances there may exist an inborn hypersusceptibility of the cell to the offending external factor.

### IMMUNE MECHANISMS

Hemolytic anemia may be caused by the injection of "natural" isoantibodies in high titer, as with the use of plasma from type O, "dangerous universal donors" possessing very high concentrations of anti-A or anti-B. Similarly, hemolytic disease of the newborn, erythroblastosis fetalis, is caused by the passive placental transfer of "acquired" isoantibodies from mothers sensitized to one or more of the fetal red-cell antigens, particularly of the Rh group. Finally, there may be spontaneously acquired an assortment of hemolytic conditions that resemble in many respects anemias produced by known antibodies and in some instances clearly involve antibodies, although usually it is not certain that these antibodies are specifically directed against the red cell. These acquired hemolytic anemias are often termed autoimmune hemolytic anemias, and, for convenience, the antibody-like substances associated with them are referred to as antibodies, recognizing that they may not be true autoantibodies, and, indeed, that they may often not be antibodies at all.

In all of these conditions, one may encounter three general categories of antibodies, as differentiated by their behavior in vitro. *Hemolysins* are antibodies that cause hemolysis of red cells in vitro by sensitizing the cells to the lytic action of serum complement. Hemolysins are present to some extent in most normal serums containing anti-A and anti-B, although they are evident by conventional testing only in about 30 percent of normal serums. They are also encountered characteristically in heteroimmune sera and occasionally in the sera of patients with acquired hemolytic anemia of the cold antibody type (see below). *Agglutinins* are antibodies that agglutinate red cells or render them agglutinable. *Complete* agglutinins, which cause red cells to clump even when suspended in physiologic saline, are found in all ABO antiserums, in most antiserums against the Rh group, and in some patients with acquired hemolytic anemia. *Incomplete* agglutinins (red-cell "coating" or sensitizing antibodies) cause agglutination only under certain conditions. They characteristically appear in the serums of subjects immunized to Rh antigens and are found adsorbed to the red cells of infants with erythroblastosis fetalis and of most patients with acquired hemolytic anemia.

Antibodies that fix complement (hemolysins) cause rapid intravascular hemolysis, and accordingly cause hemoglobinemia and hemoglobinuria. Hemolysis by complete agglutinins is somewhat slower, there is less evidence of intravascular hemolysis, and spherocytosis may be prominent. Red cells strongly agglutinated in vivo are largely sequestered in the liver, although severe agglutina-tion may cause diffuse, "embolic" blockage of blood vessels. Hemolysis in vivo by incomplete antibodies is still slower and is largely the result of filtration of the red cells by the spleen with destruction of the trapped red cells in situ.[99] Thus relatively little hemoglobin escapes into the plasma and indirect-reacting bilirubin levels are high (the pattern of so-called "extravascular hemolysis."

### SCREENING-TEST FINDINGS

In hemolytic anemias due to immune mechanisms there are no constant or specific morphologic changes. Frequently, however, spherocytosis is evident [100] and as noted earlier these cells are overhydrated "macrospherocytes," in distinction to the underhydrated "microspherocytes" of hereditary spherocytosis (Fig. 15). Consequent to the spherocytosis, formation of rouleaux is defective, and there is an increase in osmotic fragility, with a tendency toward an asymmetric "shift to the left" of the osmotic fragility curve on incubation of the red cells. Autoagglutination may be visible on examination of the blood smear, but, unless extreme, autoagglutination is difficult to distinguish from rouleaux on dried blood smears. Erythrophagocytosis may be evident, particularly in diseases such as paroxysmal cold hemoglobinuria, which involve complement-fixing antibodies. In most acquired hemolytic anemias, however, erythrophagocytes are absent. In some instances, they may appear when the buffy coat from the patient's heparinized or defibrinated blood is incubated at 37°C for 60 min in vitro before preparing the blood smears. As with the lupus erythematosus cell preparation, this phenomenon presumably depends in part on injury in vitro to the leukocytes. The presence of erythrophagocytosis is not a reliable index of acquired hemolytic anemias and may occur in certain infections unassociated with hemolysis.

141

SPECIAL SCREENING PROCEDURES FOR
DETECTING COMPLETE AGGLUTININS
IN ACQUIRED HEMOLYTIC ANEMIA

TEST FOR AUTOAGGLUTINATION

One drop or 0.1 ml of freshly drawn whole blood is placed in 10 ml of warm physiologic saline, inverted gently 2 or 3 times, and read microscopically. Agglutination is most evident in a moving-cell suspension produced by placing a large drop of the suspension on a glass slide and examining at once under a high dry lens.

INTERPRETATION

Although rouleaux of normal red cells (as in multiple myeloma) and autoagglutination (as in some cases of acquired hemolytic anemia) are difficult to distinguish with the naked eye, rouleaux of normal red cells immediately disperse upon 2- or 3-fold dilution with saline or normal plasma or with 4- or 5-fold dilution with plasma containing increased fibrinogen or other globulins. Red cells that have been agglutinated by complete antibodies, on the other hand, usually remain agglutinated in saline.

DETECTION OF WARM AND COLD
AGGLUTININS

In some patients with acquired hemolytic anemia, there may be agglutinins that, unlike isoagglutinins, clump the patient's red cells and those of persons with compatible blood types. When such agglutinins clump red cells at body temperature, a severe hemolytic process takes place. Such agglutinins are warm agglutinins. Agglutinins that operate, on the other hand, at temperatures below body temperature, cold agglutinins, are harmless except under the following conditions. (i) When cold agglutinins are present in high titer and chilling of the blood occurs, there may be peripheral vascular occlusions and acute hemolytic episodes. (ii) When the cold antibodies

have a broad thermal activity extending to peripheral body temperatures, as may be the case with very high titers of cold agglutinins, a chronic (usually mild) hemolytic anemia may develop. (iii) When, as the blood is cooled in peripheral blood vessels, antibody attaches to the red cell and (unlike the ordinary cold agglutinin) does not come off at body temperature, a hemolytic anemia will develop. Such a cold-dependent coating antibody may also act as a hemolysin, particularly at an acid pH,[101] whereas this is rarely true of warm-dependent antibodies.

**Method.** Patient's plasma may be used in place of serum, since complement is not necessary for the agglutination reaction. Normal red cells of blood group O are obtained from defibrinated blood or blood containing an anticoagulant. The cells are washed three times in 5 to 10 volumes of physiologic saline and made to a 2-percent suspension in saline. Red cells of the same blood group as the patient may be required at times. The serum is used undiluted, and after serial dilutions with saline. Equal volumes of serum and red-cell suspension are mixed and incubated at different temperatures in water baths, as indicated in Table 30. The samples are read for macroscopic agglutination after gentle mixing. During the process of reading, the temperature of the tubes must be maintained at that used in incubation by returning each tube promptly to the appropriate water bath (3–4°C, 25°C, or 37.5°C).

INTERPRETATION

The origin of cold agglutinins is unknown. They develop, frequently in high titer, in at least half of patients with virus pneumonia,[102] but only rarely are associated with hemolytic anemia in this disease. Cold agglutinins are found frequently in low or moderate concentrations in patients with acquired hemolytic anemia and must be distinguished, therefore, from other antibodies found in this

Table 30. *Demonstration of cold and warm agglutinins in serial dilutions of serum. The concentration of agglutinin is reported as the maximum final dilution of serum that gives 1+ agglutination.*

| Tube number | 1 | 2 | 3 | 4 | 5 | 6 | 7 | 8 | 9 | 10 | 11 | 12 |
|---|---|---|---|---|---|---|---|---|---|---|---|---|
| Saline (ml) | 0 | 0.5 | 0.5 | 0.5 | 0.5 | 0.5 | 0.5 | 0.5 | 0.5 | 0.5 | 0 | 0.5 |
| Serum (ml) | 0.5 | 0.5 | Contents of tube 2 mixed and 0.5 ml transferred to tube 3. Serial dilution continued through tube 10, the contents of which are mixed and 0.5 ml transferred to tube 11. | | | | | | | | | 0 |
| Suspension of 1–2 percent rbc (ml) 0.5 throughout all tubes | | | | | | | | | | | | |
| Final dilution of serum | $\frac{1}{2}$ | $\frac{1}{4}$ | $\frac{1}{8}$ | $\frac{1}{16}$ | $\frac{1}{32}$ | $\frac{1}{64}$ | $\frac{1}{128}$ | $\frac{1}{256}$ | $\frac{1}{512}$ | $\frac{1}{1024}$ | $\frac{1}{2048}$ | Control |
| *Agglutination occurring with cold agglutinins* [a] *under different conditions* | | | | | | | | | | | | |
| 1 hr at 37.5°C | 0 | 0 | 0 | 0 | 0 | 0 | 0 | 0 | 0 | 0 | 0 | 0 |
| 1 hr at 25°C | 4+ | 2+ | 1+ | 0 | 0 | 0 | 0 | 0 | 0 | 0 | 0 | 0 |
| 1 hr at 3–4°C | 4+ | 4+ | 4+ | 3+ | 2+ | 2+ | + | + | 0 | 0 | 0 | 0 |
| 24 hr at 3–4°C | 4+ | 4+ | 4+ | 4+ | 3+ | 3+ | 2+ | 2+ | + | + | 0 | 0 |
| *Agglutination occurring with a warm agglutinin* | | | | | | | | | | | | |
| 1 hr at 37.5°C | 4+ | 3+ | 2+ | + | ± | 0 | 0 | 0 | 0 | 0 | 0 | 0 |
| 1 hr at 25°C | 2+ | + | 0 | 0 | 0 | 0 | 0 | 0 | 0 | 0 | 0 | 0 |

[a] In testing for cold agglutinins, the temperature should be decreased from 37.5°C to lower temperatures since the agglutination at lower temperatures, for instance, 4°C, may not be readily reversed at higher temperature, for instance, 25°C.

condition. Rarely, intravascular hemolysis occurs with hemoglobinemia and hemoglobinuria following chilling in patients with acquired hemolytic anemia. In these cases, high concentrations of cold agglutinins and an increase in the mechanical fragility of the red cells at body temperature have been observed.[103] The Donath-Landsteiner test is negative (see below).

### SCREENING TEST FOR COLD AGGLUTININS

This test may be employed to differentiate the low concentrations of cold agglutinins (titer $< \frac{1}{32}$) found in many normal persons from higher concentrations having potential clinical significance.

**Method.** Add 0.1 ml of freshly drawn whole blood to 3 ml of 0.9-percent sodium chloride solution and place in a refrigerator over night. Examine for agglutination (i) in the cold and (ii) after warming for several minutes at 37°C.

### INTERPRETATION

The dilution selected provides a cell suspension of about 1 percent and a serum dilution of about $\frac{1}{60}$. Under these conditions, the development of strong agglutination in the cold indicates significantly increased concentrations of cold agglutinins. The actual titer (and the panagglutinating activity) of these agglutinins may then be determined as described above.

### TESTS FOR THE DETECTION OF RED CELLS COATED (SENSITIZED) WITH INCOMPLETE AGGLUTININS

The most common alteration of red cells from patients with acquired hemolytic anemia is the adsorption of antibodies onto the red-cell surface, thus sensitizing the cells in a manner analogous to the action of incomplete Rh antibodies. Such sensitized red cells are not clumped or altered in appearance and do not necessarily show abnormalities of osmotic or mechanical fragility. They are usually detected by their tendency to agglutinate under certain conditions. The most important of these conditions are (i) exposure to certain macromolecules which cause red cells to form rouleaux [104] (so-called "colloidal" or conglutinating [105, 106] media) and (ii) exposure to antiglobulin serums (the Coombs test).[107]

### THE COLLOID AGGLUTINATION TEST— DETECTION OF RED-CELL SENSITIZATION BY POLYVINYLPYRROLIDONE (PVP) OR DEXTRAN

Agents that cause normal red cells to form rouleaux and thus to sediment rapidly are hydrophilic, anisometric (elongated) macromolecules.[104] Included among such agents are fibrinogen, gamma globulin, PVP, dextran, methylcellulose, and various gums. Appropriate concentrations of these agents cause red cells to align as rouleaux. When the cells are normal, these rouleaux disperse when physiologic saline is thereafter added. However, rouleaux of red cells coated with antibody remain stuck together in clumps.

**Method.** Polyvinylpyrrolidone (PVP, viscosity grade K-30 to K-44, ideally the latter), or, if unavailable, dextran of a similar viscosity grade, is dissolved as a 5-percent solution in pH 7.4 isotonic phosphate buffer. This reagent will keep in the refrigerator for several months. To 0.5 ml of 5-percent PVP in a 12- or 15-ml test tube, add 0.1 ml of whole blood. Allow the red cells to settle in the bottom of the tube at room temperature (which may require up to an hour); then add 12–15 ml of saline, mix the contents of the tube by gentle inversion three times, and examine for agglutination. This may range from small microscopic clumps and chains (1+) to marked, grossly visible clumping, which is usually the case in acquired hemolytic anemia.

### INTERPRETATION

This simple test is highly sensitive in detecting red-cell sensitization. Unlike the Coombs test (below), it tests the stickiness of the red-cell surface, rather than the presence of globulin per se. However, in general, these tests may be interpreted interchangeably. The PVP test is equally effective in detecting red-

cell sensitization by isoantibodies, as in erythroblastosis fetalis. The PVP test and the saline test for autoagglutination may be used together in the screening and detection of acquired hemolytic anemias. High concentrations of albumin also enhance the agglutination of sensitized red cells [106] through a mechanism apparently analogous to that of agents which cause rouleaux-formation. However, despite its usefulness in the slide method for blood typing,[108] albumin has proved less sensitive and less reliable than PVP or dextran in detecting the presence of red-cell sensitization in acquired hemolytic anemia.

### DETECTION OF RED-CELL SENSITIZATION BY THE ANTIGLOBULIN (COOMBS) TEST

The method for performing the direct antiglobulin test is presented in Unit 15. It is important that the antiglobulin serum be obtained from animals (usually rabbits) sensitized to whole human serum rather than to a purified fraction of gamma globulin, since in many instances the red cells of patients with acquired hemolytic anemia are coated with a non-gamma globulin. This is true of some cases of antibody of the warm type [109] and of most cases of incomplete antibody of the cold type, where the antibody is apparently affixed to the cell surface by serum complement [104] which contains non-gamma globulin components. Thus serum prepared from animals immunized against whole human serum may be neutralized in its anti-gamma globulin activity by absorption with pure gamma globulin (Cohn Fraction II) before the Coombs test is performed. If such absorption fails to negate the agglutinating action of the serum, the protein adsorbed on the red cell may be regarded as non-gamma globulin. Since in using antiglobulin serum a prozone effect may exist, it is advisable to use several dilutions of antiglobulin serum, for example, $\frac{1}{10}$ and $\frac{1}{100}$ dilutions of serum with saline, as well as undiluted serum. The presence or intensity of agglutination of red cells by antiglobulin serum does not necessarily correlate with the severity of the hemolytic process. Thus the test may be negative or weakly positive at the onset of the hemolytic process, or may remain strongly positive after recovery.

### DETECTION OF INCOMPLETE AGGLUTININS IN THE SERUM

In many patients with active acquired hemolytic anemia, the serum contains red-cell-coating antibodies that have properties similar to those of the antibodies attached to the red-cell surface. Presumably this is so because the patient's red cells are saturated with the antibody or because their affinity for the antibodies is low. In other patients, red-cell-coating antibodies are released or eluted from the red cells only under nonphysiologic conditions, such as exposure of red-cell membranes to a pH of 3.2–3.4 [110] or to a temperature of 60°C.[97] The presence of these antibodies can then be demonstrated by incubating the suspect serum with normal compatible red cells, and then testing the cells for sensitization. Three techniques may be employed.

#### THE INDIRECT COLLOID AGGLUTINATION TEST

In each of two 12- to 15-ml test tubes, add 0.5 ml of the patient's serum to 0.1 ml of normal compatible blood or of a 50-percent washed red-cell suspension derived from compatible blood. If a titration is desired, twofold dilutions of the patient's serum in saline may also be incubated with the normal red cells. Incubate for 1 hr at 37°C, centrifuge gently, discard the supernatant solution, and add to the red cells of one tube 0.5 ml of 5-percent PVP (or dextran) and to the cells of the other, 10 to 15 ml of warm saline. The procedure is thereafter the same as described above for the colloid agglutination test and for the detection of autoagglutination.

#### INTERPRETATION

Most patients with active acquired hemolytic anemia have a positive indirect colloid-agglutination test result. This finding does not establish the diagnosis any further than does the direct test. However, if the indirect test result is positive, the patient's serum may be incubated with a panel of red cells of various types in the hope of discovering that the antibody has specificity for a certain blood type. Although almost all patients with acquired hemolytic anemia possess a nonspecific antibody, a few cases have been encountered in which antibodies were present having specificity for known antigens (usually in the Rh system) in the patient's red cells.[111] This introduces the therapeutic possibility of transfusing the patient with normal red cells lacking that factor. The finding of a positive result from the indirect colloid-agglutination test, but not from a direct test, merely indicates incompatibility with the normal red cells employed. In patients previously transfused, with or without active hemolytic disease or a positive direct colloid-agglutination test result, a positive indirect test result is quite likely to be due to isoantibodies stimulated by previous transfusions.

#### THE INDIRECT ANTIGLOBULIN (COOMBS) TEST

This test is carried out as described in Unit 15. The quantity of antibody protein may be roughly estimated by this technique by performing the indirect antiglobulin test on red cells exposed to various dilutions of the patient's serum. Also, as in the direct antiglobulin test, the nature of the antibody protein may be partially determined by using antiglobulin serum previously neutralized, or absorbed, with gamma globulin.

#### INTERPRETATION

A positive result from an indirect antiglobulin test is subject to the same interpretation as is one from an indirect colloid-agglutination test.

## THE DETECTION OF INCOMPLETE ANTIBODIES BY USING TRYPSINIZED RED CELLS

Certain proteolytic enzymes act upon the red-cell surface to render these cells hypersusceptible to the influence of antibodies. Thus antibodies that merely agglutinate normal red cells may hemolyze trypsinized red cells, and incomplete antibodies may frankly agglutinate such red cells.[112] This phenomenon may be utilized in searching for incomplete antibodies in the patient's serum.

**Method.** Crystalline trypsin is dissolved in physiologic saline to make a 1-percent stock solution which may be stored for several days at 2–4°C. A 0.1-percent solution is made from this by mixing 1 part of stock solution with 9 parts of isotonic phosphate buffer, pH 7.8. To each volume of packed, washed, O-negative red cells, add 5 volumes of trypsin solution, incubate at 37°C for 1 hr, and wash the red cells 2 or 3 times in physiologic saline before making up to a 2- or 3-percent cell suspension. To 0.2–0.5 ml of the patient's serum, and of twofold dilutions thereof, add equal volumes of trypsinized red cells. Incubate for 1 hr at 37°C and read macroscopically for agglutination or hemolysis.

### INTERPRETATION

The finding of agglutination with this technique is subject to the same interpretations as are the other methods for determining serum antibodies described above. The technique is somewhat more laborious and is less widely used than are the simpler colloid agglutination or antiglobulin methods.

## TESTS FOR THE DETECTION OF HEMOLYSINS

The occurrence in the serum of patients with acquired hemolytic anemia of factors (presumed to be antibodies) that hemolyze normal red cells at body temperature in vitro is rare. Less infrequently, however, antibodies (hemolysins) appear that are hemolytic in vitro and are active chiefly at low temperatures. Such hemolysins should be sought particularly when there is clinical evidence of cold sensitivity (as with cold agglutinins) and when there are indications of intravascular hemolysis (that is, high plasma levels of hemoglobin and methemoglobin, hemoglobinuria, and hemosiderinuria). Since fixation of the antibody usually occurs most readily in the cold and at an acid pH,[101] and since complement is required for the end point of lysis, screening tests for hemolysins should include these factors. Thus it is important to use *fresh* serum from the patient to preserve the complement activity, particularly since the complement levels in patients with hemolysinic hemolytic anemias may be already reduced, and to obtain serum from blood that was allowed to clot at 37°C rather than at room temperature.

## ACID-SERUM TEST FOR THE PRESENCE OF HEMOLYSINS

The method is that presented earlier for the detection of hemolysins by acid-serum, except that a second set of tubes is incubated at 20–25°C.

### INTERPRETATION

Unlike the findings in paroxysmal nocturnal hemoglobinuria, serum hemolysins should hemolyze normal red cells as well as the patient's cells, whereas normal serum should hemolyze neither. Furthermore, hemolysis is usually more active at room temperature than at body temperature. If hemolysins are present, their concentration may be estimated by titration of the patient's serum in fresh normal acidified serum. Usually, serum hemolysins are associated with very high levels of cold agglutinins, as in some patients recovering from virus pneumonia. Although the cold-induced ischemic symptoms (Raynaud's phenomena, peripheral gangrene) in these patients may arise solely from autoagglutination by the high concentration of cold agglutinins, it is not always certain whether the hemolytic process is due to the increased mechanical fragility of cold-agglutinated cells or to the relatively low concentrations of hemolysin. In some patients with acquired hemolytic anemia associated with high titers of cold agglutinins, the red cells may be "coated" with complement, which in turn renders them agglutinable by colloidal media and by Coombs serum. The hemolytic mechanism in such patients is presumably even more complex. In some patients, cold hemolysins, sometimes of high titer, appear without abnormal levels of cold agglutinins. These patients, unlike those described above, have a clinical picture (including the leukopenia and urticaria) that can be entirely attributed to the direct or indirect actions of hemolysins activated by cold, causing the syndrome of paroxysmal cold hemoglobinuria. As with the hemolysins associated with high-titer cold agglutinins, the serums of these patients will hemolyze normal red cells at 20°C (see above), which temperature is cold enough for the cold-dependent antibody to attach to the cell and warm enough for the consequent fixation and hemolytic action of complement. These two steps in the lysis of red cells by cold hemolysins (such as occurs in paroxysmal cold hemoglobinuria) are separately revealed in the Donath-Landsteiner reaction.[113]

## PRESUMPTIVE DONATH-LANDSTEINER TEST— A SCREENING EXAMINATION

**Method.** The presumptive Donath-Landsteiner test is performed by the simple procedure of chilling a sample of 1 to 2 ml of whole defibrinated blood at 3° to 4°C in an ice bath for 20 min, and then incubating it for 1 hr at 37.5°C. As controls, one sample of blood is centrifuged immediately after defibrination and another is incubated at 37.5°C for 1 hr without chilling. (*Precaution:* These control samples should be kept warm to avoid sensitizing cells cooled to room temperature.)

### INTERPRETATIONS AND LIMITATIONS

The possible results and their interpretations are listed below.

*Hemolysis in the chilled tube only.* This is good presumptive evidence of a cold-active hemolysin. The complete test may then be warranted.

*No hemolysis.* If no hemolysis occurs, the presumptive test result is negative and excludes the disease paroxysmal cold hemoglobinuria. It is possible, but highly improbable, that a falsely negative result will occur from a decrease in complement in fresh serum or from anticomplementary action of the serum. Guinea pig serum can be added as a source of complement, as shown in Table 31. An important cause of hemolysis, which is *not* produced by a cold hemolysin, is the mechanical destruction of red cells agglutinated by cold autohemagglutinins. Thus the agitation of chilled blood containing cold agglutinins results in significant degrees of hemolysis that may be interpreted, erroneously, to result from a hemolysin. Gentle handling of the chilled sample will prevent mechanical hemolysis. Also, the red cells will appear agglutinated after chilling.

*Hemolysis in all tubes.* Approximately the same degree of moderate hemolysis in all three tubes usually indicates either hemoglobinemia in vivo or destruction of red cells by the mechanical trauma of defibrination of blood.

### COMPLETE DONATH-LANDSTEINER REACTION

The complete test will seldom be required because the presumptive test is usually adequate. The method for the complete test is as follows:

Table 31. *Donath-Landsteiner test.*

| Tube number | 5-percent suspension washed red cells, 0.5 ml | Fresh serum [a] | Heated serum, 0.5 ml | Treatment of mixtures | Hemolysis in paroxysmal cold hemoglobinuria |
|---|---|---|---|---|---|
| 1 | P [b] | P | | | 0 |
| 2 | C | P | | Incubate 1 hr | 0 |
| 3 | P | C | | at 37.5°C | 0 |
| 4 | C | C | | | 0 |
| 5 | P | P | | | 4+ |
| 6 | C | P | | Chill 20 min at | 4+ |
| 7 | P | C | | 3°C, incubate | 0 |
| 8 | C | C | | 1 hr at 37.5°C | 0 |
| 9 | P | | P [c] | | 0 |
| 10 | C | | P [c] | Chill 20 min at | 0 |
| 11 | P | | C | 3°C, incubate | 0 |
| 12 | C | | C | 1 hr at 37.5°C | 0 |

[a] Extra complement may be added by pipetting 0.1 ml of undiluted guinea pig serum to each tube containing fresh human serum.

[b] P = Patient, C = Control.

[c] In some but not all serums, the cold hemolysin is destroyed or greatly decreased by heating. Therefore, a separate test using heated serum and *added complement* may give little or no hemolysis.

REAGENTS. (1) Patient's serum is derived from defibrinated venous blood which is kept at body temperature to prevent fixing of the hemolytic antibody to the red cells. Ideally, blood is taken with a syringe, warmed to 40°C, introduced into a tube warmed to 37.5°C in a water bath, and centrifuged at this temperature in centrifuge cups filled with warm water.

(2) Patient's red blood cells are obtained as above, washed three times with an equal volume of physiologic saline that is warmed to 37.5°C, and made to a 5-percent suspension in saline. This procedure will avoid attachment of cold autohemagglutinins.

(3) Normal serum is obtained from defibrinated venous blood of the same blood group as the patient.

(4) Normal red blood cells are prepared in a 5-percent suspension as in 2.

(5) Inactivated serum is prepared by heating it for 30 min at 56°C to inactivate the complement.

(6) Guinea pig serum is used fresh or after preservation by freezing. Lyophilized guinea pig serum occasionally is inactive for this test while showing full activity (complement) with sensitized sheep cells.

**Method.** Combinations of 0.5-ml samples of the suspensions of red cells and of serums are made and treated as indicated in Table 31. The mixtures are then centrifuged, and the supernatant serums compared for hemolysis.

INTERPRETATION. The limitations and interpretations of results are similar to those pertaining to the presumptive Donath-Landsteiner test (above).

*Demonstration of a cold hemolysin.* A positive result, which is required to identify the presence of a cold hemolysin characteristic of paroxysmal cold hemoglobinuria, is shown in tubes 5 and 6 of Table 31. If guinea pig serum is added, the hemolysis in tubes 5 and 6 may be increased. If the cold hemolysin is thermostable, then addition of guinea pig serum to tubes 9 and 10 will reestablish hemolysis.

*Evidence that the patient's red cells are normal.* Unsensitized red cells from patients with paroxysmal cold hemoglobinuria are normal when examined morphologically, by the osmotic- or mechanical-fragility tests, or by the direct Coombs test.

*Positive Coombs test result.* Red cells that have been sensitized but not hemolyzed by the cold hemolysin show agglutination in the direct Coombs test.[114] This observation may lead to the erroneous diagnosis of acquired hemolytic jaundice, which disease is *not* associated with a *cold* hemolysin.

*Paroxysmal nocturnal hemoglobinuria.* The red cells from a patient with paroxysmal nocturnal hemoglobinuria may or may not be hemolyzed by *any* fresh compatible human serum at the normal pH of the blood in tubes 1, 3, 5, and 7 in Table 31. Added guinea pig serum would enhance this hemolysis, but there would be no hemolysis in tubes 9 and 10. The hemolysis occurs only with the patient's red cells. Tests in vivo may be performed to demonstrate intravascular hemolysis by chilling and then warming the finger (the Ehrlich test), or by chilling and warming of extremities (the Rosenbach test). In the latter procedure, it is advisable to chill only one extremity initially, and only if that fails to induce hemolysis to proceed to chill all four extremities, for in some patients serious hemolytic episodes may occur from such an exposure to cold. These procedures, when they give positive results, produce hemoglobinuria, hemoglobinemia, leukopenia, and, often, a later pyrogenic reaction. Details of the tests are described elsewhere.[2] Paroxysmal cold hemoglobinuria is usually, but not always, associated with previous syphilitic infection.

### Hemolytic Anemias Associated with Methemoglobinemia and Heinz-Body Formation

#### PATHOLOGIC PHYSIOLOGY

Hemolytic anemia may occur as the apparent result of intracellular oxidation by certain chemicals or drugs. When mild, it may be measurable only by de-

termining a reduction in the levels of certain intracellular constituents, such as glutathione. With greater disturbance of red-cell oxidation-reduction mechanisms, methemoglobin may appear in the cells, with or without increased red-cell destruction. Still more severe intracellular oxidation will cause the denaturation and precipitation of hemoglobin within the cells to form stainable inclusion granules called *Heinz bodies.* Since the first two changes are reversible,[115, 116] whereas the latter is not, these alterations are not necessarily coexistent at all times. "Heinz-body anemias" may occur spontaneously, particularly in premature newborn infants, probably as an inborn error of red-cell metabolism, or, more commonly, they may be induced by exposure to certain chemicals or drugs. As pointed out by Emerson and his associates,[117, 118] the basic action of drugs that induce this type of anemia is the introduction of a reversible oxidation-reduction system into the red cell. Drugs active in this respect generally possess resonating cyclic structures and catalyze intracellular oxidation. Certain drugs (notably the antimalarial compounds pamaquine and primaquine), when given in "ordinary" therapeutic amounts, affect the red cells of normal subjects little or not at all, but do cause Heinz-body anemia in certain susceptible individuals, most of whom are Negroes. Dern and his associates have demonstrated that the red cells of these subjects are metabolically hypersusceptible to oxidant drugs,[119] apparently through a genetically determined deficiency of the oxidative enzyme glucose-6-phosphate dehydrogenase.[120]

#### SCREENING-TEST FINDINGS

Characteristically, examination of Wright's-stained smears of blood from patients with drug-induced or Heinz-body anemias reveals the presence of fragmented red cells and cells from which a "bite" appears to have been taken. Spherocytosis, basophilic stippling, and various inclusions may be encountered.

In suspected cases, a special examination should be conducted for Heinz bodies, which are not visible with ordinary Romanowsky stains. They may be visible as rounded, refractile inclusions by examination of thin blood smears or suspensions by dark-ground or phase-contrast microscopy. The particles vary in size from less than 1 $\mu$ to half the size of the cells, tend to lie in proximity to the cell membrane, and when in a wet cell suspension are subject to Brownian movements. Staining of Heinz bodies may be achieved by mixing equal volumes of blood and of 0.5-percent methyl violet in 0.85-percent sodium chloride solution in a test tube. After 10 or 15 min, one or two drops of the mixture are placed on a glass slide and covered with a glass coverslip, which is then gently blotted with a sheet of filter paper. Heinz bodies stain an intense purple, whereas Howell-Jolly bodies and siderocytes are blue-black and the reticulum of reticulocytes is pale blue. As a control, Heinz bodies may be produced in a normal blood sample by adding a small amount of acetyl phenyl hydrazine and examining the cells after the sample turns brown.

## METHEMOGLOBIN

A method for determining the presence of methemoglobin is presented in Unit 5.

## INTERPRETATION

The finding of Heinz bodies or of methemoglobinemia, or both, in patients with hemolytic anemia requires an investigation of possible exposure to the drugs and chemicals described above. At times, histories of such drug exposures may be difficult to elicit, as in infants with hemolysis induced by the skin absorption of naphthoquinone (mothballs) or the inhalation of its fumes, or in adults habituated to proprietary compounds containing acetanilid or phenacetin. Since red cells containing Heinz bodies may circulate for as long as a week or more before their removal by the spleen,[121] and since methemoglobin is converted back to hemoglobin in vivo in a matter of several hours,[116] it is not unusual to encounter Heinz bodies in affected patients in whom methemoglobin is no longer demonstrable. Such a course of events is illustrated in Table 32.[122] In

Table 32. *Effect of the administration of phenylhydrazine to a normal dog.*[a, 123]

| Day | Hemo-globin (gm/ 100 ml) | Reticu-locytes (percent) | Red cells containing Heinz bodies (percent) | Methemo-globin (percent) |
|---|---|---|---|---|
| 0 | 13.6 | 1.2 | 0 | 0.7 |
| 1 | 10.9 | 1.9 | 41 | 2.4 |
| 2 | 9.4 | 4.7 | 100 | 13.2 |
| 3 | 7.6 | 5.4 | 100 | 5.2 |
| 5 | 5.1 | 13.9 | 59 | 2.6 |
| 6 | 4.4 | 13.7 | 19 | 2.3 |
| 7 | 4.3 | 12.3 | 20 | |
| 9 | 4.8 | 19.6 | 2 | |
| 12 | 6.2 | 16.4 | 0 | |
| 14 | 7.0 | 11.0 | | |
| 17 | 7.5 | 14.0 | | |
| 22 | 8.9 | 4.0 | | |
| 28 | 10.0 | 2.1 | | |
| 35 | 10.5 | 2.9 | | |
| 42 | 12.1 | 2 6 | | |
| 49 | 13.5 | 0.5 | | |
| 63 | 13.2 | .1 | | |

[a] Dog was given 20 mg of phenylhydrazine per kilogram of body weight subcutaneously on day 0 and on day 1.

vitro tests for detecting hypersusceptibility to oxidant drugs have been described. These are based on the excessive formation of Heinz bodies [123] (or the excessive diminution of cellular-reduced glutathione) [124] when susceptible red cells are exposed to a representative oxidant drug such as acetylphenylhydrazine.

## POLYCYTHEMIA

Polycythemia exists when the blood hemoglobin concentration exceeds the upper limit of normal, which is approximately 17.5 gm/100 ml. This increase in hemoglobin concentration is usually associated with an increase above normal in hematocrit (more than 52 percent), in red-blood-cell count (more than $6 \times 10^6/mm^3$), and in total red-cell mass (more than 30 ml/kg). Despite the fact that the hemoglobin concentration is the physiologically significant parameter, most of the signs and symptoms in polycythemic patients are probably related to the concomitant increase in viscosity of whole blood and to the increase in red-cell mass. The polycythemias can be divided into relative and absolute polycythemia and classified as in Table 33.

Table 33. *Etiologic classification of polycythemias.*

| | |
|---|---|
| A. Relative polycythemia | Hemoconcentration |
| B. Absolute polycythemia | |
| 1. Secondary | |
| *a.* Tissue anoxia | High altitude |
| | Alveolar hypoventilation |
| | Chronic pulmonary disease |
| | Right-to-left shunt |
| | Methemoglobin and carboxyhemoglobin |
| *b.* Pharmacologic agents | Cobalt |
| | Testosterone |
| *c.* Neoplasm | Subtentorial tumor |
| | Renal, hepatic and uterine tumors |
| *d.* Miscellaneous | Cushing's disease |
| | Hydronephrosis |
| 2. Primary | Polycythemia vera |

### RELATIVE POLYCYTHEMIA

Relative polycythemia is frequently found in acute dehydrating illnesses and is characterized by a decrease in total plasma volume without a concomitant change in total red-cell mass. It is observed in burns and crush injuries, where there is a loss of protein-containing fluid, and in conditions of extracellular dehydration such as water deprivation, diarrhea, vomiting, excessive sweating, or polyuria. The degree of polycythemia can be used as a rough guide to the magnitude of the fluid deficit but is otherwise of little clinical significance. However, if dehydration occurs in a patient with pre-existing absolute polycythemia, the increase in blood viscosity may lead to cardiac strain or vascular thrombosis.

### ABSOLUTE POLYCYTHEMIA

Absolute polycythemia is characterized by an increased rate of red-cell production and an increase in total red-cell mass. It is found in a variety of diseases in which the oxygen transport to the tissues is impaired (secondary polycythemia) and in these diseases it presumably serves a useful purpose by facilitating the oxygen transfer. It is also found in association with certain tumors and after the administration of cobalt or testosterone. Under these conditions its physiologic significance is still unknown. Finally, it occurs as a primary or idiopathic form, polycythemia vera, a condition which at present is considered to be caused by a neoplastic proliferation of bone-marrow cells.

#### ABSOLUTE POLYCYTHEMIA SECONDARY TO TISSUE ANOXIA

Absolute polycythemia secondary to tissue anoxia is found at high altitudes where the low oxygen pressure of atmospheric air results in arterial unsaturation and impaired oxygen delivery to the tissues. An increase in number of circulating red cells along with compensatory changes in the respiratory and cardiovascular systems will permit acclimatized people to live normal, active lives even at altitudes up to 15,000 ft where the partial oxygen pressure is reduced to 90 mm-of-mercury. However, this is accomplished at a certain physiologic cost. The blood viscosity is increased, the blood volume is expanded, and both the pulmonary and the cardiac reserves are severely diminished.

Impairment of the respiratory center or mechanical interference with the chest motions leads to alveolar hypoventilation and tissue anoxia and eventually to polycythemia [125, 126] (see Unit 34). Chronic pulmonary diseases with bronchial obstruction or thickened alveolar membranes will likewise cause arterial unsaturation. However, frank polycythemia is rare in chronic pulmonary disorders, possibly because the rate of red-cell production is inhibited in patients suffering from inflammatory diseases.[127] In congenital heart disease with a right-to-left shunt, arterial blood is unsaturated and the oxygen transport suffers. Arterial unsaturation is similarly present in patients with pulmonary hemangiomata or pulmonary arteriovenous fistulas, and in some patients with Laennec's cirrhosis where vascular mediastinal anastomoses are formed between the portal circulation and the pulmonary veins.[128] Congenital methemoglobinemia and chronic exposure to carbon monoxide will reduce the oxygen-carrying capacity of hemoglobin and are frequently associated with a compensatory polycythemia.

### ABSOLUTE POLYCYTHEMIA SECONDARY TO PHARMACOLOGIC AGENTS

Cobalt, as mentioned previously under the section on histotoxic anoxia, exerts a stimulating action on the rate of red-cell production. Testosterone given in pharmacologic doses over long periods of time has been found to cause polycythemia,[129] and chronic cortisone administration may lead to a moderate increase in the hemoglobin concentration.[130]

### ABSOLUTE POLYCYTHEMIA SECONDARY TO NEOPLASMS

A considerable number of cases have been reported in which polycythemia and various tumors have occurred together. Subtentorial intracranial tumors, especially cerebellar hemangioblastomas, are not infrequently associated with polycythemia. In some cases, the polycythemia appears to be caused by a decrease in plasma volume, but in other cases the total red-cell mass has been found to be significantly increased.[131] Although it could be anticipated that the tumor might encroach upon the respiratory center, alveolar hypoventilation and arterial unsaturation have not been demonstrated, and it is uncertain at present whether the tumor produces polycythemia through a direct humoral or neurologic mechanism or whether the polycythemia is secondary to impaired respiratory function. Uterine myoma,[132] hepatic carcinoma,[133] and renal hypernephroma [134] are occasionally associated with absolute polycythemia. In a number of instances, surgical removal of a hypernephroma associated with polycythemia has resulted in a striking hematologic remission. It has been suggested that these tumors, especially the hypernephroma, may release an erythropoietically active substance.

### ABSOLUTE POLYCYTHEMIA SECONDARY TO MISCELLANEOUS DISORDERS

Polycythemia is usually thought to be a common complication of Cushing's disease. However, the ruddy, moonfaced appearance in Cushing's disease is somewhat deceiving and the hemoglobin concentration is rarely increased to more than the upper limit of normal. In a few cases, polycythemia has been found to be associated with hydronephrosis,[135] and surgical removal of the involved kidney has led to prompt hematologic remission.

### PRIMARY POLYCYTHEMIA

Polycythemia vera is a chronic illness characterized by an unrestricted and presumably purposeless proliferation of all the bone marrow elements resulting in erythrocytosis and frequently in leukocytosis and thrombocytosis.[1, 2, 136–141]

An increase in the rate of red-blood-cell production, despite normal or near normal saturation of arterial blood with oxygen, is the most striking feature of this disease and will account for many of the clinical findings. Owing to continuous overproduction of red cells with a normal life span, the red-cell count and hemoglobin concentration rise, the viscosity of the blood increases, and the red-cell mass expands from a normal of 30 ml/kg up to as high as 90 ml/kg. The increased blood viscosity is probably of importance in the frequent occurrence of vascular thrombosis. However, since vascular accidents are so much more common in polycythemia vera than in secondary polycythemia, it appears that a simultaneous increase in platelets may contribute materially to the development of these complications. An accelerated white-cell production with a moderate peripheral leukocytosis and occasional metamyelocyte and myelocyte in the smear is of diagnostic importance in polycythemia vera, but does not cause symptoms. The blood platelets are characteristically increased in number and are frequently found to be large and of abnormal appearance. The clot retraction is often poor and the clots are fragile and dissolve easily. Whether these usually minor changes in the clotting mechanism are responsible for the frequent occurrence of ecchymoses and mucous-membrane bleeding or whether this hemorrhagic tendency is caused by vascular distention is still unknown.

The pathogenesis of polycythemia vera is not clear. The production of red cells is greatly in excess of the physiologic demand for oxygen-carrying red blood cells. A slight undersaturation of arterial blood with oxygen is often found, but the saturation is rarely below 90–92 percent, as compared with the normal of 95 percent, and this slight degree of undersaturation is far too small to account for the accelerated erythropoietic activity.

The accelerated production of white cells and platelets, as well as of red cells, has led to the hypothesis that polycythemia vera is a neoplastic process involving all the cellular elements of the bone marrow and only quantitatively but not qualitatively different from myeloid leukemia, erythroleukemia, or agnogenic myeloid metaplasia.[142] This hypothesis is supported by the fact that polycythemia vera not infrequently terminates in myelogenous leukemia or agnogenic myeloid metaplasia. Recent studies of the enzyme content of leukocytes have, however, revealed a basic difference between leukemic granulocytes and granulocytes from patients with polycythemia vera or agnogenic myeloid metaplasia. In chronic myeloid leukemia, the granulocyte content of alkaline phosphatase was found to be low, while the granulocytes in polycythemia vera and agnogenic myeloid metaplasia usually contained increased amounts.[143] The belief that these diseases represent different phases or aspects of a single myeloproliferative disorder must at the present be considered an attractive but unproved working hypothesis.

### SCREENING TESTS FOR POLYCYTHEMIA

HEMOGLOBIN, HEMATOCRIT, AND RED-CELL COUNT. Hemoglobin concentration higher than 17.5 gm/100 ml; hematocrit higher than 52 percent; red-cell count higher than $6 \times 10^6$ cells/mm³

WHITE-CELL AND PLATELET COUNT. In *relative polycythemia* and *absolute secondary polycythemia,* the counts are normal; in *polycythemia vera,* the white-cell count is commonly higher than 10,000/mm³; and the platelet count is commonly higher than 300,000/mm³.

BLOOD SMEAR. Thin smears are essential because of the increased number of red cells. In *relative polycythemia* and in *ab-*

153

solute secondary polycythemia, the smear is normal. In early cases of *polycythemia vera*, the smear is normal although there may be a few metamyelocytes and a rare nucleated red cell. Platelets often appear increased in number. In late cases, there are nucleated red cells but no significant increase in the number of reticulocytes. The presence of large numbers of nucleated red cells along with anisocytosis and poikilocytosis suggests a transition of the disease into agnogenic myeloid metaplasia. There is an increase in the number of leukocytes with many metamyelocytes and myelocytes. The platelets may be strikingly increased with large and bizarre forms.

BONE MARROW. In *relative polycythemia*, the marrow is normal. In *absolute secondary polycythemia*, the marrow is normal or slightly hyperplastic, with decreased fat and usually a slight relative increase in the number of nucleated red blood cells. The marrow is hard to interpret and is rarely of diagnostic significance. In *polycythemia vera*, the marrow is hyperplastic, with normal cellular distribution except for an increase in the number of megakaryocytes. When this increase is striking, it will clearly differentiate polycythemia vera from secondary polycythemia. However, the marrow morphology often is not diagnostic.

SPECIAL TESTS

TOTAL RED-CELL MASS. The total red-cell mass can be determined by means of Evans blue dye which is bound by plasma albumin or by tagging red blood cells with radioactive phosphorus or, preferably, chromium. The *normal value* is 30 ml/kg of body weight. In *relative polycythemia*, the value is near normal. In *absolute polycythemia*, both primary and secondary, the value is increased.

ARTERIAL OXYGEN SATURATION. In *relative polycythemia*, the arterial oxygen saturation is 95–100 percent; in *absolute secondary polycythemia*, it is 60–90 percent; in *polycythemia vera*, it is 90–100 percent.

REFERENCES

1. W. B. Castle, "Disorders of the blood," in W. A. Sodeman, ed., *Pathologic Physiology: Mechanisms of Disease* (ed. 2; Saunders, Philadelphia, 1956), chap. 28.
2. M. M. Wintrobe, *Clinical Hematology* (ed. 4; Lea and Febiger, Philadelphia, 1956).
3. L. G. Lajtha, "Bone marrow cell metabolism," *Physiol. Rev. 37*, 50 (1957).
4. B. Thorell, "Studies on the formation of cellular substances during blood cell production," *Acta med. scand.*, Supp. 200 (1947).
5. J. V. Dacie and J. C. White, "Erythropoiesis with particular reference to its study by biopsy of human marros," *J. clin. Path. 2*, 1 (1949).
6. H. Wiecker, "Das Mass-Mengen- und Zeitgefüge der Erythropoiese unter physiologischen und pathologischen Bedingungen," *Schweiz. med. Wschr. 87*, 1 (1957).
7. E. E. Osgood, "Number and distribution of human hemic cells," *Blood 9*, 1141 (1954).
8. H. M. Patt, "A consideration of the myeloid-erythroid balance in man," *Blood 12*, 777 (1957).
9. D. Donohue, R. H. Reiff, M. L. Hanson, Y. Betson, and C. A. Finch, "Quantitative measurement of the erythrocytic and granulocytic cells of the marrow and blood," *J. clin. Invest. 37*, 1571 (1958).

10. W. Crosby, "The red cell and some of its problems," *Ann. Rev. Med. 8,* 151 (1957).
11. S. Granick, "The chemistry and functioning of the mammalian erythrocyte," *Blood 4,* 404 (1949).
12. B. W. Gabrio, C. A. Finch, and F. M. Huennekens, "Erythrocyte preservation: A topic in molecular biochemistry," *Blood 11,* 103 (1956).
13. R. Lemberg and J. W. Legge, *Hematin Compounds and Bile Pigments* (Interscience, New York, 1949).
14. R. L. Riley, J. L. Lilienthal, Jr., D. D. Proemmel, and R. E. Franke, "The relationships of oxygen, carbon dioxide and hemoglobin in the blood of man: Oxyhemoglobin dissociation under various physiological conditions," *J. clin. Invest. 25,* 139 (1946).
15. National Research Council Committee on Aviation Medicine, *Handbook of Respiratory Data in Aviation* (Office of Scientific Research and Development, Washington, 1944).
16. H. E. Kaufman and S. W. Rosen, "Clinical acid-base regulation. The Bronsted schema," *Surg. Gynec. Obstet. 103,* 101 (1956).
17. W. C. Grant and W. S. Root, "Fundamental stimulus for erythropoiesis," *Physiol. Rev. 32,* 449 (1952).
18. A. J. Erslev, "Effect of anemic anoxia on the cellular development of nucleated red cells," *Blood 14,* 386 (1959).
19. A. J. Erslev, "Physiologic control of red cell production," *Blood 10,* 954 (1955).
20. F. Stohlman, Jr., and G. Brecher, "Humoral regulation of erythropoiesis. III. Effect of exposure to simulated altitude," *J. lab. clin. Med. 49,* 890 (1957).
21. C. W. Gurney, E. Goldwasser, and C. Pan, "Studies on erythropoiesis. VI. Erythropoietin in human plasma," *J. lab. clin. Med. 50,* 534 (1957).
22. M. S. Sacks, "Erythropoietin" (editorial), *Ann. intern. Med. 48,* 207 (1958).
23. C. S. Houston and R. L. Riley, "Respiratory and circulatory changes during acclimatization to high altitude," *Amer. J. Physiol. 149,* 565 (1947).
24. J. Barcroft, *The Respiratory Function of the Blood* (Cambridge University Press, New York, 1925).
25. J. H. Jandl and W. B. Castle, unpublished observations.
26. A. Hurtado, C. F. Merino, and E. Delgado, "Influence of anoxemia on hematopoietic activity," *Arch. intern. Med. 75,* 284 (1945).
27. J. C. Stickney and E. J. Van Liere, "Acclimatization to low oxygen tension," *Physiol. Rev. 33,* 13 (1953).
28. E. Brown, J. Hopper, and R. Wennesland, "Blood volume and its regulation," *Ann. Rev. Physiol. 19,* 231 (1957).
29. R. J. Bing, L. D. Vandam, J. C. Handelsman, J. A. Campbell, R. Spender, and H. E. Griswold, "Physiologic studies in congenital heart disease. VI. Adaptation to anoxia in congenital heart disease with cyanosis," *Bull. Johns Hopk. Hosp. 83,* 439 (1948).
30. H. Winterstein, "Chemical control of pulmonary ventilation," *New Engl. J. Med. 255,* 217 (1956).
31. W. H. Crosby, "Treatment of haemochromatosis by energetic phlebotomy. One patient's response to the letting of 55 litres of blood in 11 months," *Brit. J. Haemat. 4,* 82 (1958).
32. D. C. Van Dyke, J. F. Garcia, and J. H. Lawrence, "Concentration of highly

potent erythropoietic activity from urine of patients with aplastic anemia," *Proc. Soc. exp. Biol.* (*N. Y.*) *96*, 541 (1957).

33. E. P. Sharpey-Schafer, "Cardiac output in severe anemia," *Clin. Sci. 5*, 125 (1944).

34. A. C. Kennedy and D. J. Valtis, "The oxygen dissociation curve in anemia of various types," *J. clin. Invest. 33*, 1372 (1954).

35. E. S. Brannon, A. J. Merrill, J. V. Warren, and E. A. Stead, Jr., "The cardiac output in patients with chronic anemia as measured by the technique of right atrial catheterization," *J. clin. Invest. 24*, 332 (1945).

36. J. D. Hatcher, "The physiological responses of the circulation to anaemia. Modern concepts of cardiovascular disease," *Amer. Heart J. 23*, 235 (1954).

37. S. Hedlund, "Studies on erythropoiesis and total red cell volume in congestive heart failure," *Acta med. scand.*, Supp. 284 (1953).

38. L. Berk, J. H. Burchenal, and W. B. Castle, "Erythropoietic effect of cobalt in patients with or without anemia," *New Engl. J. Med. 240*, 754 (1949).

39. D. Burk, J. Hearon, L. Caroline, and A. L. Schade, "Reversible complexes of cobalt, histidine and oxygen gas," *J. biol. Chem. 165*, 723 (1946).

40. H. D. van Liew, "Oxygen tension of subcutaneous gas pockets in cobalt-treated mice and adrenalectomized mice," *Proc. Soc. exp. Biol.* (*N. Y.*) *94*, 112 (1957).

41. E. Goldwasser, L. O. Jacobson, W. Fried, and L. F. Plzak, "Studies on erythropoiesis. Part V. The effect of cobalt on the production of erythropoietin," *Blood 13*, 55 (1958).

42. F. R. Birkhill, M. A. Maloney, and S. M. Levenson, "Effect of transfusion polycythemia upon bone marrow and erythrocyte survival in man," *Blood 6*, 1021 (1951).

43. J. C. Tinsley, Jr., C. V. More, R. Dubach, V. Minnick, and M. Grinstein, "The role of oxygen in the regulation of erythropoiesis. Depression of the rate of delivery of new red cells to the blood by high concentrations of inspired oxygen," *J. clin. Invest. 28*, 1544 (1949).

44. C. E. Rath and C. A. Finch, "Sternal marrow hemosiderin," *J. lab. clin. Med. 33*, 81 (1948).

45. G. Kitzes, C. A. Elvehjem, and H. A. Schuette, "The determination of blood plasma iron," *J. biol. Chem. 155*, 653 (1944).

46. T. Peters, T. J. Giovanniello, L. Apt, and J. F. Ross, "A simple improved method for the determination of serum iron. II," *J. lab. clin. Med. 48*, 280 (1956).

47. C. E. Rath and C. A. Finch, "Chemical, clinical and immunological studies on the products of human plasma fractionation. XXXVIII. Serum iron transport. Measurement of iron-binding capacity of serum in man," *J. clin. Invest. 28*, 79 (1949).

48. T. Peters, T. J. Giovanniello, L. Apt, and J. F. Ross, "A new method for the determination of serum iron-binding capacity. I," *J. lab. clin. Med. 48*, 274 (1956).

49. E. Schodt, "Observations on blood regeneration in man. III. The rise in reticulocytes in patients with hematemesis or melana from peptic ulcer," *Amer. J. med. Sci. 196*, 632 (1938).

50. J. W. Harris, J. M. Price, R. M. Whittington, R. Weisman, Jr., and D. L. Horrigan, "Pyridoxine responsive anemia in the adult human," *J. clin. Invest. 35*, 709 (1956).

51. W. B. Castle, "Development of knowledge concerning the gastric intrinsic factor and its relation to pernicious anemia," *New Engl. J. Med. 249*, 603 (1953).

52. B. Von Bonsdorff and R. Gordin, "Treatment of pernicious anemia with intramuscular injections of tapeworm extracts. Diphyllobothrium latum and pernicious anemia," *Acta med. scand. 144*, 263 (1953).

53. J. A. Halstead, "Megaloblastic anemia associated with surgically produced gastrointestinal abnormalities," *Calif. Med. 83*, 212 (1955).

54. R. M. Graham and M. H. Rheault, "Characteristic cellular changes in cells of nonhemopoietic origin in pernicious anemia," *J. lab. clin. Med. 43*, 235 (1954).

55. E. H. Reisner, J. A. Wolff, R. J. McKay, Jr., and E. F. Doyle, "Juvenile pernicious anemia," *Pediatrics 8*, 88 (1951).

56. D. L. Mollin, S. J. Baker, and I. Doniach, "Addisonian pernicious anemia without gastric atrophy in a young man," *Brit. J. Haemat. 1*, 278 (1955).

57. W. B. Castle and G. R. Minot, *Pathological Physiology and Clinical Description of the Anemias* (Oxford University Press, New York, 1936).

58. G. I. M. Ross, "Vitamin B$_{12}$ assay in body fluids," *Nature 166*, 270 (1950); A. A. Lear, J. W. Harris, W. B. Castle, and E. M. Fleming, "The serum vitamin B$_{12}$ concentration in pernicious anemia," *J. lab. clin. Med. 44*, 715 (1954).

59. S. T. Callender, A. Turnbull, and G. Wakisaka, "Estimation of intrinsic factor of Castle by use of radioactive vitamin B$_{12}$," *Brit. med. J. 1*, 10 (1954).

60. R. F. Schilling, "The effect of gastric juice on the urinary excretion of radioactivity after the oral administration of radioactive vitamin B$_{12}$," *J. lab. clin. Med. 42*, 860 (1953).

61. G. B. J. Glass, L. J. Boyd, G. A. Gellin, and L. Stephanson, "Uptake of radioactive vitamin B$_{12}$ by the liver in humans," *Arch. Biochem. 51*, 251 (1954).

62. G. M. Watson and L. J. Witts, "Intestinal macrocytic anemia," *Brit. med. J. 1*, 13 (1952).

63. C. F. Hawkins and M. J. Meynell, "Megaloblastic anemia due to phenytoin sodium," *Lancet 2*, 737 (1954).

64. J. H. Jandl and A. A. Lear, "The metabolism of folic acid in cirrhosis," *Ann. intern. Med. 45*, 1027 (1956).

65. L. J. Tepley and C. A. Elvehjem, "The titrimetric determination of 'Lactobacillus casei factor' and 'folic acid,'" *J. biol. Chem. 157*, 303 (1945).

66. H. P. Broquist, "Evidence for the excretion of formiminoglutamic acid following folic acid antagonist therapy in acute leukemia," *J. Amer. chem. Soc. 78*, 6205 (1956).

67. H. Tabor and L. Wyngarden, "A method for the determination of formiminoglutamic acid in urine," *J. clin. Invest. 37*, 824 (1958).

68. F. G. Ebaugh, Jr., C. P. Emerson, and J. F. Ross, "The use of radioactive chromium [51] as an erythrocyte tagging agent for the determination of red cell survival in vivo," *J. clin. Invest. 32*, 1260 (1953).

69. R. V. Ebert and C. P. Emerson, Jr., "A clinical study of transfusion reactions: The hemolytic effect of group O blood and pooled plasma containing incompatible isoagglutinins," *J. clin. Invest. 25*, 627 (1946).

70. C. B. Laurell and M. Nyman, "Studies on the serum haptoglobin level in hemoglobinemia and its influence on renal excretion of hemoglobin," *Blood 12*, 493 (1957).

71. F. C. Bing and R. W. Baker, "The determination of hemoglobin in minute amounts of blood by Wu's method," *J. biol. Chem.* 92, 589 (1931).
72. W. H. Crosby and F. W. Furth, "A modification of the benzidine method for measurement of hemoglobin in plasma and urine," *Blood 11*, 380 (1956).
73. N. H. Fairley, "Methaemalbumin," *Quart. J. Med. 10*, 95 (1941).
74. T. A. J. Prankerd, K. I. Altman, and L. E. Young, "Abnormalities of carbohydrate metabolism of red cells in hereditary spherocytosis," *J. clin. Invest. 34*, 1268 (1955).
75. C. P. Emerson, Jr., S. C. Shen, T. H. Ham, and W. B. Castle, "The mechanism of blood destruction in congenital hemolytic jaundice," *J. clin. Invest. 26*, 1180 (1947).
76. G. A. Daland and K. Worthley, "The resistance of red blood cells to hemolysis in hypotonic solutions of sodium chloride," *J. lab. clin. Med. 20*, 1122 (1935).
77. S. C. Shen, T. H. Ham, and E. M. Fleming, "Studies on destruction of red blood cells. III. Mechanism and complications of hemoglobinuria in patients with thermal burns: spherocytosis and increased osmotic fragility of erythrocytes," *New Engl. J. Med. 229*, 701 (1943).
78. C. P. Emerson, Jr., S. C. Shen, T. H. Ham, E. M. Fleming, and W. B. Castle, "Studies on the destruction of red blood cells. IX. Quantitative methods for determining the osmotic and mechanical fragility of red cells in the peripheral blood and splenic pulp; the mechanism of increased hemolysis in hereditary spherocytosis (congenital hemolytic jaundice) as related to the functions of the spleen," *Arch. intern. Med. 97*, 5 (1956).
79. S. C. Shen, W. B. Castle, and E. M. Fleming, "Experimental and clinical observations on increased mechanical fragility of erythrocytes," *Science 100*, 387 (1944).
80. L. Pauling, H. A. Itano, S. J. Singer, and I. C. Wells, "Sickle cell anemia, a molecular disease," *Science 110*, 543 (1949).
81. H. C. Schwartz, T. H. Spaet, W. W. Zuelzer, J. V. Neel, A. R. Robinson, and S. F. Kaufman, "Combinations of hemoglobin G, hemoglobin S and thalassemia occurring in one family," *Blood 12*, 238 (1957).
82. D. A. Rigas, R. D. Koler, and E. E. Osgood, "Hemoglobin H," *J. lab. clin. Med. 47*, 51 (1956).
83. I. C. Wells and H. A. Itano, "Ratio of sickle cell anemia hemoglobin to normal hemoglobin in sicklemics," *J. biol. Chem. 188*, 65 (1951).
84. E. W. Smith and C. L. Conley, "Filter paper electrophoresis of human hemoglobins with special reference to the incidence and clinical significance of hemoglobin C," *Bull. Johns Hopk. Hosp. 93*, 94 (1953).
85. H. J. McDonald, *Ionography, Electrophoresis in Stabilized Media* (Yearbook Publishers, Chicago, 1955).
86. H. A. Itano, W. R. Bergren, and P. Sturgeon, "The abnormal human hemoglobins," *Medicine 35*, 121 (1956).
87. H. A. Itano, "Solubilities of naturally occurring mixtures of human hemoglobin," *Arch. Biochem. 47*, 148 (1953).
88. T. H. J. Huisman and H. K. Prins, "Chromatographic estimation of four different kinds of human hemoglobin," *J. lab. clin. Med. 46*, 255 (1955).
89. J. W. Harris, "Studies on the destruction of red blood cells. VIII. Molecular orientation in sickle cell hemoglobin solutions," *Proc. Soc. exp. Biol. (N. Y.) 75*, 197 (1950).

90. M. S. Greenberg, E. H. Kass, and W. B. Castle, "Studies on the destruction of red blood cells. XII. Factors influencing the role of S hemoglobin in the pathologic physiology of sickle cell anemia and related disorders," *J. clin. Invest. 36*, 833 (1957).

91. G. A. Daland and W. B. Castle, "A simple and rapid method for demonstrating sickling of the red blood cells; the use of reducing agents," *J. lab. clin. Med. 33*, 1082 (1948).

92. K. Singer, A. M. Josephson, L. Singer, P. Heller, and H. J. Zimmerman, "Studies in abnormal hemoglobins. XIII. Hemoglobin S-thalassemia disease and hemoglobin C-thalassemia disease in siblings," *Blood 12*, 593 (1957).

93. H. G. Kunkel and G. Wallenius, "New hemoglobin in normal adult blood," *Science 122*, 288 (1955).

94. P. S. Gerald and L. K. Diamond, "The diagnosis of thalassemia trait by starch block electrophoresis of the hemoglobin," *Blood 13*, 61 (1958).

95. K. Singer, A. I. Chernoff, and L. Singer, "Studies on abnormal hemoglobins. I. Their demonstration in sickle cell anemia and other hematologic disorders by means of alkali denaturation," *Blood 6*, 413 (1956).

96. T. H. Ham, "Studies on destruction of red blood cells. I. Chronic hemolytic anemia with paroxysmal nocturnal hemoglobinuria," *Arch. intern. Med. 64*, 1271 (1939).

97. J. V. Dacie, *The Haemolytic Anemias* (Grune and Stratton, New York, 1954).

98. F. H. Gardner, "Transfer to normal red cells of an agglutinin demonstrable in the acidified sera of patients with acquired hemolytic jaundice," *J. clin. Invest. 28*, 783 (1949).

99. J. H. Jandl, A. R. Jones, and W. B. Castle, "The destruction of red cells by antibodies in man. I. Observations on the sequestration and lysis of red cells altered by immune mechanisms," *J. clin. Invest. 36*, 1428 (1957).

100. W. Dameshek and S. O. Schwartz, "Acute hemolytic anemia," *Medicine 19*, 231 (1940).

101. J. V. Dacie, "The presence of cold hemolysins in sera containing cold hemagglutinins," *J. Path. Bact. 62*, 241 (1950).

102. M. Finland, O. L. Peterson, H. E. Allen, B. A. Samper, and M. W. Barnes, "Cold agglutinins (a series of six papers)," *J. clin. Invest. 24*, 451 (1945).

103. T. H. Ham, F. H. Gardner, and P. F. Wagley, "Studies on the metabolism of hemolytic anemia and hemoglobinuria occurring in patients with high concentrations of cold agglutinins," *J. clin. Invest. 27*, 538 (1948).

104. J. H. Jandl and W. B. Castle, "Agglutination of sensitized red cells by large anisometric molecules," *J. lab. clin. Med. 47*, 669 (1956).

105. A. S. Wiener, "Conglutination test for Rh sensitization," *J. lab. clin. Med. 30*, 662 (1945).

106. L. K. Diamond and R. L. Denton, "Rh agglutination in various media with particular reference to the value of albumin," *J. lab. clin. Med. 30*, 821 (1945).

107. R. R. A. Coombs, A. E. Mourant and R. R. Race, "A new test for the detection of weak and 'incomplete' Rh agglutinins," *Brit. J. exp. Path. 36*, 225 (1945).

108. L. K. Diamond and N. M. Abelson, "The demonstration of anti-Rh agglutinin —an accurate and rapid slide test," *J. lab. clin. Med. 30*, 204, 668 (1945).

109. J. H. Vaughan, "Immunological features of erythrocyte sensitization. I. Acquired hemolytic disease," *Blood 11*, 1085 (1956).

110. P. Kidd, "Elution of an incomplete type of antibody from the erythrocytes in acquired hemolytic anemia," *J. clin. Path. 2*, 103 (1949).

111. W. Weiner, D. A. Battey, T. E. Cleghorn, F. G. W. Marson, and M. J. Meynell, "Serological findings in a case of haemolytic anaemia with some general observations on the pathogenesis of this syndrome," *Brit. med. J. 2*, 125 (1953).

112. J. A. Morton and M. M. Pickles, "The proteolytic enzyme test for detecting incomplete antibodies," *J. clin. Path. 4*, 189 (1951).

113. J. Donath and K. Landsteiner, "Ueber paroxysmalen Hämoglobinurie," *Münsch. med. Wschr. 51*, 1590 (1904).

114. A. A. Siemens, W. H. Zinkham, and P. F. Waglen, "Observations on the mechanism of hemolysis in paroxysmal (cold) hemoglobinuria," *Blood 3*, 1367 (1948).

115. E. Beutler, R. J. Dern, C. L. Flanagan, and A. S. Alving, "The hemolytic effect of primaquine. VII. Biochemical studies of drug-sensitive erythrocytes," *J. lab. clin. Med. 45*, 286 (1955).

116. H. A. Edes, C. Finch, and R. W. McKee, "Congenital methemoglobinemia. A clinical and biochemical study of a case," *J. clin. Invest. 28*, 265 (1949).

117. C. P. Emerson, T. H. Ham, and W. B. Castle, "Hemolytic action of certain organic oxidants derived from sulfanilamide, phenylhydrazine and hydroquinone," *J. clin. Invest. 20*, 451 (1941).

118. C. P. Emerson, T. H. Ham, and W. B. Castle, *The influence of resonating organic compounds on the integrity of red cells* (Conference on the Preservation of the Formed Elements and of the Proteins of the Blood; American National Red Cross, Washington, D. C., 1949).

119. R. J. Dern, I. M. Weinstein, G. V. LeRoy, D. W. Talmage, and A. S. Alving, "The hemolytic effect of primaquine. I. The localization of the drug-induced hemolytic defect in primaquine-sensitive individuals," *J. lab. clin. Med. 43*, 303 (1954).

120. P. E. Carson, C. L. Flanagan, C. E. Ickes, and A. S. Alving, "Enzymatic deficiency in primaquine-sensitive erythrocytes," *Science 124*, 484 (1956).

121. W. O. Cruz, "Acetylphenylhydrazine anemia. I. The mechanism of erythrocyte destruction and regeneration," *Amer. J. med. Sci. 202*, 781 (1941).

122. M. S. Greenberg, "Method for measuring mechanical fragility of dog red cells," *Proc. Soc. exp. Biol. (N. Y.) 89*, 320 (1955).

123. E. Beutler, R. J. Dern, and A. S. Alving, "The hemolytic effect of primaquine. VII. An in vitro test for sensitivity of erythrocytes to primaquine," *J. lab. clin. Med. 45*, 40 (1955).

124. E. Beutler, "The glutathione instability of drug-sensitive red cells," *J. lab. clin. Med. 49*, 84 (1957).

125. A. P. Fishman, G. M. Turino, and E. H. Bergofsky, "The syndrome of alveolar hypoventilation," *Amer. J. Med. 23*, 333 (1957).

126. Combined Staff Clinic, "Polycythemia," *Amer. J. Med. 24*, 132 (1958).

127. O. Ratto, W. A. Briscoe, J. W. Morton, and J. H. Comroe, "Anoxemia secondary to polycythemia and polycythemia secondary to anoxemia," *Amer. J. Med. 91*, 958 (1955).

128. P. Calabresi and W. H. Abelmann, "Porta-caval and porta-pulmonary an-

astomosis in Laennec's cirrhosis and in heart failure," *J. clin. Invest. 36,* 1257 (1957).

129. B. J. Kennedy and A. S. Gilbertsen, "Increased erythropoiesis induced by androgenic hormones," *J. clin. Invest. 35,* 717 (1956).

130. J. W. Fisher, "Increase in circulating red cell volume of normal rats after treatment with hydrocortisone or corticosterone," *Proc. Soc. exp. Biol. (N. Y.) 97,* 502 (1958).

131. G. F. Starr, C. F. Stroebel, Jr., and T. P. Kearns, "Polycythemia with papilledema and infratentorial vascular tumors," *Ann. intern. Med. 48,* 978 (1958).

132. L. Singmaster, "Uterine fibroids associated with polycythemia," *J. Amer. med. Ass. 163,* 63 (1957).

133. A. J. S. McFadzean, D. Todd, and K. C. Tsang, "Polycythemia in primary carcinoma of the liver," *Blood 13,* 427 (1958).

134. C. L. Conley, J. Kowal, and J. D'Antonio, "Polycythemia associated with renal tumors," *Bull. Johns Hopk. Hosp. 101,* 63 (1957).

135. W. M. Cooper and W. B. Tuttle, "Polycythemia associated with benign kidney lesions: report of a case of erythrocytosis with hydronephrosis with remission of polycythemia following nephrectomy," *Ann. intern. Med. 47,* 1008 (1957).

136. J. H. Lawrence, *Polycythemia: Physiology, Diagnosis, and Treatment Based on 303 Cases* (Grune and Stratton, New York, 1955).

137. G. M. Pike, "Polycythemia vera," *New Engl. J. Med. 258,* 1250, 1297 (1958).

138. J. H. Lawrence, N. J. Berlin, and R. L. Huff, "The nature and treatment of polycythemia," *Medicine 32,* 323 (1953).

139. A. Daman and D. A. Holub, "Host factors in polycythemia vera," *Ann. intern. Med. 49,* 43 (1958).

140. A. Videbaick, "Polycythemia vera: course and prognosis," *Acta med. scand. 138,* 179 (1950).

141. L. R. Wasserman, "Polycythemia vera: its course and treatment. Relation to myeloid metaplasia and leukemia," *Bull. N. Y. Acad. Med. 3,* 343 (1954).

142. W. Dameshek, "Some speculations on myeloproliferative syndromes," *Blood 6,* 372 (1951).

143. W. N. Valentine, W. S. Beck, J. H. Folette, H. Mills, and J. S. Lawrence, "Biochemical studies in chronic myelocytic leukemia, polycythemia vera and other idiopathic myeloproliferative disorders," *Blood 7,* 959 (1952).

# Unit 12

# Abnormalities of White Blood Cells

## Pathologic Physiology of the White Blood Cells

### CHEMICAL COMPOSITION AND METABOLISM OF LEUKOCYTES

In addition to a water content of 82 percent, leukocytes contain nucleoproteins, nucleic acids (DNA and RNA), phospholipids, and measurable amounts of sodium, potassium, calcium, zinc, magnesium, iron, chloride, inorganic phosphorus, and bicarbonate ion.[1] They also contain glycogen, large amounts of acid and alkaline phosphatases, and a large number of enzymes involved in metabolic reactions.[2, 3] Leukocytes removed from the circulation are very fragile and are extremely susceptible to slight trauma, changes in pH and oxygen, and $CO_2$ pressure.[4] Leukemic leukocytes do not agglutinate as readily as normal leukocytes in vitro. The same difference is also found between cancer cells and normal cells, both in vitro and in tissue culture, and may be due to changes at the cell surface or to the low calcium content characteristic of most neoplastic cells.[4]

Table 34 demonstrates the chemical differences between leukocytes in health and in disease.[5] In general, leukocytes have a high rate of both anaerobic and aerobic glycolysis and exhibit a small Pasteur effect. In this respect, they are similar to the cells of the kidney medulla, embryonic cells, brain cells, and cancer cells.[6, 7] The high rate of anaerobic glycolysis may enable the leukocyte to function in areas of lowered oxygen pressure, as in sites of inflammation. Amino-acid synthesis proceeds at a faster rate in leukemic cells than in normal cells. It is greater in chronic myelocytic leukemia and greatest in acute leukemia.[8] The

Table 34. *Changes in chemical characteristics of leukocytes in disease.*[6]

| Characteristic | Leukocytosis of infection | Polycythemia vera | Chronic leukemia | | Acute leukemia |
|---|---|---|---|---|---|
| | | | Myelocytic | Lymphocytic | |
| Aerobic glycolysis | — | — | Low | Low | — |
| Oxygen consumption | — | — | Low | Low | — |
| Lactic dehydrogenase | — | — | Low | Low | — |
| Triose phosphate dehydrogenase | — | — | Low | Low | — |
| Glycogen content | Incr. | High | Low | Very low | Very low |
| Alkaline phosphatase | High | High | Low | Very low | Very low |
| Histamine | Low | Normal or incr. | High | Low | Low |
| β-glucuronidase | — | Normal | Normal or high | Low | Very low |
| Free sulfhydryl | Normal | Normal | Normal | Low | Low |

sulfhydryl content of leukocytes is several times that of erythrocytes, and amino acids such as cystine and cysteine are incorporated at a much greater rate in leukemic cells than in normal cells.[9, 10] About one-half of the histamine of normal blood is located in the basophils, about one-third in the eosinophils, and probably most of the remaining one-sixth in the neutrophils. Lymphocytes, monocytes, erythrocytes, and platelets contain little or none. The granules of basophilic leukocytes, which are soluble in water, like the mast cells of tissue, carry an acid substance identical with or closely related to heparin. The significance of this is unknown. Electron microscopy of leukocytes has been useful in comparing morphologic with the biochemical data.[11] An example of this is the finding of an endoplasmic reticulum which is well developed in plasma cells and which characterizes secretory cells in general.[12] Certain abnormal fibrillar substances have also been found in leukemic cells by the electron microscope.[13] The exact significance of these substances is not known at the present time.

### FUNCTION AND BIOLOGIC PROPERTIES OF LEUKOCYTES

PHAGOCYTOSIS. This is probably the most important property of the leukocyte and has been used as a measure of viability.[4] Neutrophils that phagocytose bacteria and small particles are called microphages. The monocytes that characteristically engulf large bacteria, protozoa, foreign matter, and even red corpuscles are called macrophages. Through the process of phagocytosis, bacteria can be destroyed before antibodies can be formed. During phagocytosis, there is a measurable increase in anaerobic and aerobic glycolysis and an increased lipid synthesis. These findings suggest that phagocytosis is an active process requiring energy and that formation of new cytoplasmic membrane takes place by increased lipid synthesis. Particles enter the cell by invagination of the cytoplasmic membrane and appear in the cells surrounded by this membrane (pinocytosis).[14]

PRODUCTION OF ANTIBODIES. The plasma cell is the prime source of antibodies.[15] In the disease state known as hypogammaglobulinemia, or agammaglobulinemia, there is complete absence of plasma cells. This condition is characterized by repeated infections and deficient antibody production. The plasma cell may represent an altered lymphocyte, but direct evidence for establishing this fact is lacking. Lymphocytes also participate in antigen-antibody reactions since passive transfer of delayed hypersensitivity, such as tuberculin reactions, can be demonstrated by transfer of lymphocytes.[16] This suggests that lymphocytes store antibodies of the delayed hypersensitive type. According to the theory of antibody production introduced by Lederberg, groups, or clones, of lymphocytes immobilize only one strain of *Salmonella* organism when they have been previously exposed to different antigenic strains. Other groups, or clones, will immobilize other antigenic strains, but no clonal group will immobilize more than one strain.[17] Lymphocytes are rich in adenosinase, which splits adenosine and, because of this, it has been suggested that the lymphocyte is instrumental in the destruction of toxic proteins.[18] Monocytes contain many nucleases, proteinases, and carbohydrases, and also lipases. These enzymes probably enable them to digest all forms of bacteria, including those with a lipid capsule. It may explain the recognized role of the monocyte in tuberculosis and in leprosy.

PRODUCTION OF FEVER. Inflammation is characterized by migration of neutrophils to the inflammatory site through the elaboration of a substance called leukotoxine, which has been identified in exudative material.[19] Injured cells also

163

liberate a toxic substance called necrosin, found in the euglobulin substance of exudates, which, when injected into the skin, produces swelling, redness, varying degrees of central necrosis, lymphatic blockade, and endothelial vascular damage.[20] Recent evidence by Wood and Atkins indicates that leukocytes are first destroyed and then release a substance that produces fever. This substance can be transferred by serum and partially destroyed by the action of lymphocytes.[21] Steroids such as etiocholanolone and pregnanolone regularly produce fever when administered to human subjects. The fever-producing capacities of these steroids is related to a hydroxyl group on position 3 and a 5-alpha-hydrogen. Changing other parts of the molecule, such as position 11, does not alter their capacity to produce fever.[22] Basophilic leukocytes contain metachromatic granules which contain heparin and it seems plausible that they function in inflammation by delivering anticoagulants to facilitate absorption or to prevent clotting of blood and lymph in obstructed tissue.

MORPHOGENESIS AND LIFE SPAN OF LEUKOCYTES. Leukocytes, with the exception of lymphocytes, are produced by the liver and spleen in the first 3 months of fetal life and then by the bone marrow, liver, and spleen until birth, after which they are produced exclusively by the bone marrow. The mechanism of release from the production site is unknown, but after release they are sequestered and destroyed mainly by capillary beds of the lung, liver, and spleen.[23] They are also lost in the saliva, urine, and menstrual secretions, and in the contents of the respiratory and alimentary passages. Labeling of the DNA of white cells with radioactive phosphorus or $C^{14}$-labeled thymidine indicates that the bulk of labeled granulocytes remains 4 to 6 days in the bone marrow before entering the blood stream, and that their mean life span in blood is about 9 days, ranging up to 21 days.[24, 25] Others have found a mean life span of about 13 days.[26] From such measurements, the lymphocytes in chronic lymphatic leukemia seem to have a life span of 100 to 300 days,[27] whereas the life span of the normal lymphocyte may be 100 to 200 days. The life span of the eosinophil is similar to that of the neutrophil. When white cells are removed from the circulation and labeled with $Zn^{65}$, no labeled white cells can be recovered from the blood stream 30 min after readministration.[28] Transfusion of white cells has not been accomplished to date, and white cells removed from the body and stored do not live longer than 4 days.[8]

## Quantitative Abnormalities of White Cells in Disease

### TERMINOLOGY

Evaluation of the peripheral white-cell count reveals the total number of white cells circulating, the number of normal cells, and the number of abnormal cells. A reduction of the total number of white cells below 4400/mm³ is termed leukopenia. An increase above the upper range of normal, roughly 10,000/mm³, is termed leukocytosis. A marked elevation, usually above 20,000 or 30,000, is usually termed a leukemoid reaction. Leukemoid reactions may be indistinguishable morphologically from leukemia, owing to the fact that they are frequently accompanied by the appearance of immature cells in the peripheral blood and bone marrow. The course of the disease and change in the total number of white cells and the number of abnormal cells has been, in the past, the best means of distinguishing these two conditions. Determination of white-cell alkaline phosphatase (Unit 9), however, is of great value in differentiating these conditions, since the alkaline phosphatase is usually low in leukemia and usually high in conditions associated with leukemoid reactions.[5, 29]

Results of a differential white-cell count may be expressed either as the relative number of each species of white cells in percent, or as the absolute number per unit volume for each cell species. The latter figure is calculated from the white-cell count and the differential count. For example, if the white-cell count is 7000/mm³ and the differential count shows 25 percent of small lymphocytes, the absolute count of small lymphocytes is 25 percent of 7000 or 1750/mm³. In Table 15 (Unit 9) are given both percentage and absolute values for each species of white cell from counts made on 20 normal young adults.

When leukopenia or leukocytosis is found, the differential count usually indicates that the deviation from normal is predominantly due to a numerical change in one or more species of cells. Occasionally all species of white cells are involved in a proportional change, so that the differential count (in percent) is normal, although the total white-cell count is abnormally high or low. Conversely, if the quantities of two species of cells change in opposite directions (one increases while the other decreases), the total white-cell count may remain normal, but the abnormal proportions are evident in the differential count. Calculation of the absolute quantity of each cell species helps to distinguish between *relative* and *absolute* changes in the numbers of circulating leukocytes. Descriptive terms are used to describe these abnormalities and to indicate which species of cells are involved.

*Granulocytopenia.* When leukopenia is due predominantly to a reduction in neutrophils, this is termed neutropenia. When, as is commonly the case, both neutrophils and eosinophils are reduced, this is designated granulocytopenia. Varying degrees of granulocytopenia may occur following the use of various drugs

(see Table 35) and in other conditions discussed below. An extreme degree of granulocytopenia, in which granulocytes are virtually absent from the peripheral blood, is termed agranulocytosis.

*Example 1.* White-cell count, 1200/mm³; neutrophils, 6 percent; lymphocytes, 82 percent; monocytes, 12 percent. The absolute number of neutrophils is greatly reduced, to 72/mm³, and eosinophils are absent. The lymphocytes are relatively increased, but the absolute number present (984/mm³) is within normal limits.

*Lymphopenia and Moderate Neutropenia.* This type of response may occur following irradiation or after administration of drugs such as nitrogen mustard.

*Example 2.* White-cell count, 2000/mm³; neutrophils, 80 percent; lymphocytes, 10 percent; monocytes, 10 percent. The absolute number of lymphocytes is reduced to 200/mm³, and neutrophils are moderately reduced to 1600/mm³.

*Leukopenia with Extreme Increase in Number of Immature Granulocytes.* This type of change may occur in leukemia, but it is not diagnostic of leukemia since it may also occur in severe infection, widespread malignant disease, and other conditions.

*Example 3.* White-cell count, 2000/mm³; adult neutrophils, 40 percent; band forms, 35 percent; neutrophilic metamyelocytes, 8 percent; myelocytes, 5 percent; blast forms, 2 percent; eosinophils and basophils, none; lymphocytes, 10 percent. The absolute numbers of all species of cells are reduced, but the outstanding change is the increased proportion of immature granulocytes.

*Normal White-Cell Count with Relative Lymphocytosis.* This type of change is frequently seen in viral infections.

*Example 4.* White-cell count, 9500/mm³; neutrophils, 35 percent; lymphocytes, 60 percent; monocytes, 5 percent. There are both a relative and an absolute increase in lymphocytes (5700/mm³) and a normal number of neutrophils (3325/mm³).

*Leukocytosis with Increase in Mature and Immature Neutrophils.* This type of response is commonly seen in infections due to pyogenic organisms.

*Example* 5. White-cell count, 20,000/mm³; adult neutrophils, 45 percent; band forms, 25 percent; lymphocytes, 20 percent; monocytes, 10 percent. The percentage of adult neutrophils is normal but the absolute number is increased to 9000/mm³. The most outstanding change is an increase in relatively young (band-form) neutrophils to 5000/mm³.

*Leukemia.* Leukemia is a diagnostic rather than a descriptive term and should be used only when the disease process is present, as determined by characteristic morphologic changes and confirmed by the clinical course of the disease. It should be emphasized that the diagnosis of leukemia should not be made hurriedly or on insufficient evidence. Leukemia is classified as acute, subacute, and chronic, depending upon the course of the disease and the percentage of abnormal blast cells present in the peripheral blood and bone marrow. Usually in acute leukemia more than 50 percent of the immature forms present are blasts. Leukemia is further subdivided as to type of cell involved, and thus is called lymphocytic, myelocytic, or monocytic, and, rarely, basophilic and eosinophilic. In acute leukemia, the type of leukemia is indicated by the presence of the morphologically mature cells or "the company that the blast cells keep." In many instances, because of lack of mature cells, only a diagnosis of acute leukemia is possible. This is especially true in children (see p. 172).

*Shift to the Left or Right.* An increase in the number per unit volume of immature forms of neutrophils has been designated a "shift to the left." An increase in relative number of mature neutrophils is designated a "shift to the right." A shift to the right is commonly seen in pernicious anemia. These terms are based on the differential counting system of Schilling [30] and are highly arbitrary. They should be abandoned in favor of more descriptive terms.

SYMPTOMS AND SIGNS OCCURRING WITH ABNORMALITIES OF THE WHITE BLOOD CELLS

Abnormalities of the white blood cells in the peripheral blood by themselves are usually not associated with any specific symptoms or signs, in contradistinction to the pallor and weakness associated with anemia. Not uncommonly, the diagnosis of leukemia is made in patients who are symptom-free. This is especially true in chronic lymphatic leukemia, which may run a protracted course in the older individual. It is also true of granulocytopenia, which may be discovered by examination of peripheral blood and bone marrow before evidence of infection appears. In agranulocytosis or extreme leukopenia, local or generalized infection often occurs as a result of inadequate defense mechanisms. Infiltration of the bone marrow by the malignant cells of lymphoma, leukemia, or tumors, or by granulomata may be accompanied by severe bone pain, symptoms of weakness due to anemia, or bleeding due to thrombocytopenia. Infiltration of any tissue or organ by leukemic cells or lymphoma may produce symptoms and signs referable to the site involved. Joint pains accompany acute leukemia in children, presumably owing to increased marrow pressure associated with infiltrative leukemic cells.[2] Lymph nodes, spleen, kidney, skin, or the nervous system may also be involved in such diseases. In leukemia and lymphoma, symptoms of increased metabolism are usually present, indicated by an increased basal metabolic rate, fever, tachycardia, weight loss, and wasting.

### Leukopenia

Leukopenia is a term applied to a reduction in the total leukocyte count below normal. In most situations, this reduction is due to a marked decrease in the number of cells of the granulocytic series. In specific instances, the reduction is due to marked decrease in lymphocytes, as is the case following the use of ionizing irradiation or radiomimetic drugs. Lawrence and Castle have given physiologic classifications that serve as a basis for understanding certain known causes of leukopenia. These classifications are outlined below, with modifications.

DECREASED PRODUCTION OF WHITE BLOOD CELLS. *Aplasia of the Bone Marrow.* Radiation or alkylating agents in excessive dosage and chemical intoxication by benzol characteristically produce aplasia.

*Neutropenia Associated with Drugs.* Neutropenia or agranulocytosis may follow the administration of many drugs. The classical example of such a drug is amidopyrine.[31] Drugs that regularly produce leukopenia if given in sufficient dosage are listed in Table 35. In group *A*, except for unknown factors in human tolerance, a greater amount of the agent will produce a greater degree of aplasia and neutropenia. In group *B*, only a small percentage of patients develop neutropenia or agranulocytosis when the drug is administered. For example, thiouracil produced neutropenia in 3.4 percent of 781 patients.[32] In a number of instances, readministration of small amounts of the sensitizing drug is followed within 6 to 10 hr by acute agranulocytosis.[33] The present postulate is that the offending drug combines with a protein in the serum, presumably globulin, to form an antigen. Antibodies are provoked by this new antigen and become attached to the leukocytes which then become agglutinated and destroyed when the leukocyte-bound antibody and antigen come in contact. In such cases, leukocyte agglutinins have been demonstrated.[34] Serum from these patients when combined with the drug will produce loss of ameboid activity, agglutination, and lysis of normal white blood cells in comparison with control serum. This may be expressed as the "lysis index."[35] Although white cells have the

Table 35. *Agents associated with the occurrence of leukopenia.*[5]

A. Agents that regularly produce leukopenia if a sufficient dose is given
1. Ionizing radiation: roentgen rays, radioactive P, Au, etc.
2. Mustards: sulfur and nitrogen mustards, triethylenemelamine (TEM), etc.
3. Urethane, Myleran, Demecolcin
4. Benzol
5. Antimetabolites: antifolic compounds, 6-mercaptopurine, etc.

B. Agents occasionally associated with leukopenia (granulocytopenia):
   Analgesics: amidopyrine and drugs containing it (amidophen, amytal compound, causalin, cibalgin, neonal compound, neurodyne, peralga, pyraminal, yeast-vite, etc.), antipyrine, novaldin (novalgin), phenylbutazone (butazolidin)
   Antithyroid drugs: thiouracil, propylthiouracil, methylthiouracil, methimazole, carbimazole
   Anticonvulsants: trimethadione (tridione), phethenylate, phenacemide, diethazine
   Sulfonamides: sulfanilamide, prontosil, sulfapyridine, sulfathiazole, sulfadiazine, succinylsulfathiazole, sulfisoxazole (Gantrisin)
   Antihistaminics: pyribenzamine, methaphenilene (diatrin), phenothiazine
   Antimicrobial agents: organic arsenicals, chloramphenicol, thiosemicarbazone (tibione)
   Miscellaneous: dinitrophenol, chlorpromazine, gold salts, industrial chemicals
   Compounds mentioned only in one or two reports: procaine amide, barbiturates, "new allonal," acetophenetidin (phenacetin), acetanilid, pyrithyldione (presidon), quinine, cincophen, plasmochin, salol, antimony (neostibasan), bismuth, fumagillin, diamox, thioglycolic acid ("cold wave"), D.D.T.

antigens of all known blood groups, including Rh factors, this seems to be of no importance clinically in the etiology of agranulocytosis. In most cases, the marrow is hypoplastic or normal. The morphologic picture is indistinguishable from that of the hypoplastic marrow of patients who have received radiation or alkylating agents. In the case of nitrogen mustards, radiation, and radiomimetic drugs, leukopenia is accompanied first by a lymphopenia and then finally by a neutropenia which may last for several weeks. Initially, lymphopenia may be due to a loss of lymphocytes into the lymphatics rather than actual lympholysis. These agents directly affect the DNA of the cells with chromosomal damage characterized by breaks, cross linkage, and deletion.[36, 37]

*Infections.* It is probable, but not established, that granulocytopenia, neutropenia, and leukopenia, in infections by such agents as the typhoid group, certain viruses, and malaria, result from inhibition of formation of cells.

*Pernicious Anemia and Deficiency States.* In pernicious anemia and related macrocytic anemia, the leukopenia responds to treatment with liver extract or folic acid but does not respond to elevation of the hemoglobin level by multiple transfusions of blood.[38] Deficiency of $B_{12}$ produces a defect in pyrimidine synthesis with increase in enzymes such as dihydroorotic acid dehydrogynase.[39] In experimental animals, leukopenia is observed on certain purified diets that may be deficient in tryptophane, pantothenic acid, or riboflavin.[40]

REDISTRIBUTION OF WHITE CELLS IN VASCULAR CHANNELS. Redistribution of white cells in the capillaries of the lung, spleen, and other viscera may result in transient leukopenia[41] in anaphylactic shock following injection of foreign protein; in rigor following injection of typhoid vaccine; following injection of the leukopenic factor of Menkin; and following the injection of hydrophilic colloids such as gelatin, globulin, and fibrinogen. In Vejlens'[41] fundamental investigation of the effect of intravenous injection of hydrophilic colloids, he showed that there was an increase in rouleau formation causing the granulocytes to take a peripheral position in the blood flowing in capillary vessels. Following this redistribution, the granulocytes decreased in large vessels and increased in the capillaries of the spleen and lung, where they appeared as aggregates.

ABNORMAL DISTRIBUTION OF WHITE CELLS IN THE BODY. In aleukemic leukemia there may be leukopenia of the peripheral blood, with large numbers of leukemic cells in the bone marrow and other tissues. The mechanism of this bizarre distribution of cells in the body is not known. Obviously, such situations present difficult diagnostic problems.[42]

INCREASED LOSS OR DESTRUCTION OF WHITE CELLS. Experimentally, in the guinea pig, neutrophils may be destroyed promptly and in large numbers in the peripheral blood by the injection of immune antineutrophilic serum.[43] Lawrence[44] suggests that excessive loss of leukocytes from the body, as in purulent colitis, may be one factor to explain leukopenia. Wiseman and Doan,[45] Doan and Wright,[46] and others[47, 48] have described a condition of chronic neutropenia, sometimes with moderate thrombocytopenia and anemia, that is improved by splenectomy. Tagging of the red cells with $Cr^{51}$ and comparative surface counts of the spleen and liver at intervals over a 4- to 7-day period indicate the surgical benefit of splenectory in such a situation. If there is a greater than 50-percent increase in counts over the spleen as compared with the liver or precordium, this is indicative of increased splenic destruction of the red cells and splenectomy may reverse the entire blood picture.[49] Similar changes in Banti's disease and in acquired hemolytic anemia with a positive Coombs test may also be relieved by splenectomy. The extreme pancytopenia with leukopenia or agranulocytosis that occurs in certain cases of kala-azar has been interpreted as resulting from excessive removal of formed elements by the spleen.[50] The leukopenia of chronic alcoholic cirrhosis of the liver is of unknown origin.

NEUTROPENIA OF UNKNOWN ORIGIN. Agranulocytic angina associated with the menstrual cycle has been reported by Jackson *et al.*[51] Periodic (cyclic) neutropenia has been reported in both men and women[52] and is of unknown etiology. Similar cases are described in which there is a familial disposition. In all such cases, surface counting of the spleen after labeling the red cells with $Cr^{51}$ is helpful in deciding the therapeutic value of splenectomy. The neutropenia of lupus erythematosis is of unknown etiology but may be related to the lupus erythematosus phenomenon (Unit 13). Periodic disease and Mediterranean fever are usually associated with a leukocytosis that has recently been correlated with unbound etiocholanolone in the circulating blood.[53]

## Leukemoid Reactions

Changes in the white cells of the peripheral blood in nonleukemic conditions may simulate leukemia because of increase in the white-cell count or abnormal forms which suggest myelogenous, occasionally lymphatic, or, rarely, monocytic leukemia. For these changes, the descriptive terms used are "leukemoid reaction"—myelocytic or lymphocytic. These terms indicate a benign condition and should not be confused with terms used to describe a neoplastic condition such as leukemia.

### LEUKEMOID REACTIONS OF THE GRANULOCYTIC (MYELOID) TYPE

An increase in the number of immature granulocytes in the peripheral blood simulating myelogenous leukemia is usually associated with a leukocytosis which may vary from 15,000 to 50,000 white cells/mm³ and occasionally is higher than 100,000/mm³. The types of conditions associated with such a myeloid reaction are as follows:

1. *Excessive marrow response.* In infancy and childhood, the bone marrow responds so actively that immature granulocytes may be seen in the peripheral blood associated with relatively mild infections and in other conditions listed below.

2. *Infection.* In many pyogenic infections, the increase in number and immaturity of granulocytes varies with the severity of the infection. Accordingly, the changes vary from a moderate increase in band forms to a true leukemoid response.

3. *Severe malaria.*

4. *Hemorrhage,* especially into a body cavity.

5. *Thermal burns.*

6. *Severe anemia with active, acute response of the bone marrow.* A leukemoid reaction of the granulocytic type may occur in severe anemias in which there is a physiologic response of the bone marrow. It occurs in such conditions as hemolytic transfusion reaction, sickle-cell anemia, erythroblastosis fetalis, and acquired hemolytic anemia with a positive Coombs test. A few myelocytes may be present in any severe anemia.

7. *Recovery from agranulocytosis.*

8. *Myelophthisic anemia.*

9. *Neoplastic disease.* Carcinoma, especially when metastatic or necrotic, may occasionally be associated with marked leukocytosis and a leukemoid response.

10. *Extramedullary myelopoiesis.* In the normal child and adult, all erythropoiesis and formation of the granulocytic cells occurs in the bone marrow. In normal infants, both premature and full-term, there remain a few islands of blood-forming tissue in the liver and spleen. In severe anemia of infancy, such as erythroblastosis fetalis, there may be reversion to fetal extramedullary myelopoiesis in many organs, with a striking increase in the number of immature granulocytes in the peripheral blood.

11. *Myeloid metaplasia in adults.* In adults, extramedullary myelopoiesis is not normal and has been referred to as myeloid metaplasia or the myeloproliferative syndrome. This syndrome may appear *de novo* following contact with compounds containing benzol. In such cases, myelopoietic tissue is found in the liver, lymph nodes, spleen, and occasionally other organs such as the kidney. Myeloid metaplasia may follow polycythemia vera or may by itself presage a true leukemia. Myeloid metaplasia has also been reported in myelofibrosis, oste-

osclerosis of the bone marrow, myelogenous leukemia, metastatic carcinoma of the bone marrow, and Hodgkin's disease, and following nonlethal amounts of radiation. The myeloproliferative syndrome is remarkable for the many changes that occur in the peripheral blood. It may be associated with a hyperplastic marrow, a normal marrow, or a hypoplastic marrow. The peripheral blood usually is so characteristic that the diagnosis can be made by serial study. It is always accompanied by immature white cells and red cells in the peripheral blood. The red cells show marked variation in size and shape with many tear-shaped forms.[54] There may also be thrombocytopenia, and megakaryocytes may be found in the peripheral blood. The leukocyte alkaline phosphatase in myeloid metaplasia is usually very high, as it is with leukemoid reactions in contradistinction to leukemia, where it is universally low.[29] No case to date has been followed in which leukocyte alkaline phosphatase determinations have been made on the white cells during myeloid metaplasia and on the same white cells when the transition has occurred into a true leukemia.

### LEUKEMOID REACTIONS OF LYMPHOCYTIC (LYMPHOID) TYPE

The diagnosis of lymphocytic leukemia may be erroneously made in leukemoid reactions characterized by lymphocytosis, especially with abnormal forms of lymphocytes, such as are observed in infectious mononucleosis, infectious hepatitis, infectious lymphocytosis, and viral infections, and very rarely in neoplastic disease.

## Malignant Lymphoma

### CLASSIFICATION AND NATURAL HISTORY

At the present time, two major classifications of malignant lymphoma are in general use, one described by Jackson and Parker,[55] and the other by Gall and Mallory.[56, 57] The classification and their differences are listed in Table 36. Although they may all be related diseases, caused by related agents, morphologic classification has been helpful in determining prognosis and selecting the type of treatment. As with other neoplasias, the more acute and invasive lesions occur with undifferentiated and anaplastic types of cells, whereas chronicity or slow growth is associated with differentiated or mature types of cells. There may be a transition from one type of lymphoma to another at the same or different times in a patient, as described by Jackson and Parker,[55] and shown diagrammatically by Sparling, Adams, and Parker [58] and by Custer and Bernard.[59] The natural history of lymphomas varies considerably. A number of patients who have had authenticated diagnoses of Hodgkin's disease, reticulum-cell sarcoma, giant-follicle lymphoma, or lymphocytoma remain free of their disease for 15 years or more after initial treatment. In most cases, the characteristic denominator of these patients is one of local involvement without widespread dissemination at first.[60] Leukemia may accompany any one of the malignant lymphomas, and it occurs characteristically with lymphocytoma, lymphoblastic lymphoma, or, rarely, Hodgkin's disease and reticulum-cell sarcoma. It never occurs with giant-follicle lymphoma and only rarely with plasmacytoma. It occasionally occurs with mycosis fungoides.

### CLINICAL MANIFESTATIONS

The clinical manifestations of the malignant lymphoma and plasmacytoma may be indistinguishable from those of leukemia, and are so protean that they may simulate any number of disease processes, especially those of the granulomatous type which also involve the reticuloendothelial system. In some cases of plasmacytoma, a clue to the diagnosis may be obtained from electrophoresis of the serum proteins, in which a characteristic myeloma spot may be present (Unit

Table 36. *Classification of leukemia, Hodgkin's disease, and allied disorders according to the type of cell involved, as modified from Jackson and Parker* [55] *and Sparling, Adams, and Parker.*[57]

| Cell type | Comments | Disease |
|---|---|---|
| 1. Reticulum cell<br> Giant-follicle lymphoma [a]<br> Hodgkin's disease [b]<br>  Paragranuloma [c]<br>  Granuloma [d]<br>  Sarcoma<br> Reticulum-cell sarcoma<br> Histiocytic leukemia<br>  (see leukemia, below)<br>2. Lymphocytes or their precursors<br> Lymphosarcoma<br> Lymphoblastoma<br> Lymphocytoma [e]<br> Giant-follicle lymphoma | Occur largely in lymph nodes but are found also in spleen, liver, and many other organs and tissues | Hodgkin's disease and allied disorders |
| Lymphoblast<br> Lymphocyte<br>3. Granulocytes or their precursors<br> Myeloblast<br> Myelocyte<br> Eosinophil<br> Basophil | In the peripheral blood, the leukemia may be manifest, subleukemic, or aleukemic | Leukemia |
| 4. Monocytes or their precursors<br> Monoblast<br> Monocyte<br>5. Plasma cells or their precursors<br> Plasmablast<br> Plasmacytes (plasma cells) | In general, the most immature forms of cells are associated with acute leukemia, the more adult cells with chronic leukemia | Plasmocytoma, multiple myeloma |

[a] Giant-follicle lymphoma may change into Hodgkin's disease, reticulum-cell sarcoma, lymphosarcoma, or lymphatic leukemia.
[b] The origin of the Reed-Sternberg cell is in question.
[c] Hodgkin's paragranuloma may change into Hodgkin's granuloma or Hodgkin's sarcoma.
[d] Hodgkin's granuloma may change into Hodgkin's sarcoma.
[e] Lymphocytoma may be the peripheral expression of lymphatic leukemia or lymphosarcoma, or a patient with lymphocytoma may later develop lymphatic leukemia.

16). This myeloma spot may occur with the gamma globulin fraction or occasionally there may be elevations of the beta 1 and, more rarely, alpha globulins. Rouleau formations, Bence-Jones proteinuria, hypercalcemia, and hypercalciuria with multiple punched-out lesions of bone are characteristic of plasmacytoma. None of these findings are diagnostic, including Bence-Jones protein (Unit 19). The finding of a myeloma spot in an electrophoretic pattern of the serum with a serum-globulin concentration of 7 gm/100 ml or more is presumptive evidence of myeloma until proved otherwise. There is no characteristic finding in the peripheral leukocytes in the malignant lymphomas that distinguishes one from the other and the diagnosis rests on the pathologic characterization of the involved lymph nodes or other parts of the reticuloendothelial system.

## Leukemia

DEFINITION, CLASSIFICATION, AND NATURAL HISTORY. Leukemia, as defined by Jackson, may be an acute or chronic systemic disease involving primarily the blood-forming organs and characterized by a widespread, disorderly, and profitless proliferation of the leukocytes and their precursors, manifested by the presence—often in very large numbers—of immature, abnormal white cells in the peripheral blood stream, and leading, at least in the vast majority of cases, to death in a comparatively short time. Before puberty, the usual leukemia is acute and is difficult to classify as to cell type. After puberty and in the adult, the majority of leukemias are chronic and are classified on the "company that the blast cells keep" in the peripheral blood or bone marrow. The total duration of acute leukemia in the child may be less than 6 months, whereas the chronic form may extend to 3 or 4 years. Complete remissions may be obtained with the use of antifolic compounds, but as yet no cure of acute leukemia has been reported in children with the use of any agents, including total body x-ray. It seems to be well established that in mice and in fowl leukemia is due to a filterable agent, presumably a virus.

Chronic leukemia in the adult can take one of three forms—lymphocytic, myelocytic, or monocytic. Erythroblastic leukemia, or DiGuglielmo's syndrome, is a myeloproliferative disease characterized by a marked increase in erythroblasts and normoblasts in the peripheral blood and bone marrow, with invasion of the liver, spleen, and lymph nodes by these immature red cells.[61] Chronic lymphocytic leukemia may be present for many years before it is diagnosed and has a much better prognosis than chronic myelogenous leukemia. Irradiation increases the incidence of leukemia in humans, as evidenced by the dramatic increase in leukemia in atom-bomb survivors of Hiroshima.[62] Indeed, in such situations, the alkaline phosphatase of the white cells may be low and herald the onset of leukemia before the diagnosis can be made by peripheral-blood smear or bone-marrow examination.[63] Generally, the leukemic cell is metabolically more active than its normal counterpart, be it a lymphocyte or a myelocyte.[8, 39]

### GENERAL SYMPTOMS AND SIGNS OF LEUKEMIA AND LYMPHOMA

There is usually a marked increase in the basal metabolic rate in leukemia and, in some cases, in lymphoma. Murchison's fever or Pel-Epstein fever is frequent in Hodgkin's disease but is not diagnostic of the condition. Fever also occurs in other types of lymphomas, in acute leukemia, and in chronic leukemia. Loss of appetite, weakness, and wasting may occur out of proportion to other symptoms and signs. The patient with lymphoma or leukemia may have a chronic illness, an acute illness, or an overwhelming fatal illness resulting from the disease process itself. The signs and symptoms of leukemia are usually associated with the severity of the anemia and the hemorrhagic diathesis which is associated with the thrombocytopenia. There is no evidence that there is a circulating anticoagulant present in leukemia. Hemorrhage usually occurs when the thrombocytes fall below 50,000/mm³.

### LOCAL SYMPTOMS AND SIGNS OF LEUKEMIA

Many of the signs and symptoms of leukemia and lymphoma result from infiltration of the tissues, which is an outstanding feature of these diseases. Infiltration of the lymph nodes, spleen, and liver will cause enlargement of these areas with symptoms due to their enlargement. Infiltration of the bone marrow will cause changes in the peripheral blood and infiltration of the bone itself will cause pressure increase so that joint symptoms and bone pain are common. Infiltration of the surfaces of cavities will produce serous effusions.

### CHANGES IN THE PERIPHERAL BLOOD

The leukemic process may be heralded either by a decrease in the alkaline phosphatase in the white cells or by the appearance of an anemia that is resistant to therapy. Leukemia can be diagnosed, however, only by the appearance in the peripheral blood and the bone marrow of abnormal, immature white cells, and by the appearance of blast cells.[64]

### ANEMIA IN LEUKEMIA

In all forms of leukemia, survival of red cells is usually shortened, as measured either by the Ashby differential-agglutination technique or by $Cr^{51}$ tagging of red cells. As the disease progresses, the red-cell survival also seems to decrease.[65, 66] Red-cell survival can be partially, but not completely, restored by infusion of the red cells from patients with leukemia into normal individuals.[67] In some cases, there may be a positive Coombs test and a true acquired hemolytic anemia. In many cases, there may be excess destruction of red cells by the spleen, as demonstrated by a comparative difference in surface counting over the liver and spleen. A spleen-to-liver ratio of 2:1 usually indicates a need for splenectomy. Studies with $Fe^{59}$ show an accelerated plasma half-time clearance with a slowed incorporation of $Fe^{59}$ in the red cells, indicating that there is some trapping mechanism of $Fe^{59}$ in these patients, so that the cause of the anemia is twofold: shortened red-cell survival, and deficient or decreased erythropoiesis as measured by $Fe^{59}$. Acquired hemolytic anemia with a positive Coombs test in association with any of the lymphomas may be adequately treated by cortisone therapy or, in some instances, by splenectomy. Splenectomy in lymphomas such as lymphocytoma and lymphoblastoma may be followed by an overwhelming and acute manifestation of the disease with infiltration of all the organs.[68] In chronic lymphatic leukemia, there is almost always an accompanying anemia. When this disease is treated with cortisone, the anemia is reversed. Cortisone does not affect the anemia in Hodgkin's disease, lymphoblastoma, or reticulum-cell sarcoma.

### Macroglobulinemia

A new and distinct syndrome described by Wäldenstrom in 1943 may be a variant of malignant lymphoma.[69] Clinically, such patients exhibit bleeding from the mucous membranes, easy fatigability, anemia, hyperglobulinemia, and fibrinogenopenia. Bone-marrow examination, lymph-node biopsy, or autopsy demonstrates a cell which is halfway between a lymphocyte and a plasma cell. This cell is about the size of a lymphocyte, contains large cytoplasmic granules, and stains positive with periodic acid–Schiff reagent.[70] The globulins in these cases are usually gamma globulins, having the very high molecular weight of 1 million by ultracentrifuge analysis, with a Svedberg unit of 18 to 20. In most of the cases, a drop of serum in water will form an immediate white precipitate which can be redissolved in saline ("Sia Test," Unit 16). This is characteristic of the solubility of euglobulins but is not diagnostic of the syndrome and only indicates the need for ultracentrifuge measurement. Fibrinogen, rheumatoid arthritis factor, and other euglobulins will also give a positive water test.[71]

## Responses and Abnormalities of the Various White Blood Cells

### NEUTROPHILS

CHARACTERISTICS AND FUNCTIONS OF THE NEUTROPHILS. The neutrophil is an active, motile, and phagocytic cell that plays an important role in the body's defense mechanism, preventing the invasion of many varieties of bacterial agents. The neutrophil is the first leukocyte to appear and usually is the chief cellular constituent in acute inflammation. The disappearance of the neutrophils, as in agranulocytosis, is accompanied by a local or generalized sepsis in most cases. In the presence of serum antibodies and with the aid of antibiotic agents, the neutrophil may ingest, phagocytose, kill, and digest by enzymatic action many, but not all, forms of bacteria, especially those of the pyogenic group. In the absence of antibodies and without antibiotics, phagocytosis may occur by a

173

surface mechanism or it may be inhibited by substances in the slime layer of an organism such as Type 3 pneumococcus. A neutrophil ingests fragments of tissue and particulate matter and, as in lupus erythematosis, may ingest other destroyed neutrophils or portions of their nuclei and cytoplasm.[72] Mudd has found that in leukemia red-cell phagocytosis by myeloblasts is less active than by mature neutrophils from the same patient. However, no good correlation has been found in vitro between maturity of granulocytes and their phagocytic activity.

NEUTROPHILIA. An absolute and relative increase in the number of adult and band forms of neutrophils is one of the most frequent and nonspecific responses of the body.

*Physiologic Changes.* Physiologically, neutrophilia occurs after vigorous exercise, during childbirth, after repeated vomiting, after convulsions, and in the newborn infant. It is also associated with paroxysmal tachycardia.[1]

*Infection.* Infection, especially with pyogenic organisms, is classically associated with leukocytosis, neutrophilia, variable increase in band forms, and occasionally a leukemoid reaction. This may occur in acute infection within a few hours, or with chronic infection, either generalized or local. In a severe local or generalized infection thought to result from pyogenic organisms, the absence of neutrophilia may suggest a wrong diagnosis or a failure of the bone marrow to respond. Thus, in acute, severe pulmonary infection, a lack of neutrophilia may suggest a virus infection instead of one by the pneumococcus. However, if pneumococci are demonstrated in sputum and blood culture, then a lack of neutrophilia or a neutropenia suggests overwhelming infection, a toxic depression of the bone marrow, and a poor prognosis. Not all infections are associated with neutrophilia. Excep-

tions are typhoid or *Salmonella* infections, brucellosis, tuberculosis, and infections with viruses, malaria, and other metazoan agents.

*Necrosis.* Necrosis of tissue associated with infarction, trauma, thermal burns, surgical procedures without infection, and necrotic tumor tissue is typically accompanied by a neutrophilia which may be moderate or extreme. In tumor necrosis, extreme neutrophilia is not uncommon.

*Neoplastic Diseases.* Primary or metastatic tumor may be associated with variable degrees of neutrophilia and with striking elevations in some instances. Widespread tumor, especially, may be associated with a leukemoid reaction and occasionally with a marked eosinophilia. Metastatic tumors involving the bone marrow may show a so-called irritative effect, with the appearance of many immature white cells in the bone marrow and in the peripheral blood.

*Response of the Bone Marrow to Sudden Demand.* Acute hemorrhage, acute hemolytic anemia, and occasionally poisoning by carbon monoxide produce a sudden demand on the bone marrow to produce white cells. In such a situation, the earliest change in the formed elements of the peripheral blood may be leukocytosis with neutrophilia, and, in some instances, a true leukemoid reaction may ensue.

*Metabolic Diseases.* Neutrophilia may occur in metabolic abnormalities such as severe diabetic acidosis, eclampsia, prolonged diarrhea or vomiting, gout, and uremia. Leukocytosis is especially marked when pericarditis occurs with uremia. Neutrophilic increase in eclampsia is probably caused by convulsions and increased muscular activity. Leukocytosis may be especially marked in association with burns.

*Intoxications.* Poisonings with lead, mercury, illuminating gas, digitalis, and insect venoms such as that of the black widow spider are also associated with neutrophilic leukocytosis. Following injection of foreign protein, there is usually a preliminary leukopenia which is then followed by a leukocytosis. This is typical of the reaction to typhoid vaccine, which is explained by Wood as due to initial injury to the white cells by the vaccine. A release of a pyrogenic substance from the white blood cells causes fever and leukocytosis. Hemorrhage into the peritoneal cavity, pleural space, or subdural space produces extensive leukocytosis. Sudden hemolysis of red corpuscles also causes marked leukocytosis.

*Polycythemia Vera.* In most cases of polycythemia vera, there is an absolute increase in all forms of leukocytes, including the neutrophils. Alkaline phosphatase of white cells is generally increased in polycythemia vera, by comparison with stress and secondary polycythemia.[60]

ABNORMAL FORMS OF NEUTROPHILS. In many severe infections and drug reactions with fever, neutrophilic granules may be replaced by large, dark-purple granules which may fill the entire cell. These are usually referred to as "toxic granules." This abnormal granulation of the neutrophil has been confused by observers with the basophilic granulocyte. The toxic granules of the neutrophils are smaller, darker in color, and more variable in number than the normal dark-blue granules of the basophil. Other changes seen in Wright's-stained neutrophils include pyknosis of the nucleus, vacuolated areas, and irregular blue oval areas in the cytoplasm called Döhle bodies which are seen in burns and infections. With electron microscopy, abnormal fibrillar material may be seen in leukemia.[13]

A lethal anomaly of leukocytes has been described [73-76] in infants, associated with albinism, photophobia, and manifestations of lymphoma and leukemia (Chediak-Higashi syndrome). In this condition, the granulocytes and mono-

cytes contain giant cytoplasmic peroxidase-positive granules. In granulocytes, these appear as irregular, slate-green masses, similar to Döhle bodies. The condition is universally fatal and frequently associated with hepatosplenomegaly and lymphadenopathy due to malignant lymphoma.

The Pelger-Huet anomaly indicates neutrophils with rodlike or dumbbell-shaped nuclei without segmentation or lobulation. This is transmitted by a non-sex-linked dominant gene and it is observed partially or completely in many members of the same family. It is important, since it may be mistaken for an increase in the unsegmented forms of granulocytes seen in other diseases. It does not predispose to infections and has been observed mainly in Holland, Germany, and Switzerland, and among Orientals.[77] A constitutional granulation anomaly has been described by Alder, in which there is heavy azurophilic granulation of all the white cells.[78]

EOSINOPHILS

CHARACTERISTICS AND FUNCTIONS OF THE EOSINOPHILS. The exact function of the eosinophil is still not known. The eosinophil is characteristically found in abundance in the tissues in reaction to foreign protein, in allergic reactions, and in association with Hodgkin's disease. The eosinophil is less motile and more indirect in its movements than is the neutrophil, but it is phagocytic and an unusually hardy cell in anisotonic solutions.[79] The granules of the eosinophil contain iron and also phospholipids that stain with Sudan black B.

EOSINOPHILIA. Marked eosinophilia, over 50 percent, occurs in association with trichinosis and, less commonly, with widespread metastatic carcinoma. Peripheral eosinophilia is usually correlated with eosinophilia of the bone marrow. The causes of eosinophilia are parasitic infestations such as trichinosis, echi-

175

nococcus disease, *Ascaris* infection, and schistisomiasis. It is usually not associated with intestinal parasites such as enterobiasis and amebiasis.

*Allergic Diseases.* Eosinophilia may occur in malaria, all allergic disorders, bronchial asthma, urticaria, angioneurotic edema, drug fever, following the administration of hyperimmune serum, and in erythema multiforme.

*Skin Diseases.* The highest and most constant eosinophilia has been observed in pemphigus and dermatitis herpetiformis, but it may occur with scabies, psoriasis, eczema, and prurigo.

*Neoplastic Diseases.* Eosinophilia may be observed occasionally and be marked in degree in metastatic carcinoma that is widespread and also in lung cancer, stomach cancer, and Hodgkin's disease.

*Infectious Diseases.* Eosinophilia occurs most often in scarlet fever, occasionally in gonorrhea, and in leprosy. In most infections in which neutrophilia occurs, eosinophils are generally reduced in number. In Loeffler's syndrome, a peculiar type of transitory lung infiltration, eosinophilia is a characteristic finding. Tropical eosinophilia has been described in India and the South Pacific. In many instances, parasitic infestation has been demonstrated, presumably due to filarial worms.

*Miscellaneous Diseases.* Polyarteritis nodosa, pernicious anemia, and sickle-cell anemia are associated with eosinophilia.

*Familial Eosinophilia.* In a number of instances, eosinophilia has been observed in many members of the same family.[80]

### BASOPHILS

Although the tissue mast cell which contains heparin has staining characteristics similar to those of the basophilic granulocyte of blood, there is evidence that they are separate and distinct cellular entities.[81, 82] The basophil of peripheral blood does not have phagocytic or bactericidal properties. The function of the basophil is not known. The normal basophil in peripheral blood usually has a nonsegmented nucleus that has the characteristics of a band form or metamyelocyte. The blue granules filling the cytoplasm of the basophil are usually larger and more numerous than the lilac-colored granules of the neutrophil or the deep-purple toxic granules of the neutrophil. Basophilic leukocytes may be increased in chronic myelocytic leukemia, in polycythemia vera, sometimes in chronic hemolytic anemias, and following splenectomy. The number of basophils in the normal peripheral blood is low, 0–2 percent. The absence of basophils has no clinical significance. In the course of many infections, both the basophils and the eosinophils disappear during the period of leukocytosis and neutrophilia and reappear during the recovery of the patient. The number of basophils may be relatively increased, 10–40 percent, during irradiation, but the absolute number may be no greater than the pretreatment level. The type of basophil in such conditions is often bizarre.

### LYMPHOCYTES

It is known that the lymphocyte is motile. The possible conversion of lymphocytes in tissue to macrophages is reviewed elsewhere.[79] The function and purpose of lymphocytes, however, is not known, and their role in immune mechanisms is not defined. The life span of lymphocytes seems to be appreciably longer than those of the other cells and has been found to be from 100 to 300 days, as based on $P^{32}$ tagging with DNA. There seems to be a lengthening of this life span in chronic lymphatic leukemia. Biochemically, the lymphocytes take up amino acids less actively and incorporate pyrimidines less actively than leukemic cells of the granulocytic series.[8, 39] Pyogenic infections occurring with chronic lymphatic leukemia are associated with lymphocytosis even during increased cortisone therapy.[83] Lymphocytes enter the blood via the thoracic duct at a sufficiently rapid rate to replace the number of circulating lymphocytes several times over each day. Since both mature lymphocytes and granulocytes incorporate $P^{32}$ into their DNA fraction, it is difficult to interpret life spans based only on isotope data. Recent evidence suggests that the lymphocyte may be important as a precursor of other bone-marrow cells.[84] The alkaline phosphatase of the mature lymphocyte is very low, which accounts for low values seen in lymphocytosis associated with infectious mononucleosis and in lymphatic leukemia.

LYMPHOPENIA. An absolute decrease in lymphocytes is characteristic following irradiation or alkylating agents. It also follows the use of cortisone and ACTH.

LYMPHOCYTOSIS. An absolute increase in the number of lymphocytes occurs in a variety of conditions. In the normal infant or child, the absolute number of lymphocytes is significantly greater than in the adult. In acute infectious lymphocytosis, there is marked increase in the number of adult lymphocytes of normal morphology. In virus diseases, such as infectious mononucleosis, infectious hepatitis, measles, and especially German measles, there is usually a marked increase in lymphocytes. Chronic infections, such as tuberculosis, congenital syphilis, and undulant fever, may also be associated with lymphocytosis. Bacterial infections, such as pertussis, are characteristically associated with lymphocytosis. In thyrotoxicosis, there is usually an absolute or relative lymphocytosis. In such cases, it is of interest that in about 10 percent of the cases the spleen is palpable.[85] Lymphocytosis also occurs in chronic lymphatic leukemia and in maligant lymphoma of the lymphocytoma or lymphoblastoma type.

ATYPICAL AND IMMATURE LYMPHOCYTES. Atypical and immature lymphocytes or monocytes are seen regularly in infectious mononucleosis, infectious hepatitis, and virus infections due to rubeola, rubella, chicken pox, and atypical virus pneumonia. A similar response may occur in pertussis, serum sickness, and miliary tuberculosis. The number of atypical lymphocytes may be small, or so large as to suggest leukemia. In infectious mononucleosis and hepatitis, the number and variety of abnormal lymphocytes are usually greater than in any other conditions, but vary from case to case and from day to day in the same patient. In such situations, the plasma cells are frequently increased as they also are in tuberculosis. Since the finding of atypical lymphocytes is nonspecific, it is not diagnostic of infectious mononucleosis and must be combined with an increasing titer of heterophile antibody which is not absorbed by guinea pig kidney. Establishment of the diagnosis of infectious mononucleosis is important, since it usually has an excellent prognosis.[86] In fatal cases, autopsy reveals infiltration of abnormal lymphocytes throughout every organ of the body.[87] In infectious mononucleosis, the Wassermann test may give a false positive reaction.

PLASMACYTES

CHARACTERISTICS AND FUNCTION. Plasma cells are rarely found in the circulating blood and their significance is also quite obscure. They are very commonly associated with hyperglobulinemia and multiple myeloma with Bence-Jones proteinuria. The plasma cells contain large amounts of gamma globulin, and an absence of plasma cells is associated with hypogammaglobulinemia. They are distinct morphologically from the lymphocytes but are still regarded by some people as a variant of the lymphocyte. They may be increased in the peripheral blood in rubella, scarlatina, measles, and chicken pox.

PLASMACYTOSIS. An increase in the number of plasma cells in the peripheral blood may be observed in certain infections, such as pertussis, rubella, rubeola, chicken pox, bacterial endocarditis, and scarlet fever, in some cases of serum sickness, occasionally in agranulocytosis, and, rarely, as a plasma-cell leukemia accompanying plasmacytoma (multiple myeloma). Plasma cells may also occur in benign lymphocytic meningitis and occasionally in infectious mononucleosis.

### MONOCYTES

CHARACTERISTICS AND FUNCTION. The monocyte belongs to a separate and independent series of cells but has been confused at times with the myelocyte and histiocyte. Monocytes are phagocytic and show active motility when stained by supravital techniques. As reviewed by Doan and Wiseman [88] and from the work of Sabin and associates,[89] it appears that the monocyte and its forms that are found in tissue actively phagocytose the tubercle bacillus and increase in the blood in certain phases of tuberculosis and respond to chemical fractions such as the tuberculo-phosphatides.[90] Monocytes are present in large numbers in the lung during the period of resolution of lobar pneumonia, during which time there may also be monocytosis in the peripheral blood. Monocytosis in a tuberculous patient is usually an unfavorable sign. The relation of monocytes to lymphocytes is sometimes helpful in following a patient with tuberculosis. The average lymphocyte-monocyte ratio is about 2.9. An unfavorable ratio would be under 1.

MONOCYTOSIS. An absolute increase in monocytes occurs in certain bacterial infections such as tuberculosis, subacute bacterial endocarditis, brucella infections, and typhus fever. It may also occur in protozoal and rickettsial infections, such as malaria, Rocky Mountain spotted fever, kala-azar (as high as 40 percent monocytes), Oriental sore, and trypanosomiasis, and in some cases of syphilis. It also may be associated with Hodgkin's disease where it is quite common, and in tetrachlorethylene poisoning. Monocytes are also increased in monocytic leukemia. In all cases of monocytosis, phagocytosis of the red cells and leukocytes by the monocytes may be observed in the blood smear.

### HISTIOCYTES (CLASMATOCYTES, MACROPHAGES, WANDERING ENDOTHELIAL PHAGOCYTES)

CHARACTERISTICS AND FUNCTION. The histiocyte is an actively phagocytic cell of the tissue but is observed occasionally in peripheral blood and may be identified by Wright's stain. The histiocyte may contain phagocytosed red cells, white cells, or platelets. Since the histiocyte is frequently classified as a monocyte in a differential white-cell count, certain reports of monocytic leukemia probably include some histiocytic leukemias.

HISTIOCYTES IN PERIPHERAL BLOOD. Sabin and Doan [91] found histiocytes to be present in numbers up to a maximum of 4 percent in 80 percent of differential counts in a series of preparations made from 9 normal individuals. They may be increased in certain hemolytic anemias, especially erythroblastosis fetalis, in some cases of lymphoma, in severe bacterial infections such as bacterial endocarditis, and in certain parasitic diseases such as malaria and kala-azar and in some agonal states.

## REFERENCES

1. M. M. Wintrobe, *Clinical Hematology* (ed. 4; Lea and Febiger, Philadelphia, 1956).
2. W. S. Beck and W. M. Valentine, "The carbohydrate metabolism of leukocytes: A review," *Cancer Res. 13,* 309 (1953).

3. S. P. Martin, G. R. McKinney, and R. Green, "The metabolism of human polymorphonuclear leukocytes," *Ann. N. Y. Acad. Sci. 59*, 996 (1955).

4. J. L. Tullis, *Blood Cells and Plasma Proteins* (Academic Press, New York, 1953).

5. W. N. Valentine, "The Biochemistry and Enzymatic Activities of Leukocytes in Health and Disease," in L. M. Tocantins, ed., *Progress in Hematology* (Grune and Stratton, New York, 1956), vol. 1.

6. O. Warberg, "On the origin of cancer," *Science 123*, 309 (1956).

7. O. Warberg, *Metabolism of Tumors*, F. Dickens, trans. (Constable, London, 1930).

8. W. H. Baker, P. C. Zamecnik, and M. L. Stephenson, "In vitro incorporation of C–14–DL–Leucine into normal and leukemic white cells," *J. Hemat. 12*, 822 (1957).

9. A. S. Weisberger and B. Levine, "Incorporation of radioactive L–Cystine by normal and leukemic leukocytes in vivo," *Blood 9*, 1082 (1954).

10. A. S. Weisberger and L. G. Suhrland, "Comparative incorporation of S–35 L–Cystine and S–35 sodium sulfate by normal and leukemic leukocytes," *Blood 10*, 458 (1955).

11. M. Bessis, editorial, "At the level of ten angstroms," *Blood 13*, 410 (1958).

12. H. Braunsteiner, K. Fellinger, and F. Pakesch, "Demonstration of a cytoplasmic structure in plasma cells," *Blood 8*, 916 (1953).

13. J. A. Freeman and M. S. Samuels, "The ultrastructure of a 'fibrillar formation' of leukemic human blood," *Blood 13*, 725 (1958).

14. A. S. Sbarra and M. L. Karnofsky, "Biochemical events associated with phagocytosis. I. Metabolic changes during the ingestion of particles by polymorphonuclear leukocytes," *J. biol. Chem. 234*, 1355 (1959).

15. D. R. Sundberg, "Lymphocytes and plasma cells," *Ann. N. Y. Acad. Sci. 59*, 671 (1955).

16. M. W. Chase, "The cellular transfer of cutaneous hypersensitivity to tuberculli," *Proc. Soc. exp. Biol. 59*, 134 (1945).

17. G. J. V. Nossal and J. Lederberg, "Antibody production by single cells," *Nature 181*, 1419 (1958).

18. W. E. Ehrich, "The functional significance of the various leukocytes in inflammation," *Proc. Soc. exp. Biol. 74*, 732 (1950).

19. V. Menkin, *Dynamics of Inflammation* (Macmillan, New York, 1940).

20. V. Menkin, "Modern concepts of inflammation," *Science 105*, 538 (1947).

21. W. B. Wood, Jr., "The role of endogenous pyrogen in the genesis of fever," *Lancet 2*, 53 (1958).

22. A. Kappas, W. Soybel, D. K. Fukushima, and T. F. Gallagher, "Studies on pyrogenic steroids in man," *Trans. Ass. Amer. Phycns. 72*, 54 (1959).

23. H. R. Bierman, K. H. Kelly, and F. L. Cordes, "The sequestration and visceral circulation of leucocytes in man," *Ann. N. Y. Acad. Sci. 59*, 850 (1955).

24. E. E. Osgood, A. J. Seaman, H. Tivey, and D. A. Rigas, "Duration of life and of the different stages of maturation of normal and leukemic leukocytes," *Rev. d'Hemat. 9*, 543 (1954); *Acta Haemat. 13*, 153 (1955).

25. J. Ottesen, "On the age of human white cells in peripheral blood," *Acta physiol. scand. 32*, 75 (1954).

26. D. L. Kline and E. E. Cliffton, "The life span of leukocytes in the human," *Science 115*, 9 (1952).

27. B. Christensen and J. Ottesen, "The age of leukocytes in the blood stream of patients with chronic lymphatic leukemia," *Acta haemat. 13*, 289 (1955)

28. J. F. Ross, unpublished data.

29. W. N. Valentine and W. S. Beck, "Biochemical studies on leukocytes. I. Phosphatase activity in chronic lymphatic leukemia, acute leukemia, and miscellaneous hematologic conditions," *J. lab. clin. Med. 38*, 245 (1951).

30. V. Schilling, *The Blood Picture and Its Clinical Significance* (ed. 8; Mosby, St. Louis, 1929).

31. F. W. Madison and T. L. Squier, "Etiology of primary granulocytopenia (agranulocytic angina)," *J. Amer. med. Ass. 102*, 755 (1934); *J. Allergy 6*, 9 (1934).

32. F. D. Moore, "Toxic manifestations of Thiouracil therapy," *J. Amer. med. Ass. 130*, 315 (1946).

33. P. Plum, *Clinical and Experimental Investigations in Agranulocytosis* (Lewis, London, 1937).

34. S. Moeschlin and K. Wagner, "Agranulocytosis due to the occurrence of leukocyte-agglutinins," *Acta haemat. 8*, 29 (1952).

35. J. Tullis, "Prevalence, nature and identification of leukocyte antibodies," *New Engl. J. Med. 258*, 569 (1958).

36. O. S. Whitelock, ed., "Comparative clinical and biological effects of alkylating agents," *Ann. N. Y. Acad. Sci. 68*, 657 (1958).

37. A. Howard, "Ionizing radiations and cell metabolism," *Ciba Symp. 196* (1956).

38. C. S. Davidson, J. C. Morphy, R. J. Watson, and W. B. Castle, "Comparison of the effects of massive blood transfusions and of liver extract in pernicious anemia," *J. clin. Invest. 25*, 858 (1946).

39. L. H. Smith, Jr., and F. Baker, "Pyrimidine metabolism in man. III. Studies on leukocytes and erythrocytes," *J. clin. Invest. 39*, 15 (1960).

40. W. B. Castle, "Disorders of the blood," in W. A. Sodeman, ed., *Pathologic Physiology: Mechanisms of Disease* (ed. 2; Saunders, Philadelphia, 1956), chap. 28.

41. G. Vejlens, "The distribution of leukocytes in the vascular system," *Acta path. microbiol. scand.*, Suppl., *33*, 1 (1938).

42. J. Jackson, Jr., "The protean character of the leukemias and of the leukemoid states," *New Engl. J. Med. 220*, 175 (1939).

43. W. B. Chew, D. J. Stephens, and J. S. Lawrence, "Antileukocytic serum," *J. Immunol. 30*, 301 (1936).

44. J. S. Lawrence, "Leukopenia. A discussion of its various modes of production," *J. Amer. med. Ass. 116*, 478 (1941).

45. B. K. Wiseman and C. A. Doan, "A newly recognized granulopenic syndrome caused by excessive splenic leukolysis and successfully treated by splenectomy," *J. clin. Invest. 18*, 473 (1939).

46. C. A. Doan and C. S. Wright, "Primary congenital and secondary acquired splenic panhematopenia," *Blood 1*, 10 (1946).

47. T. O. Muether, L. T Moore, J. R. Stewart, and G. O. Broun, "Chronic granulocytopenia caused by excessive splenic lysis of granulocytes," *J. Amer. med. Ass. 116*, 225 (1941).

48. H. M. Rogers and B. E. Hall, "Primary splenic neutropenia," *Arch. intern. Med. 75*, 192 (1945).

49. J. H. Jandl, M. S. Greenberg, R. H. Yonomoto, and W. B. Castle, "Clinical

determination of sites of red cell sequestration in hemolytic anemias," *J. clin. Invest. 35*, 842 (1956).

50. G. E. Cartwright, H. L. Chung, and A. Chang, "Studies on the pancytopenia of kala-azar," *Blood 3*, 249 (1948).

51. J. Jackson, Jr., D. Merrill, and M. Duane, "Agranulocytic angina associated with the menstrual cycle," *New Engl. J. Med. 210*, 175 (1934).

52. H. A. Reimann and C. T. deBerardinis, "Periodic (cyclic) neutropenia, an entity," *Blood 4*, 1109 (1949).

53. P. K. Bondy, G. H. Cohn, W. Herrmann, and K. R. Crispell, "The possible relationship of etioholanolone to periodic fever," *Yale J. biol. Med. 30*, 395 (1958).

54. W. Dameshek, "Editorial—Some speculations on the myeloproliferative syndrome," *Blood 6*, 372 (1951).

55. J. Jackson, Jr., and F. Parker, Jr., *Hodgkin's Disease and Allied Disorders* (Oxford University Press, New York, 1947).

56. E. A. Gall and T. B. Mallory, "Malignant lymphoma," *Amer. J. Path. 18*, 381 (1942).

57. E. A. Gall, "The cytological identity and interrelation of mesenchymal cells of lymphoid tissue," *Ann. N. Y. Acad. Sci. 73*, 120 (1958).

58. H. J. Sparling, R. D. Adams, and F. Parker, Jr., "Involvement of the nervous system by malignant lymphoma," *Medicine 26*, 285 (1947).

59. R. P. Custer and W. G. Bernhard, "The interrelationships of Hodgkin's disease and other lymphatic tumors," *Amer. J. med. Sci. 216*, 625 (1948).

60. W. J. Mitus, I. B. Mednicoff, and W. Dameshek, "Alkaline phosphatase of mature neutrophils in various polycythemias," *New Engl. J. Med. 260*, 1131 (1959).

61. G. DiGuglielmo, "Les maladies erythremiques," *Rev. d'Hemat. 1*, 355 (1946).

62. W. C. Moloney and M. A. Kastenbaum, "Leukemogenic effects of ionizing radiation on atomic bomb survivors in Hiroshima City," *Science 121*, 308 (1955).

63. W. C. Moloney and R. D. Lange, "Cytologic and biochemical studies on granulocytes in early leukemia among atomic bomb survivors," *Tex. Rep. Biol. Med. 12*, 887 (1954).

64. G. A. Daland, *Color Atlas of Morphologic Hematology with a Guide to Clinical Interpretation* (rev. ed.; Harvard University Press, Cambridge, 1959).

65. J. G. Freymann, S. B. Burrell, and E. A. Marler, "Role of hemolysis in anemia secondary to chronic lymphocytic leukemia and certain malignant lymphomas," *New Engl. J. Med. 260*, 1336 (1959).

66. W. C. Sohier, E. Juranies, and J. C. Aub, "Hemolytic anemia, a host response to malignancy," *Cancer Res. 17*, 767 (1957).

67. G. A. Hyman, A. Gellhorn, and J. L. Harvey, "Studies on the anemia of disseminated malignant neoplastic disease. II. Study of the life span of the erythrocyte." *Blood 9*, 618 (1956).

68. R. Berlin, "Red cell survival studies in normal and leukemic subjects," *Acta med. scand.*, Suppl., 252, 1 (1951).

69. J. Waldenstrom, "Incipient myelomatosis or essential hyperglobulinemia with fibrinogenopenia—a new syndrome?" *Acta med. scand. 117*, 216 (1944).

70. R. D. Lillie, *Histopathology and Practical Histochemistry* (Blakiston, New York, 1954).

181

71. I. R. Mackay, N. Eriksen, A. G. Motulsky, and W. Volwiler, "Cryo- and macro-globulinemia. Electrophoretic, ultracentrifugal, and clinical studies," *Amer. J. Med. 20,* 564 (1956).

72. S. Mudd, M. McCutcheon, and B. Lucke, "Phagocytosis," *Physiol. Rev. 14,* 210 (1934).

73. M. D. Chediak, "Nouvelle anomalie leucocytaire de caractère constitutionnel et familial," *Rev. hemat. 7,* 362 (1952).

74. O. Higashi, "Congenital gigantism of peroxydase granules," *Tôhoku J. exp. Med. 59,* 315 (1954).

75. W. L. Donohue and H. W. Bain, "Chediak-Higashi syndrome. A lethal familial disease with anomalous inclusions in the leukocytes and constitutional stigmata," *Pediatrics 20,* 416 (1957).

76. P. Efrati and W. Jonas, "Chediak's anomaly of leucocytes in malignant lymphoma associated with leukemic manifestations," *Blood 13,* 1063 (1958).

77. N. H. Begemann and A. V. L. Campagne, "Homozygous form of Pelger-Huet's nuclear anomaly in man," *Acta haemat. 7,* 295 (1952).

78. A. Alder, "Uber konstitutionell bedingte Granulationsveränderungen der Leukozyten," *Dtsch. Arch. klin. Med. 183,* 372 (1939); *Schweiz. med. Wschr. 80,* 1095 (1950).

79. J. W. Rebuck, "The functions of the white blood cells," *Amer. J. clin. Path. 17,* 614 (1947).

80. P. R. Armand-Delille, A. R. Hurst, and V. E. Sorapure, "Familial eosinophilia," *Guy's Hosp. Rep. 80,* 248 (1930).

81. C. A. Doan and H. L. Reinhart, "The basophil granulocyte, basophilcytosis, and myeloid leukemia, basophil and 'mixed granule' types; and experimental, clinical, and pathological study, with the report of a new syndrome," *Amer. J. clin. Path. 11,* 1 (1941).

82. N. A. Michels, "The mast cells," in H. Downey, ed., *Handbook of Hematology,* vol. I (Hoeber, New York, 1938).

83. W. H. Baker, unpublished data.

84. S. Perry, C. G. Craddock, Jr., G. Paul, and J. S. Lawrence, "Lymphocyte production and turnover," *Arch. int. Med. 103,* 224 (1959).

85. J. H. Means, *The Thyroid and Its Diseases,* vol. II (Lippincott, Philadelphia, 1948).

86. J. J. Timmes, H. H. Averill, and J. Metcalfe, "Splenic rupture in infectious mononucleosis," *New Engl. J. Med. 329,* 173 (1948).

87. E. B. Smith and R. P. Custer, "Rupture of the spleen in infectious mononucleosis," *Blood 1,* 317 (1946).

88. C. A. Doan and B. K. Wiseman, "The monocyte, monocytosis, and monocytic leukosis: a clinical and pathological study," *Ann. int. Med. 8,* 383 (1934).

89. F. R. Sabin, C. A. Doan, and C. E. Forkner, "Studies on tuberculosis," *J. exper. Med. 52,* 1 (1930).

90. F. J. Anderson, "Chemistry of lipoids of tubercle bacilli," *Physiol. Rev. 12,* 166 (1932).

91. F. R. Sabin and C. A. Doan, "The presence of desquamated endothelial cells, the so-called clasmatocytes, in normal mammalian blood," *J. exper. Med. 43,* 823 (1926).

# Unit 13

# The Lupus Erythematosus Cell Test

Originally described by Hargraves in 1948,[1] the lupus erythematosus (LE) cell test has received general acceptance as a valuable adjunct in the clinical diagnosis of disseminated lupus erythematosus.[2, 3, 4] The test has also provided the starting point for extensive investigations in a number of laboratories on the pathogenesis of lupus erythematosus. It is now well demonstrated that the initial event in the LE cell phenomenon is the reaction of a factor in the gamma-globulin fraction of the lupus patient's serum with the nucleohistone of a granulocyte nucleus.[5] This reaction results in the formation of a swollen and homogeneous mass of nuclear material free of cytoplasm which is phagocytosed by a normal granulocyte to give the LE cell. Newer methods of study of the reaction of the LE factor with isolated nuclei and nucleohistone involving radioiodinated antiserums to gamma globulin, complement fixation, and hemagglutination are under investigation, but their clinical usefulness has not been evaluated.

### TECHNIQUES OF LE TEST

Many techniques of performing the LE test are presently being employed, and no single method is clearly superior in all regards.[2, 4] There are two basic methods, one using heparinized blood, and one in which the blood is permitted to clot or is defibrinated. The former method is generally considered less sensitive, while the latter method, though more sensitive, is more liable to difficulty in interpretation due to artifacts. Finally, several modifications have been developed whose purpose is to traumatize the white cells or make the nuclear material more accessible to the LE factor.

HEPARINIZED-BLOOD METHOD. Ten milliliters of venous blood from the patient is added to a tube containing 1.0 mg of aqueous sodium heparin and allowed to stand at room temperature for 30 to 60 min. One milliliter of the blood is then transferred to a Wintrobe tube and centrifuged at 1000 rev/min for 10 min. The buffy coat is pipetted off, smeared on coverslips, and stained with Wright's stain. A more concentrated preparation of buffy coat may be obtained if the original 10 ml is centrifuged for 5 min and the buffy coat so obtained is transferred to a Wintrobe tube and recentrifuged. It is important to avoid excess heparin.

CLOTTED-BLOOD METHOD. Ten milliliters of the patient's blood is permitted to clot and remain at room temperature for 1 hr. The clot is then broken up with wooden applicators, or preferably completely macerated by passing it through a fine tea sieve (30 mesh per inch). The clot fragments are permitted to stand an additional hour at room temperature and are then centrifuged and treated in the same manner as the heparinized blood.

MODIFICATIONS. (1) Zinkham and Conley[6] have introduced a modification which improves the sensitivity of heparinized blood technique. One and one-half milliliters of heparinized blood is placed in a 50-ml Erlenmeyer flask containing 15 glass beads 4 mm in diameter, and rotated in a Shen type rotater at 40 rev/min for 30 min at 37°C. The material is then transferred to a Wintrobe tube and centrifuged.

(2) Snapper[7] has described a method in which substrate slides of dried leukocytes are prepared by allowing a few drops of normal blood to clot for 1 hr within a 0.8-cm rubber ring on a glass slide placed in a Petri dish with moistened filter paper to prevent drying. The ring and clot are then slid off, and the slide is washed with serum and permitted to dry. The test is performed with a drop of the patient's finger or venous blood placed on a coverslip which is inverted over the substrate area and supported by two small pieces of No. 2 coverslips. After incubation for 2 hr at room temperature in a Petri dish with moistened filter paper, the coverslip is slid off and the slide is washed with serum and stained in the usual manner.

### INTERPRETATIONS AND LIMITATIONS

The finding of at least three classical LE cells should be required for considering any LE preparation positive, while at least 500 normal granulocytes should be counted before a smear is considered negative. Amorphous masses of purplish homogeneous extranuclear material and rosettes (amorphous masses ringed by polymorphonuclear leukocytes) are highly suggestive, but a preparation should not be considered positive in the absence of classical LE cells. Rouleau formation is a nonspecific finding. In general, the most profitable areas in which to search for LE cells are along the peripheral margins of the smear. With experience, time may be saved by using the low-power objective to locate suspicious cells which may then be definitively identified under higher powers. The LE cell is a cell usually considerably larger than an adult granulocyte. The nucleus of the LE cell has been pushed to the periphery, and the bulk of the cell is occupied by homogeneous inclusion, staining purplish with Wright's stain, and surrounded by a thin rim of cytoplasm. The inclusions may be multiple, but the homogeneous quality should be present. The LE inclusion must be differentiated from phagocytosed red blood cells and from phagocytosed nuclei which have intact chromatin structure ("tart cells" of Hargraves).[1]

Repeated LE tests can be expected to be positive in about 75–80 percent of patients with clinically typical lupus erythematosus disseminata. A single random test in a group of LE patients will probably be positive only 25–40 percent of the time, the lower figure applying to the test using heparinized blood, while the higher figure applies to the other methods described above.

Positive LE tests have been obtained in 10–20 percent of cases of rheumatoid arthritis,[8] including cases that are otherwise clinically typical. The significance of this finding is at present not clear. Positive LE preparations have also been found in allergic reactions to penicillin, the lupus-like syndrome of hydralazine toxicity, and a group of patients, usually female, with subacute hepatitis and high globulin ("lupoid cirrhosis"). Single, isolated positive tests have been found in miliary tuberculosis, reactions to tetanus antitoxin and phenylbutazone, leukemia, dermatitis herpetiformis, pernicious anemia, generalized moniliasis, myeloma, periarteritis nodosa, and thrombotic thrombocytopenic purpura. The test is usually not positive in chronic discoid lupus and in other connective-tissue diseases.

## REFERENCES

1. M. M. Hargraves, H. Richmond, and R. Morton, "Presentation of two bone marrow elements: The 'Tart' cell and the 'L. E.' cell," *Proc. Mayo Clin. 23*, 25, (1948).
2. L. Dubois and V. Freeman, "A comparative evaluation of the L. E. cell test performed simultaneously by different methods," *Blood 12*, 657 (1957).
3. A. M. Harvey, L. E. Shulman, P. A. Tumulty, C. L. Conley, and E. H. Schoenrich, "Systemic lupus erythematosus: Review of the literature and clinical analysis of 138 cases," *Medicine 33*, 291 (1954).
4. J. R. Haserick, "Evaluation of three diagnostic procedures for systemic lupus erythematosus," *Ann. intern. Med. 44*, 497 (1956).
5. G. J. Friou, "The significance of the lupus-globulin-nucleoprotein reaction," *Ann. intern. Med. 49*, 866 (1958).
6. W. H. Zinkham and C. L. Conley, "Some factors influencing the formation of L. E. cells," *Bull. Johns Hopk. Hosp. 98*, 102 (1956).
7. I. Snapper and D. J. Nathan, "The mechanism of the L. E. phenomenon, studied with a simplified test," *Blood 10*, 718 (1955).
8. I. A. Friedman, J. F. Sickley, R. M. Poske, A. Black, D. Bronsk, C. Feldhake, P. S. Reeder, and E. M. Katz, "The L. E. phenomenon in rheumatoid arthritis," *Ann. intern. Med. 46*, 1113 (1957).

# Unit 14

## Hemorrhagic Diseases

In man about 6000 ml of blood circulates under positive pressure through a vascular compartment with a surface area of over 6000 m² during more than half a century of repeated trauma. Dramatically stated, this is the problem of hemostasis. Any rupture in the continuity of a blood vessel, however small, would lead to fatal exsanguination were it not for a prompt chain of hemostatic reactions designed to seal and finally repair the defect. For most physiologic systems that have been described in man there are corresponding diseases of "too much" and "too little." This is equally true for hemostasis. Diseases associated with excessive intravascular clotting are by far the more frequent clinically, but at the present time they are not associated with reliable laboratory guides indicative of pathogenesis or suggestive of therapy. At the opposite pole are the hemorrhagic diseases, which may be associated with any defect in the complicated scheme of hemostasis leading to an increased tendency to bleed. Since the prognosis and treatment of patients with hemorrhagic diseases vary widely, it is highly important to establish the pathogenesis of the hemostatic defect. It is the purpose of this section to outline a logical approach to the problem presented by a patient with a hemorrhagic diathesis, with special attention to the methods of laboratory examination. There are several excellent monographs that can be consulted for detailed descriptions of the hemorrhagic disorders.[1-4]

### Hemostasis

A rational approach to the study of the hemorrhagic diatheses can be based only on a familiarity with the events in normal hemostasis, which will be summarized briefly in this section. Hemostasis, the prevention of the escape of blood from the intravascular compartment, depends on the controlled interplay of a large number of chemical reactions and physiologic events. The control of this chain of reactions must be precise, for it must: (a) be set in motion by any disruption of vascular integrity; (b) restrain and limit the autocatalytic reactions of coagulation within the area of usefulness; (c) allow for eventual repair of the vascular defect by lysis of the fibrin clot and reestablishment of luminal continuity; (d) not be induced inappropriately.

It is of interest that normal hemostasis is effected by an interplay of reactants and systems varying in complexity from ionized calcium to contraction of blood-vessel walls, from protein-protein interactions to protein-cell interactions. It is useful to consider hemostasis under several subdivisions which seem to have some physiologic validity and which suggest a convenient classification of the hemorrhagic disorders; these are: vascular and extravascular factors—physical defense; platelets—physical and chemical

186

defense; coagulation—chemical defense; anticoagulation and fibrinolysis—restraint and repair.

## Vascular and Extravascular Factors

It is evident that the blood vessel is the first line of defense in hemostasis. Strictly speaking, no hemorrhage occurs without rupture of a blood-vessel wall. Maintenance of normal resistance to rupture despite the stress of intraluminal pressure or extrinsic trauma is the most important vascular contribution to hemostasis. The factors that serve to maintain the integrity of the blood-vessel wall are largely unknown. Ascorbic acid, hyaluronic acid, and calcium seem to be concerned with the synthesis of capillary cement substance. The pharmacologic effects of certain agents such as corticosteroids and histamine on capillaries are easily shown clinically, but have not been defined in biochemical terms. Knowledge of hemorrhagic disorders due to diseases of blood-vessel walls is largely restricted to descriptive classification of the respective syndromes. Surrounding tissues serve to give physical support to small blood vessels and exert counterpressure during an extravascular accumulation of blood, depending upon the turgor and rigidity of the particular tissue involved.

Most blood vessels are capable of active contraction. It is probable that true capillaries do not themselves contract, but respond secondarily to the vascular tone of proximal vessels with a muscular coat.[5] The major function of this contraction is to control the distribution and pressure of circulating blood. An important secondary function is to aid in the initiation and maintenance of hemostasis after injury. Initial vasoconstriction is related to local reflexes and is generally of brief duration, but it serves to allow the formation of effective platelet plugs.[6] It is thought by some that the continuation of vasoconstriction depends on chemical pressor agents released during the process of coagulation, notably platelet serotonin. The relative importance of vasoconstriction in hemostasis is difficult to assess and seems to depend on the nature of the injury and the size of the involved blood vessel, being apparently most important at the arteriolar level.

## Platelets

Blood platelets are derived from marrow megakaryocytes and normally circulate for 8–9 days as discrete, nonnucleated tissue fragments.[7] The platelets seem to have many functions in hemostasis, all of which are imperfectly understood.

*Adhesiveness.* Platelets tend to adhere to wettable surfaces, including injured vascular endothelium, sending out numerous pseudopods of thinly spread hyaloplasm, the changes classically referred to as "viscous metamorphosis." It seems apparent that agglutinated platelets serve thereby a strictly physical function of helping to plug ruptures in the vessel wall. This may be particularly effective in smaller blood vessels, such as capillaries.

*Clot Retraction.* It is generally agreed that platelets play a major role in clot retraction, probably through the contraction of filamentous pseudopodia of intact platelets caught within the fibrin network[8] rather than by the action of some released humoral agent. Clot retraction is also influenced by a number of other factors, such as fibrinogen, thrombin, pH, and the erythrocytic mass. Its function in hemostasis is unknown.

*"Chemical Storehouse."* Recent studies have shown that the platelets contain a number of pharmacologically active amines, particularly serotonin. It has been postulated that serotonin, which was originally discovered as the vasopressor agent released from clotted blood,[9] serves to reinforce local vasoconstrictive mechanisms following injury.

The importance of this effect in hemostasis has yet to be proved.[10]

*Capillary Fragility.* All conditions that result in a marked diminution in the number of circulating platelets are associated with increased capillary fragility. When platelets are diminished immunologically, the resulting capillary damage is explained by a hypothetical common antigenicity of capillary endothelium with platelets. The same defect is found, however, when platelets are removed mechanically. The mechanism by which platelets influence the integrity of capillary endothelium is obscure.

*Coagulation.* In the absence of extravascular thromboplastic substances, platelets or platelet factors are necessary for physiologic coagulation of blood. At least four platelet factors have been partially purified: [11] factor 1, which resembles plasma proaccelerin (factor V); factor 2, which accelerates the formation of fibrin by the action of thrombin on fibrinogen; factor 3, the lipoid platelet thromboplastic factor; factor 4, an antiheparin. Of these factors, the platelet thromboplastic factor, which recent evidence suggests is a heat-stable lipid of the cephalin group,[12] seems to be of greatest importance in coagulation. Reduction in the number of platelets is generally associated with increased capillary fragility, prolongation of the bleeding time, a reduction in the amount of thromboplastin formed and to a lesser degree in its rate of formation (hence a reduced prothrombin consumption but generally a normal clotting time), and poor clot retraction.

## Coagulation

In hemostasis, coagulation of the blood represents only one phase of the defense system, as illustrated by the fact that in about 50 percent of all cases of hemorrhagic diatheses no abnormality of coagulation can be demonstrated.[13] Conversely, coagulation can be continuously compromised without hemorrhagic phenomena, as in Hageman factor deficiency.[14] Coagulation of the blood depends on the triggering of a multiphasic sequence of events with the final production of a firm fibrin polymer from fibrinogen, the only plasma clotting factor that is present in greater than trace amounts. Despite many recent advances, the initial stimulus, the exact sequence of events, the restraining reactions, and the regulation of the production and release of clotting factors are still unresolved problems. In the present context, the discussion to follow must of necessity be abbreviated and represent an eclectic choice from current leading theories.

The multiplicity of terms and nonuniformity of nomenclature make a brief initial glossary and definition of terms mandatory.

*AHF : Antihemophilic factor or globulin* (thromboplastinogen, factor VIII) —a globulin that corrects the clotting defect of human or canine hemophilia. It is present in plasma, consumed during coagulation, and thus absent from serum. It is not adsorbed by commonly used salt-adsorbing agents, and is closely associated with fibrinogen in plasma-fractionation procedures.

*PTC : Plasma thromboplastin component* (Christmas factor, factor IX)—a relatively stable beta$_2$ globulin that corrects the clotting defect of a disease clinically indistinguishable from classical hemophilia, sometimes called "Christmas disease" or hemophilia B. PTC is present in normal serum as well as plasma, and is adsorbed by a number of insoluble inorganic salts.

*PTA : Plasma thromboplastin antecedent* (plasma thromboplastic factor C)— a stable globulin, present in normal plasma and serum, which corrects the clotting defect of a small group of patients with a hemophilioid disorder. This factor has not been as well characterized as AHF or PTC. It is partially adsorbed by insoluble inorganic salts.

*Stuart factor* (Prower factor, Stuart-

Prower factor)[15]—a stable alpha globulin that closely resembles proconvertin (VII) in its physical properties, is found in both plasma and serum, and is adsorbed by certain inorganic salts and by asbestos filters. It is required for the formation of plasma thromboplastin and the action of tissue thromboplastin and Russell viper venom in the conversion of prothrombin to thrombin.

*Hageman factor* (glass factor) [14]—a heat-labile globulin that is present in both plasma and serum and is adsorbed by kaolin, glass, or quartz. The function of this factor in the early stages of blood coagulation in vitro is not clear and deficiency of it is associated with no clinical manifestations.

*Proaccelerin* (accelerator globulin, labile factor, factor V)—a labile globulin required for the conversion of prothrombin to thrombin by thromboplastin and calcium. Its activity in plasma is gradually lost on storage. During coagulation it disappears rapidly so that fresh serum is relatively devoid of it. It is not adsorbed by inorganic salts.

*Proconvertin* (serum prothrombin conversion accelerator, stable factor, factor VII)—a stable $\beta$ globulin that is recognized by its ability to correct the prolonged one-stage prothrombin times of certain coumarin-treated patients, of infants in the neonatal period, of patients with parenchymatous liver disease, and of rare patients with a congenital deficiency of this factor. It is found in serum as well as plasma and is adsorbed by insoluble inorganic salts. It is also adsorbed by asbestos (as is the Stuart factor). Proconvertin reacts with tissue thromboplastin but not with plasma thromboplastin.

*Platelet factor 3* (platelet thromboplastic factor, thromboplastic factor, thromboplastinogenase)—a heat-stable phospholipid from platelets whose exact chemical nature has yet to be defined. It serves as the platelet factor in the formation of plasma thromboplastin.

*Prothrombin*—a stable glycoprotein that has been obtained in a high state of purity, is greatly reduced in normal serum, and is adsorbed by many insoluble inorganic salts.

*Fibrinogen*—a protein with a large (molecular weight 400,000–500,000) elongated molecule, which has been highly purified and well characterized chemically and physiologically. Fibrinogen is the substrate for the proteolytic action of thrombin, by which it is transformed into fibrin.

*"Prothrombinase"* (prothrombin activator). This is a term that has been applied to the hypothetical final product of plasma thromboplastin, calcium, and the accessory substances which is able to activate prothrombin directly.[16] Its nature is far from clear, although partial separation has been reported.[17]

Some of the useful laboratory properties of these factors are summarized in Table 37.

The simplified schema of coagulation in Fig. 22 should be used as a guide in the description of the reactions of coagulation. The clotting of blood is generally presented as occurring in three stages: formation of thromboplastin, formation of thrombin, and formation of fibrin. It should be emphasized that the choice of

Table 37. *Laboratory properties of coagulation factors.*

| Factor | Plasma | Serum | Adsorbed by insoluble inorganic salts |
|---|---|---|---|
| AHF (factor VIII) | + | 0 | 0 |
| PTC (factor IX) | + | + | + |
| PTA | + | + | ± |
| Proaccelerin (factor V) | + | 0 | 0 |
| Proconvertin (factor VII) | + | + | + |
| Platelet factor 3 | 0 (not free in plasma) | 0 | 0 |
| Prothrombin | + | 0 | + |
| Fibrinogen | + | 0 | 0 |
| Stuart factor | + | + | + |
| Hageman factor | + | + | ± |

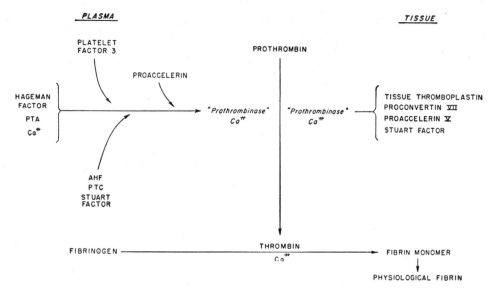

Fig. 22. A diagnostic representation of some of the stages of blood coagulation. The exact sequence of events in thromboplastin formation is not known.

these particular stages has arbitrarily evolved on the basis of convenience of laboratory tests, and in fact the reactions occur in a continuous, possibly autocatalyzed sequence.

THROMBOPLASTIN. The term thromboplastin will be used, although it is more correct to speak of "thromboplastic activity," since a number of diverse and incompletely characterized substances exhibit this activity. Two systems leading to the formation of thromboplastin must be considered: tissue thromboplastin and plasma thromboplastin. The relative importance of these two systems in hemostasis is still to be defined.

*Tissue thromboplastin.* Thromboplastic activity is found in essentially all tissues but is greatest in brain, lung, and placenta. By suitable physical and chemical means, tissue thromboplastin can be fractionated into a heat-stable lipoid substance, possibly a cephalin, which seems closely related chemically to the platelet thromboplastic factor (platelet factor 3), and a heat-labile protein or protein complex, which seems to resemble in its activity the product of the interaction of AHF, PTC, PTA, and other plasma fac-

tors.[18] Tissue thromboplastin differs from plasma thromboplastin in at least two important ways: it requires proconvertin (VII) as well as proaccelerin (V), Stuart factor, and $Ca^{++}$ for final activation to a "prothrombinase," and it is ready to act within a few seconds rather than requiring a long latent period (3–6 min) for its formation.

*Plasma thromboplastin.* The formation of plasma thromboplastin requires a series of time-consuming reactions involving the platelet factor 3, calcium, and a number of circulating proteins, of which AHF, PTC, PTA, Hageman factor, and Stuart factor would appear to be the most firmly established and clinically important.[18] Other circulating factors have been postulated as contributing to plasma-thromboplastin formation,[19, 20] but will not be discussed here. The exact sequence in which various factors interact to form plasma thromboplastin is not known. Present evidence suggests that plasma-thromboplastin formation is initiated when blood comes in contact with an activating surface, and that this first reaction involves the Hageman factor.[14, 21] The property of a surface that initiates this first phase of coagulation seems most closely related to wettability. PTA may also be concerned with the early phases of the reactions. Soon thereafter the platelets undergo the changes of "viscous metamorphosis" and liberate platelet granules containing the lipoidal factor 3. The plasma factors do not merely liberate a previously active thromboplastin from platelets, however, for platelets that are physically disrupted (as by sonic vibration) still require the presence of plasma factors to form active thromboplastin. Subsequent reactions involving AHF, PTC, Stuart factor, and $Ca^{++}$ are necessary for the formation of plasma thromboplastin. The platelet factor and AHF are used up during this series of reactions (and therefore are absent from serum); PTC, PTA, the Hageman factor, and the Stuart factor remain. The platelet factor influences the amount of thromboplastin formed but to a lesser degree the rate of the reaction. AHF influences both the rate and the completeness of the reaction.[22] Thromboplastin is formed very rapidly after a latent period of 3–6 min required by the early steps of the reaction. The resulting thromboplastic activity is unstable and largely disappears within 1 hr after clotting, probably owing to an antithromboplastin in the serum.

FORMATION OF THROMBIN. Thrombin is a proteolytic enzyme, undetectable in circulating plasma, but formed from prothrombin by the action of thromboplastin, $Ca^{++}$, and certain other essential factors. Recent evidence supports the hypothesis that plasma thromboplastin reacts with $Ca^{++}$ and proaccelerin (V) to form an unstable product called "prothrombinase," which in the presence of $Ca^{++}$ can carry out the final activation of prothrombin to thrombin alone. A seemingly similar "prothrombinase" is formed from the interaction of tissue thromboplastin, $Ca^{++}$, proaccelerin (V), proconvertin (VII), and Stuart factor. "Prothrombinase" serves to alter the stable prothrombin molecule in an unknown manner to produce the labile proteolytic enzyme thrombin.[23] Thrombin seems to have at least two actions: it forms fibrin from fibrinogen; and it catalyzes the completion of the first two stages of coagulation by speeding up the disruption of platelets and by activating proaccelerin (V). It is therefore the key substance in what has been called the "autocatalytic" or "cocatalytic" phase of coagulation during which a product of coagulation serves a feedback function to speed up the rate of its own production.[24]

FORMATION OF FIBRIN. Fibrinogen, which constitutes about 5 percent of plasma protein, is the substrate for the proteolytic action of thrombin, which removes an acidic polypeptide. The resulting fibrin monomer then polymerizes into fibrin strands.[25] In the presence of $Ca^{++}$ and an unidentified plasma factor, the initial fibrin is strengthened, probably by cross linkages of disulfide groups, to form "physiologic fibrin." [26] With the formation of a firm fibrin clot the purpose of coagulation is fulfilled.

ANTICOAGULATION AND FIBRINOLYSIS.

Under this heading will be included a brief consideration of the factors that normally prevent coagulation from occurring inappropriately, restrain it from spreading beyond the area in which it is useful, and serve to reestablish luminal continuity of the vessel—in brief, the forces of "restraint and repair." This phase of the general phenomenon of hemostasis remains the most obscure. In a broad sense, anticoagulation is largely dependent on the property of vascular endothelium that renders it inert as a stimulus to the initiation of coagulation. Failure of spontaneous coagulation to occur more frequently is also due in part to the fact that thromboplastin either is extravascular or can be formed intravascularly only through a complex, time-consuming series of reactions, of which one reactant is "locked up" within the platelets.

*Natural inhibitors.* Of the natural inhibitors of blood coagulation, perhaps the best understood relate to the inactivation of thrombin. The importance of these antithrombins is underlined by the fact that 10 ml of normal plasma can release enough thrombin to clot all of the blood in the body.[1] Some of the thrombin released during coagulation is inactivated by physical adsorption by the fibrin clot.[27] Normal plasma also contains an α-globulin antithrombin that quickly binds and inactivates circulating thrombin stoichiometrically. The sum of these reactions serves to limit thrombin activity markedly in area and time, so that it disappears promptly (10–20 min) after blood clots.

Heparin, operating in conjunction with an albumin cofactor, serves to increase the amount of thrombin adsorbed by fibrin and may influence the rate at which thrombin is inactivated by antithrombin.[28] Heparin also inhibits the formation of plasma thromboplastin, possibly by inactivation of PTC. It should be emphasized that the concentration of heparinoid substances in the blood is too low to have much effect under normal circumstances. Recent work has suggested that plasma normally contains a protein, antithromboplastin,[29] that may be responsible for the known disappearance of thromboplastin within the first hour after coagulation.

*Fibrinolysis.* Resolution of small thrombi that form during the minor injuries of daily life probably occurs constantly as a normal process. In addition, mechanisms must be available for recanalization of a larger blood vessel after hemostasis has been effected. There exists in blood and tissues an incompletely elucidated system for fibrinolysis whose current complexities are beyond the scope of this brief review.[30, 31] At the present time at least two pathways for the production of fibrinolytic activity have been described. The first of these is a local process in which an insoluble tissue activator changes the precursor profibrinolysin (plasminogen), which is found in plasma, to fibrinolysin (plasmin). Secondly, circulating profibrinolysin can be altered to fibrinolysin by a blood activator, which in turn must first be activated by a tissue or blood lysokinase. The fibrinolysin that finally evolves is not only capable of lysing a fibrin clot, but may attack, presumably by proteolysis, other coagulation factors, notably fibrinogen and proaccelerin.[32] Normal blood also contains inhibitors of both fibrinolysin and the profibrinolysin activators. These mechanisms are not normally related to hemostasis per se but are part of the processes of repair.

### The Study of Hemorrhagic Diathesis

A classification of the hemorrhagic disorders is given in Table 38. A systematic approach is necessary if an accurate diagnosis is to be made with an economical expenditure of time and effort. To a greater degree than in most varieties of disease, the differential diagnosis of a bleeding disorder depends upon the interpretation of appropriate laboratory studies. Nevertheless, as in other diseases, an accurate history and careful physical examination are of great importance and are worthy of brief comment here.

#### HISTORY

From the history the physician should obtain information about the severity of a hemorrhagic diathesis, its duration, the clinical pattern it presents (parts of the body involved, intermittency, and so forth), its possible relation to exogenous factors (such as drugs), and the presence or absence of a familial trait. Each of these categories should be kept firmly in mind and explored in detail. In addition, the history may give other informa-

Table 38. *Classification of hemorrhagic disorders.*

1. Vascular and extravascular diseases
   a. Congenital abnormalities
      Hereditary hemorrhagic telangiectasis
      Pseudohemophilia
   b. Scurvy
   c. Anaphylactoid purpura
   d. Miscellaneous: uremia, diabetes, purpura of infectious diseases, etc.
2. Platelet disorders
   a. Thrombocytopenia
      Amegakaryocytic: marrow aplasia or replacement
      Megakaryocytic: idiopathic thrombocytopenic purpura, hypersplenism, thrombotic thrombocytopenic purpura, drug-induced thrombocytopenia
   b. Thrombasthenia
   c. Thrombocythemia: polycythemia vera, idiopathic
3. Coagulation disorders
   a. Deficiency of plasma thromboplastin formation
      AHF deficiency
      PTC deficiency
      PTA deficiency
      Hageman defect
      Stuart-factor defect
   b. Deficiency of thrombin formation
      Prothrombin deficiency
      Proaccelerin (V) deficiency
      Proconvertin (VII) deficiency
      Stuart-factor deficiency
   c. Deficiency of fibrin formation
      Afibrinogenemia
      Fibrinogenopenia
4. Disorders of anticoagulation and fibrinolysis
   a. Dysproteinemias: multiple myeloma, macroglobulinemia, cryoglobulinemia, amyloidosis
   b. Parenchymal liver disease
   c. Obstetric accidents
   d. Leukemia

tion suggestive of a primary disease (such as cirrhosis) that may be associated secondarily with a bleeding tendency. In an attempt to determine the severity and duration of the disorder, one should take historical advantage of past hemostatic stresses such as menstruation, epistaxis, ease of bruising, tooth extractions, and surgical procedures. It is important to determine whether the patient has been exposed to potentially harmful drugs, chemicals, or physical agents. The family history is of particular significance in that a large proportion of hemorrhagic disorders, particularly those relating to defective plasma-thromboplastin formation, are in fact "inborn errors of metabolism."

### PHYSICAL EXAMINATION

The physical examination is rarely diagnostic of the pathogenesis of a bleeding diathesis, but it may lead to the diagnosis of a primary disease of which the bleeding diathesis is a secondary complication. In addition, the pattern of bleeding that occurs may be highly suggestive of a given hemostatic defect, such as the hemarthroses that occur in the hemophilias, the petechial and mucous-membrane bleeding of thrombocytopenia, or the follicular and perifollicular purpura of scurvy. It has been suggested that purpuric manifestations always represent vascular abnormalities, either primary or secondary to thrombocytopenia, and that bleeding into deeper tissues and joints usually is associated with coagulation defects.

### LABORATORY STUDIES

Some laboratory studies contribute primarily to the understanding of the etiology of a hemorrhagic disorder. In this section only those studies for determining the pathogenesis of a bleeding disorder will be outlined. A detailed description of these tests constitutes the section to follow.

The availability of a wide number of laboratory tests of increasing complexity demands a systematic approach to their use in the study of an individual patient. Certain relatively simple tests should be carried out initially to permit a preliminary assessment of the general type of hemorrhagic disorder to be studied. These are listed in Table 39.

Further laboratory studies will usually be indicated, depending upon the pattern of abnormalities that emerges from the initial screening tests. Some of the most frequently encountered general categories are the following.

Table 39. *Tests useful in the preliminary assessment of a hemorrhagic disorder.*

| Test | Physiologic function tested |
| --- | --- |
| Tourniquet | Blood vessel, platelets |
| Bleeding time | Blood vessel, platelets |
| Platelet count | Platelets, as physical rather than as functional units |
| Whole-blood clotting time | All three stages of coagulation, but predominantly reflects stage 1 |
| One-stage prothrombin time | Stages 2 and 3 of coagulation |
| Prothrombin consumption | Stage 1 of coagulation (if prothrombin time is normal) |
| Clot dissolution | Fibrinolysins |
| Clot retraction | Platelets |
| Fibrinogen concentration | Fibrinogen |

CLOTTING TIME PROLONGED; PROTHROMBIN CONSUMPTION DIMINISHED; ALL OTHER SCREENING STUDIES NORMAL. This condition usually indicates a defect in stage 1 of coagulation, the formation of plasma thromboplastin. Further tests are necessary to determine which of the plasma thromboplastic factors is at fault (usually as a familial hemorrhagic disorder) or to demonstrate (less frequently) the presence of a circulating anticoagulant. This information can be obtained most accurately from the thromboplastin-generation test.[33] Alternatively, much the same information can frequently be obtained more simply by appropriate modifications of the prothrombin-consumption test, to be described below.

PROTHROMBIN TIME PROLONGED; ALL OTHER SCREENING STUDIES NORMAL (INCLUDING FIBRINOGEN CONCENTRATION). This condition demonstrates the presence of an abnormality in stage 2 of clotting, the conversion of prothrombin to thrombin. Since this conversion is measured by the reaction of thrombin on fibrinogen to form visible fibrin, marked reduction in plasma fibrinogen may also prolong the prothrombin time. Further tests, to be outlined later, demonstrate whether the defect is related to deficiency of pro-thrombin, of proaccelerin (V), of proconvertin (VII), or of Stuart factor.

BLEEDING TIME OR TOURNIQUET TEST ABNORMAL. *Platelet count significantly reduced* (to less than 100,000/mm³). This will result in poor clot retraction and reduced prothrombin consumption (secondary to a deficiency of platelet thromboplastic factor). Further tests, such as bone-marrow aspiration, search for platelet agglutinins,[34] and testing of drugs,[35] taken in conjunction with the history and physical examination, may be necessary to differentiate megakaryocytic from amegakaryocytic thrombocytopenia, and various subdivisions of each.[2]

*Platelet count normal or only slightly reduced* (more than 100,000/mm³). (i) Platelet function normal (clot retraction, prothrombin consumption) but bleeding time prolonged; tourniquet test normal or abnormal; family history often positive. This suggests the diagnosis of pseudohemophilia (von Willebrand's disease).

(ii) Platelet function abnormal (clot retraction, prothrombin consumption) in spite of what would normally be an adequate number of platelets; platelets are often unusually large and may be bizarre in shape. This supports the diagnosis of thrombasthenia (thrombocytopathia).

(iii) Tourniquet test grossly abnormal, but bleeding time and platelet-function tests normal. This combination of findings is suggestive of scurvy.

RAPID LYSIS OF A NORMAL CLOT. This indicates the presence of a circulating fibrinolysin.

The foregoing categories are, of course, not all-inclusive but are merely representative of abnormalities that may be disclosed during the initial screening studies. For complete descriptions of the clinical features and laboratory abnormalities of these diseases, one of the recent monographs should be consulted.[1-4]

## Description of Screening Laboratory Tests

### TOURNIQUET TEST

The tourniquet test is a useful, though crude, index of capillary fragility as measured by the ability of the capillary to withstand the stress of intraluminal positive pressure. A number of techniques have been described, of which the following is recommended.

On the volar surface of the forearm about 4 to 5 cm below the antecubital fossa, a circular area 2.5 cm in diameter is marked off and inspected in advance for artifacts resembling petechiae. A blood-pressure cuff is applied to the upper arm in the usual manner and the blood pressure determined. The cuff is then inflated to 100 mm Hg for 10 min (unless the patient's systolic pressure is 100 mm Hg or less, in which case a pressure is selected midway between systolic and diastolic pressure). Five minutes after removal of the cuff, the number of petechiae in the marked area is counted.

INTERPRETATIONS AND LIMITATIONS. In a normal test there will be approximately 0–5 petechiae in men and 0–10 petechiae in women and children. The test is at best only crudely quantitative and may be graded on an arbitrary scale of 1+ to 4+, the latter representing confluent petechiae in all areas of the arm and dorsum of the hand.

The tourniquet test is primarily a measurement of the ability of small blood vessels to resist a standardized stress,[36] possibly reflecting their ability to resist the wide variety of traumas associated with everyday life. In brief, there are two general groups of hemorrhagic disorders in which a positive test may be found: disorders of the vessel wall without demonstrable coagulation defects, and qualitative or quantitative platelet defects. The former group is illustrated by scurvy, in which there seems to be defective synthesis of capillary cement sub-stance resulting from deficiency of ascorbic acid, with a positive tourniquet test but a normal bleeding time. A positive tourniquet test is found in about half of patients with pseudohemophilia (von Willebrand's disease) and may be found irregularly in anaphylactoid purpura (Henoch-Schönlein), the purpura of sepsis, and the purpura associated with senility, uremia, diabetes, and hypertension. Many patients with pseudohemophilia have an associated AHF deficiency.[37, 38]

Almost all conditions in which the circulating platelets are significantly reduced in number or are qualitatively defective may be associated with increased capillary fragility as measured by the tourniquet test. As noted in the introductory section, the exact relation of platelets to capillary integrity has yet to be defined.[39] In some cases this relation may represent a common antigenicity shared by capillary endothelium and platelets such that both are injured immunologically, as may be postulated in autoimmune cases of idiopathic thrombocytopenic purpura. Possibly reduction of the plugging function of the platelets in thrombocytopenia may contribute to the extravasation of blood through small capillary ruptures.

Capillary fragility may also be tested by the use of an apparatus that applies a negative pressure to an area of skin by means of a suction cup.[40] Since this technique offers few advantages over the method described above and requires a specialized apparatus that is not generally available, the various modifications of this procedure will not be presented.

### BLEEDING TIME

The bleeding time is the interval required for effective hemostasis to occur following a standardized wound of the capillary bed. Several techniques for making this determination have been described, of which the Ivy method [41] is recommended. Using a blood-pressure cuff, a pressure of 40 mm Hg is maintained about the upper arm throughout the procedure. With a Bard-Parker No. 11 blade, a puncture wound 2 mm in length and depth is made just distal to the antecubital fossa, avoiding visible subcutaneous veins. The escaping blood is adsorbed onto filter paper every 30 sec, care being taken to touch the drop but not the skin. The end point occurs when blood from the wound ceases to stain the blotting filter paper. The normal range for this method is a bleeding time of between ½ and 6½ min.

Among the most frequently used techniques is the Duke method,[42] in which a similar wound, again using a Bard-Parker No. 11 blade, is made in the dependent portion of the lobe of the ear. The bleeding time from the wound is measured as described above, with a normal range of approximately 2 to 4½ min. In general, the results are not as reproducible as in the Ivy method, and control of excessive bleeding is not as convenient.

INTERPRETATIONS AND LIMITATIONS. At best there is considerable variation in the bleeding time, perhaps largely related to the difficulty in creating a standardized wound. In general, errors in performing this test lead to values that are falsely low. At no time should a needle be used to produce the wound. To assess the significance of slight prolongation of the bleeding time, repeated tests should be performed.

As in the positive tourniquet test, an abnormally prolonged bleeding time may be found in disorders of small blood vessels without demonstrable coagulation defects, and in thrombocytopenia or qualitative platelet defects. It has been postulated that the vascular defect is predominantly that of impaired contractility. This has been demonstrated by capillary microscopy in some patients with pseudohemophilia, the most characteristic disorder in the first group.[43] A

prolonged bleeding time may also be found in senility and severe inanition. In clinical disorders associated predominantly with increased capillary fragility, such as scurvy and occasionally allergic purpura, the bleeding time is usually found to be normal. In thrombocytopenia or thrombasthenia, the bleeding time is usually prolonged. Whether this is due to absence of normal plugging by platelet aggregates or of the vasoconstrictor effect of platelet serotonin, or merely represents a parallel capillary disorder cannot be stated at this time. In contrast, coagulation disorders, however severe, are usually associated with normal bleeding times (as defined by these methods), although prolonged secondary hemorrhage from the test wound may occur later, presumably after the period of vasoconstriction has passed.

### PLATELET COUNT

The method, normal values, and interpretation of the platelet count are discussed in Unit 8. The functions of the platelets in hemostasis are complex and have been outlined earlier. The platelet count has the limitation of enumerating platelets only as physical units, although information has gradually accumulated that in rare cases platelets may be qualitatively abnormal.[44] Qualitative abnormalities may be suspected from unusual morphology (particularly giant forms), but must be demonstrated by functional tests. Thrombocytosis as well as thrombocytopenia may be associated with a bleeding tendency, the mechanism of which is obscure. The cause of a demonstrated thrombocytopenia must be determined by other appropriate studies: bone-marrow aspiration, history of drug intake, and so forth. As previously noted, thrombocytopenia is usually associated with poor clot retraction, abnormal bleeding time and capillary fragility, and normal whole-blood clotting time but reduced prothrombin consumption.

WHOLE-BLOOD CLOTTING TIME

The clotting time is defined as the time required for a firm clot to be formed in freshly shed blood placed in glass tubes. The determination of it is an empiric, arbitrary procedure which must be performed meticulously. Many techniques have been proposed, but all are subject to considerable variation and error. The following adaptation of the basic Lee-White method [45] is suggested. Following minimal stasis and an atraumatic venipuncture with a 19- or 20-gauge needle, about 2 ml of blood is drawn into one syringe and discarded. A second clean, dry syringe is then used to withdraw another 5 ml of freely flowing blood, care being taken to avoid excessive negative pressure and bubbles. The needle is removed and 2-ml samples of blood are immediately introduced into each of two chemically clean, dry, 13 × 10-mm Pyrex test tubes, the blood being allowed to run gently down the side of the tube to avoid agitation. The tubes are then placed in a water bath at 37°C. At 30-sec intervals the first tube is removed and gently tilted, the end point of coagulation being reached when the tube can be inverted without loss of contents. The second tube is then observed in the same way to the same end point. The beginning of the test is the time when blood enters the second syringe. The average time in minutes required for blood to clot in the two tubes is reported as the clotting time. If there is a difference of more than 5 min between the clotting times of the two tubes, the longer time is reported.

INTERPRETATIONS AND LIMITATIONS. The normal clotting time as determined by the foregoing method is generally found within the range of 4 to 10 min, but the normal range should be determined for the glass tubes currently in use. The technique for measuring the clotting time must be scrupulously standardized if reliable results are to be obtained, for there are many potential sources of error. Among the variables to be noted are contamination of syringe and needle with thromboplastin from tissue juice (partially controlled by the two-syringe technique), bubbling and frothing, the size, cleanliness, and surface characteristics of the glass tubes, and the temperature at which the test is performed.[46, 47] The clotting time represents the summation of all three stages of coagulation. Since the latent period in coagulation is largely the result of the time-consuming reactions involved in the formation of plasma thromboplastin, a prolonged clotting time usually reflects a defect in stage 1 of coagulation, most often a familial deficiency of a plasma globulin. A circulating anticoagulant may give a similar prolongation of the clotting time. A crude check on the differential diagnosis between these two categories can be made by repeating the determination of the clotting time after mixing the abnormal blood with an equal volume of fresh, normal plasma. In the case of deficiency of a coagulation factor, the clotting time will be corrected; in the presence of an anticoagulant, it will not. In patients with marked reduction of fibrinogen macroscopically visible, clotting may fail to occur. It must be emphasized that the whole-blood clotting-time test has many limitations both in the errors in its determination and in its nonspecificity and insensitivity. Serious hemorrhagic phenomena may occur with deficiency of a plasma thromboplastic factor (such as AHF or PTC) even if the coagulation time is normal. A normal value of the whole-blood clotting time does not exclude a coagulation defect and does not prove adequacy of plasma thromboplastin formation.

ONE-STAGE PROTHROMBIN TIME

The determination of the so-called "prothrombin time," which is really a composite function of several factors, has been one of the most important screening tests in coagulation studies since its introduction about 20 yr ago.[48] A number of minor modifications of this determination have been suggested. The following is recommended as a convenient and accurate method.

Fresh venous blood is added to 0.1 volume of isotonic sodium oxalate (1.34 percent) and mixed immediately. After centrifugation, plasma is separated, care being taken to prevent contamination by red blood cells, and used immediately or stored at 4°C until use. In any case, because of the lability of proaccelerin (V), the plasma should be tested within 5 hr of collection. The residual red cells are examined carefully for any sign of small clots, which if present will invalidate the test. Then 0.1 ml of the fresh plasma is measured into a Pyrex tube ($13 \times 100$ mm) maintained at 37° in a water bath and 0.1 ml of a thromboplastin preparation is added with mixing. Into this mixture is blown, with simultaneous mixing, 0.1 ml of calcium chloride ($0.02M$) and a stopwatch is simultaneously begun. The tube is held in the water bath until just before expected clotting (for 11–14 sec with normal plasma) and then removed, held against a good source of light, and tilted gently or flicked with a finger until the end point, the appearance of the first fibrin strands. A duplicate determination should be made, and the two should agree within 1 sec or better. There are a number of sources of tissue thromboplastin that can be used for the one-stage prothrombin time. Reliable commercial preparations are available, to which is added water or saline at the time of use. Directions are available for the preparation of potent tissue thromboplastin from rabbit or human brain.[49]

To calculate plasma-prothrombin activity in comparison with the normal expected value ("100 percent"), a curve must be available relating the prothrombin time obtained to the known concentration of the "prothrombin-time reactants" in the test. In actual practice, this relation is obtained by making prothrombin-time determinations on various dilutions of normal plasma. The curve that is obtained varies with the diluent used— saline, prothrombin-free bovine plasma, or prothrombin-free human plasma. It is recommended that barium sulfate–adsorbed human plasma be used, which will be deficient in prothrombin, proconvertin (VII), Stuart factor, and PTC. Such a curve must be determined with each newly prepared thromboplastic substance, since this crude product is one of the chief exogenous variables in the determination.

To obtain the correlation curve, pooled oxalated plasma is obtained from 5 to 7 normal subjects and divided between two tubes. To one of the tubes, 100 mg of barium sulfate is added for each 1.0 ml of plasma and the mixture is allowed to stand for about 30 min with repeated shaking. The tube is then centrifuged at 3000 rev/min for 20 min and the supernatant plasma is filtered through No. 50 filter paper to insure that all barium sulfate has been removed. Progressive dilutions of the unadsorbed normal plasma are then made with the barium sulfate–adsorbed plasma, and the respective prothrombin times are immediately determined as above. A curve relating prothrombin time to prothrombin (and proconvertin and Stuart factor) concentration can then be plotted, as shown in Fig. 23. The normal value for the prothrombin time will vary with the thromboplastin used, but generally falls within the range of 11–15 sec. It will be noted from the configuration of the curve that considerable error may be inherent in the graphic determination of prothrombin concentration from the prothrombin time in the range of 25 to 100 percent of normal because a relatively large change in concentration is reflected in a very small change in the prothrombin time. Conversely, this determination is

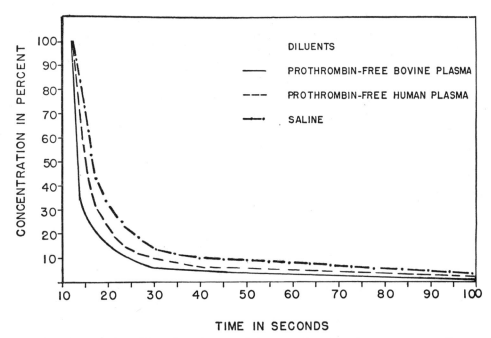

Fig. 23. Relation of "prothrombin time" (sec) to "prothrombin concentration" (percent) as determined by the one-stage method.

much more accurate at the lower concentrations.

It is important to give full emphasis to certain precautions that should be taken in determining the prothrombin time.

(i) Care must be taken to obtain venous blood uncontaminated by tissue juice and to mix it quickly with the anticoagulant. At the time the test is performed, the collection tube should be carefully examined for any evidence of clot formation.

(ii) The ratio of 1 part of 0.1M sodium oxalate to 9 parts of whole blood presupposes a normal or near-normal hematocrit. In polycythemia, correspondingly more blood should be added, and the reverse in anemia, to maintain a relatively constant plasma/anticoagulant ratio.

(iii) The prothrombin time should be tested as soon as possible because of the progressive inactivation of proaccelerin (V). During any delay the plasma should be kept at 4°C.

(iv) A new prothrombin-time concentration curve must be determined with each new batch of thromboplastin.

INTERPRETATIONS AND LIMITATIONS. In theory, the prothrombin time was initially meant to reflect prothrombin concentration, measured by its biologic activation to thrombin (following the addition of tissue thromboplastin and calcium), and the subsequent formation of visible fibrin from fibrinogen. Thus all of stages 2 and 3 of coagulation (Fig. 22) were used as a convenient assay system.

It is clear from many investigations that the one-stage prothrombin time is in effect a very complex function which reflects the velocity and amount of thrombin formation, the rate at which it is inactivated by antithrombin, the velocity of the thrombin-fibrinogen reaction, and the concentration of fibrinogen.[49] In addition, the velocity of thrombin formation is affected by the concentrations of the accessory substances proconvertin, proaccelerin, and Stuart factor. It has been estimated that the prothrombin time, measured as described above, is prolonged with concentrations of proaccelerin less than 70 percent of normal,[50] of proconvertin less than 50 percent of normal,[49] and of fibrinogen less than approximately 100 mg/100 ml.[51] The one-stage prothrombin time is therefore a crude but very useful screening test of the integrity of stages 2 and 3 of coagulation. If the result is abnormal, more specific tests will be required to define the defect more precisely.

### PROTHROMBIN-CONSUMPTION TEST

The prothrombin-consumption test is the most convenient survey method for determining the presence or absence of an abnormality in the first stage of coagulation. In essence, it measures the residual prothrombin activity in the serum, contrasted with that of the parent plasma, after coagulation has been allowed to run its course.

Venous blood, drawn with the precautions listed for the one-stage prothrombin time, is added to an oxalated tube (ten volumes of blood to one of oxalate) and an aliquot into a clean, dry test tube. From the oxalated tube a prothrombin-activity–prothrombin-time curve is obtained by determining one-stage prothrombin times on the plasma at progressive dilutions with barium sulfate–adsorbed normal plasma (as described previously). For convenience, this curve is best plotted on log-log paper, on which a straight line should be obtained. The clotted tube is immediately placed in a water bath and incubated at 37°C for 1 hr. It is then removed and centrifuged, and an aliquot of the serum is added to 0.1 volume of 0.1M sodium oxalate. The separated serum is then incubated for an additional 30 min at 37°C to insure inactivation of thrombin. After incubation, the serum is diluted with an equal volume (1:1) of normal barium sulfate–adsorbed plasma (as a source of proaccelerin and fibrinogen) and a one-stage prothrombin-time test is performed. The percentage of activity is obtained from the prothrombin-dilution curve previously determined from the plasma, and then is multiplied by a final dilution factor of

2 to obtain the percentage of the original plasma prothrombin activity remaining in serum. Prothrombin consumption is calculated as 100 percent minus the percentage of serum prothrombin, and normally is greater than 80 percent. The serum prothrombin time is normally greater than 35 sec.

INTERPRETATIONS AND LIMITATIONS. The virtually complete conversion of prothrombin to thrombin during the normal progress of coagulation is dependent on the formation of adequate plasma thromboplastin in the presence of optimal concentrations of the accessory substances required for prothrombinase formation. The measurement of the residual serum prothrombin is carried out by the addition of tissue thromboplastin and a source of proaccelerin and fibrinogen (that is, barium sulfate–adsorbed normal plasma), but requires a normal or non-rate-limiting concentration of proconvertin and Stuart factor to be present in the tested serum. If the control one-stage prothrombin time on plasma is normal, prothrombin, proaccelerin, proconvertin, Stuart factor, and fibrinogen are not limiting, and the prothrombin consumption reflects the formation of plasma thromboplastin. Defective plasma thromboplastin formation, and therefore reduced prothrombin consumption and resulting high prothrombin activity in serum, is found in two main types of hemorrhagic disorders: (*a*) deficiency of one or, rarely, two of the plasma protein reactants in thromboplastin formation, generally as familial hemorrhagic diseases (AHF, PTC, PTA, Stuart factor, or certain other postulated components as described previously); (*b*) deficiency of the platelet factor in thromboplastin formation secondary to thrombocytopenia or to a qualitative platelet defect (thrombasthenia). As will be described later, the prothrombin-consumption test not only serves as a convenient survey of the integrity of stage 1 of coagulation, but it can also be readily adapted to analyze more precisely the nature of a stage 1 defect.

### CLOT DISSOLUTION

The fibrinolytic system, previously referred to, rivals the coagulation schema in complexity. Accurate measurements of the components of this system are feasible only in laboratories specializing in research on blood coagulation.[31] For clinical purposes the following simple procedures are usually sufficient to detect the presence of circulating fibrinolysins.

*Whole-Blood Technique.* Using sterile technique, whole blood is allowed to clot in a glass tube at 37°C and then is maintained at this temperature for about 24 hr, with inspection for clot lysis at ½, 1, 2, 3, 4, and 24 hr. A normal clot will remain substantially evident during this period of time. If fibrinolysis occurs, the clot will be observed to shrink markedly with loss of its enmeshed red cells. To test for completion of fibrinolysis, the contents of the tube are poured out on a large sheet of filter paper to see if any fibrin clot remains.

*Plasma Technique.*[2] One milliliter of sterile fresh citrated plasma (5 ml of whole blood to 0.5 ml of 0.2*M* sodium citrate followed by centrifugation at 2000 rev/min for 5 min) is placed in a glass tube at 37°C and clotted with 10 units of thrombin in 0.1 ml of 0.9-percent sodium chloride solution. The tube is observed for evidence of clot dissolution during continued incubation. This test can be made more stringent by mixing 0.5 ml of the patient's plasma with 0.5 ml of fresh normal plasma prior to the addition of thrombin to insure that a normal fibrin clot is initially present as substrate for a fibrinolysin. Although slightly more complicated, the plasma technique offers an advantage in that the lysis of the clot can be seen more easily in the absence of red cells.

INTERPRETATIONS AND LIMITATIONS. Several points of technique are worth emphasizing if reliable results are to be obtained. The test for a circulating fibrinolysin should be carried out promptly, certainly within 30 min, because fibrinolysins may be rapidly inactivated by antifibrinolysins in vitro. The fibrinolytic reaction is temperature-dependent and may be significantly less active at room temperature, so the incubation should be carried out at 37°C. For practical purposes, fibrinolysins are not usually productive of a severe bleeding disorder unless they are capable of lysing a normal clot within 1 or 2 hr. Fibrinolysins attack not only the fibrin clot, but also fibrinogen and proaccelerin, so that the hemostatic defect may be complex. Circulating fibrinolysins have been found in a wide variety of conditions—shock, extensive surgery (especially of the lung, prostate, and uterus), certain obstetric disorders (premature separation of the placenta, intrauterine fetal death), liver disease, leukemia, and disseminated carcinoma. In these conditions, differentiation of fibrinolysis from the acute defibrination syndrome of excessive intravascular clotting is frequently difficult.

### CLOT RETRACTION

The mechanism by which a clot retracts and the function of this retraction in hemostasis have been widely studied but remain unclear.[8] Despite these uncertainties, however, the presence or absence of normal clot retraction may give information of clinical value. The following semiquantitative methods are suggested.[2]

*Whole-Blood Technique.* Two milliliters of whole blood is placed in a glass test tube and allowed to clot and remain in a 37°C bath over a period of 1 hr. At the end of this time, the expressed serum is carefully poured off and measured. Fifty times the volume of serum obtained is taken to represent the percentage clot retraction. The normal value is usually 20–65 percent. Occasionally the clot may stick to the wall of the tube, which artificially interferes with normal retraction. If this occurs, the clot should be separated by gently rimming the top of the clot with a platinum wire or wooden applicator. Allowance should also be made for variation in hematocrit, which profoundly influences the amount of expressible serum in the measured blood.

*Plasma Clot Retraction.* Since the number of red cells trapped in the fibrin network is one of the main variables in clot retraction, more reliable results can be obtained by the study of plasma alone. Five milliliters of whole blood is drawn into a chilled, silicone-coated syringe (preferably by the two-syringe technique described earlier) and then transferred to a chilled, silicone-coated centrifuge tube. Centrifugation is carried out at 1000 rev/min for 10 min to separate the red cells and white cells, but leaving the platelets in suspension. Two milliliters of the supernatant plasma is then transferred to a glass test tube maintained at 37°C for 1 hr, and the clot retraction is measured as described for whole blood. The normal range for plasma is 40–70 percent. The fact that the values are higher than for whole blood presumably reflects the more complete retraction in the absence of the physical interference from enmeshed red cells.

Many other methods for measuring clot retraction have been described. Tocantins' modification of Adreassen's quantitative method can also be recommended.[52]

INTERPRETATIONS AND LIMITATIONS. Clot retraction is a complex function of the amount of fibrin formed, the presence of intact platelets within the fibrin network, and the physical interference from the trapped red cells.[53] The retraction seems to be absolutely dependent on platelet function, all other factors merely influencing the extent to which the clot retracts. The test is therefore carried out mainly as a crude measure of platelet function. Clot retraction is impaired in thrombocytopenia (less than 100,000 platelets/mm$^3$) or in the presence of some qualitative platelet defects (thrombasthenia). For the reasons mentioned above, clot retraction by the whole-blood technique is reduced in polycythemia. In some varieties of thrombasthenia, there may be a reduction of the clot-retraction function independent of the platelet thromboplastic function.[44] As previously noted, the role of clot retraction in hemostasis is not understood.

FIBRINOGEN CONCENTRATION

The conversion of fibrinogen to fibrin is the final common pathway in coagulation, the prime purpose of the previous complex series of reactions. As the only protein factor in coagulation present in greater than trace amounts, its concentration can be measured with accuracy by chemical means. It is to be noted that in the final analysis almost all other coagulation factors are measured by assay systems that have as their end point the rate at which fibrinogen is converted to fibrin. Thus a normal one-stage prothrombin time already indicates that the patient's fibrinogen concentration is in excess of 100 mg/100 ml.

*Qualitative Test.*[2] A rapid qualitative index of the plasma concentration of fibrinogen can be easily and quickly obtained by adding 0.2 ml of bovine thrombin (100 units/ml) to 0.5 ml of the patient's plasma in a test tube maintained at 37°C. In the presence of a normal fibrinogen concentration, turbid solidification should occur almost immediately. In significant fibrinogenopenia, a thin, translucent gel or a delicate network of fibrin strands appears.

This test can be made much more quantitative by determining by titration the dilution of plasma at which a visible clot is produced by added thrombin.[54] A series of doubling dilutions of platelet-free citrated plasma are made from 1:2 to 1:128 in 0.5-ml volumes. To each tube add 0.1 ml of human thrombin (about

36 units/ml). Normal plasma will give a visible clot at 1:64 to 1:128. In fibrinogen deficiency, a visible clot is produced only at lesser dilutions. This test is of particular value for rapid diagnosis and following the level of fibrinogen in defibrination syndromes.

*Quantitative Test.* Blood containing citrate or oxalate anticoagulant is centrifuged at 2000 rev/min. One milliliter of the supernatant plasma is added to 25 ml of 0.9-percent sodium chloride solution, and 1.0 ml of 2.5-percent calcium chloride solution is added to initiate coagulation. If the clot is delayed in appearance, 100 units of bovine thrombin are added. After 1 hr at room temperature, the clot is filtered off, or alternatively collected on a glass rod, and washed repeatedly with distilled water. The clot can be weighed after drying, or the clottable protein can be calculated after measurement of the amount of nitrogen in the clot. The washed clot is digested with 1.0 ml of concentrated sulfuric acid over a moderate flame for 4 hr. Nitrogen is then determined by the usual micro Kjeldahl procedure. The amount of fibrinogen present in the original plasma can then be calculated from the equation:

$$\text{Fibrinogen (mg/ml)} = 6.25 \text{ N (mg/ml)}.$$

Fibrinogen may also be calculated by determining the phenolic residues of the digested clot.[2, 55]

INTERPRETATIONS AND LIMITATIONS. The normal level of circulating fibrinogen is in the range of 200 to 400 mg/100 ml in plasma. It is generally agreed that blood coagulation is not impaired unless plasma fibrinogen is reduced to a level less than 100 mg/100 ml. Indirect evidence suggests that fibrinogen is synthesized in the liver and has a half-life in the circulating blood of 24 to 48 hr. Reduction in fibrinogen may be secondary to decreased synthesis or increased utilization. Fibrinogen may be virtually absent in the rare inborn error of metabolism known as afibrinogenemia [56] or variably diminished in congenital fibrinogenopenia, presumably secondary to impaired synthesis. Decreased synthesis is also seen in a wide variety of hepatic diseases. Circulating fibrinogen may also be deficient because of excessive utilization or destruction. In the former case it is postulated that fibrinogen is used up faster than it can be replaced by extensive intravascular clotting secondary to the introduction of tissue thromboplastic substances into the blood in such conditions as obstetric abnormalities [57] or following certain surgical procedures. Fibrinogen, as well as fibrin and certain other coagulation factors, may be destroyed by fibrinolysins, as noted in the section on clot dissolution. In actual practice, it is often difficult to determine from simple laboratory procedures whether the fibrinogenopenia associated with obstetric abnormalities and surgical manipulations is the result of the release of tissue thromboplastic activity, the release of agents activating the fibrinolytic system, or a combination of the two. For a more complete discussion of this problem the reader is referred to other sources.[30, 31] Although the fibrinogen level may be somewhat elevated in certain infections and in pregnancy, no clinical significance has been associated with this other than the possible relation of fibrinogen to the erythrocyte sedimentation rate.

### Description of Follow-Up Tests

When the screening tests have been completed, it should be possible to determine whether any coagulation disorder exists in the hemorrhagic diathesis being studied, and, if present, the general nature of the derangement. Often this information suffices for effective therapy to be instituted. When there is defective generation of plasma thromboplastin, however, as reflected in reduced prothrombin consumption during coagulation (elevated serum prothrombin concentration) or when the one-stage prothrombin time is prolonged in the presence of a plasma fibrinogen concentration greater than 100 mg/100 ml, further tests are indicated to demonstrate which of a number of contributing factors is at fault.

ANALYSIS OF DEFECTIVE GENERATION
OF PLASMA THROMBOPLASTIN

When defective generation of plasma thromboplastin is indicated by a prolonged clotting time or a reduced prothrombin consumption during coagulation, the platelet count being normal or near-normal, a differential diagnosis includes the following main possibilities: classical hemophilia (AHF deficiency), "Christmas" disease (PTC deficiency), PTA deficiency, Hageman defect, Stuart-factor deficiency, presence of a circulating anticoagulant, and thrombasthenia. The rarer thromboplastic factors whose importance or even true occurrence still constitute research problems will not be discussed.

*The Thromboplastin-Generation Test.*[33] The introduction of the thromboplastin-generation test represented a major advance in the study of the coagulation disorders. In this test, an artificial coagulation system is set up, consisting of all of the known components necessary for thromboplastin generation except the substance to be tested for (AHF, or PTC, or PTA, or platelets). The patient's serum, plasma, or platelets are used as a source of this substance, incubation is carried out, and aliquots from the mixture are removed at timed intervals to test for the rate at which thromboplastin is generated. By successive substitutions of the patient's factors in an otherwise complete system, the factor at fault can be identified. Deficiency of thromboplastin formation may be present and yet be undetectable by the prothrombin-consumption test. The advantage of the thromboplastin-generation test lies in its

greater sensitivity and its adaptability for the study of individual defects. Although this test is probably the most accurate one available for the analysis of disorders of thromboplastin formation, it is described here in general terms only. The reader is referred to the original description and subsequent modifications for more details.[33]

*Cross-Correction Studies.* Perhaps the most direct method of identifying the nature of a plasma thromboplastic defect (and historically the method by which the existence of different types of "hemophilia" was discovered) is a study of the ability or inability of plasma from a patient whose defect has been previously documented as being AHF, PTC, or PTA to correct the abnormal clotting function of an unknown plasma. In practice, this is carried out by mixing equal amounts of the known and unknown plasma, recalcifying, and incubating at 37°C for 1 hr after clotting has occurred. Prothrombin consumption is then calculated as previously described. If plasma with a known defect (presumably with normal concentrations of other factors) fails to correct the abnormal prothrombin consumption of the patient's plasma, it is assumed that the patient's plasma is deficient in the same factor as the test plasma or contains an anticoagulant. This assumption is strengthened by a demonstration that plasma samples authentically deficient in the other plasma factors (AHF, PTC, or PTA) are able to correct the prothrombin consumption of the patient's plasma.

This particular test has the disadvantage that a bank of known thromboplastin-deficiency samples must be available at all times. In addition, the original differential diagnoses of the types of thromboplastin deficiency represented in this bank must be made by other methods.

*Modified Prothrombin-Consumption Test.* The prothrombin-consumption test, which was earlier described as a convenient screening test for defects in plasma thromboplastin generation, can be modified to allow definition of which component is at fault.[2] When so used, it becomes comparable to the thrombo-plastin-generation test in the information that can be obtained, although less sensitive and precise. If the prothrombin-consumption test is to be so used, the prothrombin time of the patient's plasma (that is, its response to exogenous tissue thromboplastin) must be within normal limits, since the end point of the test is a comparison of the prothrombin times of plasma and serum. To carry out this test, several preparations must be available:

(1) *Fresh platelet-rich plasma from the patient.* Blood is collected in a siliconized syringe, preferably by the two-syringe technique, in 0.1 volume of $0.2M$ sodium citrate and centrifuged for 10 min at 1000 rev/min in a siliconized tube. The supernatant, which is free of red and white cells but rich in platelets, is then separated and used as soon as possible in the test.

(2) *Normal platelet-free plasma.* Blood from a normal donor is collected as above, but centrifuged at 3000 rev/min or more for 30 min to separate all of the formed elements in the blood. The supernatant is used as soon as possible; if there is to be any delay, it should be kept in an ice bath.

(3) *AHF.* A crude source of antihemophilic factor is obtained by removing PTC from fresh, normal plasma by adsorption with barium sulfate (or calcium phosphate or aluminum hydroxide gel). Prothrombin, proconvertin, Stuart factor, and part of PTA are also removed by this procedure. Fresh blood from a normal donor is mixed with $0.1M$ sodium oxalate as anticoagulant (barium sulfate will not adsorb PTC effectively from a citrate solution) and the cells are separated by centrifugation. Barium sulfate is added to the separated supernatant plasma in the proportion of 100 mg/ml, mixed well, and incubated at $37°C$ for

15 min. The suspension is then separated by centrifugation. The supernatant "adsorbed plasma" is then used as soon as possible as a source of AHF, largely free of PTC and Stuart factor. The plasma also contains PTA.

(4) *PTC.* Plasma thromboplastin component, in contrast to AHF, does not disappear during blood coagulation. Advantage is taken of this to obtain a crude source of PTC free of AHF. Normal clotted blood is allowed to stand for several hours at $37°C$. The separated serum, rich in PTC, is then virtually free of AHF, proaccelerin, prothrombin, and thrombin, but still contains PTA and Stuart factor.

Alternatively, somewhat more reliable results are obtained by elution of PTC from the barium sulfate adsorbent used in the AHF preparation outlined above. The barium sulfate is washed with cold saline and centrifuged at 2000 rev/min for 5 min. After the saline is removed, the PTC is eluted by mixing with $0.2M$ sodium citrate in a volume 0.1 that of the original adsorbed plasma and incubating at $37°C$ for 15 min. The supernatant separated by centrifugation is rich in PTC and contains some PTA.

(5) *PTA.* Plasma thromboplastin antecedent has not been as well characterized as AHF and PTC. It is present in serum as well as plasma and seems to be only partially adsorbed by inorganic precipitates such as barium sulfate. Serum adsorbed with barium sulfate is therefore used as a source of PTA virtually free of AHF, PTC, and Stuart factor.

With these preparations of coagulation factors, a series of prothrombin-consumption tests are carried out to define the defect in thromboplastin generation. The following mixtures are made and recalcified with 0.1 ml of $0.2M$ calcium chloride. The residual prothrombin concentration is measured (as described in the prothrombin-consumption test) after incubation at $37°C$ for 1 hr after clotting has occurred.

| Patient's platelet-rich-plasma | Normal source of— | Diagnosis if prothrombin consumption of mixture returns to normal (80 percent) |
|---|---|---|
| 1. 0.5 ml | Platelet-poor plasma: 0.5 ml | Plasma component rather than platelet defect |
| 2. 0.5 ml | Fresh BaSO₄–adsorbed plasma: 0.5 ml | AHF or PTA deficiency |
| 3. 0.9 ml | Citrate eluate from BaSO₄: 0.1 ml | PTC, Stuart factor, or PTA deficiency |
| 4. 0.8 ml | Serum: 0.2 ml | PTC, Stuart factor, or PTA deficiency |
| 5. 0.8 ml | Ba₄SO–adsorbed serum: 0.2 ml | PTA deficiency |
| 6. 0.5 ml | Platelet-rich plasma: 0.5 ml | If prothrombin consumption not significantly corrected, a circulating anticoagulant is suggested |

In summary, the patient's thromboplastic defect is analyzed by the ability of various crude clotting-factor preparations to rectify the abnormal prothrombin consumption of his platelet-rich plasma in a series of replacement tests.

INTERPRETATIONS AND LIMITATIONS. The interpretations of these different methods for analysis of an unknown defect in thromboplastin formation have been described above. In the presence of a normal number of platelets, a clinically significant reduction in the formation of effective plasma thromboplastin is almost invariably due to a congenital, often familial disease characterized by failure to synthesize a normal amount of AHF, PTC, Stuart factor, Hageman factor, or PTA. Significant qualitative platelet defects or antithromboplastin anticoagulants are seen much less frequently. No diseases are known that are associated with pathologic elevation of the plasma levels of AHF, PTC, or PTA. AHF deficiency is most often associated with "classical hemophilia," with pseudohemophilia, and sometimes with the coagulation disorder associated with the introduction of tissue thromboplastin into the blood (such as the accidents of preg-

nancy). A few cases of acquired AHF deficiency have been described.[58] Of particular interest is the AHF deficiency found in certain patients with pseudohemophilia (von Willebrand's disease), but this degree of deficiency generally is not disclosed with the modified prothrombin-consumption test. In fact, it should be emphasized that an occasional patient with mild classical hemophilia may have a normal clotting time and prothrombin consumption, the defect becoming apparent only by use of the thromboplastin-generation test.

PTC deficiency simulates AHF deficiency in its clinical picture and mode of inheritance. The disorder, generally milder than classical hemophilia, is often called "Christmas disease," an eponym derived from one of the first described patients.[59] PTC is also reduced by the coumarin group of anticoagulants.[60] An occasional female carrier of Christmas disease exhibits some degree of PTC deficiency,[61] and a few cases of combined AHF–PTC deficiency are on record. Deficiency of PTA is not as frequent as that of AHF or PTC and has not been as well defined as a clinical entity. The mild hemorrhagic disorder associated with an inborn, familial, non-sex-linked defi-

206

ciency of PTA was first described by Rosenthal.[62] No other cause of clinically significant PTA deficiency has been described. Stuart-factor deficiency is described below.

As postulated 40 years ago by Glanzmann, platelets may be normal in number but abnormal in function, a condition generally called thrombasthenia or thrombocytopathia. Such qualitatively defective platelets are often exceptionally large. This rare disorder and its variations have been recently studied and reviewed by Braunsteiner.[44] Circulating anticoagulants that inhibit the effective formation of plasma thromboplastin are also found rarely, and then generally in patients with hemophilia who have received repeated treatments with AHF concentrates. A few postpartum women with circulating anti-AHF factors have been described, whose disease clinically resembles classical hemophilia,[63] and a scattering of patients with laboratory findings suggestive of pathologically increased antithromboplastin have been studied.

### ANALYSIS OF AN ABNORMAL ONE-STAGE PROTHROMBIN TIME

It has been pointed out in the discussion of the one-stage prothrombin time that this is a very complex function representing the over-all elaboration of thrombin from prothrombin and its subsequent proteolytic action on fibrinogen to produce a visible fibrin clot. When an abnormally elevated prothrombin time is noted in the presence of a fibrinogen level greater than 100 to 120 mg/100 ml, deficiency of prothrombin, proaccelerin, proconvertin, or Stuart factor must be suspected. Various combinations of these deficiencies may be found.

*Prothrombin Deficiency.*[64] A measurement of prothrombin concentration can be made by means of the one-stage prothrombin time if proaccelerin, proconvertin, Stuart factor, and fibrinogen are supplied in optimal concentrations such that prothrombin is the only "limiting" substance. In preparation for this test certain reagents must be prepared:

(1) *Source of proaccelerin.* Barium sulfate–adsorbed oxalated plasma is obtained preferably from beef blood because of its rich supply of this factor. The method of carrying out this adsorption has been previously described in the preparation of AHF.

(2) *Source of proconvertin and Stuart factor.* Normal serum is kept at room temperature for 24 to 48 hr and then oxalated (1 vol 0.1$M$ sodium oxalate to 4 vol serum).

(3) *Diluting buffer.* This consists of 0.1$M$ sodium diethylbarbiturate, 170 ml; 0.1$M$ HCl, 122 ml; 0.15$M$ NaCl, 558 ml; and 0.1$M$ sodium oxalate, 150 ml.

(4) *Thromboplastin-calcium mixture.* Equal parts of thromboplastin extract and 0.04$M$ CaCl$_2$ are mixed.

The proaccelerin and proconvertin preparations are most conveniently stored in a deep freeze after mixing in 1:1 volume ratios. In carrying out the test the normal reference plasma and the test plasma are both diluted tenfold with the diluting buffer in order to operate at an elevated prothrombin time, thus increasing the accuracy of the assay. The test is then performed much like the usual one-stage prothrombin-time test. To a tube in a 37°C bath are added 0.1 ml of the proaccelerin-proconvertin mixture and 0.1 ml of tenfold-diluted normal plasma. After temperature equilibration, 0.2 ml of the thromboplastin-calcium mixture (previously warmed to 37°C) is quickly added and the prothrombin time is determined in the usual way. This is considered to reflect 100 percent prothrombin concentration. Further dilutions of the normal plasma with the described buffer are then tested as above to construct a standardization curve relating prothrombin time to prothrombin concentration. This is most conveniently plotted on a log-log scale, where a linear relation should be obtained. The prothrombin time of the unknown plasma is then measured, after tenfold dilution with the buffer, and its prothrombin concentration determined by comparison with the standard curve. A fuller description of this test has been published by Alexander.[49]

INTERPRETATIONS AND LIMITATIONS. There is considerable variation in the "normal" level of prothrombin. In comparison with a pool of normal plasma samples, an individual specimen from a normal individual may contain from 70–120 percent prothrombin concentration. Normal plasma contains 300–350 units of prothrombin/ml,[13] one unit being the amount which, when completely converted to thrombin, will clot 1 ml of a 1-percent fibrinogen solution in 15 sec. Since partially purified human prothrombin preparations have been obtained containing about 2600 units/mg protein,[65] the actual plasma concentration of prothrombin is less than 15–20 mg/100 ml. No conditions are known with a pathologic elevation of prothrombin concentration. Deficiency of prothrombin is found as a rare congenital defect,[66] or more frequently as an acquired defect in liver disease, in vitamin K deficiency, or following the use of the coumarin group of anticoagulants. If the prothrombin concentration is greater than 20 percent of normal, there is little danger of a hemorrhagic diathesis from this abnormality alone.

*Proaccelerin (V) Deficiency* (Parahemophilia). Rather simple qualitative tests can be conveniently carried out to detect proaccelerin deficiency as a cause of an abnormally prolonged one-stage prothrombin time.

(i) Fresh normal oxalated plasma is adsorbed with barium sulfate, as previously described in the preparation of AHF, which removes prothrombin, proconvertin, and Stuart factor, but leaves fibrinogen and proaccelerin. Equal volumes of this adsorbed plasma and of the unknown plasma are then mixed and the one-stage prothrombin-time test is repeated. If there has been a marked shortening of the prothrombin time, it is assumed that the original defect was that of proaccelerin deficiency.

(ii) Sterile normal oxalated plasma is incubated at 37°C for 24 hr to inactivate proaccelerin. Then 1 vol of the plasma to be tested is added to 9 vol of the resulting proaccelerin-deficient plasma and the prothrombin time is determined in the standard manner. To express the results in a semiquantitative way, a calibration curve is then obtained by substituting various dilutions of normal oxalated plasma for the unknown plasma. The observed prothrombin times permit a correlation with proaccelerin concentration.[67, 68]

INTERPRETATIONS AND LIMITATIONS. As previously noted, the one-stage prothrombin time does not become significantly prolonged until the proaccelerin concentration becomes less than 70 percent of normal. Although it has not been demonstrated that proaccelerin and prothrombin act stoichiometrically in the formation of thrombin, reduction of either delays the appearance of thrombin to approximately the same degree. Deficiency of proaccelerin occurs in a variety of conditions. The most marked deficiencies are seen as rare congenital disorders, described under the term "parahemophilia." [69] Here, proaccelerin may occasionally be so grossly deficient as to lead to prolongation of the clotting time and reduced prothrombin consumption. Acquired proaccelerin deficiencies are almost invariably associated with abnormalities of other clotting factors in such conditions as parenchymal liver disease, leukemia, overwhelming streptococcal infection, terminal carcinoma, and extensive replacement transfusions with bank blood.

*Proconvertin (VII) Deficiency.* As in proaccelerin deficiency, simple tests are also available to determine whether a deficiency of proconvertin is a contributing cause of a prolonged one-stage prothrombin time.

(i) *Qualitative Test*.[2] Serum is obtained from normal blood 1 hr after the completion of clotting, stored in an icebox for 2–3 days, and then kept frozen at −20°C. Such serum still contains proconvertin (and PTC and Stuart factor) but is essentially devoid of prothrombin, proaccelerin, thrombin, and fibrinogen. To 0.9 ml of the abnormal plasma to be tested is added 0.1 ml of this proconvertin-containing serum, and the one-stage prothrombin-time test is repeated. If the initially prolonged prothrombin time is largely corrected (to a normal or near-normal range), it can be interpreted as demonstrating deficiency of proconvertin or Stuart factor. It should be pointed out that not uncommonly there is partial correction of the prolonged prothrombin time by the addition of serum even in the absence of proconvertin deficiency.

(ii) *de Vries Test*.[70, 2] The prothrombin times of plasma, serum, and a plasma-serum mixture are determined and compared as follows. Plasma prothrombin time is determined by adding 0.05 ml of normal oxalated plasma + 0.05 ml of saline to 0.9 ml of normal barium sulfate–adsorbed plasma (see earlier directions) and then determining the prothrombin time, which must be corrected by a dilution factor of 20 and expressed as a percentage of normal. This should be 100 percent. A similar test is carried out to determine the prothrombin time of serum, using a ratio of 3 vol of serum to 7 vol of barium sulfate–adsorbed plasma, with a dilution correction factor of 10/3 (3.33). Finally, both 0.05 ml of normal oxalated plasma and 0.05 ml of the oxalated serum are added to 0.9 ml of the adsorbed plasma, and the prothrombin time of this mixture is determined and converted by the dilution factor of 20 to percentage of normal. The proconvertin content in the serum is estimated by calculating its enhancement of the "prothrombin activity" of plasma, that is, the increase of the prothrombin activity (expressed as a percentage) beyond the activity that would be expected from simple 1:1 dilution of the plasma by an equal volume of serum with its residual prothrombin.

A sample calculation would be: plasma prothrombin activity, 100 percent; serum prothrombin activity, 20 percent (normal prothrombin utilization); anticipated from 1:1 mixture (algebraic), 60 percent; prothrombin activity of mixture, 140 percent; factor VII enhancement = (140 percent − 60 percent)/60 percent = 133 percent.

Normal values for this method of calculation have a wide range, but generally fall between 80 and 160 percent enhancement. If serum from patients with proconvertin or Stuart-factor deficiency is used, the enhancement of prothrombin activity falls far below this range. The limitations and sources of error in this test, the necessity for standardized technique for collecting blood to avoid tissue-thromboplastin contamination and frothing, and the necessity for using fresh test serum have been well summarized.[71] It is evident that serum obtained from a patient with reduced prothrombin utilization adds another source of error in that residual prothrombin is added directly to the test mixture in addition to whatever enhancement effect is obtained from activated proconvertin.

INTERPRETATIONS AND LIMITATIONS. These tests do not differentiate deficiency of proconvertin (VII) from deficiency of the more recently described Stuart factor. In contrast to deficiency of the Stuart factor, plasma deficient in proconvertin demonstrates a normal prothrombin time when Russell viper venom (Stypven) is used as a source of thromboplastin. This test is presented below. In addition, deficiency of the Stuart factor interferes with the normal formation of plasma thromboplastin, so that there is generally an associated abnormality of prothrombin consumption and of the thromboplastin-generation test. The clinical and laboratory characteristics of proconvertin (VII) have been recently reviewed.[72] A number of cases of proconvertin deficiency have been described as congenital or familial disorders, probably being transmitted as a recessive trait.[73] Deficiency of this factor may be found in the neonatal period, with liver disease, during vitamin K deficiency, and during the administration of the coumarin anticoagulants. In general, proconvertin falls more rapidly and to a greater degree than does prothrombin when these drugs are used.[74] Although a hemorrhagic tendency is produced when proconvertin is reduced to less than 10 percent of normal, this factor seems to have no role in blood coagulation initiated by plasma thromboplastin. Its obvious clinical importance, however, may furnish indirect evidence for a major role of "tissue hemostasis" in the body's defense against hemorrhage.[72]

*Stuart-Factor Deficiency.* The Stuart factor closely resembles proconvertin (VII) in its physical properties. It is present in plasma and serum, is adsorbed by inorganic precipitates and by asbestos filters, and is reduced by coumarin therapy. Advantage has been taken of the observation that the Stuart factor is required for the thromboplastic activity of Russell viper venom–cephalin [75] to develop a simple quantitative test for its assay.[76] The following reactants are placed in sequence in test tubes in a 37° water bath: 0.1 ml of Seitz-filtered ox plasma (asbestos filter pads) as a source of prothrombin, proaccelerin, and fibrinogen but free of proconvertin and the Stuart factor; 0.1 ml of 1:10 diluted plasma or serum (barbiturate buffer, previously described); 0.1 ml of Russell viper venom (Stypven 1:200,000)–cephalin (50 mg/100 ml); 0.1 ml of calcium chloride ($0.025M$) is added after a 30-sec incubation period. The time until coagulation is then determined as in the one-stage prothrombin-time test (p. 198).

Using normal plasma or serum and further dilutions of the 1:10 initial concentration ("100 percent"), a calibration curve relating Stuart factor to clotting time in seconds is obtained. On log-log paper this should give a straight line. The Stuart-factor content of the unknown plasma can then be determined in similar fashion. For details concerning the preparation of reagents and the variables involved, the original description should be consulted.[75]

INTERPRETATION. Most of the comments that have been made concerning proconvertin deficiency apply directly to the Stuart-factor deficiency. These conditions were confused until recent years. Familial deficiency of the factor has been described, probably transmitted as an autosomal recessive. Heterozygotes show lesser degrees of the deficiency.[77] The Stuart factor is also reduced by coumarin therapy and in liver disease. As has been noted, it is also involved in the generation of plasma thromboplastin, unlike proconvertin, and therefore plays a role in both "intravascular hemostasis" and "tissue hemostasis."

## REFERENCES

1. R. Biggs and R. G. Macfarlane, *Human Blood Coagulation and Its Disorders* (ed. 2; Thomas, Springfield, Ill., 1957).
2. M. Stefanini and W. Dameshek, *The Hemorrhagic Disorders* (Grune and Stratton, New York, 1955).

3. A. H. Quick, *Hemorrhagic Diseases* (ed. 2; Lea and Febiger, Philadelphia, 1957).

4. K. M. Brinkhous, ed., *Hemophilia and Hemophilioid Diseases* (University of North Carolina Press, Chapel Hill, 1957).

5. R. Chambers and B. W. Zweifach, "Vasomotion in the hemodynamics of the blood capillary circulation," *Ann. N. Y. Acad. Sci. 49*, 549 (1948).

6. M. B. Zucker, "Platelet agglutination and vasoconstriction as factors in spontaneous hemostasis in normal, thrombocytopenic, heparinized, and hypoprothrombinemic rats," *Amer. J. Physiol. 149*, 275 (1947).

7. C. H. W. Leeksma and J. A. Cohen, "Determination of the life span of human blood platelets using labelled diisoprophylfluorophosphonate," *J. clin. Invest. 35*, 964 (1956).

8. O. E. Budtz-Olsen, *Clot Retraction* (Blackwell Scientific Publications, Oxford, 1951).

9. M. M. Rapport, A. A. Green, and I. H. Page, "Partial purification of the vasoconstrictor in beef serum," *J. biol. Chem. 174*, 735 (1948).

10. J. Haverback, T. F. Dutcher, P. A. Shore, E. G. Tomich, L. L. Terry, and B. B. Brodie, "Serotonin changes in platelets and brain induced by small daily doses of reserpine," *New Engl. J. Med. 256*, 343 (1958).

11. W. H. Seegers, "Coagulation of the blood," *Advance. Enzymol. 16*, 23 (1955).

12. J. V. Garrett, "The platelet-like activity of certain brain extracts," *J. lab. clin. Med. 47*, 752 (1956).

13. B. Alexander, "Coagulation, hemorrhage, and thrombosis," *New Engl. J. Med. 252*, 432 (1955).

14. O. D. Ratnoff and J. E. Colopy, "A familial hemorrhagic trait associated with a deficiency of a clot-promoting fraction of plasma," *J. clin. Invest. 34*, 602 (1955).

15. C. Hougie, E. M. Barrow, and J. B. Graham, "Stuart clotting defect. I. Segregation of an hereditary hemorrhagic state from the heterogeneous group heretofore called 'stable factor' (SPCA, proconvertin, factor VII) deficiency," *J. clin. Invest. 36*, 485 (1957).

16. P. A. Owren, S I. Rapaport, P. Hjort, and K. Aas, "The biochemistry of thromboplastin, its formation and action," *Sang 25*, 752 (1954).

17. F. Nour-Eldin and J. F. Wilkinson, "The separation of human and bovine plasma thromboplastin with ether and a study of its properties," *J. Physiol. 132*, 164 (1956).

18. R. G. Macfarlane, "Blood coagulation, with particular reference to the early stages," *Physiol. Rev. 36*, 479 (1956).

19. F. Koller, "Le facteur X," *Rev. Hémat. 10*, 362 (1955).

20 T. H. Spaet, P. M. Aggeler, and B. G. Kinsell, "A possible fourth plasma thromboplastin component," *J. clin. Invest. 33*, 1095 (1954).

21. O. D. Ratnoff, "Hereditary defects in clotting mechanisms," *Advanc. intern. Med. 9*, 107 (1958).

22. R. G. Macfarlane and R. Biggs, "A thrombin generation test," *J. clin. Path. 6*, 3 (1953).

23. W. H. Seegers and N. Alkjaersig, "The preparation of prothrombin derivatives and an indication of their properties," *Arch. Biochem. 61*, 1 (1956).

24. A. G. Ware and W. H. Seegers, "Serum AC-globulin: Formation from plasma

211

AC-globulin; role in blood coagulation; partial purification; properties; and quantitative determination," *Amer. J. Physiol. 152*, 567 (1948).

25. L. Lorand, "Interaction of thrombin and fibrinogen," *Physiol. Rev. 34*, 742 (1954).

26. H. A. Scheroga and M. Laskowski, Jr., "The fibrinogen-fibrin conversion," *Advanc. Protein Chem. 12*, 1 (1957).

27. A. J. Quick and J. E. Favre-Gilly, "Fibrin: A factor influencing the consumption of prothrombin in coagulation," *Amer. J. Physiol. 158*, 387 (1949).

28. O. Snellman, B. Sylven, and C. Julen, "Analyses of the native heparin-lipoprotein complex including the identification of a heparin complement (heparin co-factor) obtained from extracts of tissue mast cells," *Biochim. biophys. Acta. 7*, 98 (1951).

29. L. M. Tocantins and R. T. Carroll, "Separation and assay of a lipid antithromboplastin from human brain, blood plasma, and plasma fractions," *Blood Clotting and Allied Problems* (2nd Conference of the Josiah Macy Foundation, New York, 1949).

30. T. Astrup, "Fibrinolysis in the organism," *Blood 11*, 781 (1956).

31. "Proteolytic Enzymes and Their Clinical Application," *Ann. N. Y. Acad. Sci. 68*, 1 (1957).

32. W. S. Tillett, A. J. Johnson, and W. R. McCarty, "The intravenous infusion of the streptococcal fibrinolytic principle (streptokinase) into patients," *J. clin. Invest. 34*, 169 (1955).

33. R. Biggs and A. S. Douglas, "The thromboplastin generation test," *J. clin. Path. 6*, 23 (1953).

34. J. L. Tullis, "Identification and significance of platelet antibodies," *New Engl. J. Med. 255*, 541 (1956).

35. J. F. Ackroyd, "The role of sedormid in the immunologic reaction that results in platelet lysis in sedormid purpura," *Clin. Sci. 13*, 409 (1954).

36. J. G. Humble, "The mechanism of petechial hemorrhage formation," *Blood 4*, 69 (1949).

37. B. Alexander and R. Goldstein, "Dual hemostatic defect in pseudohemophilia," *J. clin. Invest. 32*, 551 (1953).

38. K. Singer and B. Ramot, "Pseudohemophilia type B: hereditary hemorrhagic diathesis characterized by prolonged bleeding time and decrease in antihemophilic factor," *Arch. intern. Med. 97*, 715 (1956).

39. T. H. Spaet, "Analytical review: Vascular factors in the pathogenesis of hemorrhage syndrome," *Blood 7*, 641 (1952).

40. M. Stefanini and E. Petrillo, "The relative importance of plasmatic and vascular factors of hemostasis in the pathogenesis of the hemorrhagic diathesis of liver dysfunction," *Acta med. scand. 134*, 139 (1949).

41. A. C. Ivy, P. R. Shapiro, and P. Melnick, "The bleeding tendency in jaundice," *Surg. Gynec. Obstet. 60*, 781 (1935).

42. W. W. Duke, "The relation of blood platelets to hemorrhagic disease: Description of a method for determining the bleeding time and coagulation time and report of three cases of hemorrhagic disease relieved by transfusion," *J. Amer. med. Ass. 14*, 1185 (1910).

43. R. G. Macfarlane, "Critical review: Mechanism of hemostasis," *Quart. J. Med. 10*, 1 (1941).

44. H. Braunsteiner and F. Pakesch, "Thrombocytoasthenia and thrombocytopathia—old names and new diseases," *Blood 11*, 965 (1956).

45. R. I. Lee and P. D. White, "A clinical study of the coagulation time of blood," *Amer. J. med. Sci. 145,* 495 (1913).
46. A. J. Quick, R. C. Honorato, and M. Stefanini, "Value and limitations of the coagulation time in the study of the hemorrhagic diseases," *Blood 3,* 1120 (1948).
47. L. B. Jaques, "Determination of the clotting time of whole blood," in L. M. Tocantins, ed., *The Coagulation of Blood, Methods of Study* (Grune and Stratton, New York, 1955).
48. A. J. Quick, "The clinical application of the hippuric acid and the prothrombin tests," *Amer. J. clin. Path. 10,* 222 (1940).
49. B. Alexander, "Estimation of plasma prothrombin by the one-stage method," in L. M. Tocantins, ed., *The Coagulation of Blood, Methods of Study* (Grune and Stratton, New York, 1955).
50. B. Alexander and R. Goldstein, "Parahemophilia in three siblings (Owren's disease): A clinical and laboratory study elucidating certain plasma components affecting prothrombin conversion," *Amer. J. Med. 13,* 225 (1952).
51. B. Alexander, A. de Vries, and R. Goldstein, "Prothrombin: A critique of methods for its determination and their clinical significance," *New Engl. J. Med. 240,* 403 (1949).
52. L. M. Tocantins, "Measurement of the rate and extent of clot retraction," in L. M. Tocantins, ed., *The Coagulation of Blood, Methods of Study* (Grune and Stratton, New York, 1955).
53. G. Ballerini and W. H. Seegers, "A description of clot retraction as a visual experience," *Thrombosis et Diath. Haemorrhagica 3,* 147 (1959).
54. A. A. Sharp, B. Howie, R. Biggs, and D. T. Menthuen, "Defibrination syndrome of pregnancy. Value of various diagnostic tests," *Lancet 2,* 1309 (1958).
55. R. R. Holburn, "Estimation of fibrinogen in small samples of plasma (method of Ratnoff and Menzie)," in L. M. Tocantins, ed., *The Coagulation of Blood, Methods of Study* (Grune and Stratton, New York, 1955).
56. B. Alexander, R. Goldstein, L. Rich, A. G. Bolloch, L. K. Diamond, and W. Borges, "Congenital afibrinogenemia. A study of some basic aspects of coagulation," *Blood 9,* 843 (1954).
57. D. E. Reid, A. E. Weiner, and C. C. Roby, "I. Intravascular clotting and afibrinogenemia, presumptive lethal factors in syndrome of amniotic fluid embolism. II. Incoagulable blood in severe premature separation of placenta: Method of management. III. Maternal afibrinogenemia associated with long-standing intrauterine fetal death," *Amer. J. Obstet. Gynec. 66,* 465 (1953).
58. J. R. O'Brien, "An acquired coagulation defect in a woman," *J. clin. Path. 7,* 22 (1954).
59. R. G. Biggs, A. S. Douglas, R. G. Macfarlane, J. V. Dacie, W. R. Pitney, C. Merskey, and J. R. O'Brien, "Christmas disease. A condition previously mistaken for haemophilia," *Brit. med. J. 2,* 1378 (1952).
60. R. G. Biggs, "Laboratory control of anticoagulant therapy," in *Report of International Conference on Thrombosis and Embolism* (Schwabe, Basel, 1954).
61. W. R. Pitney and J. V. Dacie, "Haemophilia and allied disorders of blood coagulation," *Brit. med. Bull. 11,* 11 (1955).
62. R. L. Rosenthal, "Plasma thromboplastin antecedent (P.T.A.) deficiency in man: Clinical, coagulation, hereditary, and therapeutic aspects," *J. clin. Invest. 33,* 961 (1954).

63. H. Dreskin and N. Rosenthal, "A hemophilia-like disease with prolonged coagulation time and circulating anticoagulant," *Blood 5,* 46 (1950).

64. P. A. Owren and K. Aas, "The control of dicumarol therapy and the quantitative determination of prothrombin and proconvertin," *Scand. J. clin. Lab. Invest. 3,* 201 (1951).

65. B. Alexander, personal communication.

66. A. J. Quick, A. V. Pisciotta, and C. V. Hussey, "Congenital hypoprothrombinemic states," *Arch. intern. Med. 95,* 2 (1955).

67. P. Wolf, "A modification for routine laboratory use of Stefanini's method of estimating Factor V activity in human oxalated plasma," *J. clin. Path. 6,* 34 (1953).

68. M. Stefanini, "New one-stage procedures for the quantitative determination of prothrombin and labile factor," *Amer. J. clin. Path. 20,* 233 (1950).

69. P. A. Owren, "Parahemophilia: Haemorrhagic diathesis due to absence of a previously unknown clotting factor," *Lancet 1,* 446 (1947).

70. A. de Vries, B. Alexander, and R. Goldstein, "A factor in serum which accelerates the conversion of prothrombin to thrombin. Its determination and some physiologic and biochemical properties," *Blood 4,* 247 (1949).

71. B. Alexander, "Determination of S.P.C.A. (Convertin, Factor VII)," in L. M. Tocantins, ed., *The Coagulation of Blood, Methods of Study* (Grune and Stratton, New York, 1955).

72. B. Alexander, "Clotting factor VII (proconvertin): Synonymy, properties, clinical, and clinicolaboratory aspects," *New Engl. J. Med. 260,* 1218 (1959).

73. B. Alexander, R. Goldstein, G. Landwehr, and C. D. Cook, "Congenital S.P.C.A. deficiency: A hitherto unrecognized coagulation defect with hemorrhages rectified by serum and serum fractions," *J. clin. Invest. 30,* 596 (1951).

74. A. S. Douglas, "The coagulation defect caused by Tromexan therapy," *Clin. Sci. 14,* 601 (1955).

75. C. Hougie, E. M. Barrow, and J. B. Graham, "Stuart clotting defect. I. Segregation of hereditary hemorrhagic state from heterogeneous group hitherto-fore called stable factor (S.P.C.A., proconvertin, factor VII) deficiency," *J. clin. Invest. 36,* 485 (1957).

76. F. Bachmann, F. Duckert, and F. Koller, "The Stuart-Prower factor assay and its clinical significance," *Thrombosis et Diath. Haemorrhagica 2,* 24 (1958).

77. J. Roos, C. van Arkel, M. C. Verloop, and F. L. Jordon, "A 'new' family with Stuart-Prower deficiency," *Thrombosis et Diath. Haemorrhagica 3,* 59 (1959).

# Unit 15

# Blood Groups

Landsteiner's discovery of the basic ABO blood-group system in 1901 was the beginning of safe whole-blood transfusions.[1] During the ensuing years, with an increasing number of transfusions, reactions led to the search for other blood groups. The presence of a second major blood-group family, D ($Rh_0$) was indicated when Levine and Stetson [2] in 1939 described an atypical agglutinin that caused a severe hemolytic reaction in a recently delivered woman. This agglutinin was found to be identical to the agglutinin reacting with a factor in the red blood cells of rhesus monkeys as reported by Landsteiner and Wiener in 1940.[3] To date, nine families of blood groups have been established.[4]

Each blood-group system consists of two or more blood-group factors. Many other (minor) blood-group factors have been identified with rare antiserums from human blood. Some of these factors can be fitted into the nine blood-group systems and others have been called "private antigens" because they have been found in only a single family of humans. Although whole-blood transfusion is now a relatively safe procedure if careful attention is paid to the details of cross matching donor and recipient bloods, the occasional transfusion reaction which still occurs suggests that there are yet other problems to be solved.

In addition to making transfusions much safer, knowledge of blood-group systems has contributed to an understanding of the basic pathophysiology of erythroblastosis fetalis and its successful management.[5]

Individual blood-group factors are genetically inherited, and the genes within each of the classified blood-group systems are transmitted independently of the genes in other blood-group systems.[6] Thus the complete blood type of a person is almost as uniquely characteristic as his fingerprint. This knowledge is of increasing value in forensic medicine for solving problems of paternity or in establishing the source of blood in criminal cases. Anthropologists and geneticists have applied the study of blood types to the origin of races.

## Physiology

### NATURE OF THE BLOOD-GROUP FACTORS

The complete blood type of the erythrocyte is determined by the presence of numerous blood-group factors which occur as submicroscopic patches of specific blood-group substance in or on the envelope of the red blood cell. The chemical nature and sources of specific blood-group substances have been determined for a few of the blood-group systems.[7] A and B blood-group substances are mucoproteins. They are found in red cells and all body tissues except the nervous system. People who have secretor genes (about 76 percent in the Caucasian race) also secrete large quantities of A and B blood-group substances in body fluids (saliva, gastric juice, urine, serum, and seminal fluid).[3] A and B substances are quite widespread in nature, being found in other mammals as well as in many bacteria and plants. The common commercial source of A substance is the gastric mucosa of the hog, while the gastric mucosa of some horses provides a convenient supply of B. The chemical nature of the specific blood-group substances of other blood-group systems is still unknown. Blood-group substances of the D ($Rh_o$) and MNS systems are found only in the red blood cells of humans and some of the monkeys (for Rh). On the other hand, saliva and serum are the primary source of $Le^a$ and $Le^b$ blood-group substance of the Lewis system. They are adsorbed only incidentally on the red blood cells.

### INHERITANCE OF BLOOD GROUPS

A knowledge of some of the basic principles of genetics is necessary for understanding the fundamental problems in blood grouping.[4] Heredity is determined by units of inheritance called genes which are located in a linear order along the 23 matched pairs of chromosomes in human somatic cells. One chromosome of each homologous pair is contributed by the ovum and the other by the sperm. Each gene has specific, individual functions and each pair of genes occupy identical positions, called their locus, in their particular pair of chromosomes. Genes may exist in alternative forms, called allelomorphs. Any particular gene may have several allelomorphs, only one of which may occupy the locus for that gene. Thus, not more than two allelomorphs of any one gene can coexist in an individual. If both allelomorphs are the same, the person is homozygous for this gene; but if the genes are different, then the person is heterozygous. An individual's blood-group pattern for each of the nine blood-group systems will be determined by any of several pairs of allelomorph genes for that particular system. A simple example illustrating the inheritance of allelomorph blood-group genes is given in Fig. 24.

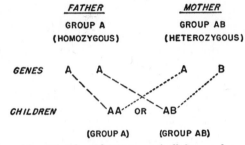

Fig. 24. The inheritance of allelomorph blood-group genes.

If both genes responsible for a characteristic or blood group can be recognized in a person, the pair of genes is called the genotype for that person, for example, the genotype AB. On the other hand, if ordinary tests cannot determine whether the genotype of a person is AA or AO, this less complete kind of genetic distinction is called group A and is labeled a phenotype.

Genes carried on different chromosomes enter into a sex cell in a chance distribution. These genes are said to segregate independently. The genes of all nine blood-group families appear to behave in this manner. Consequently, the complete blood-group pattern may have countless combinations.

### NATURE OF ANTIBODIES

The blood-group substances are antigenic. Specific antibodies are globulins that may be formed against blood-group factors not present in an individual's erythrocytes. Stimulation to the production of blood-group antibodies can result from the introduction of allelomorphs of blood-group substances via repeated transfusions, through injections of blood products, or across the placental barrier during pregnancy. Some antibodies are normally "spontaneous," occurring in humans in the absence of transfusion or pregnancy. Examples of these are anti-A, -B, -H, -M, -N, -Vw, -M$^g$, -P, -Tj$^a$, -Le$^a$, -Le$^b$, and -Wr$^a$. Antigens corresponding to some of these "spontaneous" antibodies have been found elsewhere than in human red cells. Antibodies resulting from active immunization following blood transfusion or pregnancy are called immune antibodies. Antibodies against some of the blood-group factors have been found in nature. The blood-group factor "H" of the ABO system is most easily identified by the use of an extract from seeds of the plant *Ulex europeus*. Highly diluted extracts of another seed, *Dolichos biflorus*, agglutinate A$_1$ cells, but not A$_2$. The serum of newborn babies will not contain any blood-group antibodies except in occasional cases where antibodies from the maternal blood have crossed the placenta and have entered the fetal circulation. By the age of 6 months, spontaneous antibodies, notably anti-A and -B, will have appeared in the blood of individuals who do not have the corresponding blood-group factor in their red cells.

Antibodies are classified as complete when they agglutinate saline suspensions of red blood cells containing the corresponding blood-group factor. Incomplete or blocking antibodies, on the other hand, agglutinate red cells only when suspended in serum or albumin, but not in saline. Spontaneous antibodies are complete and react more strongly at 4°C than at 37°C. Immune antibodies may be complete, but more often are incomplete. They are more active at 37°C than at lower temperatures.

### THE NATURE OF ANTIGEN-ANTIBODY REACTION

When red blood cells containing a specific blood-group factor are put with a serum containing the corresponding antibody under conditions favorable for antigen-antibody reaction, the cells are agglutinated. The blood-group factor or antigen is thus called an agglutinogen, and the antibody is termed an agglutinin.

The clumping or agglutination of the red cells indicates a positive reaction in blood-grouping laboratory tests.[9] The nature of agglutination is a matter for some speculation, though it is generally thought that a "lattice" is formed by bridges of antibody between antigens on adjacent cells. At times it may be necessary to use special temperatures, special mediums, or more complicated tests in order to bring about visible agglutination in vitro. When certain antibodies, notably those of the Duffy and Kidd systems, are mixed with red cells having the corresponding antigen, no agglutination occurs, for reasons unknown. Thus, agglutination is not an essential part of the blood-group antigen-antibody reaction in vivo. If there is no agglutination of the red cells by the usual tests in vitro, the presence of antigens and antibodies can be demonstrated by the technique of the Coombs test.[10, 11] This is based on the fact that antibodies which coat or are adsorbed on the unagglutinated red cells are globulins. Then, when an anti-human-globulin serum is added, agglutination might result from links of antiglobulin serum between antibody molecules on different cells. Specificity of the Coombs test is due to the fact that the only antibodies adsorbed on the red-cell envelope correspond to the given blood-group substance present.

Although agglutination is the chief manifestation of antigen-antibody reaction in vitro, hemolysis is the primary result of antigen-antibody reaction in vivo and, if severe enough, hemolysis leads to the serious or fatal complications of incompatible blood transfusions. In the presence of complement of fresh serum, certain blood-group antibodies act as hemolysins. When mixed with red blood cells containing the corresponding antigen, the antibody rapidly attacks the red-cell envelope and causes its rupture with liberation of hemoglobin. When performing laboratory tests for blood grouping and cross matching, hemolysis may have

217

the same positive significance as agglutination.

The quantity of specific blood-group factors contained in the envelope of the red cell may vary greatly. There is also a marked difference in the antigenicity of blood group substances. For example, A, B, and D ($Rh_o$) are strongly antigenic. $A_1$ is more antigenic than $A_2$. In the Rh system, D is much more antigenic than C or E. The titer of antibodies in the serums of individuals can also show marked variation. Weak antigens and low titers of antibodies may lead to difficulties in blood grouping and cross matching.

CLASSIFICATION OF BLOOD GROUPS

The nine blood-group systems and the large number of blood-group factors identified as of November 1959 by means of specific blood-typing reagents are listed in Table 40, together with their frequencies. The ABO groups are by far the most important potential cause of trouble and still the most frequent cause of fatal transfusion reactions. The great importance of the ABO groups depends on their strong antigenicity and the universal presence of the antibodies when the corresponding blood-group factors are absent. Pregnancy in Rh-negative mothers as well as transfusions to Rh-negative recipients give this blood-group family considerable clinical significance. The other blood-group factors are of lesser and varying importance owing to differences in frequency and in antigenicity.

THE ABO SYSTEM. The ABO group of an individual is determined by two of the four allelomorphic genes, $A_1$, $A_2$, B, and O. Table 41 shows the different combinations within the ABO system. Actually, the system is more complicated because there are other subgroups of A included in $A_2$, such as $A_3$, $A_4$, $A_5$, and so forth.

Table 40. *Blood-group factors that can be identified by specific reagents (November 1959).*[1]

| Blood-group family (system) | Blood-group factors and frequencies (percent)[2] | Number of phenotypes in each system | Number of different phenotype combinations theoretically possible (cumulative) |
|---|---|---|---|
| 1. ABO | A (45), B (14), "H" (54) | 6 | 6 |
| 2. MNS | M (79), N (71), S (55), s (89), Hu (rare), He (rare), Mi^a (rare), Vw (rare), U (almost universal), M^g (very rare), Vr (rare) | 98 | 588 |
| 3. P | P (79), Tj^a (almost universal), P^k (rare) | 4 | 2,352 |
| 4. Rh[3] | D (84), C (70), c (80), C^w (1), C^x (rare), E (30), e (98), E^w (rare), f (64), G (85), V (rare), rh_i (70), Hr_o (almost universal) | 110 | 258,720 |
| 5. Lutheran | Lu^a (8), Lu^b (99.8) | 3 | 776,160 |
| 6. Kell | K (10), k (99.8), Kp^a (2), Kp^b (99.98), Ku (99.99) | 7 | 5,433,120 |
| 7. Lewis | Le^a (21), Le^b (75) | 3 | 16,299,360 |
| 8. Duffy | Fy^a (65), Fy^b (83) | 4 | 65,197,440 |
| 9. Kidd | Jk^a (77), Jk^b (73) | 4 | 260,789,760 |
| 10. Unclassified | Levay (rare), Vel (almost universal), Ven (rare), Wr^a (rare), Be^a (rare), Rm (rare), By (rare), Yt^a (99.6), Js (rare), Di^a (rare), I (almost universal) | 2048 | Over 500 billion |

[1] Reagents are mostly of human origin, except anti-M, anti-N, anti-Hu, and anti-He, which can be produced in rabbits. The usual anti-H reagent is an extract of the seeds of *Ulex europeus*. An excellent anti-N is obtainable from the seeds of *Vicea graminea*.

[2] Frequencies are approximate, for populations of European origin.

[3] The "Rh factor," unless otherwise specified, means the factor D(Rh_o).

Table 41. *Principal genotypes in the ABO system.*

| Genotypes | Phenotypes (directly identifiable by typing tests) |
|---|---|
| $A_1A_1$ $A_1A_2$ $A_1O$ | $A_1$ |
| $A_2A_2$ $A_2O$ | $A_2$ |
| $BB$ $BO$ | B |
| $A_1B$ | $A_1B$ |
| $A_2B$ | $A_2B$ |
| $OO$ | O |

tion of serum from the various types with known red cells.

For practical purposes in the blood-typing laboratory, only anti-A and anti-B serums of strong titer are used for classifying the red cells. To confirm blood groups by identification of serum, type $A_1$ red cells are used because they give a stronger reaction with anti-A serum. The $A_1$ cells can be selected by testing group A blood with specific anti-$A_1$ serum, or, since about 80 percent of all group A bloods are of subgroup $A_1$, a pool of five random group A bloods can be used as a source of known A cells.[9] Group B cells have equal reactivity with anti-B agglutinins, so known B cells can be selected at random from group B blood.

The spontaneous antibodies of the ABO system, anti-A and anti-B, are complete antibodies and agglutinate in saline suspensions red cells containing the corresponding antigen, most actively at 4°C. In addition, the serums of many individuals will contain an incomplete or immune variety of anti-A, anti-B, or both[12] as a result of immune reaction to an A or B stimulus, for example, pregnancy in a group O mother with a group A or group B fetus, transfusion or injection of incompatible blood, or injection of materials containing specific A or B blood-group factor such as prophylactic vaccine. These immune antibodies act as isohemolysins in the presence of fresh complement. Moreover, they are not eas-

However, for typing, anti-A serum reacts with all subgroups, but more strongly with $A_1$ than with the other subgroups.

To understand the basic principles of the system, it must be realized that group O lacks A and B agglutinogens on the red cells. Group $A_1$ or $A_2$ is characterized by the presence of the corresponding antigen on the red cells and anti-B antibody in the serum. Conversely, group B has B antigen on the red cells and anti-A agglutinin in the serum. Another antigen of the ABO system, called H, has been identified in $A_2$ and O type red cells by agglutination with anti-H agglutinin obtained from the seeds of *Ulex europus,* as we have already mentioned. $A_1$ and B type red cells do not agglutinate with anti-H. The frequencies of the common types in the ABO system are shown in Table 42, along with the reaction of the red cells with specific typing reagents and reac-

Table 42. *Common types (phenotypes) in the ABO system.*

| Type (phenotype) | Approximate frequency in U.S.A. (percent) | Reactions of red cells with typing reagents | | | | Reactions of serum with known cells | |
|---|---|---|---|---|---|---|---|
| | | anti-A | -B | -$A_1$ [a] | -H [b] | $A_1$ cells | B cells |
| O | 45 | 0 | 0 | 0 | + | + | + |
| $A_1$ | 33 | + | 0 | + | 0 | 0 | + |
| $A_2$ | 8 | + | 0 | 0 | + | 0 | + |
| B | 10 | 0 | + | 0 | | + | 0 |
| $A_1B$ | 3 | + | + | + | | 0 | 0 |
| $A_2B$ | 1 | + | + | 0 | | 0 | 0 |

[a] Serum from type B persons, partially absorbed with red cells from $A_2$ donors.
[b] Extract (saline) of seeds of *Ulex europeus.*

ily neutralized by blood-group substances A and B.[13] Therefore, the presence of immune antibodies anti-A and anti-B in many group O bloods will create a danger of hemolytic transfusion reactions if group O blood is used for group A, B, or AB recipients.[14] The use of group O blood for other than group O recipients should be restricted to real emergencies, and, when group O blood is thus given, the titers of anti-A and anti-B saline agglutinins should be low. Moreover, the group O blood should preferably be tested for content of isohemolysins and immune anti-A and anti-B antibodies.

Since A and B antibodies are spontaneously present, and because of their great antigenicity, the A and B blood-group factors are of the greatest importance in transfusions of blood in humans. The majority of hemolytic transfusion reactions seen today are still the result of such incompatibility between donor and recipient. Meticulous typing of cells, back-typing of serum, and careful cross matching of donor and recipient cells and serum with respect to the ABO blood-group system is essential for safe transfusions. The ABO system is also of importance in the etiology of erythroblastosis fetalis, since incompatibilities in this system are the most frequent cause. Fortunately, most of these cases are relatively mild.

THE RH SYSTEM. The Rh system consists of a basic group of six related Rh-Hr blood-group factors. These have been designated by two different sets of symbols, D-d, C-c, E-e (Fisher and Race), or $Rh_o$-$Hr_o$, rh'-Hr', rh''-hr'' (Wiener). Many other factors ($C^w$, $c^v$, $C^v$, $C^x$, $E^v$, $E^w$, G, V, and f) have been identified and fitted into the Rh-Hr system; but they are very rarely of clinical importance.

The inheritance of Rh must be considered, not antigen by antigen, but by groups of antigens. The human rarely has as few as two of the antigens mentioned above, and commonly has six of them. Theories of the inheritance of the Rh groups has been a matter of considerable controversy. A. W. Wiener believes that a single genetic locus is involved, with many allelomorphic genes. The Fisher-Race theory holds that there are at least three sets of genes, closely connected. Regardless of which theory is correct, the pattern of inheritance, with one of the eight basic Rh gene complexes coming from each parent, is firmly established.

A second controversy involves the notation. Table 43 gives comparable terms in the Wiener and Fisher-Race system of notation. Since both nomenclatures are widely used and are applied to the different Rh-Hr typing serums released by the National Institutes of Health, all physicians and blood-bank technicians

Table 43. *Rh notation.*

| Genes | | Approximate frequency (percent) | Antigens [a] produced, Fisher-Race notation (Wiener notation in parentheses) |
|---|---|---|---|
| Wiener notation | Fisher-Race notation | | |
| $R^1$ | CDe | 41 | C (rh'), D ($Rh_o$), e (hr''), G ($rh^G$) |
| r | cde | 39 | c (hr'), e (hr''), f (hr) |
| $R^2$ | cDE | 14 | c (hr'), D ($Rh_o$), E (rh''), G ($rh^G$) |
| $R^0$ | cDe | 2 | c (hr'), D ($Rh_o$), e (hr''), f (hr), G ($rh^G$) |
| $R^{1w}$ | $C^wDe$ | 1 | $C^w$ ($rh^w$), D ($Rh_o$), e (hr''), G ($rh^G$) |
| r' | Cde | 1 | C (rh'), e (hr''), G ($Rh^G$) |
| r'' | cdE | 1 | c (hr'), E (rh'') |
| $R^z$ | CDE | 0.2 | C (rh'), D ($Rh_o$), E (rh''), G ($rh^G$) |
| $r^y$ | CdE | 0.5 | C (rh'), E (rh''), G ($rh^G$) |

[a] Wiener uses the term "factors" instead of "antigens" for these, reserving the term "antigen" for the whole antigenic complex of the red cell.

should be acquainted with the two terminologies.

The frequency of genotypes resulting from inheritance of the eight basic pairs of Rh gene complexes is presented in Table 44. This list of frequencies is of practical value in estimating the genotype of the husband of an Rh-negative woman.

The chemical nature of the Rh antigens has not been determined. The only known source of the antigens is the red blood cells of humans and some of the monkeys. The D (Rh$_0$) factor is by far

the most strongly antigenic of the Rh group and is present in about 85 percent of the white population. Therefore D (Rh$_0$) is the principal and often the only factor identified in Rh typing of red blood cells. Antigenically weak variants of the D (Rh$_0$) factor exist and can be identified with anti-D serums, by means of the indirect Coombs test. Red cells containing these weak factors are called D$^u$ variants [15] and must be considered Rh-positive. It is important to test all D (Rh$_0$)-negative bloods, in particular all

Table 44. *Frequencies of Rh genotypes (after Race and Sanger).*

| | | | Reactions of bloods with various typing serums | | | | |
|---|---|---|---|---|---|---|---|
| Fisher-Race notation | Wiener notation | Calculated frequency (percent) | Anti-C (anti-rh') | Anti-D (anti-Rh°) | Anti-E (anti-rh'') | Anti-c (anti-hr') | Anti-e (anti-hr'') |
| cde/cde | rr | 15.1020 | 0 | 0 | 0 | + | + |
| Cde/Cde | r'r' | < 0.01 | + | 0 | 0 | 0 | + |
| Cde/cde | r'r | 0.76 | + | 0 | 0 | + | + |
| cDe/cDe | $R^0R^0$ | 0.07 | 0 | + | 0 | + | + |
| cDe/cde | $R^0r$ | 1.99 | 0 | + | 0 | + | + |
| cdE/cdE | r''r'' | 0.01 | 0 | 0 | + | + | 0 |
| cdE/cde | r''r | 0.92 | 0 | 0 | + | + | + |
| CDe/CDe | $R^1R^1$ | 17.68 | + | + | 0 | 0 | + |
| CDe/Cde | $R^1r'$ | 0.83 | + | + | 0 | 0 | + |
| CDe/cDe | $R^1R^0$ | 2.16 | + | + | 0 | + | + |
| CDe/cde | $R^1r$ | 32.68 | + | + | 0 | + | + |
| Cde/cDe | $r'R^0$ | 0.05 | + | + | 0 | + | + |
| cDE/cDE | $R^2R^2$ | 1.99 | 0 | + | + | + | 0 |
| cDE/cDe | $R^2R^0$ | 0.72 | 0 | + | + | + | + |
| cDE/cdE | $R^2r''$ | 0.34 | 0 | + | + | + | 0 |
| cDE/cde | $R^2r$ | 10.97 | 0 | + | + | + | + |
| cDe/cdE | $R^0r''$ | 0.06 | 0 | + | + | + | + |
| CdE/CdE | $r^yr^y$ | < 0.01 | + | 0 | + | 0 | 0 |
| CdE/Cde | $r^yr'$ | < 0.01 | + | 0 | + | 0 | + |
| CdE/cdE | $r^yr''$ | < 0.01 | + | 0 | + | + | 0 |
| CdE/cde | $r^yr$ | < 0.01 | + | 0 | + | + | + |
| Cde/cdE | r'r'' | 0.02 | + | 0 | + | + | + |
| CDE/CDE | $R^zR^z$ | < 0.01 | + | + | + | 0 | 0 |
| CDE/CDe | $R^zR^1$ | 0.20 | + | + | + | 0 | + |
| CDE/cDE | $R^zR^2$ | 0.07 | + | + | + | + | 0 |
| CDE/CdE | $R^zr^y$ | < 0.01 | + | + | + | 0 | 0 |
| CDE/Cde | $R^zr'$ | < 0.01 | + | + | + | 0 | + |
| CDe/CdE | $R^1r^y$ | < 0 01 | + | + | + | 0 | + |
| CDE/cDe | $R^zR^0$ | 0.01 | + | + | + | + | + |
| CDe/cDE | $R^1R^2$ | 11.86 | + | + | + | + | + |
| CDE/cdE | $R^zr''$ | 0.01 | + | + | + | + | 0 |
| cDE/CdE | $R^2r^y$ | < 0.01 | + | + | + | + | 0 |
| CDE/cde | $R^zr$ | 0.19 | + | + | + | + | + |
| CDe/cdE | $R^1r''$ | 1.00 | + | + | + | + | + |
| cDE/Cde | $R^2r'$ | 0.28 | + | + | + | + | + |
| CdE/cDe | $r^yR^0$ | < 0.01 | + | + | + | + | + |

donor blood, for the $D^u$ factor. It may also be advisable to test donor bloods with anti-C (rh') and anti-E (rh") serum when it is known that a recipient is sensitized to these blood-group antigens.

Rh antibodies do not occur naturally in the serums of individuals whose red cells lack the Rh group antigens. If a transfusion or even small injections of D ($Rh_o$)-positive blood are given to one of the 15 percent of the white population who are D ($Rh_o$)-negative, an immune reaction may occur with the production of anti-D ($Rh_o$) antibodies.[16] When a D ($Rh_o$)-negative woman becomes pregnant with a D ($Rh_o$)-positive fetus, similar immunization of the mother may take place owing to passage of the antigen across the placenta.[17] In the case of pregnancy, however, the development of Rh antibodies is not generally as consistent or as strong as after transfusions.

Since anti-Rh antibodies are of the immune type, they are more reactive at 37°C. Although some anti-Rh antibodies are saline agglutinins, most are incomplete antibodies and will agglutinate only plasma or albumin suspensions of red cells carrying the corresponding antigen.[18] Some antigen-antibody reactions of the Rh system can be identified only by the Coombs test technique.

Typing of bloods with respect to Rh blood groups, most notably D ($Rh_o$), is of great importance for safe blood transfusions. Anti-D ($Rh_o$) antibodies usually cause severe hemolytic transfusion reactions when D ($Rh_o$)-positive blood is given to a sensitized D ($Rh_o$)-negative recipient who has moderate to large amounts of antibody. D ($Rh_o$) sensitization of a D ($Rh_o$)-negative mother is cause for the development of serious erythroblastosis in subsequent babies.

THE MNS SYSTEM. Four basic gene complexes, *MS, Ms, NS,* and *Ns,* exist within this system.[19, 20, 21] Other blood-group factors related to M and N have been discovered.[22, 23] Most of these are rare,

except U, which is almost universally present. M and N factors are allelomorphs. Since, as shown in Table 45,

Table 45. *The MN blood groups.*

| Geno-type | Pheno-type | Reactions with typing serums | | Frequency (percent) |
|---|---|---|---|---|
| | | Anti-M | Anti-N | |
| *MM* | M | + | − | 29 |
| *MN* | MN | + | + | 50 |
| *NN* | N | − | + | 21 |
| (Not found, in 31 years) | | − | − | 0 |

there seems to be no individual who lacks both M and N, the determination of *MN* genotypes is of value in forensic medicine and problems of paternity.

The antigens of the MNS system are found only on red blood cells, and their chemical nature is not known. Antibodies to MNS antigens have been produced in rabbits, but anti-M and a few anti-N serums have been found in humans. The MN agglutinins react with saline suspensions of red cells at room temperature, while the anti-S and anti-s antibodies are of the warm variety, more reactive at 37°C.

Although there are rare case reports of hemolytic transfusion reactions and erythroblastosis fetalis due to incompatibilities in the MNS system, these antibodies are of little clinical importance. Blood is not routinely tested for factors within the system except in problems of paternity.

THE P SYSTEM. The P system was originally based on two blood-group factors, P and p.[20] Later, another factor, $Tj^a$, was incorporated into the system.[24, 25] The present concept of the P system is presented in Table 46. Anti-P agglutinins are commonly found in the serums from P-negative individuals, but these antibodies are of the cold variety and will rarely, if ever, induce intravascular hemolysis. The P system has little clinical significance.

Table 46. *The P blood groups (after Race and Sanger).*

| Genotypes | Frequency (percent) | Anti-P$_1$ (original anti-P) | Anti-P + P$_1$ (anti-Tj$^a$) |
|---|---|---|---|
| $P_1P_1$ $P_1P_2$ $P_1p$ | 79 | + | + |
| $P_2P_2$ $P_2p$ | 21 | − | + |
| $pp$ | 0 [a] | − | − |

[a] The frequency of genotype $pp$ is given as 0 because no one of this genotype has been discovered in tests of "random" people with anti-Tj$^a$. The only Tj$^a$-negatives have been persons discovered by the presence of anti-Tj$^a$ in their serum or by tests of the close relatives of such persons.

THE LEWIS SYSTEM. The Lewis system, composed of blood-group factors Le$^a$ and Le$^b$, is not well understood.[26, 27] It is of interest because it is related to the secretor genes *Se* and *se* which are responsible for the presence or absence in saliva of A, B, and H substance of the ABO system. The antigens Le$^a$ and Le$^b$ appear to be primarily antigens of the serum and saliva, adsorbed on the red blood cells only incidentally. The secretion of Le$^a$ in the saliva is an inherited characteristic dependent on genes *L* and *l*. Persons of genotype *LL* or *Ll* are salivary secretors of Le$^a$. Persons of genotype *ll* do not secrete Le$^a$ substance. Genes *L* and *l* appear to be independent of genes Se and se. The current concept of the Lewis system is summarized in Table 47.

The antibodies, anti-Le$^a$ and anti-Le$^b$, are sometimes found in human serum, are nearly always very weak, are of the cold variety, and have not been found to cause hemolytic reactions. The Lewis system has little or no clinical significance.

THE LUTHERAN SYSTEM. This system is one of the simple blood-group systems with only two genes, *Lu$^a$* and *Lu$^b$*.[28, 29] The three genotypes and their frequency are shown in Table 48. The antibodies, anti-

Table 48. *The Lutheran blood groups.*

| Genotypes | Reactions of red cells with typing serums | | Approximate frequencies (percent) |
|---|---|---|---|
| | Anti-Lu$^a$ | Anti-Lu$^b$ | |
| $Lu^aLu^a$ | + | 0 | 0.2 |
| $Lu^aLu^b$ | + | + | 8.0 |
| $Lu^bLu^b$ | 0 | + | 92.0 |

Lu$^a$ and anti-Lu$^b$, are saline active and are of the cold variety. Although the serum titers of these antibodies are usually weak, rare cases of very high-titered serum have been discovered in patients sensitized by transfusion. The clinical importance of the Lutheran group is almost negligible.

THE KELL SYSTEM. This system is based on two genes, *K$^b$*, which produces antigens K and Kp$^b$,[30] and *K$^a$*, responsible for antigens k and Kp$^a$.[31] Table 49 shows the frequencies of the various genotypes. Blood group factors K and k have proved to be quite antigenic.[32, 33] Since 8 percent of the population is K-positive, and 92 percent K-negative, there is the probability of stimulating the production of anti-K antibodies in K-negative recipients of K-positive blood. At present, about 1 in 700 of a random patient population is

Table 47. *The Lewis blood groups (after Race and Sanger).*

| Red-cell phenotype | Frequency (percent) | Reactions of red cells with typing serums | | Substances in saliva | | | ABH secretor genotype | Le$^a$ secretor genotype |
|---|---|---|---|---|---|---|---|---|
| | | Anti-Le$^a$ | Anti Le$^b$ | A, B, or H | Le$^a$ | Le$^b$ | | |
| Le(a+b−) | 22 | + | 0 | − | + | − | *sese* | *LL* or *Ll* |
| Le(a−b+) | 72 | 0 | + | + | + | + | *SeSe* or *Sese* | *LL* or *Ll* |
| Le(a−b−) | 6 | 0 | 0 | { + | − | ? | *SeSe* or *Sese* | } *ll* |
| | | | | − | − | − | *sese* | |

Table 49. *The Kell blood groups.*

| Geno-types | Estimated frequen-cies [a] (percent) | Reactions with various typing reagents | | | | |
|---|---|---|---|---|---|---|
| | | Anti-K | Anti-k | Anti-Kp$^a$ | Anti-Kp$^b$ | Anti-Ku |
| $K^bK^b$ | 0.2 | + | 0 | 0 | + | + |
| $K^bK^o$ | 0.05 | + | 0 | 0 | + | + |
| $K^bk^b$ | 9 | + | + | 0 | + | + |
| $K^bk^a$ | 0.1 | + | Weak | + | + | + |
| $k^bk^b$ | 88 | 0 | + | 0 | + | + |
| $k^bK^o$ | 0.9 | 0 | + | 0 | + | + |
| $k^bk^a$ | 2.1 | 0 | + | + | + | + |
| $k^ak^a$ | 0.01 | 0 | Weak | + | 0 | + |
| $k^aK^o$ | 0.01 | 0 | Weak | + | 0 | + |
| $K^oK^o$ | <0.01 | 0 | 0 | 0 | 0 | 0 |

[a] The frequency of $K^o$ is estimated at 0.5 percent, but this is only approximate. $K^b$ and $K^a$ have well-established frequencies of 4.8 percent and 1.1 percent respectively in the population of Boston. Gene $K^b$ produces antigens K and Kp$^b$, $k^b$ produces k and Kp$^b$, $K^a$ produces k and Kp$^a$, $K^o$ produces no known antigens.

found to be sensitized to the K factor.[9] Anti-k antibodies have been rarely found. The antibodies of the Kell system are detected in serum medium or by the indirect Coombs test. Since anti-K antibodies have been responsible for severe transfusion reactions and erythroblastosis fetalis, the indirect Coombs test is advisable in all cross matching.

THE DUFFY SYSTEM. The Duffy system was at first based on two genes, $Fy^a$ and $Fy^b$ with three gentoypes.[34, 35] The discovery of a high incidence of Fy$^a$-negative, Fy$^b$-negative individuals in the Negro population [36] suggested the possibility of a third allele, $Fy^c$, at the Duffy locus. The frequency of the Duffy-group genotypes is shown in Table 50. The blood-group factor Fy$^a$ appears to be fairly antigenic. The antibodies of the Duffy system ordinarily are active in vitro only when the indirect Coombs test is used. Transfusion reactions and erythroblastosis fetalis have been caused by anti-Fy$^a$. This is another reason for using the indirect Coombs test for all cross matching.

THE KIDD SYSTEM. This is another simple system with two genes, $Jk^a$ and $Jk^b$, and

Table 50. *The Duffy blood groups.*

| Genotypes | Frequency (percent) | Reactions of red cells with typing reagents | |
|---|---|---|---|
| | | Anti-Fy$^a$ | Anti-Fy$^b$ |
| $Fy^aFy^a$ $Fy^aFy$ | 17 | + | 0 |
| $Fy^aFy^b$ | 49 | + | + |
| $Fy^bFy^b$ $Fy^bFy$ | 34 | 0 | + |
| $FyFy$ | [a] | 0 | 0 |

[a] This type is the most common of all in Negroes, but has not been found in whites and is presumably rare among them.

three genotypes, as shown in Table 51.[37, 38] The antibodies, anti-Jk$^a$ and anti-Jk$^b$ appear to be rare. They can be demonstrated only by the indirect Coombs test. An occasional case of erythroblastosis fetalis and of a hemolytic transfusion reaction due to these antibodies has been reported.

PRIVATE ANTIGENS. In addition to the many blood-group factors described within the nine blood-group systems, other antigens have been discovered in a single family of people. Examples of this type of blood-group antigens include Levay, Jobbins, Gr., and Becker. Increasing experience in blood grouping may place some of these private antigens within definite blood-group systems.

ERYTHROBLASTOSIS FETALIS. Erythroblastosis fetalis, a hemolytic disease of the fetus and newborn, is the result of fetal-maternal blood-group incompatibility.[5, 39] Antibody formed by the mother, sensitized by a previous incompatible pregnancy or blood transfusion, can pass

Table 51. *The Kidd blood groups.*

| Genotype | Frequency (percent) | Reactions of red cells with typing serums | |
|---|---|---|---|
| | | Anti-Jk$^a$ | Anti-Jk$^b$ |
| $Jk^aJk^a$ | 27 | + | 0 |
| $Jk^aJk^b$ | 50 | + | + |
| $Jk^bJk^b$ | 23 | 0 | + |

through the placenta into the circulation of the fetus. If the red blood cells of the fetus contain a blood-group factor corresponding to the maternal antibody, the antibody is adsorbed on the envelope of the red cell. This coating of the fetal red cells renders them vulnerable to phagocytosis and shortens the life of the red cell. When the fetus is unable to produce red cells sufficiently rapidly to keep up with red-cell destruction, the fetus becomes anemic and dies in utero. Less rapid hemolysis of red cells in utero will permit the fetus to be born alive, but there is such a rate of red-cell destruction and liberation of hemoglobin that the newborn infant becomes jaundiced. This is due to the natural inability of the newborn to conjugate such increased quantities of free bilirubin and excrete it via the bile (see Unit 24). High serum levels of bilirubin in the infant may cause brain damage, a condition called kernicterus. If, however, such a state is recognized soon after birth and exchange transfusions of blood compatible with the maternal antibody are given to the newborn, the jaundice and anemia of the infant may be controlled.

Theoretically, practically all of the known blood-group factors may, on occasion, cause erythroblastosis fetalis, but the majority of cases are due to incompatibility in the ABO or Rh systems. Although D (Rh$_o$) factor is the most important cause of severe erythroblastosis fetalis, factor A incompatibility produces the more frequent but milder manifestations of the disease. By calculation, 20 percent of mothers should have fetuses incompatible with respect to the ABO blood group. Nevertheless, the disease is clinically detectable in only 5 percent of this group. There has been no explanation of why the other 95 percent of the theoretically incompatible fetuses show no manifestations of the disease. As for the D (Rh$_o$) group, pregnancy is less dangerous than transfusion in causing sensitization. It is probable that less than 10 percent of D (Rh$_o$)-negative women are sensitized by pregnancy when the husbands are D (Rh$_o$)-positive. The first D (Rh$_o$)-incompatible pregnancy rarely results in sensitization that can be detected by tests of the serum during that pregnancy, but the anti-D antibody may be found in the mother's serum during the first few weeks postpartum after the first pregnancy. Subsequent pregnancies increase the likelihood of erythroblastosis fetalis.

### BLOOD TYPING IN DISPUTED PATERNITY AND TWINS

Evidence obtained from blood typing using the ABO and Rh systems is becoming increasingly acceptable as proof of innocence in cases of disputed paternity. A child's red blood cells can have a blood-group antigen only if either of the parents has it. If a child has a blood-group factor that is absent in the blood of the mother and the alleged father, the man is excluded. The antigens H, Le$^a$, and Le$^b$ are not used in this type of work. A second way of establishing nonpaternity is through the use of MN group typing for genetic exclusion. Reference to Table 45 shows that there is no individual who lacks both antigens M and N. Moreover, the three genotypes *MM*, *MN*, and *NN* can be proved with the use of anti-M and anti-N typing serum. The following example shows how genetic exclusion with MN typing can disprove paternity:

| Supposed Father | Mother |
|---|---|
| Type N | Type M |
| *Child* | |
| Type M | |
| Genotype *MM* | |

Since all of the supposed father's children would have to have at least one *N* gene, the child cannot be his. The occasional presence of rare blood-group factors like M$^g$ makes the exclusion of paternity by blood typing something less than 100-percent reliable. Blood types may also be useful in distinguishing non-identical twins.

## Laboratory Procedures Related to the Identification of Blood Types and Cross Matching

The basis for all laboratory procedures related to blood typing and cross matching is the agglutination that results when red cells are mixed under suitable conditions with serum containing antibodies corresponding to the blood-group antigens on the red cell.

### ABO TYPING

Except for rare and special circumstances, blood typing is limited to the ABO and Rh systems.

A saline suspension of the patient's red cells is mixed with known anti-A and known anti-B typing serum. The reaction may be carried out in a small test tube or on a glass microscope slide at room temperature. Agglutination is observed macroscopically, but if any doubt exists it is checked with a low-power ($100\times$) microscope. Confirmation of the red cell's blood group is established by serum typing where the patient's serum is mixed with saline suspensions of known $A_1$ and B type red cells. The results of serum typing are the reciprocal of those observed when the patient's cells are mixed with known A and B typing serums.

REAGENTS. (1) Clotted blood of the patient separated into clot and serum;

(2) Sodium chloride solution (0.9 percent) for making 2-percent (test tube) and 5-percent (slide) suspensions of red cells obtained from the clot with an applicator stick;

(3) Known $A_1$ and B red cells in 2-percent and 5-percent saline suspensions;

(4) Potent anti-A and anti-B typing serums. Commercial serums standardized for specificity, avidity, and titer in accordance with certain minimum requirements given by the National Insti-

tutes of Health are satisfactory. Directions accompanying the serum should be carefully followed.

**Method.** 1. *Test Tube Method.* (*a*) *Cell Typing.* Small test tubes ($7$–$8 \times 70$–$80$ mm) are used. One or two drops of a 2-percent saline suspension of red cells is placed in each of two tubes. A drop of anti-A serum is added to one tube and a drop of anti-B serum to the other. The tubes are well shaken to assure mixing and are centrifuged for 1–2 min at 1000–2000 rev/min. The cell button at the bottom is gently dislodged and agitated. A cloudy swirl of red cells indicates absence of agglutination.

(*b*) *Serum Typing.* Serum from the patient is heated to 56°C for 10 min to inactivate the complement in fresh serum which may promote hemolysis of the test red cells and lead to uncertain results in the confirmation test for the presence of antibodies in the unknown serum. A drop of this heated serum is added to each of two test tubes, one containing 2 drops of a 2-percent saline suspension of known $A_1$ cells and the other known B cells. The mixtures are shaken, centrifuged, and read for agglutination in the same way as for the cell typing.

2. *Slide Method.* (*a*) *Cell Typing.* Glass microscope slides are used. One drop of a 5–10-percent saline suspension of the patient's red cells is well mixed with one drop of anti-A typing serum on the slide. A similar preparation is made with anti-B typing serum. Agglutination will be observed usually within 1 min. and in all cases within 3 min. The presence of agglutination must be determined before the mixture begins to dry at the outer edge.

(*b*) *Serum Typing.* The confirmation test is carried out the same way with inactivated serum from the patient's blood and 10-percent saline suspensions of known $A_1$ and B cells.

INDICATIONS AND INTERPRETATION. Blood typing for ABO groups and confirmation are indicated for all patients who are to receive transfusions. Typing of both father and mother is of value in predicting the possibility of erythroblastosis fetalis in the baby. The patient's blood type as a result of observed agglutinations in the cell-typing and serum confirmation tests can be established by referring to Table 42.

LIMITATIONS AND SOURCES OF ERROR. The reliability of blood typing is disturbed by other types of agglutination which result in inconsistencies between cell typing and confirmation by serum typing. When the results of cell typing and confirmation do not agree, the patient's blood type should be based on the findings of cell typing but the cause of inconsistency should be sought for in the serum. The reason for this is that the errors are brought about by certain phenomena primarily occurring in the serum, such as rouleau formation, autoagglutination, bacteriogenic agglutinins, and specific atypical agglutinins.[9]

*Rouleau formation.* This is the appearance that red cells sometimes assume when they lie together, flat side to flat side, like a roll of coins. The cause of this phenomenon is not fully understood. It is found in serum with a high protein level, especially in the globulin and fibrinogen fractions from patients with such diseases as multiple myeloma, tuberculosis, rheumatic fever, and pneumonia. Since acceptable anti-A and anti-B typing serums do not create rouleau formation, it is only a problem in the confirmation test. Slight dilution of the serum with saline will usually break up the rouleau formation or prevent it.

*Autoagglutinins.* Small amounts of unspecific cold agglutinins that ordinarily react at low temperatures (4°C) are present in the serums from many healthy people. These agglutinins usually present no problem in blood grouping that is carried out at room temperature. Serums from patients with some diseases like acquired hemolytic anemia, virus pneumonia, cirrhosis of the liver, and Raynaud's disease will have a stronger tendency to unspecific autoagglutination. This reaction will occur even at room temperature. Depending on the quantity of cold agglutinins in the blood and the temperature at which the cells and serum are separated, the cold agglutinins may be found on the surface of the red cell or in the serum or both. This will lead to complete inconsistencies of cell typing and serum typing. The cold agglutinins can usually be removed from the red-cell surface at 37°C if there are inconsistencies.

*Bacteriologic agglutination.* Contamination of the blood specimen with bacteria may lead to unspecific agglutination in both cell typing and serum confirmation at all temperatures. No exact type determination can be made on such contaminated samples and fresh samples must be obtained.

*Specific atypical agglutinins.* Specific blood-group antibodies of the cold variety such as anti-P, and anti-Le$^a$, and anti-Le$^b$ may be present in the serum and will create errors in the serum confirmation test. Occasionally, antibodies of the warm variety such as those of the Rh system may react at room temperature and create difficulties with the confirmation test. All of these antibodies may agglutinate known A$_1$ and B test cells if these cells contain the specific antigen. When test serum shows reactions in contrast to the expected agglutination pattern of the A$_1$ and B test cells, the identity of the antibodies of the serum should be determined by testing the serum with a panel of fully typed blood cells which are available in large blood-grouping laboratories.

### Rh TYPING

Typing in the Rh system is usually limited to the D (Rh$_0$) factor. In the case of D (Rh$_0$)-negative blood donors, the D$^u$ factor is also tested for.

The commonly used Rh-Hr typing serums are of two varieties. Saline-reactive serums that contain the so-called complete antibodies will react with red cells suspended in saline, and albumin-reactive serums containing incomplete antibodies will react with red cells suspended in albumin or serum.[18] Since Rh antibodies are almost always of the warm-agglutinin type, the reactions are carried out at 37°C in test tubes or on glass microscope slides. Agglutination is observed macroscopically, or, if doubtful, is checked with a low-power microscope. Confirmation of the red cell's D (Rh$_o$) type is checked by repeating the tests with Rh typing serums of a different lot number. In the case of D (Rh$_o$)-negative blood donors, the presence of the D$^u$ factor is checked with an indirect Coombs test. This reaction depends upon the agglutination by anti-human globulin of D$^u$ red cells coated with anti-D antibody.

REAGENTS. (1) Cells from clotted blood of the patient;

(2) Sodium chloride solution (0.9 percent) for making saline suspensions of the red cells;

(3) Bovine albumin solution (15–20 percent) for albumin suspensions of the red cells;

(4) Potent anti-D (Rh$_o$) typing serums with two different lot numbers. Directions accompanying the serum should be carefully followed;

(5) Anti-human globulin (Coombs serum).

**Method.** 1. *Test Tube with Saline-Reactive Serum.* Two drops of a 2-percent saline suspension of red cells in a small test tube is mixed with 1 drop of saline-reactive D (Rh$_o$) typing serum. After incubation at 37°C for 20 min to 1 hr, the tube is centrifuged at 1000–2000 rev/min for 1 to 2 min. The cell sediment is gently dislodged and studied for agglutination.

2. *Test Tube with Albumin-Reactive Serum.* Two drops of a 2-percent suspension of red cells in 15–20-percent bovine albumin or serum is mixed in a small test tube with 1 drop of albumin-reactive D (Rh$_o$) typing serum. Incubation at 37°C, centrifugation, and investigation for agglutination are carried out in the same way as for saline-reactive serum.

3. *Slide Test.* Two drops of a heavy suspension of red cells in bovine albumin is thoroughly mixed with 1 drop of albumin-reactive slide-test anti-D (Rh$_o$) serum on a glass microscope slide. The slide is placed on the glass plate of a viewing box with a temperature of 45–50°C. After gentle rotation, the slide is observed for agglutination within 2 min, before drying occurs.

4. *Test for D$^u$ Factor.* Two drops of a 2-percent saline suspension of red cells in a small test tube is mixed with 1 drop of albumin-reactive anti-D (Rh$_o$) serum. After incubation for ½ to 1 hr at 37°C, the tube is centrifuged. The supernatant saline is poured off and the red cells are re-suspended in 0.9-percent sodium chloride solution that has been introduced via a jet stream. Again the tube is centrifuged. After the red cells have been thus washed three or four times, 2 drops of a 2-percent saline suspension of washed red cells is mixed with 1 drop of anti-human globulin (Coombs) serum. The tube is centrifuged at 1000–2000 rev/min for 1–2 min, and the cell button is gently dislodged and studied for agglutination.

INDICATIONS AND INTERPRETATION. All blood should be typed with anti-D (Rh$_o$) serum as well as for ABO blood groups. Rh typing is essential in all transfusion work and husbands of all D (Rh$_o$)-negative mothers should be typed with anti-D (Rh$_o$) serum in order to predict the possibility of erythroblastosis fetalis. Two different anti-D (Rh$_o$) serums should be used. Blood from D (Rh$_o$)-negative donors and husbands should be further investigated for the D$^u$ factor.

Interpretation of results in Rh typing

is based on a double standard. If there is any doubt about the type of a mother or a recipient of a blood transfusion, especially where there is a weakly positive $D^u$ reaction, the individual should be considered D ($Rh_o$)-negative. Conversely, if any question exists with respect to the D ($Rh_o$) and $D^u$ type of the donor or father, he should be considered D ($Rh_o$)-positive. With these precautions, transfusion reactions due to D ($Rh_o$) incompatibility can be eliminated.

LIMITATIONS AND SOURCES OF ERROR. Mixed reagents such as anti-CDE, anti-CD, and anti-DE should never be used for routine D ($Rh_o$) typing. It is advisable, however, to test D ($Rh_o$)-negative blood donors with anti-CD (anti-G) serums[40] because anti-G antibodies may be produced occasionally by D ($Rh_o$)-negative people. About 5 percent of D ($Rh_o$)-negative donors are G-positive. Anti-DE serum can be used in testing D ($Rh_o$)-negative blood for E factor. The same sources of error that have been described for ABO blood grouping apply to Rh-typing.

## Coombs Test

The Coombs test is a blood-grouping procedure, not a typing test. Coombs serum is anti-human globulin, usually prepared by immunizing rabbits against human gamma globulin, harvesting the rabbit serum, and absorbing it with normal human red cells until it no longer agglutinates normal cells. The Coombs serum is then used to test for the presence of human blood-group isoantibodies attached to human red cells.

METHOD. The technique is similar to the test for the $D^u$ factor in Rh typing. The directions furnished by the manufacturer of the serum should be followed carefully.

INTERPRETATION. In vivo coating (sensitization) of red cells by isoantibodies, in the various acquired hemolytic anemias, including erythroblastosis fetalis, is demonstrated when washed red cells from the patient are agglutinated after the addition of Coombs serum. Such testing of red cells from a patient is known as the direct Coombs test.

When uncoated (normal) red cells are exposed in a test tube to a serum that may contain blood-group isoantibodies and subsequently washed and exposed to a drop of Coombs reagent, agglutination of the cells indicates that the serum contained an isoantibody and the red cells have the corresponding blood-group factor. Use of Coombs serum to detect the presence or absence of such in vitro coating of red cells is called the indirect Coombs test.

SOURCES OF ERROR. A false positive result in the indirect Coombs test is seen when the red cells used in the test were coated in vivo. Such cells would give a positive result in the direct Coombs test. The addition of a drop of another serum would not remove the original antibodies and the Coombs test would still give a positive result, whether or not the second serum had an antibody corresponding to a factor on the red cells. Thus, a control for the indirect Coombs test is the performance of a direct Coombs test on the red cells used.

False positive results in the Coombs test may result also from improper preparation of the Coombs serum, especially failure to absorb completely the agglutinins against normal human red cells that are always present in normal rabbit serum. Excessive silica in the saline used for washing the red cells causes agglutination that may be mistaken for a positive result.

Weak or negative results in Coombs tests are regularly obtained in erythroblastosis fetalis due to anti-A or anti-B. Some Coombs serums are less likely to give negative results in these cases, but how such reagents differ from less effective reagents is not known.

## CROSS MATCHING

Even though bloods from donor and recipient have been properly tested and classified, it is still necessary to perform cross-matching tests between donor and recipient bloods. Cross matching carries with it grave responsibility because the life of the patient often depends on the accuracy of the work.

Although there is general agreement on the best techniques for ABO grouping and Rh typing, the choice of the best cross-matching procedures is subject to difference of opinion. The following procedure is recommended as one that will permit maximum reactivity of the most commonly found antibodies capable of causing hemolytic reactions.

PRINCIPLE. Cross-matching tests are designed to detect incompatibilities between the recipient's serum and the donor's red cells. This is called the major cross match. Tests for incompatibilities between the donor's serum and the recipient's red cells are called the minor cross match. Methods for both the major and minor cross-matching tests should be ones that demonstrate antigen-antibody reactions (agglutination) for saline-reactive antibodies of both the cold and warm type, for albumin-reactive antibodies, and for incomplete antibodies which can be shown only by agglutination with anti-human globulin serum (the Coombs test).

REAGENTS. (1) Clotted blood from both patient and donor separated into serum and clot and carefully labeled;

(2) Bovine albumin solution, 22 or 30 percent;

(3) Anti-human globulin serum (Coombs);

(4) Sodium chloride solution, 0.9 percent.

**Method.** 1. *Serum Cross Match (and Coombs Test)*. Two drops of serum from the patient is transferred to a small test tube. With wooden applicator sticks, small amounts of red cells from clotted donor blood are transferred to serum to make an approximate 2-percent suspension. The tube is centrifuged right away and investigated for agglutination. (All centrifugation should be carried out at 500–1000 rev/min for about 1 min.)

If no agglutination is visible, the tube is shaken and incubated at 37°C for 20 min to ½ hr, centrifuged, and investigated for agglutination.

If no agglutination is visible, the tube is filled with saline and the cells are washed 3 times with saline. The saline is discarded after the last washing and 2 drops of anti-human-globulin serum is added. After mixing, the tube is centrifuged and investigated for agglutination.

2. *Serum/Albumin Cross Match*. The serum-cell mixture is prepared as described for the serum cross match. Two drops of 22- or 30-percent bovine albumin is added to the tube. The tube is centrifuged right away and investigated for agglutination.

If no agglutination is visible, the tube is shaken and incubated at 37°C for 20 min to ½ hr, centrifuged, and investigated for agglutination.

The two cross matchings should preferably be carried out by two different technicians.

In blood-bank laboratories, where panels of red cells tested for the known blood-group antigens are available, the following screening test can be carried out. Two drops of patient's serum is mixed with 2 drops of a saline suspension of a pool of red cells from two or three bloods containing all the clinically important blood-group antigens. The tube is incubated for ½–1 hr at 37°C, and examined for agglutination. The tube is then filled with saline and the cells are washed three times with saline. The saline is discarded after the last washing and 2 drops of anti-human-globulin serum is added. After mixing, the tube is centrifuged and investigated for agglutination.

If this screening test is performed, the Coombs test part of the cross match may be eliminated except in cases where the presence of special antibodies indicates the performance of this test.

The minor cross match is considered of limited importance by many workers and is therefore optional. It can be carried out following the same principles as described for the major cross match.

INDICATIONS AND INTERPRETATIONS. The complete major cross match must be given negative results before the donor's blood can be considered safe for the recipient. Hemolysis has the same significance in indicating incompatibility as agglutination. If group O blood is being used for a group A or B recipient, the minor cross match can obviously not be expected to show compatibility.

Incompatibilities due to the important anti-A and anti-B antibodies will be detected in the serum cross match after direct centrifugation. Incubation or addition of albumin will weaken the reaction of these antibodies. The same is true of the majority of other specific blood-group antibodies of the cold variety. Most anti-Kell antibodies will also be detected in the serum cross match either after direct centrifugation or after incubation followed by centrifugation. Some anti-Kell antibodies and the majority of other antibodies such as anti-Fy$^a$, anti-Jk$^a$, and anti-S will be detected by the indirect Coombs test only. The serum/albumin test is a sensitive test for Rh antibodies. The direct centrifugation is carried out with the purpose of detecting Rh antibodies present in high titers and presenting the prozone phenomenon. The incubation followed by centrifugation will detect Rh antibodies present in low titers.

LIMITATION AND SOURCES OF ERROR. When agglutination is seen in a cross-match test, other donors must be tried and steps must be taken to identify the cause of agglutination. Nonspecific agglutination of the varieties described in the section on errors in ABO typing can create problems in cross matching. A first step in identifying the cause of trouble is to cross match the patient's serum with his own cells by the steps described above. Absence of autoagglutination by this test proves that the agglutination of donor bloods by recipient serum is due to one or more of the specific blood-group antibodies. It is very important to identify these specific serum antibodies in every case, and to type prospective donor cells for the corresponding antigens. Special techniques for studying and identifying these specific antibodies are beyond the scope of this book and are described elsewhere.[41] The use of a panel of fully typed red cells has already been mentioned.

Emergency cross matching is always a potential source of error and should be restricted to the situation where danger to the patient's life does not allow any delay. The first part (direct centrifugation) of the serum and the serum/albumin cross match can be used for emergency cross matchings. Incompatibilities due to anti-A, anti-B, the majority of anti-Kell, and high-titer Rh antibodies will be detected by this step. After the blood has been released for administration to the patient, the entire cross matching procedure is completed. If incompatibility is discovered by the additional tests, the transfusor is notified at once.

In conclusion, it should be emphasized that sensitization to all the described blood-group factors is possible. With an increasing number of blood transfusions, such sensitization even becomes probable. Consequently, it is necessary to decide whether the indications for a blood transfusion are sufficiently strong to justify exposure of the patient to blood that is not compatible for all blood-group antigens.

# REFERENCES

1. K. Landsteiner, "Uber Agglutinations Erscheinungen normalen menschlichen Blutes," *Wien. klin. Wschr. 14*, 1132 (1901).

2. P. Levine and R. S. Stetson, "An unusual case of intra-group agglutination," *J. Amer. med. Ass. 113*, 126 (1939).

3. K. Landsteiner and A. S. Wiener, "An agglutinable factor in human blood recognized by immune sera for rhesus blood," *Proc. Soc. exp. Biol. 43*, 223 (1940).

4. R. R. Race and Ruth Sanger, *Blood Groups in Man* (ed. 3; Blackwell Scientific Publications, Oxford, 1958).

5. F. H. Allen, Jr., and L. K. Diamond, *Erythroblastosis Fetalis* (Little, Brown, Boston, 1958).

6. W. C. Boyd, *Genetics and the Races of Man* (Little, Brown, Boston, 1950).

7. A. E. Mourant, *The Distribution of the Human Blood Groups* (Blackwell Scientific Publications, Oxford, 1954).

8. K. Landsteiner and J. Van der Scheer, "On the antigens of red blood corpuscles," *J. exp. Med. 41*, 427 (1925).

9. M. Grove-Rasmussen, "Characterization of erythrocytes for the purpose of transfusion," *Cyclopedia of Medicine, Surgery and Specialties* (Revision Service, S. A. Davis Co., 1914 Cherry St., Philadelphia 3, Pennsylvania, 1959), vol. 6, p. 279.

10. R. R. A. Coombs, A. E. Mourant, and R. R. Race, "A new test for the detection of weak and 'incomplete' Rh agglutinins," *Brit. J. exp. Path. 26*, 255 (1945).

11. R. R. A. Coombs, A. E. Mourant, and R. R. Race, "Detection of weak and 'incomplete' Rh agglutinins, a new test," *Lancet 2*, 15 (1945).

12. P. L. Mollison, *Blood Transfusion in Clinical Medicine* (Thomas, Springfield, 1951).

13. E. Witebsky, "Interrelationship between the Rh system and the AB system," *Blood*, Sp. Issue No. 2, 66 (1948).

14. M. Grove-Rasmussen, L. Soutter, and E. Marceau, "The use of group O donors as 'universal' donors. Dangers arising from the presence of 'immune' anti-A and anti-B in group O sera," *Proceedings, Fourth Annual Meeting of The American Association of Blood Banks* (1951), p. 27.

15. F. Stratton, "A new Rh allelomorph," *Nature 25*, 158 (1946).

16. A. S. Wiener, "Hemolytic reactions following transfusions of blood of the homologous group II," *Arch. Path. 32*, 227 (1941).

17. P. Levine, "The pathogenesis of fetal erythroblastosis," *N. Y. St. J. Med. 42*, 1928 (1942).

18. L. K. Diamond and R. L. Denton, "Rh agglutination in various media with particular reference to the value of albumin," *J. lab. clin. Med. 30*, 821 (1945).

19. K. Landsteiner and P. Levine, "A new agglutination factor differentiating individual human bloods," *Proc. Soc. exper. Biol. (N. Y.) 24*, 600 (1927).

20. K. Landsteiner and P. Levine, "Further observations on individual differences of human blood," *Proc. Soc. exper. Biol. (N. Y.) 24*, 941 (1927).

21. J. J. Walsh and C. Montgomery, "A new human isoagglutinin subdividing the MN blood groups," *Nature 160*, 504 (1947).

22. A. S. Wiener, L. J. Unger, and E. B. Gordon, "Fatal hemolytic transfusion

reaction caused by sensitization to a new blood factor U," *J. Amer. med. Ass. 153,* 1444 (1953).

23. T. J. Greenwalt, T. Sasaki, R. Sanger, J. Sneath, and R. R. Race, "An allele of the S(s) blood group genes," *Proc. Nat. acad. Sci. 40,* 1126 (1954).

24. P. Levine, O. B. Bobbitt, R. K. Waller, and A. Kuhmichel, "Isoimmunization by a new blood group factor in tumor cells," *Proc. Soc. exper. Biol. (N. Y.)* 77, 403 (1951).

25. R. Sanger, "An association between the P and Jay system of blood groups," *Nature 176,* 1163 (1955).

26. A. E. Mourant, "A new human blood group antigen of frequent occurrence," *Nature 158,* 237 (1946).

27. P. H. Andresen, "The blood group system L. A new blood group $L_2$," *Acta path. microbiol. scand. 25,* 728 (1948).

28. S. T. Callender and R. R. Race, "A serological and genetical study of multiple antibodies formed in response to blood transfusions by a patient with lupus erythematosis diffusus," *Ann. Eugen. (Lond.) 13,* 102 (1946).

29. M. Cutbush and I. Chanasin, "The expected blood group antibody anti-Lu[b]," *Nature 178,* 855 (1956).

30. F. H. Allen, Jr., S. J. Lewis, and H. Fudenberg, "Studies of anti-Kp[b], a new antibody in the Kell blood group system," *Vox Sang. (Basel)* 3, 1 (1958).

31. F. H. Allen, Jr., and S. J. Lewis, "Kp[a] (Penney), a new antigen in the Kell blood group system," *Vox Sang. (Basel)* 2, 81 (1957).

32. R. R. A. Coombs, A. E. Mourant, and R. R. Race, "In vivo isosensitization of red cells in babies with hemolytic disease," *Lancet 1,* 264 (1946).

33. P. Levine, M. Wigod, A. Backer, and R. Ponder, "A new human hereditary blood property (cellano) present in 99.8 per cent of all bloods," *Science 109,* 464 (1949).

34. M. Cutbush and P. L. Mollison, "The Duffy blood group," *Heredity 4,* 383 (1950).

35. E. W. Ikin, A. E. Mourant, H. J. Pettenkofer, and G. Blumenthal, "Discovery of the expected hemagglutinin, anti-Fy[a]," *Nature 168,* 1077 (1951).

36. R. Sanger, R. R. Race, and J. J. Jack, "The Duffy blood groups of New York Negroes. The pheno type Fy (a − b −)," *Brit. J. Haemat. 1,* 370 (1955).

37. F. H. Allen, Jr., L. K. Diamond, and B. Niedziela, "A new blood group antigen," *Nature 167,* 482 (1951).

38. G. Plant, E. W. Ikin, A. E. Mourant, R. Sanger, and R. R. Race, "A new blood group antibody, anti-Jk[b]," *Nature 171,* 431 (1953).

39. P. Levine, P. Vogel, E. M. Katzin, and L. Burnham, "Pathogenesis of erythroblastosis fetalis: statistical evidence," *Science 94,* 371 (1941).

40. F. H. Allen, Jr., and P. A. Tippett, "A new Rh blood type which reveals the Rh antigen G," *Vox Sang. (Basel)* 3, 321 (1958).

41. I. I. Dunsford and C. C. Bowley, *Techniques in Blood Grouping* (Oliver and Boyd, Edinburgh, 1955).

# Unit 16

# Proteins of Plasma and Serum

## Physiology

Though the present knowledge of plasma proteins and their relation to health and disease is appreciable, complete understanding of this field of physiology is in its infancy. The two major groups of plasma proteins, the albumins and the globulins, may be separated by means of their differing solubilities and their differential mobilities in an electric field. Each of these groups consists of an unknown number of proteins, the identity and functions of which can hardly be conjectured. By one or another technique, approximately a hundred different plasma proteins can be demonstrated. Of these, the physiologic role has been clearly demonstrated in only about a dozen. A great many empirical data have been accumulated, however, concerning the behavior of certain plasma proteins in pathologic states. For example, it is valuable to know that certain lipoproteins vary with the age and sex of the individual and with the state of the individual's health, even though the precise role and identity of the varying components are not known.

Plasma proteins have been classified in terms of three properties: solubility; mobility in an electric field; and the presence of specific nonprotein moieties. Each of these classifications stresses a different aspect of the protein's nature and the three classifications do not necessarily put the proteins in the same groups. By solubility studies, plasma proteins are separated into euglobulins, pseudoglobulins, and albumins. By electrophoresis, the same proteins are separated into alpha globulins, beta globulins, gamma globulin, and albumin. Classification by nonprotein moieties distinguishes lipoproteins, glycoproteins, mucoproteins, and phosphoproteins. There are globulins classified by solubility as euglobulins that may be alpha, beta, or gamma globulins in mobility. There are alpha and beta lipoproteins. There are euglobulin and pseudoglobulin components at each electrophoretic mobility of the globulins. There are alpha globulins that have the solubility of albumin.

There is no reason, at present, to believe that any one of these classifications is wholly preferable to another. Each has its preferred use. However, data obtained by each method can be compared only with other data similarly obtained. The best characterization, of course, applies all the classifying techniques to a single protein or group of proteins, resulting in the description, for instance, of beta$_1$-lipoprotein euglobulin. An excellent discussion of the plasma proteins in general has been provided by Hughes.[1]

## Clinical Laboratory Methods for Assessment of Plasma Proteins

### TOTAL PROTEIN

#### MICRO KJELDAHL METHOD

The total protein content of plasma is most accurately determined by the micro

Kjeldahl method. In this procedure, the protein is digested in an acid mixture and ammonia is evolved by addition of alkali to the digest. The ammonia nitrogen is measured by acidimetry or nesslerization. The nitrogen content multiplied by 6.25 gives the protein content of the sample. The factor 6.25 is the ratio of nitrogen to protein in albumin. Other plasma proteins have ratios both higher and lower than this, but they average not far from 6.25 in normal serums, although the ratio may vary appreciably in disease, as, for instance, in nephrosis when it may approach 6.7. It is nevertheless customary to use the value 6.25 arbitrarily for calculation of total plasma protein. The micro Kjeldahl procedure is a somewhat time-consuming process and requires appreciable technical skill. It is the method of reference for standardization of other methods. The procedure will not be described in detail. The total protein in normal subjects as measured by the micro Kjeldahl method ranges from 5.5 to 8.0 gm/100 ml, and averages 6.9 gm/100 ml.

THE QUANTITATIVE BIURET REACTION [2]

This test utilizes quantitative measurement of the color formation between copper and the peptide bonds of protein. Once the reagents have been prepared, performance of the test requires little time and provides a simple, direct measure of the total protein content of plasma. In contrast to the micro Kjeldahl method, the biuret reaction determines only the proteins and peptides of plasma and does not include the nonprotein nitrogenous components. The biuret test has two limitations: (i) the intensity of the color developed varies slightly from one protein to another, although it is reproducible for a given protein, and (ii) the presence of lipids may cause turbidity in the solutions and render accurate colorimetry impossible. Errors due to lipids may be avoided by prior extraction with a mixture of ethanol and di-

ethyl ether. Details of the method follow.

*Preparation of the biuret reagent.* To a solution of 30 gm of $CuSO_4.5H_2O$ in 300 ml of water, 150 ml of ethylene glycol is added, followed by 300 gm of NaOH in aqueous solution, and the whole mixture is transferred to a large Erlenmeyer flask, covered with a watch glass, and heated for 4 hr on a steam bath. The solution is filtered after cooling. The reagent should be stored in the dark.

*Procedure.* The concentration of protein in the solution to be analyzed should be 60–300 mg/100 ml; 1 ml of biuret reagent is added to 10 ml of this solution in a spectrophotometer cuvette. The mixture is allowed to stand for 20 min in the dark at room temperature (a covered water bath at 25°C is preferred) and the blue color is then read in the spectrophotometer at $550m\mu$ against a blank containing 10 ml of 0.15 M NaCl and 1 ml of biuret reagent.

If much lipid is present in the protein solution, the following procedure should be employed prior to color development. One or 2 ml of the solution to be analyzed, containing 6–30 mg of protein, is added drop by drop, with swirling, to 30 ml of alcohol-ether mixture (3:1 by volume) in a 50-ml tapered centrifuge tube. After heating to boiling and then cooling, the tube is centrifuged for 10 min and the supernatant is poured off. The extraction usually must be repeated a second time with fresh alcohol-ether. After the remaining traces of alcohol-ether have been driven off by placing the tube in a beaker of hot water, the residue is stirred with 10 ml of 0.15 M NaCl and the color is then developed by adding 1 ml of biuret reagent as before. Usually more than 2 hr is required to assure complete solution of the coagulum.

*Calculation of results.* The protein content is read from a standard curve prepared using known quantities of the protein under investigation. Duplicate determinations should agree within ± 2 percent. If the protein used for the standard curve has been analyzed by micro Kjeldahl digestion, the biuret determination can be standardized in terms of nitrogen as well as in terms of protein.

### SPECIFIC-GRAVITY METHOD

The determination of the specific gravity of plasma or serum in solutions of copper sulfate is rapid and inexpensive, and provides data that are quantitative although not highly accurate.[3, 4] One method is described below. There are also other valid techniques for the determination of the specific gravity of plasma.[5, 6]

A series of solutions of copper sulfate of known specific gravity is prepared to include the range expected in plasma or serum. Accurately prepared stock solutions or diluted solutions ready for use can be obtained commercially. The accuracy of the method depends upon the number of solutions used. For measuring the specific gravities within the plasma range, 1.015 to 1.035, 21 solutions graded at intervals of 0.001 are commonly used, corresponding to a total protein concentration of 2.8 to 10.5 gm/100 ml. This permits measurement of specific gravity with an accuracy of ± 0.004, corresponding to an error in protein content of less than ± 0.12 gm/100 ml. Care should be taken to keep the copper sulfate stock solutions covered at all times, since evaporation will increase the specific gravity of the solution and lead to error. A given standard may be used repeatedly until approximately 1/40 of its volume of blood plasma or serum has been added, that is, 100 ml of solution will serve for about 100 tests before the specific gravity is decreased by 0.0005. A duplicate standard can be prepared as a control by the addition of 1/40 of its volume of plasma, for comparison with the standards in use. The solutions in use can be renewed when the volume of precipitate equals that in the control bottle.

**Method.** A drop of plasma or serum to be tested is delivered from a height of about 1 cm into a selected solution of copper sulfate, from a medicine dropper or syringe needle. Small drops are preferable. The drop immediately becomes encased in a layer of copper proteinate that prevents any appreciable change in its specific gravity for a period of about 20 sec. The drop should penetrate 2 to 3 cm below the surface. Within 5 sec, the momentum of the fall is lost and the behavior of the drop is recorded within the next 5 to 10 sec. If the drop rises at any time, its specific gravity is less than that of the solution. If it continues steadily to fall, its specific gravity is greater. If it loses its momentum and remains suspended without falling or rising, the specific gravities are equal. The size of the drop need not be constant, since the rise or fall of the plasma depends only on its density relative to that of the solution. No temperature correction is necessary because the coefficients of expansion of the copper sulfate solution and of plasma very nearly coincide. Since convection currents in the solutions may introduce an error, the bottles containing the solution should be kept stationary and at reasonably constant temperature prior to and during the performance of the tests.

The probable extremes of the range of specific gravity of a serum can be tested and then the intermediate points tested. For example, one might find the following: 1.027+, 1.029+, 1.030−, 1.031−, where + or − indicates that the plasma has a specific gravity higher than 1.029 and lower than 1.030. By noting the relative rates of fall or rise in the two adjacent solutions, 1.029 and 1.030, an interpolation can be made. If the plasma were nearer 1.029 than 1.030, being less than 1.0295 and greater than 1.0290, it could be placed at 1.0292 or 1.0293 with an error not greater than ± 0.0002.

INTERPRETATIONS AND LIMITATIONS. When the specific gravity has been determined,

Serum or Plasma

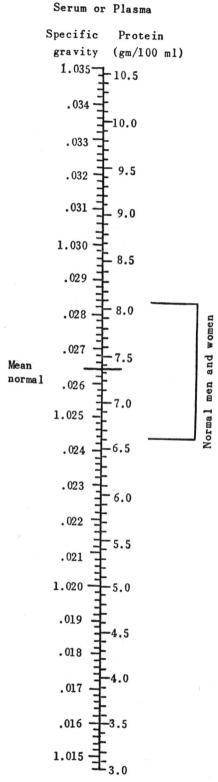

Fig. 25. Line chart for obtaining protein content of serum or plasma from its specific gravity.

the corresponding protein content can easily be read off from the line chart of Fig. 25. The line chart as reproduced has been corrected from the original publication.[4]

Attention must be paid to the anticoagulant used in collecting the sample. Heparin, 20 mg/100 ml, gives negligible errors. If oxalate is used, the specific gravity should be corrected by subtracting 0.0004 for each 100 mg of oxalate per 100 ml of blood. For the usual oxalate concentration of 200 mg/100 ml, .0008 should be subtracted. Sodium citrate or potassium oxalate alone should not be used, since they significantly alter the specific gravity of the plasma by causing a shift of fluid between cells and plasma. Serum has the advantage of requiring no anticoagulant. It is, however, devoid of one of the plasma proteins, fibrinogen.

## DETERMINATION OF TOTAL ALBUMIN AND TOTAL GLOBULIN

### SALTING-OUT TECHNIQUES

The relative amounts of total albumin and total globulin of the plasma have significance in certain clinical situations. These have most often been determined by the relatively simple salting-out techniques. For many years, the sodium sulfate system of Howe [7] was standard for this determination. With the advent of electrophoretic classification of the plasma proteins, this system came under criticism because the partition of proteins obtained did not correspond accurately to electrophoretic observations. The system was modified by Milne to provide closer adherence to the electrophoretic division of globulins from albumin. The Milne system [8] is undoubtedly the preferable one. Both systems are described below. They may both be simplified with satisfactory accuracy by substitution of the biuret for the micro Kjeldahl determination of the separated proteins. A third system involving phosphate buffers rather than sodium sulfate has been proposed by Derrien and Roche.[9] This system has the advantage of performance at a standard pH value. Derrien [10] has also described the separation of plasma into 34 components by the gradual addition of phosphate buffer under carefully defined conditions. This procedure has not received wide affirmation.

The primary problem of interpretation of data obtained by salting-out techniques stems from the fact that the degree of separation of albumins from globulins varies; pathologic serum may behave very differently from normal serum. Standardization of the particular system chosen can minimize but cannot overcome this obstacle. Primary dependence should be placed on the study of the standard and the unknown by precisely the same procedure. In order to obtain

the most reproducible and the most reliable results, the chosen technique should be performed under conditions of constant temperature, pH, and dilution. Moreover, for accurate work, the standard and the serum or plasma being measured must be prepared and handled in the same manner with respect to dilution (from the anticoagulant solution used, if any), the age of the sample (the solubility properties of some of the proteins change with time), and the method of preservation (freezing alters fibrinogen and the lipoproteins).

HOWE SODIUM SULFATE SYSTEM.[7] **Method.** Separation of plasma proteins into five fractions by the sodium sulfate system proposed by Howe is done according to the following scheme:

| Sample No. | Plasma (ml) | Reagent: 15 ml of— | *Final concentration of Reagent* (percent) | (molarity) | *Fractions precipitated* |
|---|---|---|---|---|---|
| 1 | 0.5 | 0.8-percent NaCl | — | — | — |
| 2 | .5 | 10.9-percent $Na_2SO_4.H_2O$ | 10.6 | 0.75 | Fibrinogen |
| 3 | .5 | 15.3-percent $Na_2SO_4.H_2O$ | 14.2 | 1.00 | Euglobulin, fibrinogen |
| 4 | .5 | 18.3-percent $Na_2SO_4.H_2O$ | 17.7 | 1.25 | Pseudoglobulin I, euglobulin, fibrinogen |
| 5 | .5 | 22.2-percent $Na_2SO_4.H_2O$ | 21.5 | 1.50 | Pseudoglobulin I, pseudoglobulin II, euglobulin, fibrinogen |
| 6 | .5 | 5.0-percent trichloracetic acid | — | — | Total protein |

All precipitations except Sample 6 are carried out at 37°C for 3 hr, this temperature being required for maintenance of the more concentrated sodium sulfate solutions. Precipitates may be removed by filtration or centrifugation.[11] The protein content of the filtrates is determined by the biuret reaction, or by micro Kjeldahl determination.

*Calculation of results.* If the micro Kjeldahl procedure is used to estimate

the amount of protein of a given fraction or filtrate, the values are in terms of protein nitrogen and are usually multiplied by 6.25 for conversion to protein values. If only total albumin and total globulin values are required, only Samples 1, 5, and 6 need be prepared. The concentration of the various protein fractions can be calculated by subtracting results of the determinations as follows:

| | |
|---|---|
| Sample 1 minus Sample 6 | Total protein (A) |
| Sample 5 minus Sample 6 | Albumin (B) |
| Sample 4 minus Sample 5 | Pseudoglobulin II |
| Sample 3 minus Sample 4 | Pseudoglobulin I |
| Sample 2 minus Sample 3 | Euglobulin |
| Sample 1 minus Sample 2 | Fibrinogen |
| Sample A minus Sample B | Total globulin |

MILNE SODIUM SULFATE METHOD.[8] This system varies from the Howe system in that sodium sulfate is used at a concentration of 19.6 percent for sample 4 and 26.8 percent for sample 5. The precipitate produced at 19.6 percent is believed to correspond to the beta and gamma globulins, whereas at 26.8 percent all the globulins are precipitated. The difference between the values at 26.8 percent and at 19.6 percent should thus correspond to alpha globulin. The calculations are otherwise similar to those for the Howe system.

### USE OF ORGANIC SOLVENTS

The most elaborate and carefully defined system for separation of plasma components from one another was published by Cohn and his co-workers in 1946.[12] The system involves serial reduction of the solubilities of groups of plasma proteins by manipulation of the pH, ionic strength, protein concentration, temperature, and ethanol content of the mixture. The method, which has come to be known as "cold-ethanol method 6," has become standard throughout the world for the large-scale preparation of plasma proteins. However, it is much too technical and costly for use in routine clinical studies. A description has recently been published of the fractions obtained by Method 6 and the characteristics of these fractions.[13]

A modification of the cold-ethanol system designed specifically for separation of albumin from globulin was proposed by Pillemer and Hutchinson.[14] It involves the use of methanol instead of ethanol and can be carried out simply in the laboratory if a cold bath (0° to 1°C)

is available. The separation of albumin from globulin that is achieved accords closely with the results of electrophoretic separation. The procedure is described below.

Lever and associates [15] have proposed a relatively simple modification of a cold-ethanol technique that makes possible a precise separation of beta lipoproteins from alpha lipoproteins and of beta glycoproteins from alpha glycoproteins. The system has been used to study the variations of these proteins under a variety of conditions.[16, 17]

METHANOL TECHNIQUE OF PILLEMER AND HUTCHINSON.[14] *Reagents. Methanol reagent:* 607 ml of methanol (C.P.) are added, with mixing, to 393 ml of distilled water. The mixture is cooled to 0°C and finally made up to 1 L with cold methanol.

*Acetate buffer:* 72 ml of 1 M acetic acid and 12 ml of 1 M NaOH are diluted to 1 L with distilled water.

**Method.** The serum and the reagents are maintained at 0° to 1°C in a small ice bath or by a low-temperature liquid bath. Two milliliters of serum is pipetted into a 15-ml conical centrifuge tube and 1.0 ml of acetate buffer is added with stirring. To this mixture, 7.0 ml of cold methanol reagent is added with stirring. After thorough mixing, the tube is allowed to stand for ½ hour at 0°C during which time the globulins will have precipitated, the albumins remaining in solution. The precipitate may be removed by centrifugation at 3000 rev/min, at 0° to 2°C, for 15 min, or by filtration. If filtration is used, the funnel should first be chilled. The actual filtration may be carried out at room temperature, provided sufficient filtrate for analysis is obtained in 5 to 7 min. Because of the rapid evaporation of methanol, samples should be taken for analysis promptly.

Nitrogen or biuret protein determinations are made on the filtrate and on the original serum sample. The albumin filtrates usually contain from 1.2 to 1.5 mg of nitrogen per milliliter of filtrate.

*Calculations.* 500 × mg N (or mg protein)/ml filtrate = gm albumin N (or gm of albumin)/100 ml of serum;

$$\frac{\text{gm albumin N (or gm albumin)/100 ml}}{\text{gm total N (or gm total protein)/100 ml}} = \text{percent albumin};$$

gm total N (or gm total protein)/100 ml serum − gm of albumin N (or gm of albumin)/100 ml serum = gm of globulin N (or gm of globulin)/100 ml.

It should be noted that in this system there is no correction for NPN. The nitrogen value obtained for albumin, if the micro Kjeldahl technique is used, is thus really albumin N + NPN. The biuret technique, which does not measure NPN, will yield less distortion of the albumin figure.

### OTHER TECHNIQUES

A procedure of promise is suggested by Peters's observation [18] that albumin can be extracted by ethanol from the trichloroacetic precipitate of an albumin-antialbumin complex. At 71-percent ethanol concentration, pH 2.4, 0.4 percent protein, from 88 to 92 percent of the albumin with a purity of 82–97 percent was extracted from the trichloro-acetic-precipitated proteins. It is to be hoped that further work will demonstrate that as good a separation of albumin can be had under similar circumstances from the total trichloroacetic-precipitated plasma proteins.

Another simple technique has been described for the estimation of total globulins. It is based [19] on the observation that addition of formaldehyde to solutions of serum albumin does not affect the viscosity of the mixture. With mixtures of whole serum and formaldehyde, the viscosity was found to be related to the content of the globulins. The method may be used to detect major changes in globulin concentration.

### DETERMINATION OF INDIVIDUAL PROTEINS OR GROUPS OF PROTEINS

Classification of the plasma proteins on the basis of their motion in an electric field has provided a division of the proteins into seven distinguishable groups, namely, fibrinogen, gamma globulin, $beta_1$ and $beta_2$ globulins, $alpha_1$ and $alpha_2$ globulins and albumins. This classification on the basis of electrophoretic mobility presents certain distinct advantages over earlier groupings and is at present the most commonly used system. A disadvantage of this system is that, with the probable exception of fibrinogen, each of the mobilities is common to a group of proteins.

As knowledge of the plasma proteins develops, definable and measurable characteristics of certain of them have provided a means for the measurement of the specific protein. This is obviously to be preferred when it is possible and this is the direction in which the ultimate consideration of the plasma proteins is to be sought.

### ELECTROPHORESIS

The separations of proteins according to mobility that are obtained by the moving-boundary electrophoresis techniques stemming from the original work of Tiselius [20] are undoubtedly the most satisfactory electrophoretic measurements available. The theory and practice of these techniques are discussed authoritively by Longsworth.[21]

There are even here, however, anomalies of interpretation that can distort the true picture of the quantitative relations between the plasma proteins. The primary anomaly arises from the influence of the lipid portion of the lipoproteins on the refractive index of the proteins. It has been reported by Ott and his collaborators [22] that the principal distortion occurs with the beta$_1$ lipoprotein and lesser distortions occur in the alpha$_1$ and alpha$_2$ globulin.

The development of techniques for electrophoresis with the protein placed in a structured background, such as paper or starch, has provided a simpler means of separating plasma components. These methods are satisfactory for clinical use, provided the pitfalls in the performance of the test and interpretation of results are understood.

Many varieties of apparatus for the carrying out of paper electrophoresis may be purchased. The most popular types are based on the suggestions of Durrum.[23] If cost is a major factor, a satisfactory apparatus can be constructed in any laboratory. Temperature of electrophoresis, time of electrophoresis, choice of a buffer, choice of paper, care in drying of the strips after completion of the run, and the state of the serum or plasma sample being examined all have an influence on the data obtained. These variables should all be standardized.

After completion of the electrophoresis and the drying of the paper strip, the proteins may be made visible by the application of any of a variety of protein dyes. The bands of stained protein may then be separated by cutting them out and the dye removed from the paper by elution. The eluted dye can then be estimated spectrophotometrically or colorimetrically. The ratios of the separated protein components to one another may differ when measured in this way from values obtained by moving-boundary electrophoresis. This is due to differences in the adsorption of the dye by the various plasma proteins, the highest adsorption being that of albumin. When measured by this method, the albumin of plasma may be found to present 65–80 percent of the total normal plasma

protein rather than the customary 55 percent. Amido black 10B and bromphenol blue are two commonly used dyes. Amido black 10B has been estimated by various authors to combine with albumin from 1.4 to 2.2 times its combination with globulins. Differences of dye combination among the various globulins have not been investigated.

Instruments are available for translating the color intensity of the stained protein on the uneluted paper strip into a series of curves. Such an instrument can be calibrated arbitrarily to make the curves obtained with normal plasma comparable in their relative proportions to those obtained by the moving-boundary technique. This is probably the preferable type of calibration. The instruments can also be calibrated to describe curves corresponding directly to the amount of dye bound by the band. This gives data comparable to those obtained by elution of the dye and is subject to the same criticism mentioned above for the elution techniques.

PAPER-STRIP ELECTROPHORESIS. Many varieties of buffers, papers, and stains have been suggested for carrying out the electrophoretic separation of proteins in a paper strip. Some conditions will be preferred in one laboratory and other conditions in another. Any suggestions as to desirable procedures must, to a large degree, express the personal preference of the user and should by no means be taken to exclude the possible excellence of other methods. Details of the assembly and operation of an apparatus for performance of paper electrophoresis are beyond the scope of this presentation. Reference should be made to one of the excellent manuals available [24–27] or to the operating manual received with the instrument. A very recent and excellent discussion is that of Wunderley.[28]

*Preparation of buffer.* A satisfactory buffer that is often used for paper electrophoresis of plasma is a veronal buffer, pH 8.6, 0.075 ionic strength. It can be prepared by dissolving 2.76 gm of diethyl barbituric acid and 15.40 gm of sodium diethyl barbiturate in 1 L of distilled water.

*Technique.* Satisfactory separation and definition of components is obtained by using 0.01 ml of serum or plasma and 3-mm Whatman paper strips. The power supply of the instrument should be maintained constant and a voltage regulator is usually essential. The voltage used should result in a current of 5 milliamperes, and it should be maintained for a period of 16 hr. The usual cell is so constructed that at least 8 strips can be run simultaneously. The time can, of course, be reduced by increasing the current.

Immediately following completion of the run, the strips should be dried for 30 min in an oven preheated to 120° to 130°C. It is important that the temperature throughout the oven be reasonably uniform to obtain proper drying.

*Staining of Plasma Protein Components.* For the staining of the protein bands, a solution containing 0.01 percent by weight of bromphenol blue and 3.1 percent by weight of $ZnSO_4 \cdot H_2O$ may be used. The dry mixture is dissolved in 50 ml of 95-percent ethanol and made to a volume of 1 L with 5-percent aqueous acetic acid. The strips are immersed in this dye solution for 6 hr at room temperature. They are then rinsed twice, for 6 min each time, in a solution of 5 percent by volume of glacial acetic acid (USP) or in water. This is followed by a 6-min rinse in 0.9-percent aqueous solution of sodium acetate ($1 \ H_2O$). The dyed and rinsed strips are blotted and returned to the oven at 120° to 130°C for 15 min. For the staining of the lipids and lipoproteins of plasma, a solution of Sudan black may be used in a manner similar to that described for bromphenol blue.[29] Polysaccharides may be stained with basic fuchsin.[30]

*Quantitation by Elution of Dye.* If the separated protein components are to be analyzed by spectrophotometry or colorimetry of the eluted dye, the lightest regions between bands are cut through. A section of relatively unstained paper beyond the protein pattern and of a width comparable to that of the stained section is also cut out to be used as a blank. Each segment is eluted by gentle agitation in an accurately measured volume of 0.5-percent anhydrous sodium carbonate in water. A volume should be chosen to provide a solution whose optical density may be accurately read. One must be certain that any paper fibers in the eluate have settled before measuring the optical density. A calibration curve for the colorimeter or spectrophotometer to be used must be made, using known concentrations of bromphenol blue in 0.5-percent sodium carbonate. The dye values are read at 590 m$\mu$ (or with an orange filter). The standards are read against 0.5-percent sodium carbonate solution, but the samples are read against the eluate obtained from the paper strip cut as a blank. The readings are converted to concentrations by means of the calibration curve. The concentration, in each measurement, is multiplied by the volume of the eluate to obtain the amount of bromphenol blue eluted from each segment. The amount of bromphenol blue bound by each component divided by the total dye bound (the sum of the dye bound by each component) gives the fraction of total dye bound by each component. This figure provides a measure of the distribution of the protein components of the serum or plasma but is subject to the limitation that different plasma proteins adsorb the dye with different avidities.

INTERPRETATIONS AND LIMITATIONS. Paper-strip electrophoresis, if carefully controlled, can yield accuracy of determination within 3 to 5 percent for any given electrophoretic component, and major shifts in concentration of components are readily detected. Accurate comparison of data is possible, however, only if freshly collected serum or plasma is used. This is not always feasible inasmuch as time and apparatus may not be available at the time of collection of the sample. If a delay of hours or days is unavoidable, samples should be stored in the liquid state at 0° to 2°C. Storage in the frozen state, although necessary if several days are to elapse, produces changes in several of the plasma proteins that affect their migration in the paper strip and alter the delicacy with which the interpretation of changes of concentration can be made.

A particularly advantageous attribute of the paper-strip technique is that several strips can be prepared, one of which may be stained with a protein stain, one with a lipid stain, and one with a carbohydrate stain. By this technique, it is possible to observe changes not only in proteins of a given mobility but in lipoproteins, glycoproteins, and mucoproteins within the mobility groups.

Careful paper-strip electrophoresis permits the differentiation of the following groups of proteins, listed in the order of their decreasing mobility: albumin, alpha$_1$ globulin, alpha$_2$ globulin, beta$_1$ globulin, beta$_2$ globulin, fibrinogen, gamma globulin.

STARCH ELECTROPHORESIS. Smithies [31] in 1955 described a method of zone electrophoresis using potato-starch gel as the supporting medium. A higher resolution of plasma protein fractions was obtained than by other methods of electrophoresis. The technique is of great promise, although reproducibility has been poor because of lack of standardization. A recent effort to supply such standardization is worthy of note.[32] A major application of starch electrophoresis has been the demonstration of different genetic groups of haptoglobins in normal human serum.[31, 33]

## IMMUNOELECTROPHORESIS AND OTHER IMMUNOCHEMICAL TECHNIQUES

The use of a structured base for the demonstration of individual antigen-antibody reactions was proposed by Oudin in 1946.[34] Oudin prepared gelatin tubes containing antibody. The antigens, applied in excess, diffuse into the gelatin, each antigen-antibody species forming a discrete ring or zone of precipitation. Ouchterlony [35] modified this technique by placing antigen and antibody in separate wells cut in an agar plate. As antigen and antibody diffuse into the agar, a line of precipitation forms at the juncture of their meeting. A separate line is formed for each antigen and its specific antibody.

A further refinement of these techniques, immunoelectrophoresis, arose [36] in which the antigen is first submitted to electrophoresis in a transparent gel, usually agar. The individual protein species are thus distributed in the gel. Antiserum is poured into elongated troughs made in the gel parallel to the axis of migration. When antibodies and antigens meet in suitable proportions, arcs of specific precipitation become evident.

The immunologic techniques are capable of great resolution of protein species. They are, however, subject to the serious limitation of employing a reagent, antiserum, of great variability. Few plasma proteins have been sufficiently purified to serve as specific antigens producing but a single antibody. Moreover, individual animal response to even a highly purified antigen may produce antiserums of greatly varying characteristics. The subject has been well reviewed by Grabar.[36, 37]

## CERULOPLASMIN

A blue-green copper-containing alpha globulin, ceruloplasmin,[38] which has the properties of an oxidative enzyme, can be estimated either by its characteristic light absorption at 610 m$\mu$ or by measurement of its ability to oxidize paraphenylenediamine dihydrochloride. Details of both procedures are described by Scheinberg and Morell [39] and should be consulted if the procedures are to be performed adequately.

### TRANSFERRIN

Another metal-bearing protein, beta$_1$ metal-combining protein, or transferrin, has properties that permit its direct estimation.[40] The primary function of this protein is the transport of iron in the plasma. Its estimation depends on the color formed as the protein becomes saturated with iron. The technical problems of the determination are sufficient that the original reference [40] should be consulted.

### Clinical Significance of Variations in Proteins of Blood Plasma or Serum

In general, the several components of plasma appear to vary independently and widely in disease. Only the major and well-established variations will be considered here, both because these are the most valuable for clinical assessment and because the true significance of the many reports of minor variations of plasma proteins in specific syndromes are difficult to evaluate until confirmed by repeated observation. Authoritative discussion of many aspects of variation in plasma proteins is provided in *The Plasma Proteins,* edited by Putnam.[41]

### PHYSIOLOGIC VARIATIONS IN SERUM PROTEIN CONCENTRATION

In the first 2 years of life, the distribution of the plasma proteins (as measured by electrophoresis) differs somewhat from the normal distribution of later life. As the antibody received from maternal sources disappears in 1 to 4 months, a decrease in the relative amount of gamma globulin is noted in the plasma. There-

after, the gamma globulin increases gradually to reach an adult normal relative value by the end of the first year. Alpha and beta globulins are relatively elevated in the newborn and approach adult values at the end of the second year.[42, 43] In old age, available data suggest a somewhat lower value for total protein than for the earlier years. The albumin tends to be relatively lower, and the globulin concomitantly higher than during the vigorous years.

Total protein may be elevated with essentially normal distribution of the various individual proteins due to dehydration. This may result from insufficient water intake or from an abnormal water loss from vomiting, diarrhea, hyperthermia, shock, diuresis, or burns. In burns, although hemoconcentration is often seen, it is equally likely that the relative albumin content of the plasma may drop.

### HYPOGAMMAGLOBULINEMIA

A deficiency in the synthesis of gamma globulin is usually manifested clinically by recurring severe bacterial infections.

*Congenital agammaglobulinemia* is a hereditary disorder occurring predominantly in males, and apparently transmitted as a sex-linked recessive characteristic. The deficiency in plasma gamma globulin is due to an almost total failure to synthesize gamma globulins or to respond to antigenic stimulation by forming antibodies. There is an associated paucity of the cells involved in the formation of these proteins. Thus plasma cells are absent, and lymphoid tissues are generally deficient. Most patients with congenital agammaglobulinemia have gamma globulin concentrations of less than 50 mg/100 ml, and some have no detectable circulating gamma globulin.[44] Electrophoresis of serum proteins usually demonstrates the deficiency in gamma globulin, although immunochemical measurement is more reliable. There is usually a low or absent titer of isohemagglutinins.

*Acquired agammaglobulinemia* clinically resembles the congenital form, except for its appearance later in life and its equal sex distribution. It may result from granulomatous disease involving lymphoid tissues. It also occurs in association with thymoma or in the absence of any recognizable cause. The defect in gamma globulin synthesis is usually less severe in the acquired than in the congenital form.

*Transient hypogammaglobulinemia* may occur during infancy if there is a delay in development of the ability to synthesize gamma globulin after the decay of antibodies acquired by placental transfer during the latter months of pregnancy. Low gamma globulin, together with increased beta globulin, is found in dystrophia myotonica.

### NEPHROTIC SYNDROME

The nephrotic syndrome, with the cardinal signs of proteinuria, hypoproteinemia, hyperlipemia, and edema, occurs in a wide variety of conditions that have in common a rapid urinary loss of protein due to increased glomerular permeability. In many instances, especially in children, hypoproteinemia is due as much to an increased rate of protein catabolism as to the urinary loss of protein. The hyperlipemia in this syndrome is due chiefly to an increase in the plasma concentration of low-density beta lipoproteins. The serum concentrations of albumin and gamma globulin are reduced, and, as seen in paper electrophoresis, alpha$_2$ and beta globulins are elevated. Electrophoretic characteristics of the urinary proteins are discussed in Unit 19.

### SERUM PROTEIN CHANGES IN LIVER DISEASE

Chronic liver disease is usually associated with a reduced serum concentration of albumin and an increase in gamma globulin. The increased globulin concentration is due to an increase in synthesis and is correlated with an in-

crease in plasma cells in the bone marrow. The highest increases occur in postnecrotic and "lupoid" cirrhosis. Moderate increases occur in acute hepatitis, and small increases may be seen in obstructive jaundice. A deficiency in fibrinogen and other proteins involved in coagulation may occur in severe liver disease. (See Units 14 and 24.)

### HYPOALBUMINEMIA

In addition to nephrotic syndrome and chronic liver disease, a decreased albumin concentration is seen in a variety of other conditions. Nutritional deficiency or protein starvation results in hypoalbuminemia. Globulins are usually not diminished and may be increased. A similar pattern is seen in widespread carcinoma, sprue, and many other chronic wasting diseases. Hypoalbuminemia due to an increased rate of protein catabolism may occur in diseases of the gastrointestinal tract, notably in hypertrophic gastritis and ulcerative colitis. It may also occur in the absence of any recognizable cause. Acute infections may cause moderate reduction in serum albumin.

### HYPERGAMMAGLOBULINEMIA

The wide variety of conditions which may cause hyperglobulinemia, with a predominant increase in gamma globulin, are summarized in Table 52 from Gross, Gitlin, and Janeway.[45] The most marked increases are seen in chronic granulomatous infections of long duration. The rise in gamma globulin in these conditions represents both specific antibodies and nonspecific gamma globulin. Chronic bacterial infections may be associated with increases in beta globulin, gamma globulin, or both.

### MULTIPLE MYELOMA

Hyperglobulinemia is present in approximately two-thirds of patients with multiple myeloma. In a somewhat larger fraction, electrophoresis of serum dem-

Table 52. *Conditions in which hypergammaglobulinemia has been noted.*[45]

I. Infections
  A. Bacterial
    1. Streptococcal, especially in subacute bacterial endocarditis, rheumatic fever and acute glomerulonephritis
    2. Severe staphylococcal infections
    3. Advanced tuberculosis, pulmonary and extrapulmonary
    4. Lepromatous leprosy
  B. Spirochetal
    1. Syphilis (all three stages)
  C. Viral
    1. Lymphogranuloma venereum [a]
    2. Infectious mononucleosis
    3. Psittacosis
  D. Rickettsial
    1. Typhus
  E. Fungal
    1. Histoplasmosis
  F. Protozoal
    1. Kala-azar [a]
    2. American mucocutaneous leishmaniasis
    3. Malaria
  G. Helminthic
    1. Visceral larva migrans (toxicara canis or catis) [a]
    2. Trichinosis
  H. Chronic infection [a] of nonspecific etiology

II. Hyperimmunization [a]

III. Liver Disease
  A. Portal cirrhosis [a]
    1. Laënnec's cirrhosis
    2. Postnecrotic cirrhosis
  B. Acute viral hepatitis
  C. Toxic hepatitis (such as that from arsenic)
  D. Chronic liver disease in young women with extreme hypergammaglobulinemia ("lupoid hepatitis") [a]
  E. Cholangiolitic hepatitis
  F. Biliary cirrhosis (late)

IV. Severe Malnutrition
  A. Kwashiorkor
  B. Nutritional-recovery syndrome [a]

V. Neoplasms
  A. Multiple myeloma [a]
  B. Leukemia (monocytic, chronic myelogenous and chronic lymphatic)
  C. Lymphomas
    1. Hodgkin's disease
    2. Lymphosarcoma
    3. Reticulum-cell sarcoma
  D. Primary carcinoma and sarcoma, with or without metastases

VI. Paraproteinemias and Dysproteinemias
  A. Macroglobulinemia [a]
  B. Cryoglobulinemia [a]
  C. Benign hyperglobulinemic purpura [a]
  D. Amyloidosis

VII. Diseases Possibly Associated with Hypersensitivity
  A. Connective-tissue diseases ("collagen" diseases)
    1. Disseminated lupus erythematosus [a]
    2. Scleroderma [a]
    3. Rheumatic fever
    4. Rheumatoid arthritis
    5. Ankylosing spondylitis
    6. Periarteritis nodosa
    7. Sjögren's syndrome
  B. Others
    1. Serum sickness
    2. Acquired immune hemolytic anemia
    3. Autoimmune thyroiditis; Hashimoto's disease
    4. Erythema nodosum

VIII. Granulomas
  A. Sarcoidosis [a]
  B. Chronic beryllium poisoning

IX. Dermatologic Disorders
  A. Pemphigus vulgaris (late)
  B. Extensive dermatitis (such as exfoliative dermatitis)
  C. Burns

[a] Often associated with striking elevations of gamma-globulin fraction.

onstrates an abnormal globulin component. This may appear with any of the globulins from alpha to gamma$_2$, but is most commonly seen in the gamma$_2$ position. This "myeloma protein" shows a high degree of homogeneity and appears discrete and sharply outlined when seen in paper electrophoresis. The myeloma proteins differ among different patients, and the proteins that appear in serum are a separate species from the Bence-Jones proteins that may appear in the urine (see Unit 19). Similar serum globulins occasionally occur in certain lymphomatous diseases.

### MACROGLOBULINEMIAS

The macroglobulins consist of proteins with a molecular weight in excess of 1,000,000, and a sedimentation constant of 20 or more. Normally, these comprise 3 to 5 percent of the total serum proteins. In Waldenström's macroglobulinemia, these proteins comprise 20 percent or more of total proteins.[46] Definitive diagnosis of this disease can be made only by ultracentrifuge analysis of serum. The solubility of macroglobulins in electrolyte solutions and their precipitation by dilution forms the basis of a simple test by which large quantities of macroglobulins can often be demonstrated. A rapid erythrocyte sedimentation rate and demonstration of high serum viscosity also suggest the diagnosis.

WATER-DILUTION TEST FOR MACROGLOBU-LINEMIA (SIA TEST). Into a test tube filled with distilled water, 1 drop of serum is allowed to drop from a pipette. Normally, this disperses and either becomes invisible or produces a slight haziness. When macroglobulins are present in high concentrations, a heavy precipitate forms and drops to the bottom of the tube. This protein is collected by centrifugation, redissolved in 0.85-percent sodium chloride solution, and again reprecipitated by addition of distilled water to confirm its identity as macroglobulin.

INTERPRETATIONS AND LIMITATIONS. When positive, the test strongly suggests, but does not prove, the presence of macroglobulins, since false positive reactions can occur. It is usually negative when small or moderate amounts of macroglobulin are present, and is not consistently positive even in the presence of large quantities of macroglobulin.

### CRYOGLOBULINEMIA

Cryoglobulins are a group of proteins that precipitate from cooled serum and redissolve on warming. Cryoglobulinemia most commonly occurs in patients with multiple myeloma, but may occur in a wide variety of other conditions, or by itself. Cryoglobulins may be detected by any of a variety of tests based on the effects of temperature on their solubility. A simple and useful test is to determine the erythrocyte sedimentation rate at 37.5°C and at 10°C. In the cold, red cells do not sediment at all, owing to precipitation and gel formation by cryoglobulins, whereas, when warmed to 37.5°C, the sedimentation rate is usually abnormally rapid. This response is the reverse of that seen with cold agglutinins.

### REFERENCES

1. W. L. Hughes, Jr., Chap. 21, in H. Neurath and K. Bailey, eds., *Proteins: Chemistry, Biological Activity, and Methods* (Academic Press, New York, 1954), vol. IIB.
2. J. W. Mehl, "The biuret reaction of proteins in the presence of ethylene glycol," *J. biol. Chem.* 157, 173 (1945).
3. R. A. Phillips, D. D. Van Slyke, V. P. Dole, K. Emerson, Jr., P. B. Hamilton, and R. M. Archibald, *Copper-Sulfate Method for Measuring Specific Gravities of Whole Blood and Plasma* (United States Navy Research Unit at the Hospital of the Rockefeller Institute for Medical Research, 1943–1944; republished by the Josiah Macy Foundation, New York, 1945).
4. P. B. Hawk, B. L. Oser, and W. H. Summerson, *Practical Physiological Chemistry* (ed. 12; Blakiston, Philadelphia, 1947), pp. 546–556.
5. B. M. Kagan, "A simple method for the estimation of total protein content of plasma and serum. I. A falling-drop method for the determination of specific gravity," *J. clin. Invest.* 17, 369 (1938).
6. O. H. Lowry and T. M. Hunter, "The determination of serum protein concentration with a gradient tube," *J. biol. Chem.* 129, 465 (1945).
7. P. E. Howe, "The use of sodium sulfate as the globulin precipitant in the

determination of proteins of the blood," *J. biol. Chem. 49,* 93 (1921); *57,* 235–241 (1923).

8. J. Milne, "Serum protein fractionation: comparison of sodium sulfate precipitation and electrophoresis," *J. biol. Chem. 169,* 595 (1947).

9. Y. Derrien and J. Roche, *C. R. Soc. Biol. (Paris) 142,* 1042 (1948).

10. Y. Derrien, *C. R. Soc. Biol. (Paris) 139,* 909 (1945).

11. G. R. Kingsley, "A rapid method for the separation of serum albumin and globulin," *J. biol. Chem. 133,* 731 (1940).

12. E. J. Cohn, L. E. Strong, W. L. Hughes, Jr., D. J. Mulford, J. N. Ashworth, M. Melin, and H. L. Taylor, "Preparation and properties of serum and plasma proteins. IV. A system for the separation into fractions of the proteins and lipoprotein components of biological tissues and fluids," *J. Amer. chem. Soc. 68,* 459 (1946).

13. R. B. Pennell, "Separation of plasma proteins by precipitation methods," in F. Putnam, ed., *Plasma Proteins* (Academic Press, New York, 1959).

14. L. Pillemer and M. D. Hutchinson, "The determination of the albumin and globulin contents of human serum by methanol precipitation," *J. biol. Chem. 158,* 299 (1945).

15. W. F. Lever, F. R. N. Gurd, E. Uroma, R. K. Brown, B. A. Barnes, L. Schmid, and E. Schultz, "Chemical, clinical and immunological studies on the products of human plasma fractionation. XL. Quantitative separation and determination of the protein components in small amounts of normal human plasma," *J. clin. Invest. 30,* 99 (1951).

16. W. F. Lever and N. Hurley, "The plasma glycoproteins and lipoproteins," in J. L. Tullis, ed., *Blood Cells and Plasma Proteins* (Academic Press, New York, 1953).

17. D. P. Barr, E. M. Russ, and H. A. Eder, "Protein lipid relationships in plasma," in J. L. Tullis, ed., *Blood Cells and Plasma Proteins* (Academic Press, New York, 1953).

18. T. Peters, Jr., "The isolation of serum albumin from specific precipitates of serum albumin and its rabbit antibodies," *J. Amer. chem. Soc. 80,* 2700 (1958).

19. S. Foster and F. Biguria, "Estimation of serum globulin by measurement of viscosity of formalin-treated serum," *J. lab. clin. Med. 28,* 1634 (1943).

20. A. Tiselius, *Nova Acta Reg. Sci., Upsala* (IV) 7, 4, (1930); *Trans. Far. Soc. 33,* 524 (1937).

21. L. G. Longsworth, "Moving boundary electrophoresis-theory" and "Moving boundary electrophoresis-practice," chaps. 3 and 4 in M. Bier, ed., *Electrophoresis* (Academic Press, New York, 1959).

22. H. Ott, H. Huber, and G. Körver, "Comparison of the electrophoresis methods of Tiselius, Antweiler and Turba," *Klin. Wochschr. 30,* 34 (1952).

23. E. L. Durrum, "A microelectrophoretic and microionophoretic technique," *J. Amer. chem. Soc. 72,* 2943 (1950).

24. R. J. Block, E. L. Durrum, and G. Zweig, *A Manual of Paper Chromotography and Paper Electrophoresis* (Academic Press, New York, 1955).

25. M. Lederer, *An Introduction to Paper Electrophoresis and Related Methods* (Elsevier, Amsterdam, London, New York, 1955).

26. H. J. McDonald, *Ionography-Electrophoresis in Stabilized Media* (Year Book, Chicago, 1955).

27. G. E. W. Wolstenholme and E. C. P. Miller, eds., *Paper Electrophoresis* (Ciba Foundation Symposium; Little, Brown, Boston, 1956).

28. C. Wunderly, "Paper electrophoresis," chap. 5 in M. Bier, ed., *Electrophoresis* (Academic Press, New York, 1959).

29. B. Swahn, "Localization and determination of serum lipids after electrophoretic separation on filter paper," *Scand. J. clin. Lab. Invest. 4,* 98 (1952). "Blood Lipids," *ibid. 5,* Supplement 9, 5 (1953).

30. E. Köiv and A. Grönwall, "Staining of serum-bound carbohydrates after electrophoresis of serum on filter paper," *Scand. J. clin. Lab. Invest. 4,* 244 (1952).

31. O. Smithies, "Zone electrophoresis in starch gels: group variations in the serum proteins of normal human adults," *Biochem. J. 61,* 629 (1955).

32. J. H. Pert, R. E. Engle, Jr., K. R. Woods, and M. H. Sleisenger, "Preliminary studies on quantitative zone electrophoresis in starch gel," *J. lab. clin. Med. 54,* 572 (1959).

33. O. Smithies and N. F. Walker, "Notation for serum-protein groups and the genes controlling their inheritance," *Nature 178,* 694 (1956).

34. J. Oudin, "Method of immunochemical analysis by specific precipitation in gelled medium," *C. R. Acad. Sci. (Paris) 222,* 115 (1946).

35. O. Ouchterlony, "Antigen-antibody reactions in gels," *Acta path. microbiol. scand. 26,* 507 (1949).

36. P. Grabar and C. A. Williams, "Immuno-electrophoretic analysis of mixtures of antigenic substances," *Biochim. biophys. Acta 17,* 67 (1955).

37. P. Grabar, "Immunochemical Methods in Studies on Proteins," in C. G. Anfinsen, Jr., M. L. Anson, K. Bailey, and J. T. Edsall, eds., *Advances in Protein Chemistry,* vol. 13 (Academic Press, New York, 1958).

38. C. G. Holmberg and C. G. Laurell, "Investigations in serum copper. II. Isolation of a copper-containing protein and a description of some of its properties," *Act. chem. scand. 2,* 550 (1948).

39. I. H. Scheinberg and A. G. Morell, "Exchange of ceruloplasmin copper with ionic $Cu^{64}$ with reference to Wilson's disease," *J. clin. Invest. 36,* 1193 (1957).

40. C. E. Rath and C. A. Finch, "Chemical, clinical and immunological studies on the products of human plasma fractionation. XXXVIII. Serum iron transport. Measurement of iron-binding capacity of serum in man," *J. clin. Invest. 28,* 79 (1949).

41. F. W. Putnam, ed., *The Plasma Proteins* (Academic Press, New York, 1960).

42. J. Gras, "Normal proteinogram, physiological variation and mechanism of regulation," in *Proteinas Plasmaticas* (Editorial JIMS, Barcelona, 1956), chap. 4.

43. R. Caspani, M. Negri, and C. Sticca, "L'elettroforesi su carta delle sieroproteine; osservazione nel bambino sano con particulare riguardo all'eta del lattante," *Minerva pediat. (Torino) 5,* 198 (1953).

44. C. A. Janeway, "Hypogammaglobulinemia and agammaglobulinemia," in *Les Gamma-Globulines et la Médecine des Enfants* (Masson, Paris, 1955), p. 201.

45. P. A. M. Gross, D. Gitlin, and C. A. Janeway, "The gamma globulins and their clinical significance. III. Hypergammaglobulinemia," *New Engl. J. Med. 260,* 122 (1959).

46. J. Waldenstrom, "Abnormal proteins in myeloma," *Advance. Intern. Med. 5,* 298 (1952).

# Unit 17

# Laboratory Evaluation of Inflammation and Necrosis

A wide variety of tests have been designed for the purpose of detecting abnormalities in the blood associated with inflammatory and necrotic processes in tissues. The most widely used and most generally useful of these tests is the determination of the erythrocyte sedimentation rate. A number of other tests also give abnormal results following acute or chronic inflammatory processes, and together with the erythrocyte sedimentation rate constitute the so-called acute-phase reactants. Among these are the determination of C-reactive protein, serum hexosamine, serum mucoprotein, and serum nonglucosamine polysaccharides. Other tests, such as serum glutamic oxaloacetic transaminase (SGOT) are slightly more specific, in that they reflect especially damage to certain tissues. As a group, these tests have no common physiologic or theoretical basis. Some involve measurement of enzymes liberated by damaged tissues; others involve detection of qualitative or quantitative changes in proteins or other serum components; and others appear to involve antigen-antibody reactions. All of them show abnormal responses in the presence of tissue destruction or inflammation, and none is wholly specific for a single disease entity.

A few of the most widely used tests of this type are presented below. In general, they are useful, when negative, for excluding certain diagnoses, and, when positive, in supporting diagnostic impressions gained from other clinical data.

The measurement of serum enzymes has been increasingly employed in recent years in the diagnosis and evaluation of myocardial infarction. Because these enzymes may be liberated by a variety of tissues, the tests must be considered nonspecific but they can be of considerably more value when other possible sources of increased serum enzyme levels have been excluded.

The Congo-red test is not a measure of inflammatory or necrotic changes, but is useful in detecting the presence of amyloid in tissues. It is included in this unit for purposes of convenience.

### Erythrocyte Sedimentation Rate

Subsequent to the investigations of Fahraeus [1] in 1921 on the factors active in the sedimentation of erythrocytes in plasma, the erythrocyte sedimentation rate gradually came into general use as one indication of the presence of tissue damage of various types. It has been utilized in many diseases: chronic infections like tuberculosis; infarctions, as of the myocardium; neoplasms; and the various so-called generalized connective-tissue diseases such as rheumatic fever and rheumatoid arthritis. Of normal physiologic states, pregnancy only has been shown to elevate the sedimentation rate. The sedimentation of erythrocytes is preceded by aggregation of individual cells into rouleaux. Fahraeus concluded that the aggregation of erythrocytes and the rate of sedimentation are affected by the number of red cells per cubic millimeter, the type and amount of individual protein fractions in the plasma (especially fibrinogen), the fat content of the blood, the temperature of the plasma, the diameter and length of the tube used for the determination, the degree of deviation of the tube from a vertical position, the anticoagulant used, and the length of time between aspiration of the blood and determination of the sedimentation rate.[2, 3] Many methods for determination of the erythrocyte sedimentation rate have been described, varying chiefly in the size of the tube, the anticoagulant, the frequency of readings, and the presence or absence of a correction for anemia. Three commonly used methods are the Westergren,[4] the Wintrobe-Landsberg,[4–6] and the Rourke-Ernstene.[7] They are outlined here in detail to indicate the differences in technique. The multiplicity of methods has caused confusion, and makes interpretation of figures possible only if one knows the method used.

The sedimentation tube has a length of 120 mm, an internal diameter of 4.0 mm, is graduated in 2-mm divisions from 0 to 100 mm, and contains 1.2–1.25 ml. The most satisfactory anticoagulant is heparin. An amount of heparin solution is measured such as to give a final concentration of 2.5 mg of heparin per 100 ml of whole blood, or 0.015 ml of heparin solution for 3.0 ml of blood. It has also been shown that dry oxalate mixture, 200 mg/100 ml of blood, is satisfactory as an anticoagulant (see Unit 3). In a small percentage of patients, the oxalate mixture falsely slows the sedimentation rate. In such cases, the correct rate can be obtained only by the use of heparin. The test should be started within 6 hr after the blood is drawn when heparin is used, and within 3 hr when oxalate mixture is used. The temperature of the room during the measurement should be approximately 25°C. The

blood sample is mixed and the sedimentation tube is filled to the zero mark by means of a pipette drawn out to a diameter and length that will allow insertion to the bottom of the tube. The tube is placed in a vertical position in a rack. Six or eight readings are taken at regular intervals during the first hour of the settling, the level of the top of the column of red cells and the time being recorded, until the readings indicate a decreased rate of settling owing to packing of the rouleaux. The rate of sedimentation during the period of constant fall is calculated either from inspection of the data or by plotting the curve as shown in Fig. 26. The sedimentation tube is then centrifuged for 30 min at 3000 rev/min and the hematocrit reading is made. From the chart shown in Fig. 27, the sedimentation rate is corrected to a hematocrit value of 45 percent and reported as the corrected sedimentation rate in millimeters per minute. The normal range is from 0.05 to 0.35 mm/min.

The Wintrobe tube has a length of 120 mm, an internal diameter of 2.5 mm, is graduated from 0 to 105 mm for the height of the blood column, and contains slightly less than 1.0 ml. The anticoagulant used is the dry mixture of ammonium and potassium oxalate, 200 mg/100 ml of whole blood (see Unit 3). The blood sample is mixed and the Wintrobe tube is filled with it to a height of 100 mm. The blood should be used within 3 hr of the time of its collection. For the determination, the room temperature should be not less than 22°C. A single reading of the depth of settling is taken at the end of 1 hr. The method of timing of sedimentation at 1 hr is an arbitrary choice based on convenience. It does not give a *rate* of sedimentation, as obtained in the Rourke-Ernstene method. However, readings at 15-min intervals are

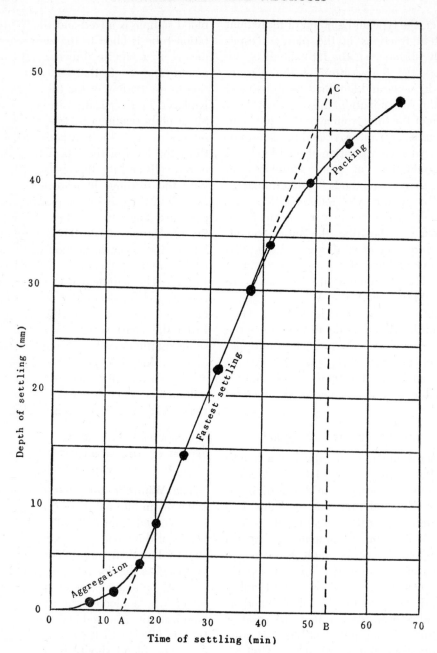

Fig. 26. Curve of sedimentation of red cells in plasma, showing periods of aggregation, of fastest (constant) settling rate, and of packing. For the Wintrobe-Landsberg method,[5, 6] the depth of settling in millimeters is recorded only once, at the end of 1 hr. For the Rourke-Ernstene method,[7] the rate of settling during the period of fastest (constant) settling is obtained (sedimentation rate) in millimeters per minute from the slope of the line $AC$, viz., $BC/AB$.

*Example:* In the figure, $BC/AB = 48/38$, or 1.26 mm/min. After obtaining the hematocrit, the rate is corrected (corrected sedimentation rate) by reference to Fig. 27. [Reproduced by permission from D. R. Gilligan, "The rate of sedimentation of erythrocytes," *The Cyclopedia of Medicine, Surgery, and Specialties* (Davis, Philadelphia, 1939).]

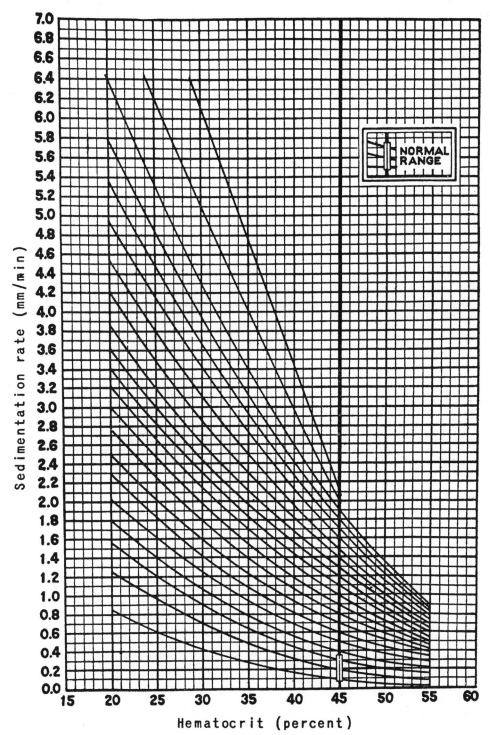

Fig. 27. Reference chart for correction of the sedimentation rate for the hematocrit, using the Rourke-Ernstene method.[7] The rate of settling (sedimentation rate) during the period of constant fall (Fig. 26) is corrected from the observed hematocrit of the blood sample to the sedimentation rate that corresponds to a hematocrit of 45 percent ("corrected sedimentation rate" or C.S.R.). The normal range is shown by the blocked area on the vertical line for 45-percent hematocrit.

*Example.* If the uncorrected sedimentation rate is 1.26 mm/min (Fig. 26) and the hematocrit is 30 percent, the point represented by these two values is located on the chart. The curve nearest to this point is followed to the point at which it intersects the vertical line corresponding to a hematocrit of 45 percent, and the corrected sedimentation rate is read from the ordinate. In this instance, the corrected sedimentation rate is 0.5 mm/min. [Reproduced by permission from D. R. Gilligan, "The rate of sedimentation of erythrocytes," *The Cyclopedia of Medicine, Surgery, and Specialties* (Davis, Philadelphia, 1939).]

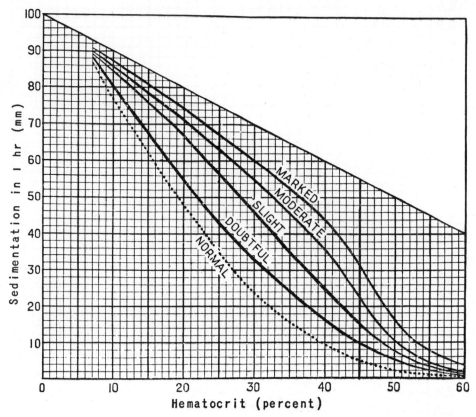

Fig. 28. Reference chart for correction of the depth of sedimentation in 1 hr for the hematocrit, using the Wintrobe Landsberg method.[5, 6] The chart is the modification from Hynes and Whitby.[8]

The sedimentation in 1 hr is corrected from the observed hematocrit of the blood sample to sedimentation that corresponds to a hematocit of 45 percent. The normal range for the corrected sedimentation in 1 hr is 0 to 10 mm.

To correct for a hematocrit above or below 45 percent, find the junction of the line represented by the observed sedimentation in 1 hr and that of the observed hematocrit; the point will fall in one of the five zones which indicate the approximate degree of increase in the rate. To correct to a hematocrit of 45 percent, the nearest appropriate curve is followed to the point where it intersects the line corresponding to 45 percent; the corrected sedimentation in 1 hr is then read from the ordinate.

*Example 1.* If the observed sedimentation is 50 mm and the observed hematocrit is 25.0 percent, then the sedimentation in 1 hr corrected to a hematocrit of 45 percent is approximately equal to 11 mm.

*Example 2.* If the observed sedimentation is 8 mm and the observed hematocrit is 56.0 percent, then the sedimentation in 1 hr corrected to a hematocrit of 45 percent is approximately equal to 30 mm.

helpful in giving some indication of the rate. The hematocrit is then determined by centrifugation at 3000 rev/min for 30 min and the observed rate is corrected from the observed hematocrit to that of 45 percent with the aid of the chart shown in Fig. 28 from Hynes and Whitby[8] and used as described by Whitby and Britton.[9] The results are outlined by the five zones (labeled "normal," "doubtful," "slight," "moderate," and "marked" in Fig. 28)[3] which represent averages and indicate roughly the degree of elevation of sedimentation at the end of 1 hr for different hematocrit values. The upper limit of normal is considered to be 10 mm settling in 1 hr after correction to a hematocrit of 45 percent.

### WESTERGREN METHOD [4]

The Westergren "tube" is a pipette filled from the bottom. It is 300 mm in length, 2.5 mm in internal diameter, is graduated from 0 to 200 mm, and contains about 1.0 ml. The anticoagulant is an aqueous solution of 3.8 gm of sodium citrate/100 ml; 0.2 ml of the anticoagulant is added for every 0.8 ml of whole blood, making a final concentration of 760 mg of sodium citrate per 100 ml of mixture and a dilution of 20 percent of the blood with an aqueous solution. The citrated blood is mixed and drawn up into the Westergren tube, which is then placed vertically in a stand of special construction that closes the bottom of the pipette by a rubber stopper and holds the tube firmly against the stopper by means of a spring. The depth of settling of the top of the red blood cell column is measured at the end of 1 hr. The author reports that the normal range for men is 1–3 mm and for women 4–7 mm in 1 hr. Although methods for correction of the effect of varying concentrations of red cells have been suggested, they have been discarded. When the specified anticoagulant is used, the sedimentation rate is not influenced by changes in the concentration of red cells as much as it is in methods using anticoagulants that do not dilute the whole blood.[10]

FACTORS AFFECTING THE ERYTHROCYTE SEDIMENTATION RATE. The many factors that affect the settling velocity of red cells must be realized. For instance, the longer the column of blood, the higher the settling velocity; reduction of the internal diameter of the tube to less than 2.5 mm decreases the rate of settling; dilution of blood by aqueous solutions such as anticoagulants reduces the settling velocity significantly; prolonged standing of blood—for more than 3 hr—is associated with slowing of the settling; an increase in temperature increases the sedimentation rate; moderate inclination of the tube from the vertical may cause a large increase in the sedimentation rate; the rate of fall of microcytic red cells is significantly lower than that of normocytic red cells; macrocytic red cells fall somewhat more rapidly than do normal cells; the lower the concentration of red cells suspended in plasma, the more rapid the settling velocity.

In vitro experiments have proved that an increase in the concentration of fibrinogen or of globulin in any individual plasma increases the sedimentation rate of the red cells in that plasma. Fibrinogen has been found to have a greater effect than globulin. In general, in vivo, the higher the concentration of fibrinogen, the faster the sedimentation rate, and, to a much lesser extent, abnormally high concentrations of globulins cause increase in the sedimentation rate. However, increased rates may be found with normal fibrinogen and globulin concentrations. No absolute correlation occurs between the sedimentation rate and any of the plasma-protein fractions.[3]

COMPARISON OF METHODS. The sedimentation rate, as measured by the Rourke-Ernstene method, has been shown to have the most nearly linear correlation with plasma fibrinogen,[10] and its correlation with other indicators of activity clinically has been judged to be closest. It should be pointed out, however, that the performance of this method is time-consuming and requires the preparation of the heparin solution every few weeks. The Wintrobe method, especially when modified to give readings every 15 min, is a simple and adequate screening procedure. The Westergren method is a distinctly satisfactory screening procedure and has been widely employed. The normal value for the sedimentation rate differs with the method used. Opinion varies considerably as to whether or not the upper limit of normal is different in males and females and whether or not it increases in old age. There is no conclusive evidence that females have a higher corrected rate than males or that the normal rate is higher in persons over 60.

INTERPRETATIONS AND LIMITATIONS. Increase in sedimentation rate of erythrocytes apparently represents a nonspecific response to tissue damage. The value of the sedimentation rate is in the indication of the presence of disease of such types as chronic infections, infarctions, neoplasms, and rheumatic diseases. In addition, to some extent it measures the severity of the process. In the majority of cases, it can be used as one indication of the subsidence of the inflammation and may be of considerable aid in determining the necessary duration of treatment.

Sedimentation rate may be elevated under certain conditions where tissue necrosis or inflammation is not apparent, at least by other criteria. Examples of this are the poorly understood dysproteinemias and paraproteinemias. Conversely, in some situations the sedimentation rate may not be elevated even though tissue damage is present. Examples of this are some cases of trichinosis, and cases of abruptio placenta associated with afibrinogenemia. In some cases of acute myocardial infarction and acute rheumatic fever associated with congestive heart failure, sedimentation rate may not be increased.

### Latex Fixation Test for Rheumatoid Arthritis

The past 30 years have seen the development of a number of tests for the study of serologic reactions in rheumatoid arthritis. These include agglutination of streptococci,[11-13] collodion particles,[14] and amboceptor-sensitized sheep red blood cells.[15, 16] The latter have utilized human serum gamma globulin spectrally adsorbed to cells, for example,

the Fraction II test of Heller,[17] the sensitized Rh-positive cell of Waller and Vaughn [18] incorporated in a suspension of particles such as latex [19, 20] or beutonite,[21] or used alone as antigen in a precipitation test.[22] None of these tests is specific for rheumatoid arthritis. Nevertheless, the relatively high frequency with which these tests give positive results in peripheral rheumatoid arthritis, and the relative infrequency with which the results are positive in most other disease states, has encouraged their use in clinical diagnosis.

Although it has not been definitely established that the tests measure an antigen-antibody reaction, the various methods for testing serums for the so-called "rheumatoid factor" utilize immunologic principles in design and each test can be analyzed accordingly. In each test it is clear that a substance present in rheumatoid serums—which has been called "rheumatoid factor"—behaves like an antibody directed against an antigen, or reactant, which is human serum gamma globulin, slightly denatured. This denaturation has been demonstrated by Christrom [23] and is characterized by an aggregation of the low-molecular-weight gamma globulin of normal human serum. The gamma globulin with a Svedberg sedimentation constant of 7–S, when slightly denatured, aggregates into larger particles having sedimentation constants varying between 30 and 40–S. This slightly aggregated human serum globulin (or antigen) contains (or is) the reactant prepared by differential precipitation. When this aggregated human serum globulin is coated on the surface of a tannic-acid-treated red blood cell or is present in solution, it will combine with "rheumatoid factor" in a manner similar to an antigen-antibody reaction. As a result, the coated red blood cells will be agglutinated by serum with high titer of "rheumatoid factor." On the other hand, if the aggregated gamma globulin reactant is present in solution, precipitation will occur on contact with "rheumatoid factor." If latex particles are included in the reaction system, they will provide a sensitive indicator of precipitation. Although aggregation has not been demonstrated to occur on the surface of amboceptor-sensitized red blood cells, it is believed that the reaction is basically the same in those tests that utilize antibody-sensitized cells.

**Method.** *Reagents.* (1) Polystyrene latex particles of uniform size, approximately 0.8 $\mu$ in diameter; the stock solution is made in concentration such that when diluted 1:100 and examined in a 13 × 13 × 100-mm square cuvette at 650 m$\mu$ in a Coleman spectrophotometer, light transmission is 5 percent.

(2) Glycine saline buffer made up of 0.1$M$ glycine adjusted to pH 8.2 with sodium hydroxide, to which is added 10 gm of sodium chloride per liter of buffer.

(3) Lyophilized human serum gamma globulin.

*Procedure.* The stock solution of latex particles is diluted 1:100 in the glycine saline buffer. Gamma globulin is dissolved in this diluted latex suspension in a final concentration of 250 $\mu$g/ml. The test serum, after heating at 56°C for 30 min,[24] is titrated by two-fold dilutions from 1:20 through 1:5120. An equal volume of latex gamma globulin reagent is added to the titrated diluted serum tubes. The tubes are mixed, incubated at 56° for 1½ hr and centrifuged at 2300 rev/min for 3 min, and agglutination is read. Agglutination in a final serum dilution of 1:80 or higher titer is considered a positive result. Not all preparations of lyophilized gamma globulin appear equally suitable for antigen in this test. However, it has been found that if an unsuitable preparation is obtained, it may be made suitable by heating the solution at 63°C for 10 min. Any particulate matter formed by heating is removed before making the final latex globulin reagent solution.

INTERPRETATIONS AND LIMITATIONS. A positive result in the latex test occurs in approximately 70 percent of patients with peripheral rheumatoid arthritis, with variations from one laboratory to another ranging from approximately 60 percent to 75 percent.[25-28] At the same time, normal control individuals will have positive test results less often than 3 percent if the test is being satisfactorily performed. It is thus clear that a positive result is fairly strong evidence that the serum is not from an entirely healthy person. However, it has not been found that positive results are confined to individuals with rheumatoid arthritis. Among the connective-tissue group of diseases, significant numbers of patients with lupus erythematosus disseminata, dermatomyositis, and scleroderma will have positive test results.[25-28] Among other diseases, sarcoidosis,[29] certain forms of chronic liver disease,[29] syphilis,[30] leprosy, and kala-azar[29] have been reported to give positive results in a variable but significant proportion of tests. The use of the test as a diagnostic tool is limited by the absence of specific tests for these other chronic inflammatory conditions. Furthermore, it has not yet been established as a reliable means of differentiating the various connective-tissue diseases.[31]

### C-Reactive Protein

The C-reactive protein was first detected in the serum of patients with pneumonia. It is a beta globulin that is precipitated by the somatic "C" polysaccharide of pneumococci. It is detected by the capillary precipitation test of Anderson and McCarty[32] which utilizes a specific antiserum obtained from rabbits sensitized with crystalline C-reactive protein.

INTERPRETATIONS. The presence of C-reactive protein in the serum is always abnormal, but may be due to any of a large number of inflammatory or necrotic disease processes. The greatest usefulness of the test is in the exclusion of active rheumatic fever. Except in some cases of chorea, C-reactive protein is always present in the serum during acute rheumatic fever and its absence virtually excludes the diagnosis.[33] In contrast to the sedimentation rate, it is not suppressed in the presence of congestive heart failure. The C-reactive protein reflects changes in rheumatic activity more promptly than the sedimentation rate, and usually becomes negative before the sedimentation rate returns to normal. Following cessation of suppressive therapy, the C-reactive protein usually does not show a "rebound" phenomenon.[34]

In addition to rheumatic fever, the C-reactive protein test also gives a positive result in many infections and in the presence of necrosis, inflammation, and some granulomatous diseases.[35] In acute myocardial infarction, the result usually becomes positive in 24 to 48 hr and becomes negative again after 1 to 2 weeks. Although it is regularly positive in transmural infarctions, it may be negative in the presence of small infarcts or during the early stages of infarction.

### Serum Enzyme Determinations

In myocardial necrosis there is increased cell-membrane permeability, permitting outward leakage of intracellular enzymes. Enzymes in high concentration in cardiac muscle will therefore give rise to significant serum elevations. Since there is no enzyme unique to the myocardium, elevated levels of these enzymes are of diagnostic assistance only if other possible sources for such elevations are excluded.

SERUM GLUTAMIC OXALOACETIC
TRANSAMINASE (SGOT)

PRINCIPLE. Serum glutamic oxaloacetic transaminase catalyzes the transfer of an amino group from aspartic acid to alpha ketoglutaric acid to form glutamic and oxaloacetic acids. It is present in all tissues and in especially generous quantities in the myocardium, skeletal muscle, brain, liver, and kidneys, in descending order of concentration.[36] Experimentally, it has been shown that there is a progressive decrease in the transaminase activity of infarcted myocardium in 7 to 9 days to only 2 to 10 percent of normal values, with a corresponding rise in serum transaminase concentration. It has been estimated that necrosis of 1 gm of myocardium will suffice significantly to raise the serum level of SGOT.[36] Necrosis of any tissue, especially those that are transaminase-rich, may lead to increased SGOT levels, with the exception of the brain, where an effective blood-brain barrier results in normal or near-normal serum levels in the presence of high cerebrospinal-fluid values.

METHOD.[37] The determination uses a double enzyme system, the first of which is the catalysis of the aspartic alpha ketoglutaric system by SGOT to form oxaloacetic and glutamic acids. In the presence of malic dehydrogenase and reduced diphosphopyridinenucleotide, oxaloacetic acid is converted to malic acid and the reduced diphosphopyridinenucleotide is oxidized. This oxidation can be measured photometrically. The enzyme is stable in serum stored at 0–5°C up to 2 weeks, and is not affected by freezing. However, hemolysis will increase the serum enzyme concentration by variable amounts.

INTERPRETATION AND LIMITATION.[38] Following myocardial infarction, SGOT activity begins to increase in about 6 hr, reaching a peak in 24 to 48 hr—the peak elevation being from 2 to 15 times the normal value—usually returning to normal in 3 to 4 days, but occasionally not until the 7th day after infarction. It follows, therefore, that a normal level of SGOT determined 3 days after infarction does not rule out myocardial infarction. This accounts for a sizable portion of the so-called "false negatives" reported in the literature. However, in well-studied series, the incidence of false negatives has been variously reported as 0–2.4 per cent. The elevation of the SGOT has experimentally and clinically been found to bear a rough correlation to the amount of muscle infarcted. SGOT activity exceeding 350 units in myocardial infarction is usually a grave prognostic sign. Secondary rises after a previous decline to normal levels are indicative of further infarction.

The curve of SGOT activity plotted against time is rather characteristic, with a sharp rise to a peak within 24 to 48 hr, and a rapid descent to normal levels within a period of days. The upper limit of normal for SGOT activity is about 40 units/ml but values slightly in excess of this cannot be considered significant. Normal SGOT values within 6 to 48 hr following the acute episode make recent myocardial infarction extremely unlikely. Elevated levels provide valuable confirmatory evidence, but demand careful exclusion of other possible causes of such elevation [39] (see Table 53).[40]

1. Acute pericarditis may be associated with elevated SGOT levels in up to 75 percent of reported series, but the values seldom exceed 100 units and usually remain elevated for more than the initial several days.

2. In congestive heart failure, values as high as 2000 units have been reported,[41] presumably due to hepatic congestion, and, in some instances, central hepatic necrosis.

3. Following pulmonary infarction, SGOT usually remains normal but may be elevated. Occasional early rises may be due to acute hepatic congestion. A late rise may occur at about the 5th to 7th day, probably from the infarcted lung itself, but the values seldom exceed 100 units. Because of the late rise in SGOT in pulmonary infarction, reports purporting to show normal SGOT values in this condition should be regarded with caution.

Table 53. *Diseases in which normal serum glutamic oxaloacetic transaminase levels are maintained.*[40]

| *Infectious conditions* | *Degenerative conditions* | *Neoplastic conditions* |
|---|---|---|
| Pneumonia | Cerebral thrombosis | Carcinoma |
| Tuberculosis | | Melanoma |
| Cystitis | Cerebral arteriosclerosis | Osteogenic sarcoma |
| Pyelonephritis | | |
| Empyema | Cerebral hemorrhage | Lymphoma |
| Wound infection | | Teratoma |
| Cholecystitis | Multiple sclerosis | Neurofibroma |
| Hydrops of gall bladder | | Mesenchymal tumor |
| | Muscular dystrophy | |
| Acute cholangitis | Nephrosclerosis | *Congenital conditions* |
| | Osteoporosis | |
| Thrombophlebitis | Osteoarthritis | Heart disease |
| | Pulmonary fibrosis | |
| Cellulitis | | *Miscellaneous conditions* |
| Gastroenteritis | Senile brain atrophy | |
| Subacute bacterial endocarditis | | Psychoneurosis |
| | *Allergies* | Pulmonary infarction |
| Perinephric abscess | Dermatitis | Anemia |
| | Hay fever | Intestinal obstruction |
| | Asthma | |
| *Metabolic conditions* | Urticaria | Pemphigus |
| | | Acute renal shutdown |
| Hyperthyroidism | *Collagen diseases* | Duodenal ulcer |
| Hypothyroidism | Rheumatoid arthritis | Hypertension |
| | | Aortic aneurysm |
| Addison's disease | Acute rheumatic fever without carditis | |
| Panhypopituitarism | Chorea | |
| Uremia | Disseminated lupus erythematosis | |
| Uremic pericarditis | Periarteritis nodosa | |
| Ureteral calculus | | |

4. Controversy exists with regard to the SGOT levels in severe and prolonged coronary insufficiency. Experimentally,[42] prolonged myocardial ischemia without necrosis in dogs does not cause increased SGOT levels and it is therefore reasonable to suppose that in these conditions elevation in SGOT denotes otherwise undetectable myocardial necrosis.

5. Extremely high values of SGOT are found in hepatocellular disease and the test is also useful as a liver-function test (see Unit 24). Since large amounts of glutamic oxaloacetic transaminase are excreted by the biliary tract, acute chole-

cystitis or chololithiasis may give rise to elevated SGOT levels so that this determination does not necessarily differentiate between coronary and biliary-tract disease.

SERUM LACTIC DEHYDROGENASE (SLD)

PRINCIPLE. Serum lactic dehydrogenase reduces alpha keto and alpha-gamma diketo acids in the presence of reduced diphosphopyridinenucleotide. It is present in all tissues, but especially in kidney, heart, and skeletal muscle, in decreasing order of concentration.

METHOD.[43] Sodium pyruvate is reduced by lactic dehydrogenase to lactate in the presence of reduced diphosphopyridinenucleotide (DPNH). The rate of the concomitant oxidation of reduced DPNH can be measured photometrically.

INTERPRETATIONS AND LIMITATIONS. The mean activity of serum lactic dehydrogenase (SLD) in the normal adult is 400 $\pm$ 120 units/ml, with a normal range of 200 to 680 units/ml. The enzyme is stable for at least 24 hr at 4°C. Hemolysis of even slight degree may significantly affect the level of SLD. At room temperature, hemolysis may increase the SLD activity by as much as 25 percent in 1 hr.[44] Oxalated plasma shows less SLD activity than the corresponding serum, for reasons not entirely clear.

A rise in SLD begins in about 6 to 12 hr after myocardial infarction, rising to a peak in 24 to 48 hr—the peak elevation being 2 to 8 times normal levels—returning to normal levels in 5 to 6 days. SLD levels of over 3500 units/ml are considered to be of grave prognostic significance.

The elevations of SLD generally parallel those of SGOT, except that (1) in myocardial infarction, an elevated SLD usually persists through the 6th day after infarction, and in 30 percent of cases it may persist through the 10th day;[45] (2) some cases of leukemia, disseminated carcinoma, and lymphoma have been reported to cause elevations of SLD activity; (3) SLD is not increased in obstructive jaundice, unlike SGOT; (4) like SGOT, SLD may occasionally be elevated in congestive heart failure.

SERUM ALDOLASE (FRUCTOALDOLASE) [46]

PRINCIPLE. Fructoaldolase catalyzes the splitting of one fructose diphosphate into two triose phosphates.

METHOD. A known quantity of fructose diphosphate is added to 1 ml of serum and the amount of triose phosphate formed is determined colorimetrically.[47]

INTERPRETATION AND LIMITATION. The normal range is from 3.0 to 10.5 units, without significant age or sex difference. Normal values are encountered in most acute and chronic inflammatory diseases, postoperative patients, nonmalignant blood dyscrasias, uremia, and most metabolic disorders. Elevated values are seen in myopathies, especially in progressive muscular dystrophy in children, and in degenerative anterior-horn-cell diseases such as myotonia congenita and Tay-Sachs disease. Muscle wasting not of neurologic origin does not raise the serum aldolase level. Elevated levels have also been observed in massive pulmonary infarction, extensive peripheral gangrene, acute hepatitis, severe pneumonia, acute pancreatitis, and hemolytic anemia. Many cases of delirium tremens and myxedema also show elevations of serum aldolase.

In myocardial infarction,[48, 49] the peak values are reached in 24 to 48 hr with values ranging from 19 to 112 units, followed by a rapid decline to normal levels in 4 to 5 days.

Because of the much greater concentration of serum aldolase in the red cells than in serum, any hemolysis will give rise to serious errors. If the serum is separated immediately, it can be stored for hours at room temperature and for weeks under refrigeration without affecting the determinations.

## Congo-Red Test for Amyloid Disease [50, 51]

Amyloidosis occasionally develops in patients with rheumatoid arthritis and allied diseases, tuberculosis, and prolonged bacterial infections, notably osteomyelitis. It is one of the chief causes of death in leprosy and in paraplegic individuals who develop intractable sepsis. It may accompany multiple myeloma. In the above-mentioned cases it is usually manifested by proteinuria and hepatosplenomegaly. In many individuals it develops without known predisposing disease. In these cases it may be manifested by nephrotic syndrome, polyneuropathy, purpura, cardiomegaly and cardiac failure, or hepatosplenomegaly. Because of a large degree of overlap between the clinical manifestations of primary and secondary amyloidosis, differentiation of these syndromes on the basis of organ involvement alone is not reliable. Although the diagnosis is most accurately established by biopsy of a parenchymal organ, two tests have proved helpful in confirming its presence—the Congo-red test and the gingival biopsy. The Congo-red test is based on the fact that, for reasons that are not entirely understood, Congo red disappears more rapidly from the serum of most patients with amyloidosis than from that of normal individuals.

**Method.** Prior to use, it is advisable to recrystallize the Congo red dye under sterile conditions.

The test is performed with the patient fasting. After an initial blood specimen has been obtained for a blank, 10 ml of 1-percent Congo red is injected intravenously. Blood is drawn at 4 min and at 60 min after injection, from a vein other than that used for the injection. After clotting, and separation of the clot, aliquots of the serums from the three specimens are diluted 1:10 with 0.9 percent

sodium chloride solution or with acetone and are read in a colorimeter, the pre-injection specimen being used as a blank. If saline is used as the diluent, the serums are read at 560 m$\mu$ (optimal for hemoglobin) and 510 m$\mu$ (optimal for Congo red). If analysis of the 4- or 60-min sample indicates that the reading at 560 m$\mu$ is greater than $\frac{1}{8}$ of the reading at 510 m$\mu$, it is concluded that sufficient hemolysis has occurred to render the test invalid. The other aliquots of the serums are therefore diluted 1:10 with acetone, which precipitates the hemoglobin, and centrifuged. The specimens are read at 510 m$\mu$. Occasionally the acetone method yields inconsistent results, for reasons that are not clear. Repetition of the test, with a fresh bottle of acetone, usually produces more consistent results. Because of these difficulties in interpretation, both the saline and acetone methods should, ideally, be used. Once the readings have been obtained, an estimate of "percentage remaining in plasma" is obtained by the following formula:

$$\frac{\text{Reading of the 60-min sample}}{\text{Reading of the 4-min sample}} \times 100$$
$$= \text{percentage of dye remaining in plasma.}$$

INTERPRETATION AND LIMITATIONS. The test as described above is a crude one. The assumptions that 4 min is the optimal mixing time and that the dose should be standard for all patients rather than based on surface area are not absolutely valid. Nevertheless, the results have proved to be very helpful. Normal individuals customarily exhibit dye retention in the plasma of 65 to 90 percent. Patients with severe amyloidosis frequently exhibit retention in the plasma of less than 10 percent. Retention of less than 20 percent in the plasma is strong indication that amyloidosis exists. Values of less than 40 percent make one suspicious. Patients with rheumatoid arthritis frequently exhibit values ranging between 50 and 65 percent. Loss of the Congo-red dye in the urine, even in patients with massive proteinuria, is rarely, if ever, great enough to influence the results of the test.

A positive result in the Congo-red test, that is, less than 20-percent retention, seldom occurs in conditions other than amyloidosis. On the other hand, in many patients with amyloidosis, especially of the idiopathic or so-called primary sort, the test gives borderline or negative results.

Since gingival biopsy with the use of formalin fixation and methyl-violet or crystal-violet stain also indicates the presence of amyloidosis in many of the patients with the disease, and since the results of the two tests do not always correlate in individual amyloid patients, a higher incidence of positive results can be obtained by using both tests together than by using either one alone.

## REFERENCES

1. R. Fahraeus, "The suspension stability of the blood," *Acta med. scand. 55,* 1 (1921).
2. M. A. Adams and A. N. Ballou, "A comparison between the values for plasma or serum protein as obtained by the specific gravity and the micro-kjeldahl methods," *J. lab. clin. Med. 31,* 507 (1946).
3. M. W. Ropes, E. Rossmeisl, and W. Bauer, "The relationship between the erythrocyte sedimentation rate and the plasma proteins," *J. clin. Invest. 18,* 791 (1939).
4. A. Westergren, "The technique of the red cell sedimentation reaction," *Amer. Rev. Tuberc. 14,* 94 (1926).
5. M. M. Wintrobe and J. W. Landsberg, "A standardized technique for the blood sedimentation test," *Amer. J. med. Sci. 189,* 102 (1935).
6. M. M. Wintrobe, *Clinical Hematology* (ed. 4; Lea and Febiger, Philadelphia, 1956), p. 314.
7. M. D. Rourke and A. C. Ernstene, "A method for correcting the erythrocyte sedimentation rate for variations in the cell volume percentage of blood," *J. clin. Invest. 8,* 545 (1930).
8. M. Hynes and L. E. H. Whitby, "Correction of the sedimentation rate for anemia," *Lancet,* 2, 249 (1930).
9. L. E. H. Whitby and C. J. C. Britton, *Disorders of the Blood. Diagnosis, Pathology, Treatment and Technique* (ed. 7; Blakiston, Philadelphia, 1953), p. 756.
10. T. H. Ham and F. C. Curtis, "Sedimentation rate of erythrocytes. Influence of technical, erythrocyte and plasma factors and quantitative comparison of five commonly used sedimentation methods," *Medicine 17,* 447 (1938).
11. R. L. Cecil, E. E. Nicholls, and W. J. Stainsby, "Characteristics of streptococci isolated from patients with rheumatic fever and chronic infectious arthritis," *Amer. J. Path. 6,* 619 (1930).
12. E. E. Nicholls and W. J. Stainsby, "Streptococcal agglutinins in chronic infectious arthritis," *J. clin. Invest. 10,* 323 (1931).
13. M. H. Dawson, M. Olmstead, and R. H. Boots, "Agglutinating reactions on rheumatoid arthritis: I. Reaction with streptococcus hemolyticus," *J. Immunol. 23,* 187 (1932).
14. A. D. Wallis, "Rheumatoid arthritis. II. Non-specific serological reactions," *Amer. J. med. Sci. 212,* 716 (1947).
15. E. Waaler, "On occurrence of factor in human serum activating specific ag-

glutination of sheep blood corpuscles," *Acta path. microbiol. scand. 17,* 172 (1940).

16. H. M. Rose, C. Ragan, E. Pearce, and M. O. Lipman, "Differential agglutination of normal and sensitized sheep erythrocytes by sera of patients with rheumatoid arthritis," *Proc. Soc. exp. Biol. (N. Y.) 68,* 1 (1948).

17. G. Heller, A. S. Jacobson, M. H. Kolodny, and W. H. Kammerer, "The hemagglutination test for rheumatoid arthritis. II. The influence of human plasma fraction II (gamma globulin) or the reaction," *J. Immunol. 72,* 66 (1954).

18. M. V. Waller and J. H. Vaughn, "Use of anti-Rh sera for demonstrating agglutination activating factor in rheumatoid arthritis," *Proc. Soc. exp. Biol. (N. Y.) 92,* 198 (1956).

19. J. M. Singer and C. M. Plotz, "The latex fixation test. I. Application to the serological diagnosis of rheumatoid arthritis," *Amer. J. Med. 21,* 888 (1956).

20. C. M. Plotz and J. M. Singer, "The latex fixation test. II. Results in rheumatoid arthritis," *Amer. J. Med. 21,* 893 (1956).

21. J. Bozicevich, J. J. Bunim, J. Freund, and S. B. Ward, "Beutonite flocculation test for rheumatoid arthritis," *Proc. Soc. exp. Biol. 97,* 180 (1958).

22. W. Epstein, A. Johnson, and C. Ragan, "Observations on a precipitin reaction between serum of patients with rheumatoid arthritis and a preparation (Cohn Fraction II) of human gamma globulin," *Proc Soc. exp. Biol. 91,* 235 (1956).

23. C. L. Christrom, "Characterization of the 'reactant' (gamma globulin factor) on the F II precipitin reaction and the F II tanned sheep cell agglutination test," *J. exp. Med. 108,* 139 (1958).

24. A. F. Shubart, A. S. Cohen, and E. Calkins, "Latex-fixation test in rheumatoid arthritis. I. Clinical significance of a thermolabile inhibitor," *New Engl. J. Med. 261,* 363 (1959).

25. J. W. Thomas, H. S. Robinson, J. P. Gofton, M. Stuckey, and R. Lamont-Hoves, "The latex fixation test on rheumatoid arthritis," *Canad. med. Ass. J. 76,* 621 (1957).

26. H. A. Feldman, T. W. Mou, and H. Wadsworth, "The epidemiology and serology of rheumatoid arthritis," *Arch. intern. Med. 101,* 425 (1958).

27. H. Bartfeld, E. Mahood, and E. F. Hartung, "Evaluation of hemagglutination tests in the diagnosis of rheumatoid arthritis," *Ann. rheum. Dis. 17,* 83 (1958).

28. R. M. Pike, S. E. Sulkin, H. C. Coggeshall, and M. L. Shultze, "A trial of the latex fixation test for rheumatoid arthritis," *Amer. J. clin. Path. 30,* 28 (1958).

29. H. G. Kunkel, H. J. Simon, and H. Fudenberg, "Observations concerning positive serological reactions for rheumatoid factor in certain patients with sarcoidosis and other hyperglobulinemic states," *Arthritis and Rheumatism 1,* 289 (1958).

30. A. Pettier and C. L. Christian, "The presence of the 'rheumatoid factor' in sera from patients with syphilis," *Arthritis and Rheumatism 2,* 1 (1959).

31. E. Calkins and A. F. Shubart, personal communication.

32. H. C. Anderson and M. McCarty, "Determination of C-reactive protein in the blood as a measure of the activity of the disease process in acute rheumatic fever," *Amer. J. Med. 8,* 445 (1950).

33. G. H. Stollerman, S. Glick, D. J. Patel, I. Hirschfeld, and J. H. Rusoff, "Determination of C-reactive protein in serum as a guide to the treatment and management of rheumatic fever," *Amer. J. Med. 15,* 645 (1953).

34. H. F. Wood and M. McCarty, "Laboratory aids in the diagnosis of rheumatic fever and in evaluation of disease activity," *Amer. J. Med. 17*, 764 (1954).
35. R. J. Roantree and L. A. Rantz, "Clinical experience with the C-reactive protein test," *Arch. intern. Med. 96*, 674 (1955).
36. I. Nydick, F. Wroblewski, and J. S. LaDue, "Evidence for increased SGOT activity following graded myocardial infarcts in dogs," *Circulation 12*, 161 (1955).
37. A. Karme, F. Wroblewski, and J. S. LaDue, "Transaminase activity in human blood," *J. clin. Invest. 34*, 126 (1955).
38. F. Wroblewski, "Clinical significance of serum enzyme alterations associated with myocardial infarction," *Amer. Heart J. 54*, 219 (1957).
39. J. J. Sampson, "Serum transaminase and other enzymes in acute myocardial infarction," *Progr. cardiovasc. Dis. 1*, 187 (1958).
40. F. G. Conrad, "Transaminase," *New Engl. J. Med. 256*, 602 (1957).
41. C. H. DuToit, "Usefulness of serum transaminase determinations in diagnosis of myocardial infarction," *Proc. New Engl. cardiovas. Soc. 14*, 36 (1955–56) (Mass. Heart Ass., 1956).
42. I. Nydick, P. Ruegsegger, F. Wroblewski, and J. S. LaDue, "Variations in SGOT activity in experimental and clinical coronary insufficiency, pericarditis, and pulmonary infarction," *Circulation 15*, 324 (1957).
43. F. Wroblewski, P. Ruegsegger, and J. S. LaDue, "Serum LDH activity in acute transmural myocardial infarction," *Science 123*, 1122 (1956).
44. K. M. Hsieh and H. T. Blumenthal, "Serum lactic dehydrogenase levels in various disease states," *Proc. Soc. exp. Biol. 91*, 626 (1956).
45. W. E. C. Wacker, D. D. Ulmer, and B. L. Vallee, "Metalloenzymes and myocardial infarction. II. Malic and lactic dehydrogenase activities and zinc concentrations in serum," *New Engl. J. Med. 255*, 449 (1956).
46. J. A. Sibley and G. A. Fleischer, "The clinical significance of serum aldolase," *Proc. Mayo Clin., 29*, 591 (1954).
47. J. A. Sibley and A. L. Lehninger, "Determination of aldolase in animal tissues," *J. biol. Chem. 177*, 859 (1949).
48. B. W. Volk, S. Losner, S. M. Aronson, and H. Lew, "Serum aldolase level in acute myocardial infarction," *Amer. J. med. Sci. 232*, 38 (1956).
49. S. Losner, B. W. Volk, and S. M. Aronson, "Diagnostic aids in acute myocardial infarction: Clinical and experimental," *Amer. Heart J. 54*, 225 (1957).
50. P. S. Unger, M. Zuckerbrod, G. J. Beck, and J. M. Steele, "Study of the disappearance of Congo red from the blood of nonamyloid subjects and patients with amyloidosis," *J. clin. Invest. 27*, 111 (1948).
51. N. Trieger, A. S. Cohen, and E. Calkins, "Gingival biopsy as a diagnostic aid in amyloid disease," *Arch. oral Biol. 1*, 187 (1959).

# Unit 18

# Extravascular Fluids

## PLEURAL, PERICARDIAL, AND PERITONEAL FLUIDS

A wide variety of pathologic conditions may be associated with the accumulation of fluid in the body cavities. Frequently the history and physical examination provide sufficient information to lead to a correct diagnosis. The examination of the fluid itself may yield a specific diagnosis or alert the physician to the type of disease process present.

### THE FORMATION AND CHARACTERISTICS OF TRANSUDATES AND EXUDATES

TRANSUDATES. Under normal conditions, fluids move between the vascular and extracellular compartments of the body. According to the Starling equilibrium, the interchange of fluid between the blood and tissue spaces is controlled by the balance between the capillary blood pressure, forcing fluid into the tissue spaces, and the osmotic pressure of the plasma proteins, retaining fluid in the vascular compartment. Small molecules such as water, electrolytes, and crystalloids diffuse rapidly back and forth. The concentration of these substances in the extravascular fluids approaches that of the blood as modified by the Donnan equilibrium. The large protein molecules diffuse to a very limited extent at usual plasma flow rates. Experimentally, both the amount of capillary filtrate and its protein concentration can be altered in a number of ways. Increased capillary hydrostatic pressure increases the capillary filtrate and its protein concentration. Decreased plasma osmotic pressure due to hypoalbuminemia increases the filtrate. Both decreased plasma flow and anoxia increase the diffusion of protein across the capillary membrane. Vasodilation also favors edema formation. There are also regional differences in the permeability of capillaries to protein. The capillaries of the liver and intestine are the most permeable and very sensitive to changes in pressure.[1-4]

The lymphatics also have an important role in returning interstitial fluid and protein to the plasma. Obstruction of the lymphatics may lead to excessive accumulation of interstitial fluid.

Disease states may produce excessive accumulation of fluid in the tissues and body cavities by altering the normal mechanisms that control the movement of fluids between the vascular and extravascular compartments. The localization and the characteristics of this fluid will vary according to the way these normal mechanisms are disrupted. There is also an increase in the total body fluid through renal retention of sodium and water which is controlled by a variety of hemodynamic and hormonal mechanisms. It may be difficult to determine which factor is primary in causing the transudation. Congestive heart failure, cardiac tamponade, venous obstruction, cirrhosis of the liver, acute and chronic

265

renal failure, and hypoproteinemia all produce serous effusions primarily by transudation.

A fluid that is produced by transudation is usually clear and straw-colored, with a low protein content and specific gravity. There is no fibrinogen and no clot formation. There are nearly the same concentrations of sugar, nonprotein nitrogen, urea, inorganic ions, and other freely diffusible substances as in the blood plasma. Since inflammation is absent, the cellular content of such fluid is low and the mononuclear cells predominate.

EXUDATES. Exudates are formed by inflammatory or neoplastic processes that damage and disrupt capillaries and lymphatics. Characteristically, exudates have a high specific gravity that corresponds to the concentrations of protein and nonprotein solutes, both of which approach the levels observed in the plasma. Usually, exudates contain fibrinogen and therefore clot readily when removed from the body. No clot forms, however, if defibrination occurs in a body cavity. There may be a decrease in the concentration of sugar and chloride in exudates, compared to those of

plasma. The sugar concentration of exudates may be greatly reduced or absent as the result of glycolytic action in such instances as bacterial infection and high concentrations of leukocytes. The number and type of cellular elements depend upon the disease process causing the tissue injury. In many instances, blood vessels are ruptured, with resulting contamination of the exudate with red blood cells.

While a typical exudate may be easily differentiated from a typical transudate (Table 54), not infrequently the various diseases produce fluids that have values that overlap. This limits the diagnostic value of examination of the fluid in the individual case. However, a fluid whose characteristics vary grossly from those expected from the clinical diagnosis should alert the physician to the possibility of an error in diagnosis. In addition, bacteriologic studies and cytologic examination for tumor cells may yield a specific diagnosis.

### SEROUS EFFUSIONS IN THE ABDOMINAL CAVITY

Congestive heart failure, constrictive pericarditis, obstruction to the inferior vena cava and hepatic vein, cirrhosis of

Table 54. *Comparison of unmodified transudate and typical exudate.*

| Pathologic physiology and characteristics of fluids | Unmodified transudate | Typical exudate |
|---|---|---|
| Protein content: | | |
| Range (gm/100 ml) | 0.4 ± 0.2 | Approaches the protein content of blood plasma, 6.0 ± 1.0 gm/100 ml; may be modified by infectious agents and destruction of tissue |
| Fibrinogen and clot | None | Present |
| Dializable substances: | | |
| Concentration | Approaches that of blood plasma as modified by Donnan equilibrium | Approaches that of blood plasma as modified by Donnan equilibrium, as well as by infectious agents and destruction of tissue |
| Glucose | Equivalent to plasma | Frequently decreased to absent owing to glycolysis |
| Specific gravity | 1.010 ± 0.002 | Approximately 1.020 and above |
| Cells: | | |
| White blood cells | Few (lymphocytes) | Many to frank pus |
| Red blood cells | Rare | Variable from few to bloody |
| Fixed tissue cells | Rare | Variable |

Table 55. Data from Paddock [17] representing examinations of 1300 fluids from the records of four different hospitals. It was not possible to control the methods used. Therefore, these data are necessarily crude.

| Diseases affecting pleural or peritoneal cavity | Pleural fluids | | | | | Peritoneal fluids | | | | |
|---|---|---|---|---|---|---|---|---|---|---|
| | No. of cases | Specific gravity or protein concentration (gm/100 ml) | White-cell count (cells/mm³) 1000 to 5000 | White-cell count (cells/mm³) 5000 or more | Red-cell count, more than 10,000 cells/mm³ | No. of cases | Specific gravity or protein concentration (gm/100 ml) | White-cell count (cells/mm³) 1000 to 5000 | White-cell count (cells/mm³) 5000 or more | Red-cell count, more than 10,000 cells/mm³ |
| | | | Percentage of cases | | (These data do not exclude bloody taps) | | | Percentage of cases | | (These data do not exclude bloody taps) |
| Cardiac failure (75% from right chest) | 313 | 1.004–1.020 (av. 1.010) | 9 | 1 | 10 | 100 | 1.006–1.018, 1.016 or more, 34 percent cases | 10 | | 10 |
| | 29 | 0.2–3.6 (av. 1.6) | | | | 21 | 1.5–5.3 (av. 3.7) | | | |
| Nephrosis | 16 | 1.001–1.008 (av. 1.006) | | | | 17 | 1.003–1.012 (av. 1.007) | | | |
| | 10 | 0.1–1.0 (av. 0.4) | | | | 9 | 0.1–0.9 (av. 0.3) | | | |
| Cirrhosis of liver | 21 | 1.004–1.019 (av. 1.010) | 18 | 7 | 30 | 270 | 1.002–1.016 (av. 1.009) | 9 | | 1 |
| | 5 | 0.6–3.2 (av. 1.8) | | | | 69 | 0.6–3.2 (av. 1.2) | | | |
| Pulmonary infection | 100 | 1.010–1.042 (av. 1.019) | 25 | 60 | 30 | 21 | (av. 1.020) | 70 | | 7 |
| Tuberculosis | 290 | 1.010–1.024 (av. 1.020), 1.016 or less, 10 percent cases (see column 8) | 50 | 20 | 10 | | | | | |
| | 8 | 2.7–5.1 (av. 4.2) | | | | | | | | |
| Neoplasm | 123 | 1.010–1.020 (Even distribution) | 30 | 10 | 65 | 60 | 1.010–1.020 (Even distribution) | 35 | 15 | 20 |
| | 9 | 2.1–4.6 (av. 3.4) | | | | 15 | 1.5–4.2 | | | |

the liver, nephrosis, and other hypoalbuminemic states produce ascites mainly by transudation (Table 55). The dynamics of ascitic-fluid formation in cirrhosis has been extensively studied.[5-7]

Ascites occurring during the course of liver disease implies hepatocellular failure and portal-vein hypertension. The failure of liver cells to produce albumin to maintain the normal plasma osmotic pressure, together with the portal hypertension, causes fluid transudation into the abdominal cavity. In this condition there is marked retention of sodium and water. It has been postulated that the segregation of fluid in the abdominal cavity causes a decrease in "effective" circulating blood volume. This stimulus sets into action homeostatic mechanisms to maintain an "effective" blood volume and prevent hypovolemia. An increased urinary excretion of aldosterone is found in this condition, which is probably in part a response to this stimulus and related to the associated sodium and water retention. The role of antidiuretic hormone is at present not clear. The retained sodium and water, however, fail to correct the circulating volume as the retained fluid continues to be segregated in the abdominal cavity. This results in continuing ascites unless the cycle is interrupted by reduction in portal pressure, restoration of normal osmotic pressure, or therapeutic measures promoting sodium excretion. Experimentally, ascites has been produced by inducing portal-vein hypertension and hypoalbuminemia. It has also been produced by constriction of the thoracic inferior vena cava above the hepatic vein. This leads to hepatic congestion and an ascitic fluid high in protein. It is thought that the ascitic fluid is due to an overflow of hepatic lymph. This may be of importance in the ascites of congestive heart failure and hepatic venous obstruction. The importance of this mechanism in the usual type of cirrhosis has yet to be shown.

Studies with tritium-labeled water indicate that the ascitic fluid is in dynamic equilibrium with the plasma. Albumin and globulin also participate in the exchange between blood and ascitic fluid.

"Ascitic fluid in cirrhosis is clear, straw-colored, green or bile-stained. The protein content is usually low, 1 to 2 gm/100 ml. The concentration is directly proportional to that in the blood. Values in the ascitic fluid up to 3.5 gm/100 ml are reported usually in patients with subacute hepatitis or hepatic vein occlusion with relatively high serum protein values. The electrolyte concentrations in the ascitic fluid are those of other extracellular fluids. The fluid usually contains 20–100 cells/mm[3], mainly endothelial. Irritation of the peritoneum following paracentesis may result in the appearance of polymorphonuclear leukocytes and lymphocytes in the ascitic fluid." [6]

Ascitic fluid having the high protein content of an exudate may be produced by neoplasm involving the abdominal viscera and lymphatics. A variety of infections, perforations of the gastrointestinal and biliary tract, and pancreatitis are other common causes of abdominal fluid having the characteristics of an exudate. The value of the routine and some special examinations in differentiating these fluids is discussed in subsequent sections.

### SEROUS EFFUSIONS IN THE PLEURAL CAVITY

The commonest cause of pleural effusion produced mainly by transudation is congestive heart failure. Cirrhosis of the liver and nephrosis are less common causes.[8]

Neoplasms of various types are the commonest cause of pleural effusions produced mainly by exudation. Bronchial carcinoma, breast carcinoma, lymphomas, and leukemias are the commonest malignant lesions producing effusions. Tuberculosis is probably the most frequent bacterial infection producing pleural effusion. Other causes include pulmonary infarction, postpneumonic serous effusion, trauma, idiopathic pleuropericarditis, lupus erythematosis, and subdiaphragmatic abscess.[9]

### SEROUS EFFUSIONS IN THE PERICARDIAL CAVITY

Little has been written concerning pericardial fluid. Hydropericardium may appear during congestive heart failure. Pericardial fluids having the characteristics of an exudate have been reported in tuberculosis, idiopathic or benign pericarditis, polyserositis, rheumatic pancarditis, pyogenic infections, malignant diseases, and trauma.[10–12]

### COLLECTION OF THE FLUID

The fluid is collected under aseptic conditions. Sufficient fluid should be taken for determination of specific gravity, quantitative protein, white- and red-blood-cell count and smear, cell block, and Papanicolau cytologic examinations. All examinations should be performed while the fluid is as fresh as possible. This is particularly true of the cytologic examination, where deterioration of the cells and coagulation of the fluid may make a satisfactory examination impossible.

Since immediate examination of the fluid is not always possible, an anticoagulant should be added to the fluid. Aqueous sodium citrate may be made up into a stock solution containing 20 gm of citrate per 100 ml. This solution then is added 1 ml to each 10 ml of the serous fluid. Small quantities of fluid may be drawn up into a heparinized syringe to prevent clotting. Oxalates should not be used, since they distort cellular morphology.[13]

### GROSS EXAMINATION OF SEROUS EFFUSIONS

The following features of the fluid should be observed and recorded:

(i) Amount of fluid.

(ii) Color and general appearance—record whether the fluid is clear or turbid, thin or thick, colorless or colored, for example, straw-colored, bloody, purulent.

(iii) Odor—describe the odor, if present, or indicate its absence.

(iv) Clot—record the absence or presence of clot.

Fluids that result primarily from transudation are usually clear and straw-colored. In the presence of jaundice they may be bile-stained. If the fluid is bloody, one should attempt to determine whether this was due to a traumatic tap. If the bleeding was due to rupture of small vessels by the tap, there is frequently progressive clearing as the fluid continues to drain. A uniform distribution of blood throughout the specimen usually indicates another process. In the absence of trauma, neoplasm, with its associated necrosis and invasion of blood vessels, is the most frequent cause of a bloody effusion.[12]

A milky serous effusion may be due to the mixture of chyle with the effusion. The commonest cause of a milky (chylous) effusion is neoplasm. While the presence of chyle probably contributes to the milky appearance, there is no parallelism between gross milkiness and fat content.[14] It is possible that necrotic debris contributes to this appearance.

In some instances, a milky fluid has been reported in the absence of an increased fat content (pseudochylous). In these cases, the opalescence is due to a lecithin-globulin complex. There seems to be no specific etiology associated constantly with this type of fluid.[15]

Fluids having a foul odor are usually associated with infection or neoplasm. A fluid that clots indicates the increased fibrinogen content of an exudate. Mucinous effusions may occasionally be seen. These have always been associated with neoplasm.[16]

## DETERMINATION OF THE SPECIFIC GRAVITY OF SEROUS EFFUSIONS

The specific gravity of serous effusions has been used clinically to determine whether the fluid is the result of transudation or exudation. A specific gravity below 1.016 generally has been considered characteristic of a transudate, and one above this, characteristic of an exudate. The specific gravity has been shown to be directly proportional to the protein content of the fluid.[17] However, in the routine laboratory examination of these fluids, a discrepancy between the specific gravity and protein content occurs so frequently as to limit its value. The protein content of the serous fluid is generally considered to be a more accurate indicator of the underlying disease process.[9]

The specific gravity of serous effusions is determined in the same way as that of urine (Unit 19), and the determination is subject to the same errors.

### PROTEIN CONTENT OF SEROUS EFFUSIONS

Those fluids that are produced primarily by transudation usually have a lower protein content than those produced by exudation. While there are frequent exceptions to the average, a value that grossly deviates from that expected from the clinical diagnosis should alert the physician to the possibility of an error in the diagnosis.

A study of protein content of pleural fluids [18] found that most of the fluids due to congestive heart failure had a protein content of less than 3.0 gm/100 ml, while those due to cancer and tuberculosis had more than 3.0 gm/100 ml. Those fluids due to pulmonary infarcts, pneumonia, and lupus erythematosus usually had the high protein content of an exudate.

Peritoneal fluids in general show the same type of relation.[12] The average protein concentration of fluids due to neoplasm and tuberculosis is above 3.0 gm/100 ml; in cirrhosis, the average value is 1.2 gm/100 ml. However, in abdominal fluid secondary to congestive heart failure or hepatic-vein occlusion, the fluid is usually 3.0 gm/100 ml or above.

A more detailed analysis of serous fluids has been made by protein electrophoresis, salting-out methods, and mucoprotein determination. These methods show characteristic patterns for different diseases. However, there is considerable overlap in values obtained with the various diagnostic categories which limits their usefulness in the individual case.[14, 19–21]

### QUANTITATIVE DETERMINATION OF PROTEIN

The concentration of protein in body fluids may be determined by the same chemical, physical, and immunological methods that are employed for blood plasma.

### THE CYTOLOGY OF SEROUS EFFUSIONS [13, 22]

Pleural fluid obtained from normal people contains 1700–6200 cells/mm$^3$. These cells are mostly large mononuclears with a smaller number of mesothelial cells and lymphocytes.[23] Fluids produced by transudation usually have a low cell count. The cells are mainly mesothelial cells and lymphocytes. Polymorphonuclear leukocytes and red blood cells are uncommon.

The total and differential white-blood-cell counts of serous effusions have generally been of little value in establishing the etiology in the individual case, except in nontuberculous infected fluids where polymorphonuclear leukocytosis is the rule.[12] The cells occurring in serous effusions in disease states are listed below.

### THE CELLS OF EFFUSIONS

MESOTHELIAL CELLS. These cells form the lining of the serous cavities. Mesothelial cells shed into the serous cavities are frequently rounded up and undergoing active multiplication. These may be difficult to tell from macrophages which are also present.

LYMPHOCYTES. Lymphocytes are present in every serous effusion. They predominate in most tuberculous effusions, in some cases of malignant disease, and, rarely, in postpneumonic effusion. The cells are similar to those seen in lymphoid tissue and, rarely, to the mature type seen in the peripheral blood.

PLASMA CELLS. These occur in small numbers and seldom predominate. There seems to be no specific disease process associated with these cells. The plasma cells are morphologically the same as those in the peripheral blood and may include the less mature "Turk cell."

NEUTROPHIL POLYMORPHONUCLEAR CELLS. These cells are found in almost every serous fluid. In inflammatory exudates and especially bacterial exudates, they are abundant. They resemble the neutrophils of the blood, but undergo degenerative changes. "Lupus erythematosus" cells may be demonstrated in pleural and pericardial fluid in disseminated LE [24] (see Unit 13).

EOSINOPHIL POLYMORPHONUCLEAR CELLS. These are frequently found in effusions and not uncommonly may represent 10 percent or more of the total present. These cells in excess of 20 percent in pleural fluid have been associated with pneumothorax, postpneumonic effusion, malignant disease, infarct, "vasculitis," rheumatic pericarditis, and parasitic disease. Peritoneal eosinophilia has been reported in malignant disease, vasculitis, and parasitic infection. A number of cases of eosinophilic pleural and peritoneal effusions have occurred without being explained.[25-28]

### RED-CELL CONCENTRATION

The determination of the red-blood-cell concentration of serous fluid gives circumstantial evidence as to the etiology of the fluid. Pleural fluids with a red-cell count of over $100,000/mm^3$ are, in the absence of trauma, most likely due to a neoplastic process. Peritoneal fluids generally have a lower concentration of red blood cells than pleural fluids due to the same etiology. This is probably a result of the dilution of the red blood cells with a greater quantity of fluid. Pleural and peritoneal fluids having a concentration of less than 10,000 red blood cells per cubic millimeter are not characteristic of any specific disease entity.

Bloody effusions may not clot unless the fluid has been withdrawn soon after the bleeding. This has been shown to be due to intrapleural clotting and defibrination rather than to any specific anticoagulant.[29]

### CELL COUNT AND DIFFERENTIAL COUNT OF WHITE CELLS

The cell count for serous fluids is performed on a hemocytometer as described in Unit 4, except that the technique is adapted for values from 1 or 2 cells to many thousands of cells per cubic millimeter. For identification of cells and accurate determination of the differential count a film, stained with Wright's stain, is prepared from a centrifuged sample of fluid, the cells being resuspended in serum or bovine albumin.

METHODS FOR CELL COUNTS. The cell count should be made as soon after removal of the fluid as possible, since cells may disintegrate. The cell counts should be made from the fluid containing an anticoagulant, since clot formation removes a large proportion of the cells. The methods of counting cells will vary with the number of cells in the serous fluid.

*Method for Low White-Cell Counts.* Many extravascular fluids will have white-cell counts of from 10 to 500 cells/$mm^3$, with or without the presence of red cells. Such fluids are clear or have only faint turbidity. The cell count is determined by transferring directly an undiluted drop of well-mixed fluid to one counting chamber of a hemocytometer and counting all the cells in all nine large squares of the chamber. Since this represents a volume of 9/10 mm³, the result is multiplied by the fraction 10/9 to convert the number of cells counted to the number per cubic millimeter.

*Example 1.* In a transudate, a total of 270 cells is counted in nine large squares. The corrected count is 270 × 10/9 = 300 cells/mm³.

*Method for High White-Cell Counts.* The white-cell count is determined as described in Unit 4 for values of 1000 or more white cells per cubic millimeter.

*Method for Counting a Mixture of White Cells and Red Cells.* Many serous fluids contain both red cells and white cells and it is essential to determine these values separately. In grossly bloody fluids, a red-cell count and a white-cell count are made in the usual manner. If only moderate numbers of red cells and white cells are present, they may be determined as follows. A total cell count is observed on undiluted serous fluid as described above. A second count of white cells only is performed on a sample in which the red cells are hemolyzed by glacial acetic acid, as described below. The difference between the two counts represents the red-cell count.

The procedure for performing the white-cell count is as follows. A white-cell pipette is filled to the 1.0 mark with glacial acetic acid that contains a few drops of methylene blue (to aid in seeing the height of the column of acid in the pipette). The pipette is then filled to the 11 mark with the serous fluid, producing a dilution of the serous fluid in the pipette of 9/10. The sample is well mixed and tranferred immediately to the counting chamber of a hemocytometer, and the white cells are counted. The white-cell count is corrected for dilution by multiplying by 10/9. The

preparation in the counting chamber is subsequently used for estimating the differential count of white cells as described below.

*Example 2.* For a fluid, transferred directly to a counting chamber, the total cell count (red and white cells) for nine large squares (0.9 mm³) is 450. To convert to 1.0 mm³, this is multiplied by 10/9, giving 500 cells/mm³. When the fluid is diluted 9/10 with glacial acetic acid, as described above, the white-cell count in nine chambers is 162. This is multiplied by 10/9 to correct for the dilution, giving 180, and then again by 10/9 to convert the volume to 1.0 mm³, giving 200 white cells/mm³. Thus the total cell count of 450 cells/mm³, minus 200 white cells/mm³, leaves 250 red cells/mm³.

*Example 3.* If a fluid is moderately bloody, the total cell count will be made, with Gower's solution and an appropriate dilution, such as 1/10, using a white-cell pipette. The cell count on each of five groups of 16 small squares is 25, 20, 30, 27, 22. The sum is 124. This result obtained in five small squares (0.02 mm³) is multiplied by 50 to obtain the number in 1.0 mm³, namely, 6200 cells. This is multiplied by 10 to correct for the dilution, giving 62,000 cells/mm³.

METHODS FOR DIFFERENTIAL CELL COUNTS. *Method for Estimating Differential Count of White Cells in the Counting Chamber.* A rough estimate of the differential count of white cells in serous fluids may suffice for some clinical purposes. The use of dilute solutions of methylene blue, Unna's stain, is frequently recommended but is of little merit since the staining of white cells is too faint. The differential count may be estimated more satisfactorily in the counting chamber on the sample of serous fluid treated with glacial acetic acid as described above. Acetic acid hemolizes the red cells and delineates the shape and size of the nucleus from the cytoplasm of white cells sufficiently to permit rough accuracy in distinguishing three types of cells: polymorphonuclear leukocytes, lymphocytes, and large mononuclear cells. Enough cells are counted to estimate the proportion, in percent, of the different types of cells. The method is a crude screening procedure but has value as such. For example, it is possible to recognize immediately a large number of polymorphonuclear leukocytes, in contrast to a predominance of lymphocytes.

*Stained Films of Cells from Extravascular Fluids.* It is frequently difficult to obtain satisfactory stained films of cells from extravascular fluids, apparently because of irregular staining reactions of the low-protein medium. This may be improved remarkably by suspending the cells in a small quantity of serum from the patient or in bovine albumin. A sample of 5–10 ml of serous fluid is centrifuged, the supernatant fluid is discarded, and the sediment is resuspended in 0.2–0.5 ml of cell-free serum from the patient or bovine albumin. Films are then made from the mixture, as described for a blood film (Unit 9). These films may be stained with Wright's stain, Gram's stain, or a dilute aqueous solution of methylene blue. If a proper thin film is made, Wright's stain is entirely satisfactory for the differential count of leukocytes and the estimation of the ratio of red cells to white cells.

### CYTOLOGIC DIAGNOSIS OF MALIGNANT DISEASE

Malignant disease involving the serous cavities frequently can produce an effusion into which are shed tumor cells. Malignant disease may also produce an effusion without direct involvement of the cavity. In this instance, tumor cells may not be present in the effusion.

The sediment of effusions may be studied for malignant cells by the cell-block method. This method consists in sectioning the centrifuged deposit after fixation for microscopic study. The Papanicolaou method is being widely used for this purpose also.

In the cell-block or histologic method, the diagnosis is usually made from cell aggregates and seldom from the individual cells. These sections are comparable to tissue sections. In the Papanicolaou method, malignant cells even in the absence of cell aggregates may be recognized by a number of features. By using both methods one increases the percentage of accuracy and positive yield. Some tumors are associated with a higher proportion of positive results. Ovarian carcinoma produces an effusion that yields a high percentage of positive results, whereas a lower percentage is obtained in carcinoma of the lung. Lymphomas may occasionally be diagnosed by this method.

In chronic effusions of a benign nature, mesothelial cells undergoing active regeneration are shed into the effusion. These cells may be difficult to differentiate from malignant cells and may rarely be the cause of a false positive result. In proved cases of malignant disease with effusion, about 70 percent yield positive findings for malignancy by cell-block or Papanicolaou cytologic examination of the effusion. False positive reports occur in less than 1 percent in most series.[13, 30–35]

It is important that the fluid collected for cytologic examination be studied as fresh as possible, for the cells degenerate with standing. The fluid should also have sodium citrate added, since clotting may make examination of the fluid difficult or impossible (p. 269).

### LIPID CONTENT OF SEROUS FLUID

Chyle is a modification of lymph that differs chiefly in that it may contain 5–15 percent of emulsified fat and has a milky appearance. Chyle occurs in the lymphatics draining the small intestine after a fatty meal. This chyle is carried from the intestines via the cisterna chyli and eventually to the thoracic duct from which the lymph is poured into the blood stream.

Obstruction and rupture of these lymphatics may cause a loss of chyle into the serous cavities. The resulting effusion is milky and is termed chylous. The commonest cause for this type of fluid is lymphatic obstruction due to neoplasm; less frequently, it comes from surgical or other trauma and tuberculosis. The effusion that results is due not only to chyle but to the mixture of chyle with the other products of the inflammatory or neoplastic exudates.[36-39]

The chief way to determine the presence of chyle in the effusion is to demonstrate an increase in the lipid content of the fluid. If the fluid is milky, this may be easily determined by making the fluid alkaline to litmus paper and adding ether. If the milky appearance is due to fat, it should clear. A quantitative chemical analysis can be performed. In a study of ascitic fluid, it was found that cancerous ascites had 0.35 gm of fat or more per 100 ml. Ascitic fluid due to cirrhosis had less than this level.[14] The fat content of ascitic fluid in other conditions has not been adequately studied.

The other criteria for chylous fluid will vary according to the varying amounts of chyle, lymph, and inflammatory and neoplastic exudates present. These characteristics have been given for chylous fluid: (1) it has a milky appearance; (2) it does not change in appearance on standing but frequently forms a creamy top layer; (3) it has no odor; (4) it is sterile; (5) it resists putrefaction; (6) it is finely emulsified; (7) it has an alkaline reaction; (8) its specific gravity is greater than 1.012; (9) its fat content is 0.4–4.0 percent; (10) its protein content is variable; (11) it contains 7.04 percent of solids; (12) a smear shows varying numbers of leukocytes, mainly lymphocytes; (13) shaking with ether after the addition of alkaline causes the fluid to clear. A sudan III stain of the fluid will also show the presence of fat particles. Several quantitative methods for determining the fat content of serous effusions have been used.[14, 39]

## BACTERIOLOGY

The bacteriologic examination of serous fluids is discussed in Unit 26 on infectious diseases. This examination is of first importance since it may reveal the etiologic agent in instances of infection. The procedures of preparation of stained films, culture, immunologic study, and inoculation of the guinea pig are important in analysis of serous fluids resulting from infection.

### MISCELLANEOUS DETERMINATIONS

AMYLASE. Peritoneal-fluid amylase has been reported as an aid in diagnosis of acute pancreatitis. The peritoneal-fluid level of amylase is higher than the blood level in pancreatitis and remains significantly elevated for 2–3 days longer than the blood level.[40]

BILIRUBIN. Analysis of a fluid for bilirubin may aid in the diagnosis of a perforation or a comunication involving the biliary tract. A quantitative analysis for bilirubin may be performed using the same method as for blood.

CHOLESTEROL EFFUSIONS. This fluid is described as being filled with golden, glittering particles that microscopically consist of cholesterol crystals in suspension. Most of the fluids have been found years after a bout of untreated pleuritis, peritonitis, or pericarditis; in some, tubercle bacilli have been demonstrated.[41-44]

GLUCOSE. Determination of the glucose content of serous effusions is seldom made. It is said to be of some help in distinguishing tuberculous and nontuberculous pleural effusions.[45]

ACIDITY. The gross appearance of a fluid may suggest the presence of gastric content due to perforation or communication with the stomach. A qualitative and quantitative determination for acid content may be made by the same methods as for determining gastric acid content.

# CEREBROSPINAL FLUID

## PHYSIOLOGY OF FORMATION AND CONTENT OF CSF

The cerebrospinal fluid (CSF) has many of the characteristics of an ultrafiltrate of plasma. However, it differs in some respects from other extravascular fluids, especially as regards its formation, circulation through special anatomic channels, and mode of absorption.[46] The cerebrospinal fluid is a clear, colorless fluid that fills the ventricles of the brain and the subarachnoid spaces of the brain and spinal cord. The total quantity formed in the adult during a single day is estimated to be 45 to 130 ml. The normal cellular content and the chemical composition of fluid drawn from the lumbar subarachnoid space are given in Table 56.[46, 47] From these data it is evi-

Table 56. *Normal values for cerebrospinal fluid obtained by lumbar puncture.*

| | |
|---|---|
| Initial pressure (horizontal position) | 70–180 mm $H_2O$ |
| Cell count | 0–5/mm³, lymphocytes or mononuclear cells |
| Bilirubin | 0 |
| Calcium | 4.5–5.5 mg/100 ml |
| Chloride | 120–130 mEq/L, as $Cl^-$ |
| Cholesterol | 0.06–0.22 mg/100 ml |
| Creatinine | 0.4–1.5 mg/100 ml |
| Glucose | 50–75 mg/100 ml |
| Magnesium (average) | 3.3 mg/100 ml |
| Nonprotein nitrogen | 12–30 mg/100 ml |
| Protein | 14–45 mg/100 ml |
| Potassium | 3.5–5.0 mEq/L |
| Urea nitrogen | 6–15 mg/100 ml |

dent that cerebrospinal fluid differs from blood plasma in having no bilirubin, extremely low cholesterol, low protein, and less sugar, calcium, and nonprotein nitrogen, but more chloride. The fluid is formed by a process of secretion from the epithelial cells of the choroid plexuses of the lateral, third, and fourth ventricles and by dialysis from the blood vessels of the choroid plexuses and pia of the brain and spinal cord. Most of its components are derived from blood plasma. In addition, some substances presumably come from the brain tissue during its metabolism, but relatively little is known about them. Plasma constituents vary as to the site and mode of entry and of concentration in different parts of the cerebrospinal-fluid spaces. Sodium and chloride enter the ventricles through the choroid plexuses at a concentration that can be accounted for only by secretion. Evidence that this process is not simply one of diffusion comes from the fact that these ions do not pass from the ventricle to the blood stream. These ions also enter the cisternal and subarachnoid spaces even after they have been artificially isolated from the ventricles. Water diffuses into all of the cerebrospinal-fluid spaces at the same time, the amount being determined by the content of ions. Blood proteins are selectively filtered out by the vascular endothelium (6500 or 7000 mg/100 ml to 30 mg/100 ml), and this difference requires certain adjustment of Na, K, Cl, and bicarbonate in accordance with the Gibbs-Donnan equation. The cells and part of the protein of the cerebrospinal fluid are derived from ependymal and pial surfaces, that is, along the Virchow-Robin spaces. This point has been verified by studies of radioactive iodinated albumin which has been shown to pass more readily from the blood stream to the cisterna magna and subarachnoid space than to the ventricular. Accordingly, the lumbar fluid contains more cells and has a higher protein content than that from the brain (28 mg of protein per 100 ml in lumbar fluid, as compared with 20 mg/100 ml in cisterna magna, and 10 mg/100 ml in ventricles). Thus one should not think of the cerebrospinal fluid as flowing from the ventricles into the subarachnoid spaces, like urine down the ureter, but rather as both a flow and a diffusion of ions, the concentration of which determines the pressure at any point in the cerebrospinal fluid pathway. The hydrostatic pressure is so great that obstruction at some point in the ventricles or subarachnoid space may cause hydrocephalus of such degree as virtually to destroy the brain. If obstruction is complete, death occurs within a few hours.

The surfaces of the cerebral hemispheres and to a lesser extent of the brain stem and spinal cord are the sites of cerebrospinal-fluid absorption and probably a small amount is also absorbed from the ventricular walls themselves. The mechanism of absorption is unknown. If one assumes that the arachnoidal villi are capable of transferring protein from the cerebrospinal fluid into the veins, the movement of water molecules would follow, in order to maintain the balance between hydrostatic and osmotic forces. This hypothesis would account for the opposite effect—an elevation of intracranial pressure that accompanies a high protein level in the cerebrospinal fluid (higher than 500–1000 mg/100 ml).

The only known function of the cerebrospinal fluid is a mechanical one, to provide a protective water jacket for the brain and spinal cord. No specific metabolic activity has been discovered, though the fluid may aid in the removal of certain waste products from the perivascular spaces and surface of the brain.

### INDICATIONS FOR EXAMINATION OF THE CEREBROSPINAL FLUID

The cerebrospinal fluid is obtained for examination by a needle puncture of the lumbar subarachnoid space below the caudal end of the spinal cord, at the interspaces between lumbar vertebrae 2–3, 3–4, or 4–5. Occasionally a puncture of the cisterna magna, or, as a special surgical procedure, of the occipital horn of the lateral ventricle, is necessary. Under proper conditions of asepsis, a lumbar puncture can be performed safely in all cases except those with obviously elevated intracranial pressure or skin sepsis in the lumbar region.

The examination of the cerebrospinal fluid is of value in the diagnosis and treatment of neurologic diseases, particularly those listed in Table 57. It is especially useful in the diagnosis of inflammatory diseases and hemorrhage in the meninges. The existence of increased intracranial pressure can also be confirmed by lumbar puncture but caution must be exercised because of the danger of provoking a fatal herniation of the temporal lobe or cerebellum. Although lumbar puncture is regarded by many physicians as an essential part of the neurologic examination, it should be realized that it is only an accessory method in diagnosis and often does not contribute conclusive data. The procedure should include measurement of the spinal-fluid pressure, and removal of fluid for inspection, cell counts, determination of protein content, serologic examination for syphilis, and under certain circumstances bacteriologic examination, and measurement of glucose content. With suspected compressive lesions or tumors of the spinal cord, the dynamic changes in cerebrospinal-fluid pressure upon compression of jugular veins and compression of the abdomen should also be tested.

### PATHOLOGIC PHYSIOLOGY OF CEREBROSPINAL FLUID

ELEVATION OF THE CEREBROSPINAL-FLUID PRESSURE. The normal pressure of the cerebrospinal fluid (CSF), which ranges from 50 to 180 mm-of-water, is maintained by the hydrostatic pressure in the capillaries and other small vessels in the brain. In circulatory collapse this pressure falls. With uncomplicated arterial hypertension it rises, but only slightly because the capillary pressure, even in severe hypertension, is increased relatively little. The cerebrospinal-fluid pressure becomes elevated whenever there is an increase in the contents of the cranial

| Diseases affecting cerebrospinal fluid (lumbar puncture) | Initial pressure, patient in horizontal position (mm of spinal fluid) | Appearance | Number of cells/mm$^3$ | Protein (mg/100 ml) | Glucose (mg/100 ml) | Colloidal gold | Comment |
|---|---|---|---|---|---|---|---|
| *Normal cerebrospinal fluid* | | | | | | | |
| NORMAL Ventricular Cisternal Lumbar | 70–180 | Clear colorless no clot | 0–3 0–5 0–5 | 5–15 10–25 15–45 | 55–85 50–80 50–80 | 0000000000 or 000100000 0012100000 | Sugar values apply to fasting normal subjects |
| *Aseptic meningeal reaction* to brain abscess, sinus thrombosis, epidural abscess, subdural empyema | | | | | | | |
| Aseptic meningeal reaction | 130–750+, usually increased | Clear, cloudy or turbid; may be xanthochromic | Usually 5–500 Occasionally 2000 | 20–200+ | 40–110, usually normal | Variable | Meningeal reaction to a septic focus in dura, cranium, or in brain; neutrophils often predominate, especially if cell count high; sugar usually normal |
| *Septic meningeal reaction* to pyogenic organisms | | | | | | | |
| Acute purulent meningitis | Normal to 500; usually elevated; rarely over 500, except with cerebellar pressure cone | Opalescent to purulent, faint yellow coarse clot | 500–20,000, chiefly neutrophils | 50–1500 | 0–45 (may be normal if antibiotics given) | Variable, rarely first zone | Rarely white count below 100; sugar nearly always reduced; organisms in sediment and culture |
| *Tuberculous meningitis.* Note the importance of the sugar concentration. When low, it suggests infection in contrast to an aseptic meningeal reaction. The predominance of lymphocytes and decreased sugar are important in the diagnosis of tuberculous meningitis | | | | | | | |
| Tuberculous meningitis | 150–500 | Opalescent, faint yellow, delicate clot | 25–500, chiefly lymphocytes | 45–500+ | 0–45 | Usually mid zone or normal | Sugar usually falls progressively; tubercle bacilli in clot, sediment |
| *Syphilitic infections* of brain and spinal cord. Note the difficulty of distinguishing syphilitic meningitis from other forms of meningitis and the importance of the Wassermann reactions in the spinal fluid, the colloidal-gold curve, the lymphocytosis, and elevated protein in all forms of active neurosyphilis | | | | | | | |
| Acute syphilitic meningitis (untreated) | Usually increased; occasionally normal; rarely elevated up to 400 or more if hydrocephalus is present | Clear and colorless, rarely xanthochromic | 25–500, chiefly lymphocytes | 45–300 | Usually normal; rarely decreased | First zone, 40%; mid zone, 55%; normal, 5% | Wassermann positive in CSF and blood; difficult at times to differentiate from tbc meningitis, brain abscess |
| Dementia paralytica (untreated) | Normal | Normal, clot rarely present | 15–150+, chiefly lymphocytes | 50–300 | Normal | First zone, occasionally mid zone | Serologic tests for syphilis positive in CSF and blood; CSF findings may occur in any form of neurosyphilis |
| Tabes dorsalis (untreated) | Normal | Normal | 10–80+ | 25–100+ | Normal | Mid zone or first zone | Serologic tests for syphilis practically always positive in CSF; normal fluid not uncommon in "burnt out" cases; findings depend on degree of accompanying syphilitic meningitis |
| Meningovascular neurosyphilis | Normal | Normal | 6–100, 55%; normal, 45% | 45–150, 70%; normal, 30% | Normal | Normal, 35%; first zone, 15%; mid zone, 50% | Serologic tests for syphilis give positive results in CSF and blood in active stages; other findings depend on degree of accompanying syphilitic meningitis |
| *Virus infections* of brain and spinal cord. Note that in the virus infections the sugar level of the cerebrospinal fluid is normal, that the cellular reaction is almost exclusively lymphocytic, and that the protein level seldom is found initially above 100 mg/100 ml. The Wassermann reaction is negative | | | | | | | |
| Acute anterior poliomyelitis | Usually normal; may be elevated | Clear or slightly opalescent; colorless or faint yellow; may be clot | 10–500+ lymphocytes and neutrophils | 20–350; often progressive increase | Normal | Normal or mid zone | Cell count rarely normal, usually under 300 with progressive decrease in total cells and percent of neutrophils; protein usually increased for several weeks |
| Herpes zoster | Normal | Normal | 0–500, often increased | 20–110 | Normal | Usually normal | Cells practically all lymphocytes, appearing early and persisting several weeks; protein increase may persist several months |

| Diseases affecting cerebrospinal fluid (lumbar puncture) | Initial pressure, patient in horizontal position (mm of spinal fluid) | Appearance | Number of cells/mm³ | Protein (mg/100 ml) | Glucose (mg/100 ml) | Colloidal gold | Comment |
|---|---|---|---|---|---|---|---|
| Mumps meningitis | Normal or slightly increased | Normal or opalescent | 0–2000+, chiefly lymphocytes | 20–125 | Normal | Usually mid zone | Lymphocytes increased in many cases of mumps even in absence of meningeal signs |
| Other virus infections: choriomeningitis; encephalitis due to equine, St. Louis, and other viruses | Normal or increased | Normal or slightly turbid | 10–3000, usually less than 200 | 20–200+ | Normal | Normal or mid zone | Lymphocytes predominate in choriomeningitis excess of polychromatophilic cells, occasionally in equine type |
| Postinfectious encephalomyelitis | *Postinfectious encephalomyelitis* 80–450; often slightly increased | Normal | 25–1000, chiefly lymphocytes | 15–75 | Normal | Normal or slight change | Cells rarely exceed 200 |

*Vascular accidents.* CSF is of aid in differential diagnosis of vascular disease of the brain. It should be stressed that brain hemorrhage, hemorrhagic infarcts due to embolism, subarachnoid hemorrhage from aneurysm will all produce a bloody CSF

| | | | | | | | |
|---|---|---|---|---|---|---|---|
| "Bloody tap" | Normal or low | Bloody with clot; supernatant fluid colorless | Many red blood cells and white cells in same proportion as those in blood | Normal or increased, depending on amount of blood | Normal | Normal, unless red blood cells over 20,000 | Variation in amount of blood in different tubes clotting may occur; approximately 1 wbc added with every 500 rbc and mg of protein/100 ml with 1000 rbc |
| Cerebral thrombosis | Normal, 75%; 180–400, 25% | Normal | Normal, 75%; 6–50, 25% | Normal, 60%; 46–100+, 40% | Normal | Usually normal | Pressure over 200 or a protein greater than 100 mg suggests the possibility of brain tumor |
| Cerebral hemorrhage | Normal, 20%; 180–300, 40%; over 400, 40%. | Normal, 15%; bloody, 75%; xanthochromic, 10% | Many red blood cells, 75% | 20–2000, usually increased | Normal | Variable | The elevated pressure and the blood are the important changes but do not distinguish brain hemorrhage from head injury and subarachnoid hemorrhage |
| Subarachnoid hemorrhage (primary) | 110–700+, usually increased | Bloody, xanthochromic within 12–24 hr; no clot | Many red blood cells | 20–1000+, usually increased | Normal | Variable | Must be distinguished from "bloody tap"; white cell count may increase 24 to 48 hr |
| Cerebral trauma | 0–500, usually increased | Normal, bloody or xanthochromic | Often many red blood cells | 20–1000+, increased if bloody | Normal | Variable | Normal in concussion nearly always bloody with brain laceration |
| Subdural hematoma | 180–600+, 80%; normal, 20% | Normal, bloody only in cases with associated contusion | Normal (red blood cells with contusion) | Normal or slightly elevated | Normal | Variable | Fluid may be bloody after injury but quite normal in patients dying of epidural or subdural hematoma |

*Tumors.* The cellular reaction to tumors of the brain and cord is usually lymphocytic, but highly variable. The presence of increased protein in conjunction with increased pressure is of the greatest value

| | | | | | | | |
|---|---|---|---|---|---|---|---|
| Brain tumor: subtentorial | 150–800+, usually above 220 | Clear, occasionally xanthochromic | Normal, 80%; 6–25, 15%; 26–150, 5% | 30–500 (see comment) | Normal | Variable; normal, 30%; first zone, 10% | Cells chiefly lymphocytic pressure cone may develop; protein varies with type of tumor, high in acoustic neuroma |
| supratentorial | 150–800+, usually above 220 | Clear, occasionally xanthochromic | Normal, 70%; 6–25, 20%; 26–150+, 10% | 20–300 (see comment | Normal | Variable; normal, 40%; first zone, 2% | Cells chiefly lymphocytic rarely over 100; increased protein related to invasion of the ventricular walls or meninges |
| Cord tumor | Normal or low | Clear, colorless or xanthochromic, clot often present if protein over 500 | Normal, 60%; 6–100, 40%; chiefly lymphocytes | 36–45, 15%; 46–3500; 85% | Normal | Variable | Complete or partial subarachnoid block practically always present; yellow fluid with high protein may show spontaneous clotting (loculation block may occur in Pott's disease, fracture or location of vertebra acute and chronic meningitis, epidural abscess, |

Table 57. *Cerebrospinal fluid in differential diagnosis* (*modified from Merritt and Fremont-Smith* [46]) (*continued*).

| Diseases affecting cerebrospinal fluid (lumbar puncture) | Initial pressure, patient in horizontal position (mm of spinal fluid) | Appearance | Number of cells/mm³ | Protein (mg/100 ml) | Glucose (mg/100 ml) | Colloidal gold | Comment |
|---|---|---|---|---|---|---|---|
| | | | *Other Abnormalities* | | | | |
| Epilepsy (idiopathic) | Normal | Normal | Normal | Normal | Normal | Normal | Brain tumor should be suspected when pressure is above 200 or protein is greater than 100 gm/100 ml |
| Multiple sclerosis | Normal | Normal | Normal, 70%; 6–40, 30% | Normal, 75%; 45–130, 25%; increase in gamma globulin in 75–80% of cases | Normal | Normal or slight change, 50%; first zone, 25%; mid zone, 25% | Slight lymphocytosis in 30%; negative test for syphilis with abnormal colloidal-gold curve is evidence for multiple sclerosis |
| Polyneuritis (spinal-fluid changes differ in the various types of polyneuritis) | Normal | Normal; xanthochromic if protein is markedly elevated | Normal | 20–1500 | Normal | Variable | In alcoholic polyneuritis, polyarteritic polyneuritis, beri-beri, porphyric polyneuritis, and arsenical polyneuritis the protein is usually normal; in diphtheritic and diabetic polyneuritis the protein is moderately elevated, 50–300; in acute infectious polyneuritis, very high protein levels may occur; with increased protein, fluid is often xanthochromic, rarely clots spontaneously; colloidal gold may show any type of curve; pressure increased with respiratory paralysis |
| Lead encephalopathy | Increased | Normal or slightly yellow | 0–100, increased usually, lymphocytes predominate | 20–100 | Normal | Variable | Pressure nearly always increased; lead is present in the fluid |

cavity, that is, the brain tissue, the cerebrospinal fluid, and blood. Accordingly, the CSF pressure closely parallels that of the jugular vein and is, therefore, elevated in heart failure or obstruction of the superior mediastinum and of the jugular veins, because of the increased venous pressure. Tumors, abscesses, and other space-consuming lesions raise intracranial pressure by increasing the volume of brain tissue and by obstructing the flow of cerebrospinal fluid, thus producing hydrocephalus. Except when there is herniation of the brain into the notch of the tentorium or into the foramen magnum, this intracranial pressure is freely transmitted to all parts of the spinal and cranial subarachnoid space and can, therefore, be measured through a lumbar-puncture needle.

When the lumbar puncture is done to determine the CSF pressure, the following steps are advised. The patient should lie on his side with his head on the same horizontal level as the sacrum (elevation of the head will cause an elevation of lumbar pressure). A water manometer, preferably the Ayer type, should be used. The pressure should be measured before any fluid has escaped or has been withdrawn. The patient should be relaxed, since nervous tension, breath holding, and straining elevate the pressure markedly. The legs should be straightened if the patient is obese because pressure of the thighs against the abdomen can raise the intraspinal pressure. Jugular compression in cases of raised intracranial pressure or of tumors of posterior fossa is contraindicated because of the danger of herniation of the brain, and, unless there is need of verification of the pressure, the procedure should be undertaken only with caution.

BLOCK IN THE SPINAL SUBARACHNOID SPACE. The testing of the dynamics of the CSF should be employed only when lesions of the spinal cord or spinal roots are suspected. A block in the subarachnoid space of the spinal canal can be tested by lumbar puncture or by combined lumbar and cisternal puncture. As stated above, there is normally free communication between the cranial and spinal subarachnoid space. Compression of both jugular veins, which increases the volume of blood within the cranial cavity, will promptly raise the intracranial pressure. This is immediately transmitted to the lumbar subarachnoid space and through the lumbar-puncture needle to the manometer. The pressure rises by 100 to 300 mm-of-water within 20 sec and usually falls to the original level within another 20 sec after the release of the jugular veins. This is called Queckenstedt's phenomenon. With spinal subarachnoid block, as produced by tumor or fracture-dislocation of a vertebra, the rise is slight and much slower than normal.

With combined cisternal and lumbar punctures, normal pressure changes appear only in the cisternal manometer. Abdominal pressure and straining, on the other hand, elevate the CSF pressure by producing congestion of the spinal veins. The rise and fall of spinal subarachnoid pressure obtained by this maneuver is as prompt as that which follows jugular compression. Sometimes the CSF pressure does not rise upon compression of the jugular veins because the point of the needle is touching the meninges. To avoid this error, the patency of the manometric system should always be tested by abdominal compression. The compression of one jugular vein at a time is of relatively little value, although it has been suggested as a test of thrombosis of the lateral sinus. Failure of the CSF pressure to rise with compression of a thrombosed jugular vein is called the Tobey-Ayer test. If the jugular veins cannot be located, a blood-pressure cuff is wrapped around the neck and quickly inflated to 40 mm-of-mercury, held for 20 sec, then released. An increase in total protein, sometimes to several thousand milligrams per 100 ml with xanthochromia and spontaneous clotting, accompanies a partial subarachnoid block (Froin's syndrome).[48]

EFFECT OF INFECTION ON CEREBROSPINAL FLUID. Inflammatory diseases of the nervous system and particularly of the meninges produce characteristic abnormalities in the cerebrospinal fluid.[49-52] Purulent meningitis, which is essentially an empyema of the subarachnoid space, causes alterations in CSF similar to those occurring in other infected body cavities. The pressure is usually elevated because of the increased rate of CSF formation, congestion of meningeal blood vessels, and at times interference with CSF circulation and absorption. Leukocytosis, predominantly of neutrophils, is presumably due to the presence of chemotactic substances in the subarachnoid spaces. The blood proteins, albumin, globulins, and fibrinogen exude through inflamed meningeal blood vessels in abnormal quantities. The sugar is decreased owing to the glycolytic action of bacteria and, to a slight degree, of cells. The chloride concentration may be decreased when there is a decrease in serum chloride concentration, or through the Donnan effect as the result of an increase in the protein content of the CSF.

The number of cells, the type of cells, the degree of change in protein and sugar values, special tests like the Wassermann reaction, and above all the presence of the causative organisms in films and cultures permit an exact diagnosis of the etiology of the meningitis.

XANTHOCHROMIA IN CEREBROSPINAL FLUID. Normally the CSF is colorless, containing no bilirubin. Xanthochromia is a general term indicating a yellow color of the CSF. There are at least three mechanisms that produce xanthochromia. (i) In subarachnoid hemorrhage, bilirubin is formed from hemoglobin within 3 to 4 hr after a vascular accident. This pigment gives an indirect diazo reaction (van den Bergh).[47] Oxyhemoglobin (tested by benzidine) and methemoglobin (brown to black color) also form to varying degrees. The bilirubin of the CSF increases for the first 4 to 7 days and then decreases until, by the 10th to 20th day, depending on the amount of blood, the fluid is usually clear. However, with large subarachnoid hemorrhages, enough serum enters the subarachnoid space to give some coloring to the CSF immediately. In normal premature infants, there is regularly an increase in bilirubin (indirect diazo reaction) in the CSF that lasts for several weeks.[47] (ii) Bilirubin appears in the CSF in severe jaundice, particularly of the obstructive type. The presence of bilirubin in the CSF under these conditions is comparable to the passage of conjugated bilirubin into the urine (see Unit 24). (iii) In the CSF with high protein content, as in Froin's syndrome,[47, 48] there is xanthochromia. Almost any fluid with a protein content of over 150 mg/ 100 ml will be faintly yellow. The pigment is probably bilirubin.

In the examination of xanthochromic CSF, it is of practical value to attempt to differentiate between the pigments from hemorrhage, jaundice, and high protein content. The finding of oxyhemoglobin or methemoglobin by spectrographic analysis, or, in the instance of oxyhemoglobin, by the benzidine test, is of value in establishing the existence of recent hemorrhage. These techniques (Units 5 and 11) are applicable to the CSF. Also, bilirubin can be detected by spectrophotometer and the wavelength at which the pigments are seen serves to distinguish the bilirubin bound to protein from the unconjugated forms that enter the CSF when the serum bilirubin is greatly elevated, as in jaundice due either to biliary obstruction or to hepatocellular disease. The van den Bergh test can be adapted for purposes of measuring the relatively small quantities of pigment in the CSF. The total protein measurement provides the clue usually to faintly yellow fluids when its concentration is high and bilirubin and other blood pigments are absent.[53]

### LIMITATIONS AND INTERPRETATIONS IN THE RESULTS OF LUMBAR PUNCTURE

The pathologic physiology of changes in pressure in the CSF has already been discussed, and the variety of changes observed in disease of the brain and spinal cord are indicated in Table 57. Common sources of error in measurement or in the interpretation of pressure of the CSF and blood are as follows.

ELEVATION OF CEREBROSPINAL-FLUID PRESSURE. Since an elevation of CSF pressure is significant evidence for disease of the central nervous system, it is important to recognize the conditions in which the pressure is falsely elevated: (*a*) if the patient's head is elevated above the horizontal level of the lumbar region; (*b*) if the patient is not relaxed and thereby increases the venous pressure by straining; and (*c*) if the venous pressure is increased as in heart disease or obstruction to the superior vena cava.

LOW CEREBROSPINAL-FLUID PRESSURE. Low pressure of the CSF but with some response to jugular compression may occur in circulatory collapse or from measurement of the pressure after removing the CSF or when the CSF has continued to leak from a previous tap.

Low pressure of the CSF that fails to respond to jugular compression may be falsely interpreted as resulting from block under the following conditions: (*a*) the operator may be unsuccessful in occluding the jugular veins so that no rise occurs in pressure; (*b*) the manometer system may not be patent, the point of the needle being occluded by contact with a solid structure such as the meninges or a nerve root.

BLOOD IN THE CEREBROSPINAL FLUID. A "bloody tap" resulting from injury of a meningeal vessel may be mistaken for subarachnoid hemorrhage (see Table 57). With a bloody tap, the pressure is often low, and the CSF is not evenly mixed with blood and tends to clear progressively as it is collected in separate small samples. If much blood is present, the CSF clots but the supernatant fluid after centrifugation is clear and colorless. Conversely, in subarachnoid hemorrhage the distribution of blood is uniform and the supernatant fluid after centrifugation shows xanthochromia. The blood does not clot because it is defibrinated within the subarachnoid space.

SIGNIFICANCE OF CLOTTING. When the CSF is bloody, a sample should be centrifuged immediately and the supernatant fluid examined for xanthochromia. A few red cells (50 to 100/mm³) may be found in apparently nontraumatic lumbar punctures and can usually be disregarded. Red cells may be mistaken for lymphocytes in the counting chamber and a false lymphocytosis reported. Since a lymphocytosis of 5 to 100 cells/mm³ has an important clinical significance, the results of a chamber count should be confirmed by examining a stained film of the fluid (p. 273).

In tuberculous meningitis, a delicate weblike clot forms frequently in spinal fluid but may also be observed in syphilitic meningitis, aseptic meningeal reaction, poliomyelitis, and brain tumor. A coarse fibrin clot may be found in fluids that are also grossly purulent. Jellylike clots occasionally form in spinal fluid containing high levels of protein, as obtained in cases of subarachnoid block or polyneuritis. The clotting of CSF from a bloody tap and the lack of clotting in subarachnoid hemorrhage are discussed above.

TESTS FOR PROTEIN CONTENT OF
CEREBROSPINAL FLUID

PANDY TEST FOR CEREBROSPINAL FLUID. Pandy's solution is a saturated aqueous solution of carbolic acid that precipitates both albumin and globulin. To perform the test, 1.0 ml of Pandy's solution is placed in a small test tube, 1 drop of cerebrospinal fluid is added, and the results are read immediately. In a normal fluid only the faintest opalescence is observed. In a fluid with an increased protein content, a smokelike white cloud develops immediately wherever the drop comes in contact with the acid. When there is only a slight increase in protein content of the fluid, it is difficult to estimate the concentration by this rough screening test.

ROSS-JONES TEST FOR GLOBULINS IN CEREBROSPINAL FLUID. This is a crude qualitative test for the presence of globulins. Approximately 0.5 ml of cerebrospinal fluid is placed in a small tube and 0.5 ml of a saturated solution of ammonium sulfate is carefully underlaid with a pipette to prevent mixing. If globulins are present, a turbid white ring appears within approximately 2 min. The precipitation of globulins is produced by approximately half-saturated ammonium sulfate solution that occurs at the junction of saturated ammonium sulfate and cerebrospinal fluid. The test should be read after 2 min against a black background with indirect light to detect the fine colloidal ring of precipitate at the interface when the result is positive. The test differs from the Pandy test in that it is quite specific for globulins which are present in significant amounts only in abnormal cerebrospinal fluids.

QUANTITATIVE DETERMINATION OF PROTEIN. The concentration of protein in body fluids may be determined by the same chemical, physical, and immunochemical methods as are employed for blood plasma, including the separation of albumin and globulin (see Unit 16).

ELECTROPHORESIS OF CEREBROSPINAL FLUID. In multiple sclerosis, the cerebrospinal fluid usually shows an increase in the gamma globulin fraction.[54] The electrophoretic method for the determination of proteins, as described by Kunkel and Tiselius,[55] seems to be well adapted for the study of cerebrospinal fluid. The technique is similar to that used for the plasma proteins (Unit 16). The CSF should be concentrated prior to electrophoresis by dialyzing it in a Visking casing against 25-percent polyvinyl pyrrolidone in barbital buffer. A rough estimate of the globulin content in the cerebrospinal fluid can be made by the zinc sulfate test, as described by Donovan et al.[56]

CELL COUNT AND DIFFERENTIAL COUNT
OF WHITE CELLS

The cell count for CSF and the fluids of other body cavities is performed on a hemocytometer as described in Unit 4. The differential count may be crudely performed by examining the cells in the hemocytometer. This method is not reliable and for exact identification of cells and accurate determination of the differential count a film, stained with Wright's stain, should be prepared from a centrifuged sample of fluid, the cells being resuspended in serum. The cell counts should be made promptly after the fluid has been obtained. Cells are counted in the manner described for serous effusions in body cavities (p. 271). Anticoagulants are usually unnecessary.

CONCENTRATION OF GLUCOSE IN
CEREBROSPINAL FLUID

The glucose concentration of CSF may be measured by any of the methods used to determine blood sugar. It is usually 10–20 mg/100 ml lower than the concentration in venous blood, which should be measured at the same time for comparison. A semiquantitative test for CSF glucose content is described below. This is of occasional value in rapidly detecting gross deviations from the normal when quantitative determinations are not readily available.

SEMIQUANTITATIVE METHOD FOR ESTIMATION OF GLUCOSE IN CEREBROSPINAL FLUID. Into each of five small test tubes, 1.0 ml of Benedict's qualitative sugar reagent is introduced (see Unit 19). CSF is added with a serologic pipette, 0.05 ml (1 drop) being introduced into the first tube, 0.10 ml into the second, 0.15 ml into the third, 0.20 ml into the fourth, and 0.25 ml into the fifth. The tubes are heated in a gently boiling water bath for 5 min and allowed to cool. The qualitative Benedict's reaction for a normal spinal fluid will usually show a color change to faint green, greenish-yellow, or olive in the fourth and fifth tubes and sometimes in the third tube. Such a reaction indicates a sugar level of 50 mg/100 ml or more. The absence of a reduction reaction in the fifth tube denotes a pathologically decreased concentration of sugar and is of significance. Such a lowered sugar level might be produced by low blood glucose concentration or by the presence of bacteria or other infectious agents in the CSF. A reduction reaction occurring in the fifth tube but not in the fourth tube is a borderline result and usually corresponds to a sugar value of from 40 to 60 mg/100 ml. If this test is done carefully, the results are reliable, but they should not supplant the more accurate quantitative analysis by the standard sugar methods or by the Somogyi method. If the fluid contains an increase in protein but no sugar, there may be a deep purple, violet, or pink-violet color resulting from the biuret reaction of protein with copper.

### TESTS FOR SYPHILIS ON CEREBROSPINAL FLUID

The complement-fixation or precipitin tests for the reagin of syphilis may be performed qualitatively and quantitatively on both the cerebrospinal fluid and the blood serum of a patient suspected of syphilis.[57] In syphilis of the central nervous system, the Wassermann test may give a positive result in the spinal fluid and a positive or a negative one in the blood serum. A strongly positive Wassermann-test result in syphilis of the central nervous system may occur in cerebrospinal fluid that shows a normal cell count or a normal protein content, or both. A positive result obtained on spinal fluid rarely occurs in the absence of neurologic syphilis. Rare exceptions are leprosy, trypanosomiasis, and yaws (frambesia). False positive Wassermann reactions may occur, rarely, if negative spinal fluid is contaminated by blood that is Wassermann positive (from subarachnoid hemorrhage or a bloody spinal tap).

### TEST OF CEREBROSPINAL FLUID WITH COLLOIDAL GOLD

The test of CSF with colloidal gold demonstrates the presence of abnormal proteins.[58] The procedure depends upon changes in color as well as precipitation produced by the addition of varying dilutions of cerebrospinal fluid to a colloidal solution of gold. The changes that occur in the colloidal gold apparently result from qualitative and quantitative alterations in the proteins of the CSF. The normal protein content of CSF produces no change. Qualitatively, the globulins produce maximum change in the colloidal gold, whereas albumin appears to have protective action in preventing changes in the colloidal gold. Quantitatively, the total protein concentration may be significantly elevated without affecting the colloidal gold, provided the ratio of albumin to globulin is high. Experimentally, if such a fluid is diluted

before testing, the protective action of albumin may be so reduced that the remaining globulins may produce change in the colloidal gold. This colloidal-gold test serves as an indirect method for detecting protein changes in CSF. It is usually performed in a special laboratory that is equipped to prepare and use the solution of colloidal gold under standardized conditions. The pH of the reaction mixture should be adjusted to 7.4 to prevent false positive results.[58] The test and the interpretation of results are outlined below.

**Method.** Ten clean, dry tubes are placed in a rack. Cerebrospinal fluid is added and diluted serially with aqueous sodium chloride, 0.85 gm/100 ml, from 1:10 to 1:5120. An equal volume of a solution of colloidal gold at pH 7.4 is added to each of the tubes, which are then covered and allowed to stand at room temperature over night. The changes produced in the color of the colloidal-gold solution are read and graded from 0 to 5 by the following arbitrary scale: 0, no change in the red color of the solution; 1, very slight change to a deeper red; 2, lilac color; 3, blue color; 4, blue with some precipitation of colloidal gold; 5, complete precipitation of the gold with clear, colorless supernatant fluid.

INTERPRETATION. In a normal cerebrospinal fluid there should be no change in the color of the solutions in any tube. A 1 or 2 change in the colloidal gold occurs occasionally in the third through the fifth tubes in cerebrospinal fluids that show no other abnormalities. In reporting the results of the test, the appearance of the colloidal gold in each tube is graded and recorded from left to right, from the lowest dilution to the highest dilution of the spinal fluid. Usually the results are reported as a curve with 0 on the base line and the numbers, up to 5, plotted on the ordinate. The tubes are indicated in order of dilution from left to right on the abscissa. These methods of reporting have given rise to the arbitrary terms "first-zone curve" (5543210000 or 4443210000), "mid-zone curve" (0012332000), or "end-zone curve" (0001123333). These types of curves have been found by Merritt and Fremont-Smith [46] to occur as follows.

*First Zone.* Changes are observed frequently in CSF containing increased globulins in such conditions as syphilis of the central nervous system and in multiple sclerosis. These changes may occur rarely in acute purulent meningitis, tuberculous meningitis, brain tumor, brain abscess, acute encephalomye-litis, aseptic meningeal reaction, or polyneuritis, or in fluids contaminated by blood due to cerebral hemorrhage or cerebral trauma.

*Mid Zone.* Changes are found in any abnormal fluid, especially those containing increased albumin and globulin. Therefore these results have no definite value in differential diagnosis.

*End Zone.* Changes are ordinarily found in fluids with a high protein content of 500 mg/100 ml or more, such as occurs in acute purulent meningitis, or subarachnoid block (Froin's syndrome) from any cause, and extravasation of blood into the subarachnoid space.

## SYNOVIAL FLUID

### NORMAL SYNOVIAL FLUID [59]

The synovial cavity is a mesodermal space, lined by flattened mesenchymal cells, rather than a true membrane; its fluid is embryologically and in many other respects analogous to the extracellular fluid or its histologic counterpart, the "intracellular matrix." Histologic, physiologic, and chemical studies bear out this analogy. Histologically, the cells of the synovial fluid consist of lymphocytes, monocytes, polymorphonuclear leukocytes, and clasmatocytes. The latter cells are identical with the histiocytes or wandering macrophages of loose connective tissue. Physiologically, only a few facts are known. Studies of the passage of substances across the blood-synovial-fluid barrier indicate fairly free diffusion of water and small molecular substances. Proteins enter the fluid and leave in a manner analogous to extracellular fluid; they enter by diffusion, but leave by way of the lymph. When particulate matter is injected into the joint, or accumulates as cellular detritus, it is removed primarily through a process of phagocytosis.

Normal synovial fluid is a clear amber fluid that does not clot on standing. Chemically, it closely resembles edema fluid or lymph. Except for calcium, which exists in joint fluid in increased concentration, presumably owing to its binding by the mucopolysaccharides, the electrolyte concentrations of synovial fluid and plasma are related in accordance with the Gibbs-Donnan equilibrium. The proteins of the synovial fluid have been shown to be identical with those of the plasma, although there are certain differences in concentration. The one chemical characteristic of the synovial fluid that differentiates it sharply from serum is hyaluronic acid, which is thought to be responsible for its viscosity. Hyaluronic acid can readily be precipitated as a protein complex, which is referred to by the term "mucin." Whether or not this complex is present in vitro is subject to discussion. There is considerable evidence that the hyaluronic acid is synthesized by the mesenchymal cells which line the synovial cavity.

### METHODS OF OBTAINING AND ANALYZING SYNOVIAL FLUID

OBTAINING SYNOVIAL FLUID. The analyses that are commonly carried out on synovial fluid for diagnostic purposes are as follows: cell count, differential count, estimation of the amount of clot, if present,[59] and of the amount and quality of "mucin," and glucose concentration (to be compared with simultaneous blood-glucose determination). In addition, bacteriologic culture and guinea pig inoculation may be carried out if indicated.

The fluid is withdrawn in a sterile syringe; a needle with a stylet is preferable, but not essential. Since the fluid may, on occasion, be so viscous that it will not pass through a No. 19 needle, attempts at aspiration should not be abandoned until a No. 15 needle has been used. The needle is customarily inserted approximately 2 cm medial or lateral to the patella. It may then be passed into the suprapatellar pouch, or posterior to the patella.

When the fluid is obtained, 2–4 ml should be placed in a "double oxalate" tube containing 3 mg of ammonium oxalate and 2 mg of potassium oxalate for 5 ml of blood or fluid. If smaller amounts of fluid are to be used, part of the oxalate should be discarded. The fluid should be mixed with the oxalate with great thoroughness, since its extreme viscosity tends to prevent satisfactory mixing. Two or 3 ml of fluid are cultured. Two to 5 ml are placed in a tube containing 5 mg of potassium oxalate and 5 mg of sodium fluoride for glucose determination. The remainder of the fluid, ideally 2 ml or more, is placed in a test tube or, better, a centrifuge tube for clot and mucin estimation.

CELL COUNTS. With normal synovial fluid, or that from effusions due to trauma, the cell count should be made directly on the undiluted fluid. With more cellular effusions, the count is carried out in the same manner as a white-blood-cell count except that the diluting medium consists of 0.85-percent sodium chloride solution with a little (approximately 0.09 percent) methylene blue added. Acetic acid, which is used in blood-counting solution for white cells, is not used for synovial fluid because the acid usually results in precipitation of the mucin in the pipette. The solution used for counting red cells in peripheral blood is not used for synovial fluid since the sodium sulfate exhibits the same effect. Both red-cell and white-cell counts can be performed with the saline–methylene blue diluting mixture and the same chamber.

DIFFERENTIAL COUNT. After the tube containing synovial fluid and oxalate is shaken thoroughly, a minute drop is placed on a coverslip, and a very thin smear is drawn, using a second coverslip, in the same manner used in preparing a blood film (Unit 9). The film is stained with Wright's stain and a differential count is performed. A total of 100 white cells should be examined. Polymorphonuclear leukocytes often exhibit signs of "irritation," with laking or extrusion of the nucleus, and vacuoles and other phagocytized substances in the cytoplasm. Clasmatocytes are irregularly shaped, with small, irregular nuclei and vacuolated cytoplasm containing ingested particulate matter.

EXAMINATION FOR CLOTTING. The fluid without anticoagulant should be examined after 1 hr at room temperature for the presence of a fibrin clot. In normal fluid, no clot is seen. Occasionally the entire fluid has formed a large clot. This is arbitrarily given a grade of 4+, and intermediate degrees of clotting are assigned the grades of 1+, 2+, and 3+ respectively.

EXAMINATION OF MUCIN. The character of the "mucin" is assayed by the following method. The fluid is centrifuged (approximately 2200 rev/min for approximately 10 min) to precipitate cells, debris, and clot, if any has formed. To 1 ml of the clear supernatant is added 4 ml of distilled water. Enough acetic acid is then added to make the final concentration 1 percent (0.13 ml of 7N acetic acid). The solution is stirred well and examined. With normal synovial fluid, a tight clump of ropey material will have formed, surrounded by clear fluid. Upon reexamination 24 hr later, after repeated shaking, the tight coagulum is unchanged. In this instance, the mucin is described as "good." This is taken to indicate that the hyaluronic acid was normally polymerized. In many disease states, however, a different reaction is observed: (i) a good, tight coagulum may form initially, in a slightly cloudy fluid, only to loosen in appearance upon shaking 15 min later; (ii) a thin, shreddy coagulum, surrounded by slightly turbid fluid, may form initially and upon shaking 15 min later may entirely disperse; (iii) no coagulum may form at all, and irregular flecks of mucin may be scattered throughout a murky suspending medium. In these instances, the mucin is described as "fair," "poor," or "very poor," respectively. The exact chemical change that is responsible for these alterations in the precipitation of mucin is not known. It is probably related to depolymerization of the long-chain hyaluronate molecules.

GLUCOSE CONTENT. Normally, the concentration of glucose in the synovial fluid is approximately 10 mg/100 ml lower than that of the blood. It is very difficult to evaluate unless the patient is fasting at the time of aspiration to permit adequate equilibration between fluid and blood. Synovial-fluid sugar determinations should be performed by the Somogyi or macro Folin methods. The micro Folin method may give excessively high values.

INTERPRETATIONS AND LIMITATIONS. The average value for each of the foregoing characteristics, together with the minimum and maximum values one may expect to see, are recorded in Table 58, both for the fluids of normal individuals and for those in various disease states. Synovial-fluid findings alone seldom establish a diagnosis. Thus, rheumatoid arthritis, gouty arthritis, and infectious arthritis may be manifested by identical fluid findings except that cultures in the latter condition are often, but not always, positive. The greatest diagnostic value of synovial-fluid analysis is in differentiating an effusion due to rheumatoid arthritis or infection from that due to a mechanical cause, such as trauma or neuropathy (as in a Charcot joint). In the former instance, there is usually an elevated cell count (chiefly polymorphonuclear cells), and there may be poor mucin; the concentration of glucose may be 20 mg/100 ml or more below that of the blood, and the fluid may clot. In effusions due to a mechanical cause, there is usually only slight deviation from normal.

Occasionally the fluid findings present evidence that provides material assistance in differentiating among the various inflammatory diseases. For example, a white-blood-cell count of 75,000/mm³ or more is most unusual in diseases other than infectious arthritis, especially when accompanied by a differential count that is high in polymorphonuclear cells. Similarly, a decrease in glucose concentration in the synovial fluid to less than 30 mg/100 ml is strong evidence for an infectious process, particularly tuberculosis. It may occur, however, in rheumatoid arthritis of greater than one year's duration. Bloody effusions are of diagnostic importance, provided they do not reflect a "bloody tap." Erythrocyte counts of 200,000/mm³ or more are rarely seen except in hemophilic arthritis, traumatic arthritis with hemorrhage, or hemorrhagic villo-nodular synovitis. Patients with lupus erythematosus disseminata characteristically have effusions that are clear, very viscous, with very good mucin and very few polymorphonuclear cells. In any case in which infectious arthritis is a possibility, cultures should be obtained. When tuberculous arthritis is suspected, the fluid should be inoculated into a guinea pig.

Table 58. *Characteristics of synovial fluids in the normal and in certain diseases of joints.*

| Joint disease (etiology) | Appearance | Clot | Leukocytes (no./mm³) | Neutrophils (percent) | Mucin [a] | Glucose difference [b] (mg/100 ml) |
|---|---|---|---|---|---|---|
| Normal | Clear | 0 | 13–180 (av. 63) | 0–25 (av. 6.5) | Good | 10 |
| *Group 1. Joint diseases, without infection, associated with trauma* | | | | | | |
| Traumatic | Clear | 0–2+ | 200–5800 (av. 1680) | 0–36 (av. 10) | Good (usually) to fair (rarely) | 0–20 (av. 7) |
| Degenerative | Clear | 0–2+ | 70–1950 (av. 520) | 0–58 (av. 8) | Good (usually) to fair (rarely) | 6 |
| *Group 2. Joint diseases, usually distinguishable from Group 1, of unknown or infectious origin* | | | | | | |
| Rheumatic fever | Slightly turbid | 0–3+ | 1000–63,000 (av. 10,000) | 8–98 (av. 46) | Fair to good | 6 |
| Gout | Turbid | ±–2+ | 1000–31,000 (av. 14,000) | 48–94 (av. 83) | Poor to fair | 0–41 |
| Rheumatoid | Clear to turbid | 0–3+ | 600–66,000 (av. 14,000) | 5–96 (av. 65) | Poor (usually) to fair (rarely good) | 0–88 (av. 31) |
| Tuberculous | Turbid | 0–2+ | 2500–105,000 (av. 23,500) | 29–96 (av. 67) | Poor (usually) to fair | 0–108 (av. 57) |
| Gonorrheal | Turbid | 0 to 3+ | 1500–108,000 (av. 14,000) | 2–96 (av. 65) | Poor to fair | 0–97 (av. 26) |
| Septic | Very turbid | 2+–3+ | 25,000–213,000 (av. 65,000) | 75–100 (av. 95) | May progress from good to poor | 40–122 (av. 71) |

[a] *Good:* firm clot, clear supernatant; *Fair:* clot somewhat softer, supernatant somewhat turbid; *Poor:* flocculant precipitate, turbid supernatant.

[b] Refers to difference between sugar concentration in joint fluid and fasting blood, taken at the time of joint tap.

Because of its ready availability, and the fact that it is frequently of diagnostic assistance, synovial fluid should be examined in every case of arthritis of unknown etiology, manifested by effusion. It is often worth while to attempt aspiration in cases that present with a hot, tender joint, not completely explained by other known diseases, whether or not an effusion is evident on clinical grounds, in order to obtain material for culture.

## REFERENCES

1. E. H. Starling, "On the absorption of fluids from the connective tissue spaces," *J. Physiol. 19*, 312 (1895).
2. E. M. Landis, "The passage of fluid through the capillary wall," *Harvey Lect.* 32, 70 (1936).
3. J. R. Pappenheimer, "Passage of molecules through capillary walls," *Physiol. Rev. 33*, 387 (1953).
4. J. P. Peters, "Water balance in health and disease," in G. G. Duncan, ed., *Diseases of Metabolism* (ed. 3; Saunders, Philadelphia, 1952).

5. R. E. Hyatt and J. R. Smith, "The mechanism of ascites," *Amer. J. Med. 16,* 434 (1954).

6. S. Sherlock, *Diseases of the Liver and Biliary System* (ed. 2; Blackwell Scientific Publications, Oxford, 1958).

7. H. P. Wolff, K. R. Koczorelt, and E. Buckborn, "Aldosterone and antidiuretic hormone in liver disease," *Acta endocr. 27,* 45 (1958).

8. H. C. Hinshaw and H. L. Garland, *Diseases of the Chest* (Saunders, Philadelphia, 1956).

9. E. C. Lenallen and D. T. Carr, "Pleural effusion: A statistical study of 436 patients," *New Engl. J. Med. 252,* 79 (1955).

10. P. H. Wood, *Diseases of the Heart and Circulation* (ed. 2; Lippincott, Philadelphia, 1956).

11. A. M. Harvey and M. R. Whitehill, "Tuberculous pericarditis," *Medicine 16,* 45 (1937).

12. F. Paddock, "The diagnostic significance of serous fluids in disease," *New Engl. J. Med. 223,* 1010 (1940).

13. A. I. Spriggs, *The Cytology of Effusions in the Pleural, Pericardial and Peritoneal Cavities* (Heinemann Medical Books, London, 1957).

14. R. A. Rovelstad, L. G. Bartholomew, J. C. Cain, B. F. McKenzie, and E. H. Soule, "The value of examination of ascitic and blood for lipids and for proteins by electrophoresis," *Gastroenterology 34,* 436 (1958).

15. R. L. M. Wallis and H. A. Shölberg, "Chylous and pseudochylous ascites," *Quart. J. Med. 3,* 301 (1910); *4,* 153 (1911).

16. S. Amberg and N. M. Keith, "Mucin in the pleural fluid," *Proc. Mayo Clin. 8,* 181 (1933).

17. F. K. Paddock, "Relationship between specific gravity and protein content in human serous effusions," *Amer. J. med. Sci. 201,* 569 (1941).

18. D. T. Carr and M. Power, "Clinical value of measurements of concentration of protein in pleural fluid," *New Engl. J. Med. 259,* 926 (1958).

19. J. A. Loetscher, Jr., "Electrophoretic analysis of the proteins of plasma and serous effusions," *J. clin. Invest. 20,* 99 (1941).

20. E. Taipole and E. Hokkanen, "The mucoprotein levels of ascitic and pleural fluids and their clinical significance," *Acta med. scand. 155,* 3 (1955).

21. I. Spak, "On the clinical value of paper electrophoresis and determination of mucoprotein in ascitic fluid," *Scand. J. clin. Lab. Invest. 10,* 34 (1958).

22. G. Wihman, "A contribution to the knowledge of the cellular content in exudates and transudates," *Acta med. scand. 205,* 30 (1948).

23. S. Yamada, "Uber die Seröse flüsigkeit im Pleurahöle der gesunden Menschen," *Z. ges. exp. Med. 90,* 342 (1933).

24. A. J. Seaman, "Demonstration of L. E. cells in pericardial fluid," *J. Amer. med. Ass. 149,* 45 (1952).

25. N. E. Clarke, "The etiology of eosinophilic pleural effusion," *J. Amer. med. Ass. 79,* 1591 (1922).

26. J. D. Rolleston, "A case of eosinophilic ascites," *Brit. med. J. 1,* 238 (1914).

27. F. G. MacMurray, S. Katz, H. J. Zimmerman, "Pleural fluid eosinophilia," *New Engl. J. Med. 243,* 330 (1950).

28. R. F. Robertson, "Pleural eosinophilia," *Brit. J. Tuberc. 48,* 111 (1954).

29. M. D. Denney and L. R. Minot, "The coagulation of blood in the pleural cavity," *Amer. J. Physiol. 39,* 455 (1916).

30. N. C. Foot, "Identification of types and primary sites of metastatic tumors from exfoliated cells in serous fluid," *Amer. J. Path. 30,* 661 (1954).
31. O. Saphir, "Cytologic diagnosis of cancer from pleural and peritoneal fluids," *Amer. J. clin. Path. 19,* 309 (1949).
32. E. Sattenspiel, "Diagnosis of cancer in transudates and exudates. A comparison of the Papanicolaou method and paraffin block technique," *Surg. Gynec. Obstet. 89,* 478 (1949).
33. C. B. Chapman and E. J. Whalen, "The examination of serous fluids by the cell block technique," *New Engl. J. Med. 237,* 215 (1947).
34. M. Leichling, "Carcinoma diagnosed by examination of pericardial fluid," *New Engl. J. Med. 247,* 884 (1952).
35. G. G. Graham, J. R. McDonald, O. T. Clagatt, and H. W. Schmidt, "Examination of pleural fluid for carcinoma cells," *J. thorac. Surg. 25,* 366 (1953).
36. W. M. Yater, "Non-traumatic chylothorax and chylopericardium," *Ann. intern. Med. 9,* 600 (1935).
37. M. A. Brescia, "Chylothorax: Report of a case in an infant," *Arch. Pediat. 58,* 345 (1941).
38. A. M. Olsen and G. T. Wilson, "Chylothorax," *J. thorac. Surg. 13,* 53 (1944).
39. W. R. Bloor, "The determination of small amounts of lipid in blood plasma," *J. biol. Chem. 77,* 53 (1928).
40. L. M. Keith, R. M. Zollinger, and R. S. McCleery, "Peritoneal fluid amylase determinations as an aid in diagnosis of acute pancreatitis," *Arch. Surg. 61,* 930 (1950).
41. A. Merrill, "Cholesterol pericarditis," *Amer. Heart J. 16,* 505 (1938).
42. T. M. Curran, "Cholesterol pleural effusion," *Edinb. med. J. 55,* 252 (1948).
43. O. Creeck, W. M. Hicks, H. B. Snyder, and E. E. Erickson, "Cholesterol pericarditis," *Circulation 12,* 193 (1955).
44. A. E. W. Ada, O. R. Jones, and S. D. Sheeran, "Cholesterol pericarditis," *J. thorac. Surg. 20,* 28 (1950).
45. W. L. Calnan, "Comparison of glucose content of tuberculous and non-tuberculous pleural effusions," *Brit. med. J. 1,* 1239 (1951).
46. H. H. Merritt and F. Fremont-Smith, *The Cerebrospinal Fluid* (Saunders, Philadelphia, 1937).
47. A. Cantarow and M. Trumper, *Clinical Biochemistry* (ed. 5; Saunders, Philadelphia, 1955).
48. D. Denny-Brown, *Handbook of Neurological Examination and Case Recording* (Harvard University Press, Cambridge, 1946).
49. H. H. Merritt and M. Moore, "Acute syphilitic meningitis," *Medicine 14,* 119 (1935).
50. J. H. Dingle, "Medical progress. The encephalitides of virus etiology," *New Engl. J. Med. 225,* 1014 (1941).
51. J. H. Dingle and M. Finland, "Diagnosis, treatment, and prevention of meningococcic meningitis," *War Med. (Chicago) 2,* 1 (1942).
52. T. W. Farmer and C. A. Janeway, "Infections with the virus of lymphocytic choriomeningitis," *Medicine 21,* 1 (1942).
53. L. J. Barrows, F. T. Hunter, and B. Q. Banker, "The nature and clinical significance of pigments in the cerebrospinal fluid," *Brain 78,* 59 (1955).
54. E. Roboz, W. C. Hess, and F. M. Forster, "Quantitative determination of gamma globulin in cerebrospinal fluid: Its application in multiple sclerosis," *Neurology 3,* 419 (1953).

55. H. G. Kunkel and A. Tiselius, "Electrophoresis of proteins on filter paper," *J. gen. Physiol. 35,* 89 (1951).

56. A. M. Donovan, J. M. Foley, and W. C. Moloney, "The precipitation of cerebrospinal fluid globulin by zinc sulfate," *J. lab. clin. Med. 37,* 374 (1951).

57. J. H. Stokes, H. Beerman, and N. R. Ingraham, *Modern Clinical Syphilology* (ed. 3; Saunders, Philadelphia, 1944).

58. C. Lange and A. H. Harris, "The significance of the pH in the colloidal gold reaction," *J. lab. clin. Med. 29,* 970 (1944).

59. M. W. Ropes and W. Bauer, *Synovial Fluid Changes in Joint Disease* (Harvard University Press, Cambridge, 1953).

# Unit 19

## Examination of the Urine

The urinalysis is a composite examination that is usually carried out with a single specimen of urine. The urinalysis should be performed and recorded in a systematic sequence. The observations and simple laboratory tests which are included in the urinalysis provide qualitative or semiquantitative information about the following characteristics of the urine: (1) appearance; (2) bile pigment; (3) pH; (4) specific gravity; (5) protein; (6) sugar; (7) ketone bodies; and (8) the urine sediment.

The urinalysis is an integral part of the basic examination of patients in all branches of medicine. It can be performed with a minimum of equipment and provides a wide range of information quickly and inexpensively. Many substances are measured in urine in addition to those included in the urinalysis. Often, collections of urine must be timed in order to obtain quantitative information about rates of excretion. The use and interpretation of many of these examinations are described below. The measurement in urine of electrolytes, hormones, and certain other substances is discussed in other units.

### Collection and Preservation of Urine Samples

Ideally, urine for examination should be fresh, well concentrated, and of acid pH. Casts and red cells are poorly preserved in dilute or alkaline urine. In addition, the presence of small amounts of protein, sugar, and other substances may be overlooked when testing is done on dilute urine. In general, samples having a specific gravity of less than 1.010 are not satisfactory for examination. When disease is present which prevents adequate concentration or acidification of the urine, examination of a fresh specimen is of paramount importance. It has been suggested that the addition of sodium chloride crystals or a few drops of concentrated hydrochloric acid may prevent loss of formed elements.[1] After urine has stood for a few hours at room temperature, bacterial contamination destroys its usefulness for examination. Samples can be kept for 24 to 36 hr in a refrigerator, but examination of the sediment in such samples is less satisfactory, since crystals often appear or increase in number at low temperatures.

To preserve the formed elements in a 24-hr urine sample, a few drops of concentrated formaldehyde may be added to the collection flask.[2] The presence of formaldehyde may give a positive reaction in the nonspecific reducing methods for detection of urine sugar. Commercially available preservative tablets are satisfactory for use with small samples of urine when a considerable delay between collection and examination cannot be avoided. These tablets elevate the specific gravity of the sample by a predictable amount, but do not interfere in the other routine tests. They are widely used by insurance companies.

When 24-hr urine specimens are collected for chemical determinations, the choice of preservative is often dictated by the requirements of the test. A few drops of toluol may be used when urine is to be analyzed for protein or creatinine, or when a quantitative determination of glucose is to be made. Concentrated hydrochloric acid is required when calcium or catechol amines are to be determined. Sodium carbonate must be used when coproporphyrins are to be measured, but is unsatisfactory for determinations of urinary lead excretion. Many of these special requirements are summarized in Table 3, Unit 1.

Urine specimens from female patients often contain cellular elements from the vulva and vagina as contaminants. By cleansing and spreading the vulva and obtaining a "clean-catch" midstream specimen, this contamination can usually be avoided. The same technique should be used to obtain urine for bacteriologic examination. Bladder catheterization should be avoided whenever possible.[3]

## Appearance

Normal urine varies in color from faint yellow to amber, depending on whether the sample is dilute or concentrated. The main urinary pigment is called urochrome. This comprises several substances that have not been chemically characterized. A fraction of the urochrome can be precipitated by saturating urine with ammonium sulfate. Another reddish pigment of unknown composition, termed uroerythrin, coprecipitates with urates in acid urine.

Although freshly voided normal urine is usually clear, turbidity may be present in alkaline urine owing to the presence of amorphous phosphate crystals. Abnormal appearance of a urine sample may be due to the presence of formed elements which can be removed by centrifugation. If an abnormal color remains in the supernatant, this may be due to certain exogenous substances excreted in the urine or to endogenous abnormal pigments. The exogenous substances that commonly produce highly colored urine are listed in Table 59. Many of them behave as pH indicators. The naturally occurring (endogenous) abnormal urinary pigments include hemoglobin, myoglobin, bile pigments, certain indoles, porphyrins and their derivatives, homogentisic acid, and melanogen. Methods

Table 59. *Common exogenous urinary pigments.*

| Substance | Source | Color of urine | |
| | | Acid | Alkaline |
| --- | --- | --- | --- |
| Beets | Food | Red | Yellow |
| Anthracine derivatives yielding chrysophanic acid (aloe, cascara, rhubarb, and senna) | Cathartics | Yellow-brown | Red-violet |
| Antipyrine | Analgesic | Red (pH changes not known) | |
| Congo red | Test dye | Yellow | Red |
| Hedulin | Anticoagulant | Colorless | Red |
| Phenol | Poisoning | Colorless | Gradual oxidation of hydroquinone to olive to black pigment |
| Phenolphthalein | Cathartic | Colorless | Red |
| Phenolsulfonphthalein | Test dye | Colorless | Red |
| Bromsulfalein | Test dye | Colorless | Red |
| Pyridium | Analgesic | Red | Colorless |
| Santonin | Antihelminthic | Yellow | Pink |
| Thymol | Antihelminthic | Colorless | Thymol hydroquinone turns olive on oxidation |

for identifying these substances are described below (p. 323). Not infrequently, in attempts to identify an abnormal urinary pigment, all of these substances may be excluded by appropriate tests, and explanation of the abnormal color is still lacking.

### Tests for Bile Pigments

The metabolism of the bile pigments and tests for their detection are discussed in Unit 24. Qualitative testing for bile in the urine is a part of the routine urinalysis.

#### FOAM TEST

Urine is shaken in a test tube and inspected. A distinctly yellow or brownish foam indicates the presence of both bile pigments and bile acids. The test is crude but fairly specific.

#### HARRISON-FOUCHET METHOD [4]

This method makes use of the principle that bilirubin in urine is precipitated with barium salts. The color development depends on the production of blue and green derivatives on oxidation of bilirubin (the Gmelin reaction).

*Reagents.* (1) Fouchet's reagent: Dissolve 25 gm of trichloracetic acid in 100 ml of water. Add 10 ml of 10-percent $FeCl_3$. (2) 10 gm of $BaCl_2 \cdot H_2O$ in 100 ml of water.

**Method.** Measure 10 ml of urine into a test tube. Add 5 ml of barium chloride solution. Mix by tapping; filter through Whatman No. 2 filter paper. Unfold the paper and invert on another dry filter paper, gently transferring the precipitate. Add 1 or 2 drops of Fouchet's reagent. A green or blue color indicates the presence of bilirubin.

INTERPRETATION. This method is the most reliable qualitative test available for detection of bilirubin in urine. It will detect bilirubin at a concentration of 3 mg/100 ml.

#### MODIFICATIONS OF THE HARRISON SPOT TEST

A simplification of the Harrison spot test employs strips of heavy filter paper, impregnated with barium chloride, and dried. These are dipped in urine and removed, and Fouchet's reagent is applied to the area corresponding to the upper border of the urine. A green color is indicative of bilirubin. Considerable sensitivity is lost by this method, but it is useful in detecting gross bilirubinuria. A similar method employing a diazo dye is available under the name "Ictotest" (Ames Co., Elkhart, Ind.).

### Measurement and Significance of Urine pH

#### PHYSIOLOGY

A full discussion of the factors that influence renal acid-base regulation is beyond the scope of this book.[5] It is now generally accepted that hydrogen ion is excreted by the renal tubule in exchange for sodium ion. The concentration of free hydrogen ion in the urine is limited to a pH range of 4.5 to 8.0. Random specimens of urine are usually somewhat acid, since metabolism of normal diets yields from 50 to 150 mEq of free hydrogen ion per day. Because of the presence of phosphate salts and other buffers in the glomerular filtrate and of ammonia formed by the tubular cells, this large daily load of acid is excreted at an average pH above 4.5. When larger acid loads are imposed (as in diabetic acidosis), the kidney normally responds by increasing the tubular formation and excretion of ammonia. The total daily excretion of acid may be estimated as the sum of the titratable acidity and the ammonia content of a 24-hr urine sample, but this is seldom necessary for clinical purposes. Urine pH may be measured quickly and conveniently with Nitrazine indicator.

**Method.** A strip of Nitrazine paper is immersed in the urine and the color that immediately appears is compared with a reference color chart. The method is accurate to within 0.5 pH unit, and is satisfactory for clinical purposes.

### INTERPRETATION AND LIMITATIONS

As emphasized elsewhere, the pH of the urine influences the preservation of formed elements in the sediment. In addition, knowledge of urine pH sometimes gives important clues in diagnosis, especially when urine pH is "inappropriate" with respect to the pH of blood (see below). It must be emphasized that the pH is a measure of free hydrogen ion and does not reflect the total daily acid excretion. In renal insufficiency, the ability to excrete acid is reduced, owing chiefly to impairment in ammonia excretion, but the ability to excrete a highly acid urine is often preserved even in frank renal failure.

It is not uncommon for random samples of urine to be alkaline, especially following a heavy meal. Constantly alkaline urine may occur normally owing to ingestion of an alkaline ash diet or large amounts of alkaline salts. Otherwise, the presence of constantly alkaline urine may be due to the presence in the urine of urea-splitting organisms or to certain disease states discussed below.

URINE PH IN RENAL TUBULAR ACIDOSIS AND POTASSIUM DEFICIENCY. Renal tubular acidosis is characterized by hyperchloremic acidosis with inability to form a highly acid urine.[6] In some cases the urine may be persistently alkaline; in others it may fall below 7.0; but it always remains inappropriately high with respect to the associated systemic acidosis, seldom dropping below 6.5 or 6.0 throughout the 24-hr cycle.

In potassium deficiency from any cause, a systemic alkalosis develops and the pH of the urine tends to rise. At the same time, there is an increase in renal bicarbonate reabsorption, and urine pH, although not highly acid, is often inappropriately low with respect to the associated alkalosis. This has been called "paradoxical aciduria." In primary aldosteronism, urine pH is usually relatively alkaline.[7, 8]

ALKALINE URINE DUE TO UREA-SPLITTING ORGANISMS. Some strains of *Proteus, Pseudomonas, Staph. albus,* and other urinary-tract pathogens break down urea to form ammonia. Since under normal circumstances only trace quantities of ammonia are found in alkaline urine, the presence of large amounts of ammonia in an alkaline urine may be taken as presumptive evidence that such an organism is present. Confirmation depends on bacteriologic studies.

*Tests for Ammonia in Urine.* A sample of urine is heated gently while a strip of pink litmus paper is held in the mouth of the tube above the liquid. As ammonia is evolved, the paper will turn blue.

*Interpretation and Confirmatory Tests.* The test is extremely sensitive, and even the small amount of ammonia normally present in alkaline urine may cause a slight or transient change in color. To be considered a positive result, definite and permanent color change should occur. Where doubt exists, the urine sample may be boiled, and the pH measured after the ammonia has evolved. A drop in pH after boiling confirms the presence of ammonia. The presence of bicarbonate in normally alkaline urine may be demonstrated by adding a few drops of concentrated hydrochloric acid to the sample and watching for bubbles of free carbon dioxide to rise.

## Specific Gravity and Osmolality of Urine

### OSMOLALITY VS. SPECIFIC GRAVITY

The degree to which a solution is osmotically concentrated is best expressed in terms of osmolality. The osmolality of a solution depends on its total concentration of osmotically active particles, regardless of the mass or chemical properties of the constituent solutes. When a single molecular species is present in solution, a close correlation exists between the number of particles (osmolality) and the density (specific gravity). In a solution of variable and complex composition such as urine, the correlation will be less close, since specific gravity is determined by the mass of the constituent solutes, rather than the number of particles. It has long been customary to measure the concentration of urine by its specific gravity because of the ease and simplicity of this measurement and because simple methods of directly measuring osmolality have not been generally available.

The osmolality of urine (or other fluids) may be calculated from the freezing point, since the freezing point is depressed below that of water by 1.86 C deg for each 1000 milliosmols per liter of solution. Rapid methods for measuring the freezing point of biologic fluids are now available for use in hospitals and are preferable to measurement of specific gravity when precise information is desired, as in urine-concentrating tests (Unit 20).

The relation between urine osmolality and specific gravity for subjects on normal diets is illustrated in Fig. 29.[9] A fairly good correlation is evident, although

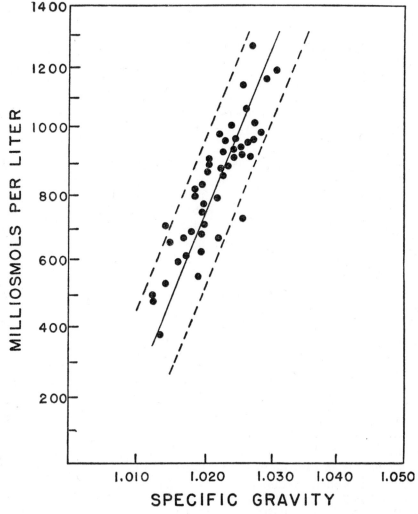

Fig. 29. Osmolality *vs.* specific gravity (adapted from Dustan and Corcoran [9]).

there is considerable vertical scatter in the data. For example, a specific gravity of 1.020 may represent variations in osmolality of from 550 to 900 mOsm/L. Further variability occurs in subjects on special diets. Sodium restriction decreases specific gravity in relation to osmolality.

### MEASUREMENT OF URINE SPECIFIC GRAVITY

**Method.** The urinometer is a hydrometer adapted to the observation of specific gravity of urine at 20°C. A correction should be made if the urine is distinctly warm or cold, 0.001 being subtracted or added for each 3 C deg below or above 20°. Urinometers should be calibrated by floating in distilled water and are usually accurate to within ±0.002. The urinometer must be floated in a vessel large enough to prevent adherence at the sides.

INTERPRETATIONS AND LIMITATIONS. The specific gravity of random samples of urine varies widely, depending on the state of hydration of the subject. A specific gravity as high as 1.038 may occur in dehydrated normal subjects. Extremely high specific gravity suggests the presence of solutes not normally present in urine, such as glucose or Diodrast. When such substances are present, specific gravity is poorly correlated with osmolality. Protein raises specific gravity by 0.001 for each 0.4 gm/100 ml. Corrections need to be made, therefore, only when large amounts of protein are present. Glucose increases the specific gravity by 0.001 for each 0.27 gm/100 ml.

Knowledge of specific gravity is of aid in evaluating the significance of the routine urinalysis, since all substances are present in lower concentration in dilute urine. Tests of urine-concentrating ability are discussed in Unit 20. In general, these tests are unnecessary when a specific gravity of 1.025 or above is found in a random specimen.

## Proteinuria

### PHYSIOLOGY OF PROTEINURIA

#### FILTRATION AND REABSORPTION OF PROTEIN

A small amount of protein, probably less than 30 mg/100 ml,[10, 11] is normally present in glomerular filtrate. Nearly all of this is reabsorbed by the tubules,[12–14] leaving the urine free of protein as measured by the usual clinical tests. Normal urine does, however, contain a small amount of protein. The quantity detectable in concentrates of urine from normal subjects ranges from 30 to 50 mg/24 hr, averaging 39 mg/24 hr.[15] "Proteinuria" denotes the presence of protein in urine in sufficient quantity to be detected by clinical tests, and implies greater than normal excretion of protein.

Immunologic and electrophoretic studies have shown that urine protein is identical with plasma protein. All the electrophoretically separable components of serum are usually represented in urine protein, although they occur in different proportions than in the serum. It is inferred that protein which appears in the urine ordinarily enters by way of filtration at the glomerulus. The only important exception to this is when gross bleeding occurs in the lower urinary tract.

The mechanism of proteinuria in disease has long been a subject of controversy. The two most prevalent hypotheses are (a) that increased leakage of protein through the glomerular membrane results in an abnormally high concentration of protein in glomerular filtrate, the maximum rate of protein reabsorption is exceeded, and the remainder is excreted in the urine; and (b) that normal amounts of protein are filtered at the glomerulus, but the ability of the tubules to reabsorb it is diminished or absent. The problem of the relative importance of filtration and reabsorption of protein has not been resolved. However, recent studies indicate that leakage of protein through the glomerulus is increased at least in those situations where massive proteinuria occurs.[16-18]

### KINDS OF PROTEIN IN THE URINE

Urinary protein usually contains the same five electrophoretic components normally found in the serum. The small quantity of protein in concentrates of urine from normal subjects shows a uniform electrophoretic pattern, with relatively more globulin and less albumin than the serum ($A/G = 0.51$).[15] By contrast, electrophoresis of urine from subjects with proteinuria shows a predominance of albumin (50–80 percent).[17] Electrophoresis of the serum during severe proteinuria reveals a pattern that is the mirror image of the pattern in the urine, with marked reduction in the concentration of components (for example, albumin) that predominate in urine, and preservation of components (for example, alpha$_2$ globulin) which are excreted less rapidly.

Under certain conditions, proteins may appear in the urine that are not normally found in the serum. The most important of these are the Bence-Jones proteins, which may be excreted by patients with multiple myeloma. It is often stated in textbooks of clinical pathology that cleavage products of proteins ("proteoses") occur in the urine in certain diseases and as a result of contamination of the urine by prostatic secretions. Pseudo-Bence-Jones protein (discussed below) and nucleoprotein may also rarely occur in the urine. The significance of these abnormal constituents and the methods for their detection need to be reexamined with the aid of modern techniques.

### FACTORS INFLUENCING THE RATE OF PROTEIN EXCRETION IN DISEASE

The rate of loss of protein in the urine depends on the interrelation of several factors, all of which must be evaluated in interpreting the significance of changes in protein excretion in disease.

These are: (*a*) the permeability of the glomerulus to protein; (*b*) the serum level of protein, especially albumin; (*c*) the glomerular filtration rate; and (*d*) the rate of reabsorption of protein by the tubules. Moderate rates of proteinuria do not affect serum protein concentration. However, if glomerular permeability is greatly increased, the ensuing large urinary losses of proteins may result in a drop in serum protein concentration. This will proceed until a new equilibrium is reached, with less protein excreted, since less is filtered. Changes in filtration rate have a direct effect on protein excretion. If the glomerular filtration rate falls, less protein will be filtered and excreted. Conversely, a rise in the filtration rate may increase protein excretion.

Although a decrease in the rate of urinary protein excretion is usually interpreted as an indication of favorable progress in renal disease, this is true only if it is due to healing of damaged glomerular capillaries. It may be of unfavorable significance if it is due to a drop in glomerular filtration rate or to a decreased serum level of albumin. These factors are especially important in evaluating the course of patients with the nephrotic syndrome.

## QUALITATIVE TESTS FOR PROTEINURIA

The tests usually used for routine urinalysis depend on the precipitation of protein by heat or by a strong acid. The amount of protein present is estimated from the density of a ring of precipitated protein and is usually graded from 1+ to 4+. A faint trace of white precipitate, seen when viewed against a black background, is graded as ± or "trace." The tests differ in sensitivity, as noted below, and a 1+ reaction has a different quantitative significance depending on which test is used. When a substantial amount of protein is present, no exact quantitative significance can be attached to the result. Nevertheless, careful grading in "pluses" gives clinically useful information concerning the relative amount of protein present.

The following scheme is recommended to standardize the recording of qualitative protein tests:

No turbidity 0

A faint ring of precipitate visible against a black background ±

A definite but small ring of precipitate through which print can be read 1+

A dense ring of precipitate that is not opaque when viewed from above (black lines on a white background are still visible) 2+

A dense ring of precipitate that is opaque when viewed from above (black lines on a white background are not visible) 3+

A dense, opaque ring with flocculent precipitate 4+

Tests that use a tablet or "stick" have recently been introduced for the detection of urine protein. These depend on the presence of an indicator in the testing device which changes color when protein is adsorbed. Preliminary trials indicate that they are considerably less sensitive than the older tests.

### NITRIC ACID TEST (HELLER TEST)

**Method.** Approximately 2 ml of concentrated nitric acid (technical grade may be used) is poured into a test tube. Approximately 5 ml of clear urine is carefully poured down the side of the container so that it overlies the acid. Turbid urine should be filtered or centrifuged before analysis. After 3 min, the zone of contact between the acid and the urine is inspected for a white ring of precipitated protein. Observation is best made against a dull black background. If a ring is present, its intensity is graded according to the scheme outlined above from 1+ to 4+. Dark-colored

rings of changed pigment are disregarded.

INTERPRETATION AND LIMITATIONS. The nitric acid test will detect protein concentrations of 15mg/100 ml immediately, and, if allowed to stand 30 min, concentrations of 10 mg/100 ml may be detected.[19] It is therefore a less sensitive test than the heat and acetic acid test or the sulfosalicylic acid test. The test gives a maximum degree of precipitation at protein concentrations of 300 to 400 mg/100 ml, and larger amounts are not distinguishable. All proteins present in the urine, including Bence-Jones protein, are regularly precipitated by this test.

### HEAT AND ACETIC ACID TEST

**Method.** Turbid urine should be filtered or centrifuged before analysis. A Pyrex test tube is filled to about ⅔ of its capacity with clear urine. The upper portion (about 1 in.) is heated to boiling over a small flame and compared with the unboiled lower portion. Then 1 to 3 drops of 3-percent acetic acid is added, and the upper portion is boiled a second time. During the initial boiling of alkaline urine, phosphates may precipitate, but they will be redissolved by addition of the acetic acid. The precipitate of protein is observed against a black background and its intensity graded from 1+ to 4+ as described above.

A modification of this test involves addition of approximately 2 ml of saturated sodium chloride solution which prevents the precipitation of mucin (glycoprotein) if this is present in increased amounts.

INTERPRETATION AND LIMITATIONS. The heat and acetic acid test is the most sensitive of the qualitative tests, and will detect protein at a concentration of 2–3 mg/100 ml. Because of its sensitivity, it may detect the small quantity of protein in concentrated samples from normal subjects. For example, if a normal subject excretes 40 mg of protein in a 24-hr volume of 1000 ml, the concentration in a sample of this urine will be 4 mg/100 ml, just detectable by the heat and acetic acid method. Nevertheless, urine from normal subjects rarely contains a detectable amount of protein, and a positive test result warrants further investigation.

Since the heat and acetic acid test involves the rapid boiling of a small volume of urine, Bence-Jones protein may easily be overlooked when this method is used. For this reason, the nitric acid test, although less sensitive, is slightly preferable as a routine procedure. Both tests should be made where any doubt exists as to the existence of proteinuria.

### SEMIQUANTITATIVE MEASUREMENT OF PROTEIN BY THE SULFOSALICYLIC ACID METHOD

Sulfosalicylic acid precipitates protein from urine with an even turbidity that is roughly proportional to the concentration of protein in a solution. The turbidity may be measured by direct visual comparison with turbidity standards in an illuminated comparator rack, or by using a photoelectric colorimeter as a nephelometer. The turbidity standards may be purchased or prepared [20] and correspond to protein concentrations of from 5 to 100 mg/100 ml. By proper dilution of the urine, a high protein concentration may be brought within the range of the standards.

**Method.** Turbid urine should be filtered or centrifuged before analysis. Two and one-half milliliters of urine is measured in a pipette and placed in a test tube that has the same dimensions as the turbidity standards. Then 7.5 ml of an aqueous solution of sulfosalicylic acid, 3 gm/100 ml, is added and mixed by inversion. After 10 min, the turbidity of the unknown sample is matched against that of the standards. If the turbidity of the sample is too great, the

urine is diluted, preferably with protein-free urine, and the procedure repeated; the final reading is multiplied by the dilution factor.

INTERPRETATION AND LIMITATIONS. The sulfosalicylic acid method will detect protein at a concentration of 5 mg/100 ml or slightly less. All proteins present in the urine, including Bence-Jones protein, are precipitated. As a quantitative method, its accuracy has been estimated at ± 20 percent. It is somewhat cumbersome for use as a routine test, but it is valuable when semiquantitative information is desired.

### TESTS FOR BENCE-JONES PROTEINURIA

#### DIAGNOSTIC SIGNIFICANCE OF BENCE-JONES PROTEIN

In multiple myeloma, characteristic abnormalities of protein metabolism may be detectable in serum (Unit 16), urine, or both. In the urine, an abnormal protein with unique heat-solubility properties, known as Bence-Jones protein, is detectable in approximately 50 percent of patients with this disease. Some 18 percent of these patients have Bence-Jones proteinuria despite a normal or nondiagnostic serum electrophoretic pattern.[21] The source and significance of the protein abnormalities seen in multiple myeloma are debated. Both the serum abnormalities and Bence-Jones proteinuria may also be seen, although rarely, in patients with malignant lymphoma,[22] lymphatic leukemia,[22] and primary amyloidosis.[23] When Bence-Jones proteins, isolated from the urines of different patients, are analyzed and compared, it is found that the molecular weight and certain other properties exhibit considerable variability. However, each patient excretes a single homogeneous protein with consistent physical properties.[23] Recent studies indicate that Bence-Jones proteins may be formed *de novo* by abnormal or neoplastic cells.[23] They are of small molecular size, and consequently may leak through the glomerular capillaries in substantial quantities in the absence of any renal abnormality.

### METHODS OF IDENTIFYING BENCE-JONES PROTEIN

Identification of Bence-Jones protein depends on the fact that it precipitates from urine at a temperature of 45–65°C, but redissolves at or just below the boiling point, and precipitates once again during cooling. Its identification is easy if it is the only protein present in the urine, but becomes more difficult when other proteins are also present. A complete scheme for the qualitative analysis of urine proteins is described by Jacobson and Milner.[24] The methods outlined below have been modified from those of Jacobson and Milner and of Snapper *et al.*[25] It is well to begin with the simple exclusion tests, proceeding sequentially with the more involved methods to a point where Bence-Jones protein can be either definitely excluded or positively identified.

EXCLUSION TESTS FOR BENCE-JONES PROTEIN. *Ring Test with Nitric Acid.* Although the presence of Bence-Jones protein may be overlooked when testing is done with heat and acetic acid, it is regularly precipitated, along with other proteins, by nitric acid. If the ring test with nitric acid gives a negative result, no Bence-Jones protein is present.

*Bradshaw Test.* Bence-Jones and certain other proteins are precipitated by concentrated hydrochloric acid. A ring test is made in the same manner described for nitric acid, and is examined for a precipitate after 5 min. If the result is negative, no Bence-Jones protein is present.

ANALYTIC SCHEME FOR IDENTIFYING BENCE-JONES PROTEIN. Urine for analysis should be fresh and free from bacteria. Turbid urine should be centrifuged or filtered. All heating should be done in a water bath and temperatures should be measured with a mercury thermometer placed in the urine sample. The following sequence of procedures should be pursued until Bence-Jones protein is identified or excluded.

**Method.** *Stage 1.* To 10 ml of appropriately diluted urine in a test tube, add 2 ml of saturated sodium chloride solution. Then add 3-percent acetic acid drop by drop to adjust the pH to about 5.0 as measured by Nitrazine paper. Adjustment of pH is necessary to assure maximum precipitation of Bence-Jones protein. Heat in a water bath while agitating the urine gently with the thermometer. If Bence-Jones protein is present, coagulation starts at a temperature of 45° to 55°C, and usually becomes maximal between 55° and 65°C. When the temperature approaches the boiling point, this protein goes into solution. Apparent clearing may occur during boiling, owing to the separation of albumin and globulin into small, dense particles. If this occurs, turbidity immediately reappears when the tube is shaken.

*Interpretation.* If turbidity is present at 55° to 70°C and dissolves completely at 100°, the presence of Bence-Jones protein is established. If no turbidity appears below the boiling point, Bence-Jones protein is not present. If the precipitate forms but does not dissolve with boiling, this may be due to the coagulation of albumin and globulin, appearing as Bence-Jones protein dissolves, or, less commonly, to the presence of pseudo-Bence-Jones protein. This poorly characterized protein is formed at times by the action of bacteria on ordinary urine proteins. At other times its origin is obscure.[24] It resembles Bence-Jones protein in being precipitated below 70°C, but differs in that it is insoluble at the boiling point and in the presence of nitric acid.

*Stage 2.* If several abnormal proteins

are present together, they can usually be differentiated by the following procedure. To 10 ml of appropriately diluted urine, add 2 ml of saturated sodium chloride solution and acidify with 3-percent acetic acid to pH 5 (Nitrazine paper). Then heat the sample for 10 min at 60°C, centrifuge, and remove the supernatant. The heat and acetic acid test should then be made on the supernatant, to detect the presence of albumin and globulin. The precipitate, containing Bence-Jones or pseudo-Bence-Jones protein, or both, is resuspended in 10 ml of normal urine. Ten drops of concentrated nitric acid is added and the sample is placed in a boiling-water bath for 10 min. If Bence-Jones protein only is present, the coagulum will dissolve on boiling. Failure to dissolve indicates the presence of pseudo-Bence-Jones protein. The sample is then filtered hot, using a heated funnel to prevent rapid cooling. If both abnormal proteins are present, the pseudo-Bence-Jones protein will be removed by filtration and Bence-Jones protein will precipitate in the filtrate during cooling.

Occasionally, urates present in the filtrate may precipitate during cooling and simulate a positive reaction at this stage. The addition of 1 ml of 25-percent sulfosalicylic acid will dissolve a precipitate of urates, but will intensify a precipitate of Bence-Jones protein.

*Interpretation.* Complete clearing during boiling with nitric acid and reappearance of turbidity in the filtrate during cooling establish the presence of Bence-Jones protein. Other proteins simultaneously present are also identified as described.

DETECTION OF BENCE-JONES PROTEIN
BY ELECTROPHORESIS OF URINE
PROTEINS

Bence-Jones proteins have an electrophoretic mobility similar to the globulins. However, their mobilities are variable as measured in urine samples from different patients. Mobility is also different (generally more rapid) from that of the abnormal globulin detectable in the serum. The abnormal spot detectable in the urine is characteristically homogeneous and sharply outlined. When only Bence-Jones protein is present in the urine or when other proteins are present in moderate amounts, the characteristic discrete and dominant globulin spot is virtually diagnostic.[21] The presence of a large amount of albumin and globulin may, however, obscure the pattern. Electrophoresis is probably at least as reliable as the precipitation methods for the presumptive recognition of Bence-Jones protein.

If the qualitative nitric acid test shows 2+ or more protein present, electrophoresis can be carried out on untreated urine. If less protein is present, the urine should be concentrated by dialysis against 25-percent polyvinal pyrrolidone in the electrophoresis buffer.[21]

PROTEINURIA IN NORMAL SUBJECTS

Except during gross bleeding into the lower urinary tract, protein enters the urine by way of filtration at the glomerulus. Proteinuria therefore usually signifies a disorder at the renal level, but it does not necessarily signify renal disease. Proteinuria may occur in normal subjects in a variety of circumstances. When proteinuria is found, it is the physician's responsibility to determine whether it is benign, or whether disease is present.

In general, proteinuria in normal subjects is not constant, but transient or intermittent, whereas in renal disease constant proteinuria is the rule. An exception to this is chronic pyelonephritis, where proteinuria may be intermittent until extensive renal damage has occurred. Proteinuria in normal subjects is usually small in amount (less than 1 gm per day). It may be accompanied by some increase in excretion of formed elements in the urine as measured by quantitative counts but is not usually accompanied by large numbers of granular or cellular casts, or large numbers of red cells.

Transient proteinuria may occur in normal subjects following violent exertion [26, 27] or immersion in cold water,[26] during severe emotional stress,[28] following syncope,[28] subarachnoid hemorrhage,[26] and epileptic seizures [26] and in subjects receiving intravenous epinephrine and nor-epinephrine.[28] Some degree of renal ischemia is probably common to all these situations.[28] Proteinuria is also common during fever from any cause.[29] In normal subjects, the proteinuria that occurs in these situations disappears promptly when the cause is removed.

### Orthostatic Proteinuria

In certain normal subjects, proteinuria may occur during ordinary daily activities, but urine formed while the subject is recumbent is free of protein. Although this form of proteinuria is clearly related to postural factors, its exact mechanism is controversial. Bull [30] has given evidence that it may be related to increased renal venous congestion due to compression of the inferior vena cava by the liver in the erect posture. Others [31] have noted that many patients who exhibit the phenomenon show evidence of vasomotor instability. The amount of protein excreted is greatest in the erect lordotic posture.[30, 31] However, proteinuria may be induced in many normal subjects by a position of exaggerated lordosis,[30] and subjects with orthostatic albuminuria do not have an increased lumbar lordosis.[30] The condition is fairly common, occurring in approximately 3 percent of normal subjects.[31] It is most common in the second and third decades, and may persist or disappear with age. Although it is usually benign, studies have shown that severe and constant orthostatic proteinuria may be associated with organic pathology, including anom-

alies of the genitourinary tract, pyelonephritis, and hypertension.[31] Postural effects may also influence the rate of protein excretion in patients with established renal disease,[26] although in these patients the urine does not become protein-free during recumbency. The rate of protein excretion in orthostatic proteinuria is usually less than 1.0 gm/day. There may be an increase in the excretion of formed elements, but large numbers of granular casts and red cells are not seen.

### TESTS FOR ORTHOSTATIC PROTEINURIA

To establish a diagnosis of orthostatic proteinuria it is necessary to show that the urine formed while the patient is in the recumbent posture is regularly free of protein. The demonstration that lordotic posture will produce proteinuria is of much less importance, since this posture will also increase proteinuria in renal disease and may induce proteinuria in normal subjects whose urine is otherwise constantly protein-free.

**Method.** The patient takes only the usual amount of fluid. Three samples of urine are collected, and examined for pH, specific gravity, formed elements, and protein.

*First sample* (recumbent). One hour after retiring, the patient voids while recumbent and discards the urine. This assures that no urine formed while still erect will be included in the sample. He remains in bed throughout the night. In the morning he voids while still in bed and saves the urine.

*Second sample* (lordotic). On arising the patient stands for 30 min with the back flat against a wall. The sample is collected as soon thereafter as possible.

*Third sample* (ordinary activity). The patient pursues his ordinary activities and saves the next spontaneously voided sample of urine.

INTERPRETATION. In orthostatic proteinuria the sample obtained during recumbency should be free of protein. The lordotic sample usually contains the greatest amount of protein, although this is of no diagnostic significance. The samples obtained during ordinary activity give an index of the constancy and severity of the proteinuria. Absence of proteinuria should be accepted only when the samples tested are well concentrated (specific gravity 1.016 or above). To establish the diagnosis, the test should be repeated several times.

### QUANTITATIVE TESTS FOR PROTEINURA

Knowledge of the rate of urinary protein excretion is of value in following the course of renal disease, and in planning and evaluating therapy. The protein content must be determined in a sample of urine collected over a measured interval of time. Usually a 24-hr urine sample is used. The rate of excretion is calculated as follows:

Protein concentration (gm/L) × urine volume (L/day) = protein excretion (gm/day).

METHODS FOR QUANTITATIVE URINE PROTEIN DETERMINATION. The Kjeldahl method is by far the most accurate method available for quantitative protein determinations but is time consuming and requires the facilities of a chemical laboratory. Several simpler methods are available, although none is entirely satisfactory. The semiquantitative sulfosalicylic acid method has been previously described. There are several sedimentation methods which depend on the estimation of protein content from the height of a column of precipitated protein. They are notoriously unreliable since the height of the column may be markedly influenced by the size of the flocculent particles and the density with which they are packed. The most reliable of these methods is that of Shevky and Stafford.[32, 33] A method that is rapid and reliable at protein concentrations above 200 mg/100 ml is described by Chinard.[34]

### URINARY PROTEIN EXCRETION IN DISEASE

RATE OF EXCRETION IN RENAL DISEASE. In disease of the kidneys, the rate of protein excretion tends to remain constant from day to day,[2] although the degree of constancy is limited by the accuracy of the method used to measure it, and variations of ± 20 percent are common. Serial determinations of the rate of protein excretion are valuable in following the course of renal disease, especially in patients with the nephrotic syndrome. Physiologic factors influencing the rate of excretion of protein in disease have been discussed above (p. 298).

In the diagnosis of renal disease, measurements of the rate of protein excretion are of limited value. Approximate figures for the expected range of excretion in various diseases are summarized in Table 62, together with other data obtained from the urinalysis. Considerable overlap between different diseases is apparent, and exceptional rates of excretion frequently occur.

URINARY-TRACT INFECTIONS. Clinical evidence [2] indicates that infection confined to the lower urinary tract does not usually result in proteinuria, even though the urinary sediment many contain large numbers of leukocytes. The presence of proteinuria in urinary-tract infections therefore implies that the kidney is involved in the inflammatory process. On the other hand, the absence of proteinuria does not give assurance that the kidney is not involved, since proteinuria in chronic pyelonephritis is not a constant finding except in its late stages.

PROTEINURIA IN CONGESTIVE HEART FAILURE. Some degree of proteinuria is almost always present in congestive heart failure and may occur even when failure is compensated. In general, the degree of proteinuria is correlated with the severity of the cardiovascular status. Abnormalities in the sediment are also seen in congestive failure. When congestive failure becomes superimposed on renal disease, protein excretion is often increased.

### Sugar (Reducing Substances) in Urine

A search for glucose is a part of every routine urine examination. Glucose is the commonest reducing substance found in the urine, and its presence there may be the first hint of diabetes mellitus.

In the past, the urine has been tested by any of a variety of nonspecific tests for the presence of reducing substances. If such a substance was found in the urine, it was likely (on statistical grounds) to be glucose. Attention was then focused on the blood sugar and glucose-tolerance tests. If the results of these proved to be normal, it then became necessary to determine, by specific tests, the nature of the reducing substance in the urine. Other reducing sugars such as fructose or galactose, and other reducing substances such as ascorbic acid, antibiotics, and glucuronides, may also occur in the urine. With the introduction in 1956 of an easily performed specific enzyme test for glucose, this detection process has been simplified.[35] By the routine use of this enzymatic test for glucose as the initial screening procedure, urinary reducing substances other than glucose will not be found. The older methods of detection are still useful, however, since they can provide semiquantitative estimates of the amount of reducing substance (glucose) present.

### SCREENING TESTS FOR URINARY REDUCING SUBSTANCES

#### SPECIFIC ENZYME TESTS FOR GLUCOSE

A specific enzyme, glucose oxidase, can catalyze the oxidation of glucose

with oxygen to gluconic acid and hydrogen peroxide. The hydrogen peroxide formed in the presence of other enzymes and appropriate dyes gives an easily discernible color reaction. By impregnating an absorbent paper with these enzymes and other reagents, specific tests for glucose have been developed. These depend upon the appearance of a color when fresh urine comes in contact with the paper.[35] Two such papers are manufactured commercially, "Tes-Tape" (Eli Lilly Co., Indianapolis, Ind.) and "Clinistix" (Ames Co., Elkhart, Ind.).

**Method.** A strip of the test paper of the appropriate length is moistened in a sample of fresh urine and observed for a change in color. If glucose is present, a green color will develop with Tes-Tape and a blue with Clinistix.

INTERPRETATIONS AND LIMITATIONS. The test is specific for glucose. No substance has been found that will give a false positive result. The test is extremely simple. The test end of the paper may be either dipped into the urine sample, held momentarily in the urinary stream, or merely moistened with a drop of urine. Almost no equipment, therefore, is needed. Color development will be noted with a glucose concentration as low as 0.1 gm/100 ml of urine. Thus the test is more sensitive than the Benedict's reaction. There is disagreement among workers concerning whether or not the depth of the color reaction in these specific enzymatic tests is proportional to the concentration of glucose in the urine.[36-38] The majority feel that these tests have not proved useful in semiquantitative estimations of glucosuria. This would seem especially so when large amounts of glucose are present in the urine. The test is, therefore, not recommended for urine tests in the patient with labile diabetes, where quantitation may be necessary. Because of its specificity, sensitivity, and ease of performance, it is useful as a screening test for the detection of diabetes.

### NONSPECIFIC TESTS FOR GLUCOSE

BENEDICT'S QUALITATIVE TEST. The reactive element in Benedict's qualitative sugar reagent is a soluble blue copper-carbonate-citrate ion. When compounds with one or more free aldehyde or ketone groups are heated in this solution, the soluble cupric ions are reduced to the cuprous form and precipitated as yellow or red cuprous oxide. A finely divided yellow precipitate, in small amounts, viewed through the blue solution will impart a green color to the mixture.[39]

**Method.** Five milliliters of Benedict's qualitative sugar reagent and 8 drops of urine are mixed in a test tube and placed in boiling water for 5 min. The test is read in terms of the color and precipitate, as indicated in Table 60.

INTERPRETATIONS AND LIMITATIONS. Because it will give a positive reaction with a number of reducing agents besides glucose, the Benedict qualitative test is a nonspecific one. Usually these other substances are present in only small amounts, and any reduction accompanied by a yellow precipitate is almost always caused by glucose. Though the reagent itself is inexpensive, the amount of accessory equipment and the time involved must be taken into consideration in the over-all cost. When other reducing substances are not present, a trace

reaction indicates glucose in a concentration of 0.25 gm/100 ml of urine. When carefully performed, the Benedict's qualitative test is a semiquantitative one for glucose, again in the absence of other reducing substances. Accordingly, it can be used by the patient with diabetes mellitus to estimate the amount of his glycosuria. By appropriate reduction in the number of drops of urine used in the test, concentrations of glucose above 2 gm/100 ml of urine can be estimated.

USE OF A SINGLE TABLET FOR THE DETECTION OF URINE SUGAR—CLINITEST. The Clinitest tablet (Ames Co., Elkhart, Ind.) is an ingenious combination of copper sulfate, anhydrous sodium hydroxide, citric acid, and sodium bicarbonate. On addition to diluted urine, boiling is produced by the heat of the solution of the anhydrous sodium hydroxide and the neutralization between the sodium hydroxide and the citric acid. The reaction for copper is comparable to that described for the Benedict's qualitative test.

**Method.** Five drops of urine and 10 drops of water are mixed in a test tube. One reagent tablet is added and the solution is allowed to boil without agitation. The new color is recorded 15 sec after the boiling has ceased. The results roughly parallel those of the Benedict's test, as shown in Table 60.

INTERPRETATIONS AND LIMITATIONS. The properties of specificity and quantitation of the Clinitest tablet and Benedict's

Table 60. *Color reactions for different urinary sugar concentrations.*

| Reagent | Urinary sugar concentration (gm/100 ml) | | | | | | |
|---|---|---|---|---|---|---|---|
| | 0 | 0.25 | 0.5 | 0.75 | 1.0 | 1.5 | 2.0 or more |
| Benedict's | Blue | Green | Green with yellow precipitate | | Yellow to olive | Brown | Orange to red |
| | 0 | trace | + | | 2+ | 3+ | 4+ |
| Clinitest | Blue | Green | Green with yellow precipitate | Olive | Brown | | Orange |
| | 0 | trace | + | 2+ | 3+ | | 4+ |

qualitative sugar reaction are alike. Although the tablet is more expensive than the Benedict reagent per test, an external source of heat is not needed and the time required is less. The tablets will decompose and give unreliable test results when exposed to air and moisture. Users of this testing method must be warned of the blackened appearance of the deteriorated test tablet and should be instructed in the precautions of capping and storage in dry places necessary to avoid early spoilage of their supply.

USE OF A DRY POWDER CONTAINING BISMUTH OXIDE—GALATEST. This test (Denver Chemical Manufacturing Co., New York) depends upon the reduction of powdered bismuth oxide to black metallic bismuth by urinary reducing substances. It is largely being replaced by the enzymatic tests for urinary glucose which are not only specific as to glucose but are easier to perform.

DIFFERENTIATION OF VARIOUS URINARY REDUCING SUBSTANCES

When the initial screening test is a nonspecific one, such as the Benedict's qualitative test, and the reducing substance found proves not to be glucose by specific enzyme test, its exact nature should be determined.

Besides glucose, the following reducing sugars may appear in the urine: fructose; galactose; lactose; and pentose (xylose). Essential fructosuria and pentosuria are extremely rare and benign conditions.[40] There is a danger in their being confused with the glycosuria of diabetes mellitus. Fructose as well as glucose may occur in the urine of diabetics. Galactose is found in the urine of infants suffering from congenital galactosemia, a potentially fatal disease. Early recognition of galactosemia is of immense importance.[41] Lactose appears in the urine of women at term and during lactation.

Nonsugar reducing substances that may appear in the urine include preservatives such as chloroform and formaldehyde; ascorbic acid; creatinine in increased concentrations; protein in large amounts; penicillin and streptomycin; and homogentisic acid. The presence of this last substance is diagnostic of alkaptonuria. Glucuronic acid, which can be found in the urine following the administration of such substances as salicylates, acetanilid, and chloral hydrate, also has reducing properties.

By the appropriate use of a modified Benedict's test, followed by specific testing for the various sugars, an accurate differentiation among these substances can be accomplished.

**Method.** A schema for identifying sugars in urine is shown in Fig. 30.

(*a*) The modified Benedict's test consists of reduction with Benedict's qualitative reagent at 55°C for 10 min. This separates fructose and pentose from the other nonglucose reducing substances, since only these two sugars accomplish reduction under these conditions. Urine that contains galactose, lactose, and nonsugar reducing agents will remain blue.[42, 43]

(*b*) The presence of pentose is established by the orcinol–hydrochloric acid reaction (Bial's test).[39]

(*c*) The presence of fructose is confirmed by the resorcinol–hydrochloric acid reaction (Seliwanoff's reagent).[39]

(*d*) Lactose and galactose are detected by the mucic acid test by mixing 50 ml of urine and 12 ml of concentrated nitric acid in a 150-ml beaker. The mixture is placed in a boiling-water bath until the volume is reduced to about 10 ml. This is then cooled, 10 ml of water is added, and the solution is allowed to stand over night. A fine white precipitate of mucic acid crystals which can be seen under the microscope will appear if lactose or galactose is present.

(*e*) Lactose is differentiated from galactose by the phloroglucinol–hydrochloric acid reaction (Tollen's test). To

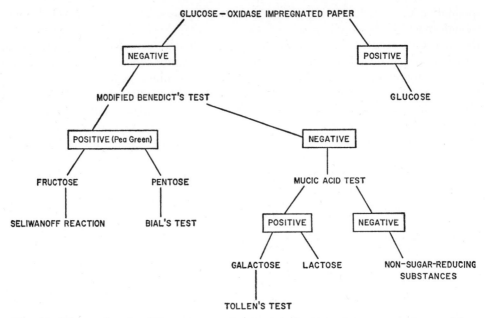

Fig. 30. Schema for the differentiation of urinary reducing substances as detected by routine Benedict's test or by Clinitest. Because of its clinical importance, steps leading to the identification of galactose are described in detail in the text.

equal volumes of urine and hydrochloric acid (specific gravity 1.09), a small amount of phloroglucinol is added and the mixture is heated in a boiling-water bath. Galactose, pentose, and glucuronic acid will all give a red color.[39]

The enzyme defect in congenital galactosemia can be demonstrated directly using whole blood, but requires specialized techniques.[41] Paper chromotography has been used as a method of separating sugars.[43, 44] Polariscopy and testing with phenylhydrazine can also be employed in such a differentiation.[43]

### QUANTITATIVE TESTS FOR URINARY GLUCOSE

A number of methods for determining urinary glucose quantitatively are available.[39, 45, 46] Such information may be very useful clinically, especially in the regulation of patients with labile diabetes and in diabetes associated with a low renal threshold for glucose, such as may occur in pregnancy. A simple method devised by Somogyi can be carried out without special equipment.[46] This test depends upon the development of a yellow to brown color upon the caramelization of glucose in a hot alkaline solution. The color reaction is quantitative and can be compared with the color developed by solutions containing known concentrations of glucose. Color standards in a comparator block are available commercially.

**Method.** The alkali solution is made by dissolving 10 gm of anhydrous sodium carbonate in distilled water and bringing the volume to 100 ml. Ten milliliters of this solution is mixed with 1 ml of clear urine in a test tube of standard size for the comparator block. The mixture is placed in boiling water for 8 min and the color that develops is compared with that of the standards in a comparator block.

INTERPRETATIONS AND LIMITATIONS. The test is not specific for glucose and so has the same limitations as those discussed under the Benedict's qualitative test for glucose. The color cannot be judged for low concentrations of glucose (less than

0.3 gm/100 ml). For values from 0.6 to 7.0 gm/100 ml the agreement of the Somogyi method with other methods is of the order of ± 25 percent or less.[47] Description of the technique of quantitative methods used to determine urinary glucose is beyond the scope of this manual.

## Urinary Ketone (Acetone) Bodies

The ketone bodies—acetone, acetoacetic acid, and β-hydroxybutyric acid—appear in the blood and are excreted in the urine as the result of increased fat catabolism (see Unit 28). They appear during the ingestion of high-fat, low-carbohydrate diets, in starvation, and in diabetic ketoacidosis. In fresh urine containing ketone bodies, the concentration of acetoacetic acid is 5 to 15 times that of acetone. The concentration of β-hydroxybutyric acid is usually 2 to 4 times that of the acetoacetic acid.[48] On standing, the latter two substances are decarboxylated to form acetone.

The nitroprusside reaction ("acetone test") tests for both acetone and acetoacetic acid. However, acetoacetic acid will yield a positive color reaction about 20 times more intense than acetone in equal concentrations. The ferric chloride test ("diacetic test") is specific for acetoacetic acid but is some 20 times less sensitive than the nitroprusside test for detecting this substance. It would, therefore, be more rational to consider the ferric chloride test simply a less sensitive test for "ketone bodies" than the nitroprusside test. Its usefulness accordingly lies in the fact that a positive ferric chloride reaction would indicate a more severe degree of ketonuria than a positive nitroprusside reaction—a well-established clinical observation. The expressions "acetone test" and "diacetic test" are so embedded in medical terminology that the physician must be familiar with them. At the present time, there is no simple method to test for β-hydroxybutyric acid.

## METHODS OF TESTING FOR KETONE BODIES

NITROPRUSSIDE REACTION. *Rothera Test.* A number of different modifications of this procedure are available. A commonly used one employs a stable, dry, pulverized mixture containing 5 gm of sodium nitroprusside mixed with 200 gm of ammonium sulfate. Approximately 1 gm of this preparation is added to 5 ml of fresh urine and shaken gently to dissolve. One to 2 ml of full-strength ammonium hydroxide is layered over this mixture by dropping bottle or medicine dropper. A reddish-brown ring develops in a few minutes at the interface in the presence of ketone bodies. The color of the ring is recorded according to intensity (pink 1+ to dark purple-red 4+). A faint brown ring is of no significance. A more precise method has been described in which 5 ml of fresh urine is saturated with ammonium sulfate and 10 drops of 2-percent sodium nitroprusside is added and mixed. Ten drops of concentrated ammonium hydroxide is layered over the mixture, and the color development is observed after 15 min and recorded as above.[48]

*Nitroprusside Tablets—Acetest* (Ames Co., Elkhart, Ind.). Acetest is a stable, noncaustic tablet containing sodium nitroprusside, glycine, disodium phosphate, and lactose, which will give a color reaction in contact with fluids (urine, plasma, or serum) containing acetone or acetoacetic acid. The technique of the test is to place the tablet on white paper and add a drop of urine to its surface. In the presence of acetoacetic acid or acetone, color will develop, the intensity of which is read at 30 sec. This intensity is roughly proportional to the concentration of acetone bodies. A color chart is provided with the tablets. Trace color reactions are frequently of no significance clinically.[49]

*Nitroprusside Powder—Acetone Test Denco* (Denver Chemical Manufacturing Co., New York). This is a powder of

309

sodium carbonate, ammonium sulfate, and sodium nitroprusside, the use of which is very similar to that of the Ace-test tablet. A drop of urine is added to a small amount of powder on white paper. Acetoacetic acid or acetone will cause the development of a purple color. A color chart is provided with the powder. The substance will also yield trace color reactions of no significance.

FERRIC CHLORIDE TEST FOR ACETOACETIC ACID. Ferric chloride solution is made by dissolving 10 gm of ferric chloride in 100 ml of distilled water. This solution is added to 5 ml of urine in a test tube, drop by drop, with agitation of the tube until the precipitate of ferric phosphate that usually forms redissolves. A deep Bordeaux red color develops if aceto-acetic acid is present.

*Interpretations and Limitations.* This test gives positive results in the presence of a number of other substances, the most important of which are salicylates. If a positive result is obtained, the urine must be boiled vigorously for approximately 15 min. With boiling, the aceto-acetic acid will be oxidized to acetone and the sample will no longer give a positive reaction. The salicylates will remain unchanged in solution and continue to give a red color.[48]

## Examination of the Urine Sediment

### GENERAL CONSIDERATIONS

The centrifuged sediment contains all the insoluble materials that have accumulated in the urine in the process of glomerular filtration and during passage of the fluid through the tubules of the kidneys and lower urinary tract. Intelligent examination of this material demands an awareness of the dynamic nature of the process of urine formation and knowledge of the implications of qualitative and quantitative changes in the exfoliations of the kidney and urinary tract. For certain formed elements, notably casts, the site of origin can definitely be identified as the kidney. For others, such as white blood cells and red blood cells, definite localization is not possible, unless these cells are found trapped within the matrices of casts. When renal disease is present, it is often possible to surmise, from examination of the urine sediment, the nature of the pathologic process in the kidney and its degree of activity.

Localization of disease in the lower urinary tract may be aided by use of fractional urine collection. The information obtained by the qualitative examination of the unstained sediment may be supplemented, where indicated, by the use of quantitative methods, stains, and other special examinations.

### COLLECTION OF URINE FOR EXAMINATION OF SEDIMENT

Urine for examination of sediment should be fresh (preferably still warm from voiding), well concentrated and of acid pH, since hyaline casts and erythrocytes dissolve rapidly in dilute and alkaline solution. Ideally, the specimen for examination should be the first morning urine passed after a 12- to 18-hr period of fluid deprivation. Tests of concentrating ability (Unit 20) therefore provide an ideal opportunity for sediment examination.

### FRACTIONAL COLLECTION OF URINE: THE TWO- AND THREE-GLASS TESTS

Fractional collection of urine may help in determining the site of origin of cells in the urine sediment, especially in males.

**Method.** Three collection flasks are provided. The patient voids the first 30 ml into the first flask; then, without interrupting the stream, he collects the majority of the bladder contents in the second flask, switching to the third flask to collect the final 20 or 30 ml at the end of micturition. Equal volumes of the three specimens are promptly centrifuged and the sediment is examined.

*Interpretation.* In males, the first specimen contains material washed out of the anterior urethra. The third specimen may contain cellular elements squeezed out of the prostate at the end of urination. If cells are present in all three flasks, it indicates that their source is proximal to the vesical neck, that is, in the bladder or upper urinary tract.

In the *two-glass test,* the presence of cells in the first glass only indicates anterior urethritis.

## QUALITATIVE EXAMINATION OF THE URINE SEDIMENT

### DIRECT EXAMINATION OF UNSTAINED SEDIMENT

The simplest and most widely used method of examining urinary sediment is the direct examination of the unstained material. Ten to 15 ml of urine is centrifuged in a conical tube for 5 min. The supernatant is decanted and the sediment resuspended in the remaining fluid by finger flicking. A drop of this concentrated sediment is then transferred to a slide and a coverslip is added. The specimen is examined under reduced light with the use of an Abbe condenser and diaphragm. The entire specimen should be first examined under low power. This assures that casts and rare elements will be located. Identification of individual elements is aided by changing from low to high power and by varying the focus and light intensity. After the entire specimen has been scanned and the sparser elements enumerated, an examination is made under high-power magnification of 15 or more representative fields for the purpose of identifying and enumerating cells and other small elements, as well as the more numerous casts.

### CONVENTIONS FOR RECORDING THE FREQUENCY OF FORMED ELEMENTS IN THE URINE

Although the direct examination of the unstained sediment, as described above, is a qualitative examination, knowledge of the relative frequency of various types of cells and casts is extremely valuable and some convention is necessary for quantitating the approximate frequency of the scantier elements as well as those that appear in every high-power field. Quantitation of other elements such as crystals and bacteria is less feasible and a general estimate of their frequency ("occasional," "few," or "many") is usually sufficient.

When cells or casts are present in all or nearly all fields under high magnification, their frequency should be recorded as the number per high-power field. When an element fails to occur in each field but appears as often as once in each two or three fields, its frequency may be recorded as 0–1 per high-power field. The following scheme is recommended for recording the frequency of elements that occur less frequently than once in three high-power fields: 1–2 per coverslip, rare; 2–10 per coverslip, occasional; more than 10 per specimen but less than 1 per high-power field, frequent.

### USE OF STAINS IN EXAMINATION OF URINE SEDIMENT

Many staining techniques have been designed for use with urine sediments. Although each technique has its adherents, none has supplanted the direct examination of the unstained sediment for routine use. A variety of staining techniques are described by Schreiner.[1] The most useful stains are those that serve special purposes, such as the identification of "granular motility cells" or erythrocytes in casts. Stains may also be used in preparing permanent mounts of urine sediment.

STERNHEIMER-MALBIN STAIN.[50] This supravital stain was designed for the identification of "granular motility cells" with special staining characteristics (see p. 314). It has also become increasingly popular in recent years as a general-purpose stain for identification of formed elements.

*Reagents.* Solution A: methylrosaniline (crystal violet), 3.0 gm; 95-percent ethanol, 20 ml; ammonium oxalate, 0.8 gm; distilled water to make a total volume of 80 ml.

Solution B: Safranine-O, 0.25 gm; 95-percent ethanol, 10 ml; distilled water to make a total volume of 100 ml.

*Technique.* Mix 3 parts of Solution A and 97 parts of Solution B; filter and store in a dropper bottle. One drop of the stain is added to the reconstituted sediment in the centrifuge tube; microscopic examination should be done promptly.

*Interpretation.* Ordinary polymorphonuclear leukocyte nuclei stain orange-purple. "Granular motility cells" are colorless or stain light blue. Hyaline casts stain pink to purple, epithelial cells dark purple, erythrocytes faint lavender, bladder epithelial-cell nuclei blue, and vaginal epithelial-cell nuclei purple.

BENZIDINE-NITROPRUSSIDE STAIN.[51] This stain is useful for differentiating erythrocytes from yeast and identifying red blood cells and heme pigments.

*Reagents.* (1) Benzidine-nitroprusside reagent: Dilute 1 ml of 1-percent aqueous benzidine to 6 ml with distilled water; then add 1 ml of 2-percent sodium nitroprusside, and bring the volume up to 10 ml with distilled water. This is stable for 2 weeks or more and should be discarded when a precipitate forms.

(2) Three-percent hydrogen peroxide: Dilute superoxol 1 to 10. This is stable for 3–4 days.

*Technique.* To 1 drop of sediment on a slide, add 1 drop of benzidine nitroprusside reagent; mix thoroughly, then add 1 drop of peroxide and mix again. If the specimen is alkaline, add 1–2 drops of 10-percent nitric acid. Specimens of high specific gravity and those with preservatives added should be stained for 5 to 8 min. Others may be examined after 2 min.

*Interpretations and Limitations.* Erythrocytes usually stain deep purple but are sometimes pale blue. Yeast cells are either unstained or show a faint blue-green iridescence. Leukocytes stain pale gray. Hyaline casts are unstained. The granules of granular casts have a deep purplish-blue color. Casts containing heme pigments are homogeneously dark purple or blue. Since the granules in casts are stained by this method, the presence of blue color must be interpreted with caution when the method is used for identification of red-cell casts.

### USE OF POLARIZED LIGHT

Lipid droplets containing cholesterol esters are anisotropic in polarized light. The presence of these droplets may be identified by observing the sediment while using one polarizing film in the condenser and another in the ocular lens. With high-power magnification and bright illumination, one of the polarizing filters is turned to produce maximum darkening of the field. Anisotropic fat droplets show up brightly and appear to be divided into four quadrants, giving the appearance of a Maltese cross. Crystals, hair, and clothing fibers also show up brightly with this technique, but do not exhibit division into quadrants.

### QUANTITATIVE EXAMINATION OF URINARY SEDIMENT

#### GENERAL CONSIDERATIONS

When the sediment is examined qualitatively, only a crude estimate can be made concerning the abundance of formed elements in the urine. The number of cells and casts seen will depend not only on their rate of excretion, but also on the concentration (osmolality) of the urine sample, the volume of urine centrifuged, and the residual volume into which the sediment is resuspended after decanting. Quantitative examination of the sediment as developed by Addis [2] eliminates these variables. A timed specimen is obtained and the formed elements are counted in a hemocytometer using a volume of urine representing the quan-

tity formed in 1/5 hr. By applying correction factors, figures are obtained for the 24-hr rate of excretion of the various formed elements.

### TECHNIQUE OF THE ADDIS COUNT

A timed specimen of urine is obtained representing an interval of at least 4 hr but preferably 8 or 9 hr. An overnight specimen is ideal. The volume of the

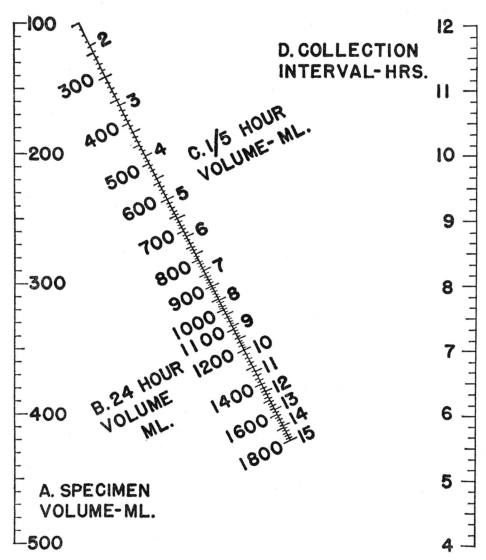

Fig. 31. Nomogram for calculating the 1/5-hr urine volume.[32] Lay a transparent ruler on the nomogram so that it intersects scale *A* at the observed volume and scale *D* at the collection interval. The 24-hr volume and the 1/5-hr volume are read at the point where the ruler intersects scales *B* and *C*. If an observed value is not included on scales *A* or *D*, divide it by 2, and multiply the result by 2. (From R. W. Lippman, *Urine and the Urinary Sediment*, 1952. Courtesy of Charles C Thomas, Publisher, Springfield, Illinois.)

sample is measured in a graduated cylinder and the volume representing the urine excreted in $\frac{1}{5}$ hr is calculated or obtained by reference to a nomogram [33] (Fig. 31). This volume of urine is then measured into a 15-ml conical tube and centrifuged for 5 min at 2000 rev/min. The supernatant is withdrawn, leaving 0.5 ml in the tube. The sediment is resuspended in this volume and thoroughly mixed. A drop of this suspension is transferred with a pipette to the chamber of a standard hemocytometer. Microscopic examination is then made under reduced light. Casts are counted under low-power magnification in six contiguous large squares representing 0.0006 ml of urine. The number of casts seen, multiplied by 100,000, represents the number of casts excreted per 24 hr. Erythrocytes, leukocytes, and tubular epithelial cells are then counted under "high dry" magnification in 13 contiguous medium-sized squares representing 0.00006 ml of urine. The number of each cell type, multiplied by 1,000,000, represents the number excreted per 24 hr. If the $\frac{1}{5}$-hr volume exceeds 15 ml, half the volume may be used and the figures doubled.

INTERPRETATIONS AND LIMITATIONS. Quantitative counts of urine sediment represent rates of excretion and make possible direct comparisons between examinations done at different times and in different patients. The technique has its greatest usefulness in following the course of patients with known renal disease, especially glomerulonephritis, where the rates of excretion of cells are valuable indices of the activity of the disease. The quantitative technique should not be substituted for the qualitative examination, since, in the limited quantity of material examined, important abnormalities may be overlooked. The use of large "correction" factors also introduces an artificial variability into the results, especially when the numbers of elements actually counted are small.

SIGNIFICANCE OF CELLS IN THE
URINE SEDIMENT

LEUKOCYTES. The white blood cells that appear in urine are predominantly polymorphonuclear neutrophils. Morphologically, leukocytes may be difficult or impossible to distinguish from renal tubular epithelial cells either in the stained or the unstained sediment and the two types of cell often have to be grouped together in recording results. The presence of increased numbers of leukocytes in the sediment is often indicative of urinary-tract infection, especially when clumping of the cells occurs. Occasional white cells are frequently found in normal urine sediment. Rates of excretion of up to 650,000 or 1,000,000 cells/24 hr [33, 52] have been considered normal in the past. However, it has been emphasized recently [53, 54] that in chronic pyelonephritis active infection may be present without significant pyuria. This disease may therefore escape detection if the presence of increased numbers of white cells in the sediment is used as the sole criterion of diagnosis. Bacteriologic studies represent the most reliable method of detection (Unit 26). The presence of granular motility cells in the sediment may also suggest the diagnosis.

Increased numbers of leukocytes and epithelial cells occur in glomerulonephritis and other diseases not associated with bacterial infection. Contamination of urine specimens with cells from the vulva and vagina can usually be avoided by obtaining a "clean catch" midstream specimen.

GRANULAR MOTILITY CELLS ("Glitter Cells"). Large leukocytes exhibiting active Brownian movement of their cytoplasmic granules have been termed granular motility cells or glitter cells. The presence of these cells in the urine sediment was thought by Schilling (1908) [55] to denote active pyelonephritis as opposed to infection elsewhere in the urinary tract. With the Sternheimer-Malbin supravital stain (p. 312) granular motility cells stain differently from ordinary leukocytes. The nature of the changes that give rise to these special characteristics is obscure. The active granular motility is apparent only in a dilute medium and is inhibited when the concentration of the urine exceeds 600 mOsm/L.[56] The special staining characteristics are not altered by changes in osmolality. Recent studies support the contention that the presence of these cells in the urine sediment often denotes chronic pyelonephritis.[50, 54, 56] However, they are often absent from the urine of patients with this disease. Furthermore, typical granular motility cells may be found in vaginal secretions, prostatic fluid, and biologic fluids from other sites more remote from the genitourinary tract.[56]

ERYTHROCYTES. Erythrocytes, like leukocytes, may enter the urine from any part of the urinary tract. In the urine, red blood cells act as osmometers and alter in size and appearance depending on the osmolality of the urine. In concentrated urine they lose their usual biconcave contour and become small and crenated. In dilute urine, they may appear large and swollen, or they may rupture leaving only a ring of stroma, or "ghost cell." Red blood cells in the urine must be differentiated from yeast cells. The latter are ovoid, rather than round, and may show buds. Where differentiation is difficult, the benzidine-nitroprusside stain may be of value (p. 312). Erythrocytes are less commonly seen in normal urine sediment than are leukocytes, although the frequency with which they are seen probably depends on the diligence with which they are sought. Maximum excretion rates ranging from 130,000 to 600,000 cells/24 hr [33, 51] are reported in normals.

Increased numbers of red cells may appear in the urine following violent physical exertion [57] and during the acute febrile phase of streptococcal infections [58]

without signifying disease of the kidneys or urinary tract. A variety of hemorrhagic diseases may result in hematuria. Gross or microscopic hematuria of renal origin is almost always found in glomerulonephritis and other vascular renal diseases associated with glomerulitis. It is a common but not constant finding in subacute bacterial endocarditis. Intermittent or constant hematuria is usual in severe hypertension and may also occur following renal infarction or when a tumor of the kidney is in communication with the urinary collecting system. Hematuria associated with pyuria commonly occurs in tuberculous pyelonephritis. Hematuria may also signify infection, infarction, or neoplasm of any part of the lower urinary tract and is usually present when a stone is traversing the ureter.

EPITHELIAL CELLS. Cells of the renal tubular epithelium are round, mononuclear, and generally larger than leukocytes. They may occasionally be seen in urine from normal subjects. Their presence in the urine in increased numbers signifies degenerative exfoliation of the tubular epithelium and may be seen in glomerulonephritis and other vascular nephritides, following exposure to nephrotoxic substances, or during acute infections involving the renal medulla. When intense degenerative changes occur, whole sheets of epithelial cells may appear in the sediment or may be identified in casts. A moderate increase in excretion of epithelial cells may occur in orthostatic proteinuria. When both epithelial cells and leukocytes are present in a sample of urine, characteristic members of both cell types usually can be identified but it is often impossible clearly to differentiate all members of the two groups. In such cases, it is preferable to count and record them together.

Large numbers of renal tubular epithelial cells are usually excreted in the urine of patients with massive proteinuria from any cause, whether or not other features of the nephrotic syndrome are present. Many of these cells contain droplets of lipid and often are so heavily laden with lipid that cellular architecture is obscured. In the past, these fat-laden epithelial cells have been called "oval fat bodies." Under polarized light many of the fat droplets are anisotropic, indicating the presence of cholesterol esters. The pathogenesis of the "fatty degeneration" of tubular epithelial cells in the nephrotic syndrome is uncertain; it is probably linked causally to the associated proteinuria.

Large squamous epithelial cells are often seen in urine sediment, especially in samples from female patients. These cells have their origin in the vagina and lower urinary tract. For practical purposes, their presence may be ignored.

### SIGNIFICANCE OF CASTS IN URINE SEDIMENT

SIGNIFICANCE AND PATHOGENESIS OF CASTS. Casts represent protein coagula formed in the lumina of the renal tubules and subsequently washed into the urine. For casts to form, protein must be present in tubular urine in sufficient concentration and under conditions favorable to coagulation. In histologic sections of the kidney, casts are rarely found in the proximal tubule or thin limb of the loop of Henle. They first appear in the ascending limb of the distal tubule and increase in frequency in the distal convolution and the collecting tubules.[59] It is in these sites that the final reabsorption of water occurs to produce an osmotically concentrated urine.[60] The concentration of unreabsorbed urine protein is therefore greatest in this region of the nephron and the rate of flow is slowest. Experimental data concerning the physicochemical conditions that favor or inhibit the coagulation of protein in tubular urine are scanty. Data of Oliver[61] indicate that the solubility of naturally occurring protein in urine is influenced by

a variety of factors, including the concentrations of urea and electrolytes, the pH of the urine, and the concentration of a nondialyzable heat-resistant substance bearing some resemblance to chondroitin sulfuric acid.

Casts are usually classified descriptively as hyaline, cellular, granular, or waxy. It is probable that all types have a common mode of origin in the coagulation of unreabsorbed protein in the tubular lumen. Within this coagulum may be trapped the cells, bacteria, crystals, and other debris present at the site of formation. When cells are trapped in large quantities, the cast may appear to be made up entirely of them and the protein matrix is obscured. When cells are scantier, they may appear as inclusions within the substance of an otherwise homogeneous cast. When no cells or debris are present, the coagulum alone forms a clear "hyaline" cast. From clinical observations, Addis[2] concluded that cellular casts undergo progressive changes after formation, with disintegration of the cells and dispersion of cellular contents giving rise first to coarsely granular, then to finely granular, and finally to waxy casts. This concept is reasonable but lacks any direct experimental confirmation.

HYALINE CASTS. Hyaline casts are homogeneous cylindrical structures of low refractile index, best seen under reduced light. Small numbers of hyaline casts are seen in normal urine and large numbers appear in the urine of normal subjects following strenuous exercise.[57, 62] They are seen in increased numbers when proteinuria is present from any cause, including postural and febrile proteinuria. Hyaline casts should be carefully inspected for inclusions, since the presence of formed elements within the casts indicates that these are derived from the kidney rather than the lower urinary tract.

RED-BLOOD-CELL CASTS. The term "red-cell cast" is usually applied to casts that are densely packed with erythrocytes so that no hyaline matrix is visible. In some instances the individual red cells may be distinguished within the cast; in others, the cast is homogeneous with no discernible cellular structure. Recognition in both instances depends on the characteristic rufous-orange color of the contained heme pigment, best identified by increasing the light transmission through the cast. Bile-stained granular casts have a somewhat similar appearance, but may usually be distinguished by detecting bile in the urine. The presence of red-cell casts is characteristic of diseases associated with glomerulitis, such as glomerulonephritis, focal embolic glomerulitis, lupus erythematosus disseminata, and polyarteritis nodosa. Red-cell casts may also be seen in the first urine passed following an ischemic injury to the kidney due to hypotension. In this circumstance their presence usually presages the onset of acute renal failure. Casts containing heme pigment are also seen in the urine following intravascular hemolysis. Typical red-cell casts may be seen occasionally in all diseases associated with hematuria of renal origin. The presence of hyaline casts with red-cell inclusions implies renal hematuria of lesser degree.

WHITE-BLOOD-CELL CASTS. In acute or chronic pyelonephritis, casts may appear that are densely packed with leukocytes. Hyaline casts containing leukocytes, bacteria, or both usually have a similar significance. Differentiation of leukocytes from epithelial cells may be aided by use of the Sternheimer-Malbin supravital stain, especially if granular motility cells are present.

EPITHELIAL-CELL CASTS. With exfoliation of the renal tubular epithelium, variable numbers of epithelial cells may appear as inclusions in hyaline casts. These may be difficult or impossible to distinguish from leukocytes. With intense exfoliative changes, casts densely packed with epithelial cells appear. Occasionally, two rows of apposed epithelial cells may be recognized, representing the lining tubular epithelium. Epithelial cell casts may appear following exposure to nephrotoxic agents and in chronic glomerulonephritis and other vascular nephritides. In the nephrotic syndrome, epithelial-cell casts containing anisotropic fat droplets are frequently seen. In early acute glomerulonephritis, casts containing both epithelial cells and red blood cells are regarded by Addis [2] as characteristic.

GRANULAR CASTS. Granular casts are thought to represent cellular casts that have undergone degenerative changes after formation. They are of higher refractive index than hyaline casts but are best identified in subdued light. Coarsely granular and finely granular casts are usually reported separately. They are rarely seen in normal urine but may be seen in variable numbers in orthostatic proteinuria and in congestive heart failure as well as in any of the acute or chronic renal diseases.

WAXY CASTS. These are thought by Addis [2] to represent a final degenerative end product in the evolution of cellular casts. They are homogeneous or very finely granular in texture and of higher refractive index than hyaline casts. They often show cracks and fissures. They do not occur in normal urine and are most often seen in chronic renal disease of long duration. They also appear during the diuretic phase following acute renal failure.

BROAD CASTS. Casts of wide diameter appear in the urine in far-advanced chronic renal disease [2] and during recovery from acute renal failure. They are probably formed in the distal collecting tubules where the convergent outflow of a number of contributing nephrons ordinarily prevents the precipitation of protein. When function is reduced or absent in a sufficient number of tributary nephrons, conditions are favorable for cast formation in these sites. Broad casts are usually cellular, granular, or waxy. They are from two to six times as wide as ordinary casts and can usually be identified by direct comparison with other casts in the same urine sample.

"FATTY CASTS." In the nephrotic syndrome, lipid droplets may be seen within epithelial-cell or granular casts. These inclusions may be rare or conspicuous enough to give the appearance of a "fat-stuffed" cast. The presence of anisotropic lipid may be identified by the use of polarized light (p. 312).

PIGMENTED CASTS. When bile is present in the urine, casts, cells, and cellular debris are stained a uniformly greenish-yellow color. On casual inspection, bile-stained casts resemble red-blood-cell casts. The similar staining of cells and cellular debris may aid in differentiation. Tests for bile are usually positive. Very dark or black casts containing calcium salts may appear in the urine of patients with nephrocalcinosis. Black casts may also appear in melanuria.[59] In patients with hemoglobinuria or hemochromatosis, hemosiderin may appear within casts as yellowish globules. Its presence can be identified by the Prussian blue reaction (Unit 9).

### CRYSTALS IN URINE SEDIMENT

The crystals that may appear in normal urine are listed in Table 61 and Figure 32. They can be conveniently divided into those which appear in acid urine and those which appear in neutral or alkaline urine. Increased quantities of crystals may occur in patients who tend to form kidney stones. The recognition of

cystine crystals is of considerable importance, since they occur only in patients with aminoaciduria. Sulfonamide crystals may appear in the urine of patients receiving sulfadiazine but only rarely appear when the more soluble sulfonamide drugs are used.

### MISCELLANEOUS FINDINGS IN URINE SEDIMENT

BACTERIA. Rod-shaped bacilli are easily identified in the unstained urine sediment. Cocci are less easily recognized. Bacteriologic examination of the urine is discussed in Unit 26. The presence of bacteria in a gram stain of the unsedimented clean voided morning urine indicates active urinary-tract infection.[53]

YEAST. Yeast cells are commonly found in urine samples, especially from diabetic patients. They have no pathologic significance but may be confused with erythrocytes. Yeast cells are ovoid, rather than round, and vary somewhat in size. They reproduce by budding and the presence of buds is helpful in identification. They are insoluble in acids and alkalis and do not take the benzidine-nitroprusside stain (p. 312).

MUCIN. A small amount of mucin is often present in the urine sediment of normal subjects. It is presumably secreted by the mucous membrane of the lower urinary tract and appears in the urine sediment as a diffuse, translucent, uneven background material, occasionally taking the form of shreds. An increase in mucin commonly accompanies inflammatory disease anywhere in the urinary tract.

TRICHOMONADS. Trichomonas vaginalis is a common vaginal contaminant in the urine of female subjects. Trichomonads occasionally invade the lower urinary tract of male or female subjects and produce an inflammatory reaction. They may be recognized as unicellular organisms with flagellate motility and are usually somewhat larger in size than leukocytes.

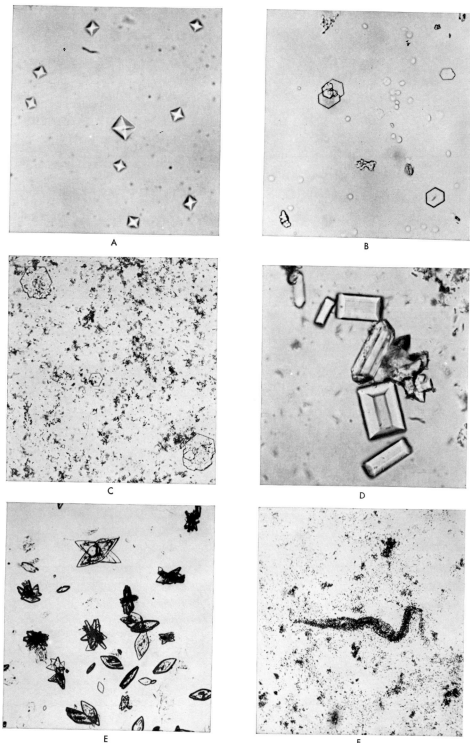

Fig. 32. Stone-forming elements in the urine. (*a*) Calcium oxalate crystals, usually found in concentrated acid hypercalciuric (and hyperoxaluric) urine; crystals are birefringent. (*b*) Cystine crystals at pH 4.5. Cystine is less soluble in acid urine and crystals may be elicited in cystinuric urine by acidification with glacial acetic acid and cooling overnight in a refrigerator. (*c*) Cystine crystals at pH 7.5 (with amorphous phosphates in background). The crystals are thin plates with color and typically hexagonal; they are diagnostic of cystinuria. (*d*) Triple phosphate crystals at pH 7.5 (magnesium, ammonium, and calcium phosphate), typically found in urinary sediment of pyelonephritis with urea-splitting urinary infection. (*e*) Uric acid crystals at pH 4.5. These are the most pleomorphic of the common crystals. They are yellowish brown in color, and may produce brick red sediment when plentiful. (*f*) Amorphous phosphates and calcium phosphate cast at pH 7.5. The granules are brown-black and with distinct structure under the light microscope. The finding suggests hypercalciuria. (Photographs by Philip H. Henneman, M.D., Endocrine and Metabolism Laboratories, Massachusetts General Hospital.)

Table 61. *Crystal forms found in urinary sediments of normal urine [from M. R. Mattice,* Chemical procedures for clinical laboratories (*Lea and Febiger, Philadelphia, 1936*), *with permission].*

| Sediments | Urine reaction | Forms | Usual size | Chemical behavior |
|---|---|---|---|---|
| Calcium oxalate | Neutral, alkaline, or acid, but usually acid | Octahedral or envelope form with highly refractive center<br>Dumbbell type | Octahedra, small as a rule, about the size of rbc; seen as points of light under low power | Insoluble in acetic acid; soluble in strong HCl; insoluble in NaOH |
| Uric acid | Acid | Yellow or brown-red rhombic prisms, wedges, rosettes, irregular plates, somewhat oval forms with pointed ends; the rhombic plates may be colorless, although uric acid crystals are recognized largely by color | Large "brick dust" can be detected macroscopically; colorless forms tend to be smaller than pigmented | Soluble in NaOH, in ammonia with subsequent formation of ammonium urate crystals; insoluble in acetic acid and HCl |
| Sodium urates [a] | Acid | Amorphous; light or dark-brown granules in mosslike arrangement<br>Crystalline; colorless needles or fan-shaped clusters | Recognizable under low power | Dissolve on heating; soluble in NaOH, HCl, or acetic acid with formation of uric acid crystals in 10 to 20 min |
| Ammonium urates | Alkaline (free ammonia) | Opaque, yellow crystals, smooth and spherical or covered with spicules, "thorn-apples" | Easily recognized under low power | Soluble in acetic acid like sodium urates |
| Ammonium magnesium phosphate (triple phosphate) | Alkaline; also in slightly acid urine if there is an abundance of ammonium salts | "Coffin lids"; square prisms that can be distinguished from calcium oxalate by the size and highly refractive center of the latter as well as by chemical means; irregular prisms; disintegrating prisms; feathery, leaflike forms | Very large | Soluble in acetic acid |
| Calcium carbonate | Usually alkaline | Dumbbells, single or clustered | Smaller than calcium oxalate | Soluble in acetic acid with evolution of $CO_2$ |
| Calcium phosphate [b] (stellar phosphate) | Alkaline | Amorphous; colorless globules or granules single or clustered<br>Crystalline; wedge-shaped, single or rosettes | Recognizable under low power | Soluble in acetic acid |

[a] Calcium, magnesium, and potassium urates are amorphous. They are found in concentrated urine of strong acidity.

[b] Phosphate crystals resembling thin broken sheets of ice are frequent in urine of mild reaction.

HEMOSIDERIN. In patients with hemoglobinuria or hemochromatosis, hemosiderin may appear in the urine sediment, either free or in casts or epithelial cells. Hemosiderin appears as yellowish-brown spheroids and may be identified by the Prussian blue reaction (Unit 9).

CONTAMINANTS. A great variety of contaminants find their way into urine samples. Hairs, shreds of clothing, and talcum-powder crystals are common examples. Talc crystals resemble calcium oxalate crystals but have softer margins, are less uniform in size and shape, and have a highly refractile center. Spermatozoa are frequently found in the sediment of male subjects.

DIAGNOSIS AND EVALUATION OF
RENAL DISEASE BY MEANS OF
URINE SEDIMENT

The interpretation of urinary abnormalities is to some extent empirical and must always be evaluated in the light of other clinical data. Nevertheless, both qualitative and quantitative examinations of sediment often provide important information concerning the nature and intensity of pathologic processes in the kidney. The numbers of red blood cells and casts excreted in the urine provide rough but useful indices of the activity of diseases such as glomerulonephritis. Similarly, the activity of degenerative processes in the tubules is roughly reflected by the rate of excretion of epithelial cells. The quantity of leukocytes in the urine may reflect the intensity of urinary-tract infections, although, as emphasized elsewhere, the absence of pyuria does not exclude active infection. It is often possible to detect clinically important changes in rates of excretion of formed elements by careful qualitative examination of sediment alone. Use of the Addis count is helpful in detecting more subtle changes and is especially valuable in following the course of patients with glomerulonephritis. Knowledge of renal function, as measured by creatinine or urea clearance, is also necessary for the interpretation of changes in the rates of excretion of protein and formed elements, since excretion rates usually decline as renal failure supervenes.

Characteristic findings in a variety of renal diseases are given in Table 62. The quantitative excretion rates for protein and formed elements are representative values and must not be regarded as limits. Exceptions are common and considerable overlap among the different disease entities is apparent. The findings in chronic glomerulonephritis have been arbitrarily divided into three "stages,"[2] although no true division exists and transitional states may be observed. Urinary findings in the nephrotic form of chronic glomerulonephritis are similar to those seen in nephrotic syndrome due to any other cause and etiologic diagnosis may be difficult or impossible without the aid of renal biopsy. In lupus erythematosus disseminata, polyarteritis nodosa, and other forms of diffuse vasculitis involving the kidney, the urine sediment frequently resembles that seen in one or more of the "stages" of glomerulonephritis. The urine sediment in these diseases sometimes contains at one and the same time the characteristic findings of all three "stages" of chronic glomerulonephritis.[63] This has been called a "telescoped sediment."[2] The pathologic significance of this is not clear. It is not a pathognomonic finding, since similar sediments have been observed in glomerulonephritis and subacute bacterial endocarditis.[64]

### Cytologic Examination of the Urine for Detection of Malignant Disease

The Papanicolaou technique for cytologic diagnosis of urinary-tract malignant disease has been in use for over 10 years. Reports concerning its reliability are conflicting,[65] but up to the present time the method appears to be less useful in detecting early and curable cancer in the urinary tract than in other sites.[65, 66] The early reports on the use of the method indicated a high percentage of false positive results and of unsatisfactory specimens.[65, 67] With refinements in technique and in the criteria for recognition of malignant cells, these percentages have been improved. Best results are obtained with epithelial tumors of the renal col-

320

Table 62. *Representative findings in renal disease.*

| Disease | Protein (gm/24 hr) | Erythrocytes ($10^6$/24 hr) | Leukocytes and epithelial cells ($10^6$/24 hr) | Abnormal elements [a] | Casts [a] | Remarks |
|---|---|---|---|---|---|---|
| Normal | 0–0.05 | 0–0.130 | 0–0.650 | | Hyaline, 2000/24 hr | Casts more common in older age group |
| Orthostatic protein-uria | 1.0 | 0–0.130 | 0–3.0, epithelial | | Variable hyaline and granular | Protein absent and casts and epithelial cells diminished or absent during recumbency |
| Acute glomerulo-nephritis | 0.5–5.0 | 1–1000 | 1–400 | | *Rbc casts, mixed rbc and epithelial cell casts,* hyaline and granular casts | "Coffee-colored urine" due to hemoglobin derivatives |
| Chronic glomerulo-nephritis | | | | | | |
| Latent stage | 0.1–2.0 | 1–100 | 1–20 | | *Rbc casts,* hyaline and granular casts | Rbc casts may be rare |
| Nephrotic form | 4.0–40.0 | 0.5–50 | 20–1000 | Fat-laden epithelial cells | *Epithelial-cell casts, "fatty casts,"* granular and hyaline casts | Anisotropic fat droplets in epithelial cells and casts |
| Terminal stage | 2.0–7.0 | 0.5–10 | 1–50 | | *Broad casts, waxy casts,* epithelial-cell, granular and hyaline casts | |
| Lupus erythematosus disseminata | 0.5–20+ | 1–100 | 1–100 | Fat-laden epithelial cells [a] | *Rbc casts,* hyaline cellular and granular casts, *"fatty casts," "waxy casts," "broad casts"* | Variable sediment |
| Acute pyelonephritis | 0.5–2.0 | 0–1 | 20–2000 | Bacteria | *Wbc casts,* hyaline and granular casts containing bacteria | |
| Chronic pyelonephritis | 0–5.0 | 0–1 | 0.5–50 (often in clumps) | Bacteria, *granular motility cells* | *Wbc casts,* hyaline and granular casts containing bacteria | Casts often scanty or absent; bacilliuria, pyuria, and proteinuria may be intermittent |
| Renal tuberculosis | 0.1–3.0 | 1–20 | 1–50 | Tubercle bacilli | Wbc casts, hyaline granular casts | Microscopic hematuria more prominent than in nontuberculous infection |
| Acute tubular necrosis | | | | | | |
| Ischemic phase | Amount varies with urine volume | Usually abundant | Variable—may be abundant | | *Rbc casts early,* epithelial cells, hyaline and granular casts | Rbcs and rbc casts more prominent after ischemic injury; epithelial cells and casts more prominent after exposure to nephrotoxins |
| Diuretic phase | 0.5–10.0 | 0–1 | 1–100 | | Broad casts; waxy casts; epithelial-cell, granular and hyaline casts | |
| Accelerated hypertension | 1.0–10.0 | 1–100 | 1–30 | | Rbc casts (sometimes), hyaline and granular casts | |
| Toxemia of pregnancy | 0.5–10.0 | 0–1 | 1–5 | | Hyaline and granular casts, occasional epithelial-cell and fatty casts | Hypertension usual; azotemia absent |
| Intercapillary glomerulonephrosis | 2.0–20.0 | 0–1 | 1–30 | Fat-laden epithelial cells | Epithelial cell and "fatty" casts; hyaline and granular casts | Often coexists with chronic pyelonephritis and nephrosclerosis |

[a] The more characteristic findings are italicized.

lecting system. Recent data from a laboratory specializing in the use of cytologic methods [68] indicate that in malignant diseases of the bladder, ureters, and renal pelvis, correct positive results are obtained in approximately 62 percent, and 18 percent are read as suspicious. In malignant disease of the prostate, cytologic examinations are read as positive in 15 percent and suspicious in 21 percent, and in malignant disease of the kidney approximately 8 percent are read as positive and 25 percent as suspicious. In this series, there were approximately 1 percent false positive results and 8 percent were read as suspicious when no malignant disease was present. False positive results may occur in chronic cystitis and when renal calculi are present. Variations in the reliability of the method probably represent differences in interpretation of the observed changes.[68] The technical details of cytologic examination are beyond the scope of this manual.[69]

### Aminoaciduria

GENERAL CONSIDERATIONS. Amino acids are actively reabsorbed by the renal tubule and do not normally appear in the urine in large amounts. However, normal urine contains small amounts of glycine, taurine, and histidine, and varying quantities of many other amino acids.[70] The $\alpha$-amino nitrogen ordinarily accounts for less than 1.5 percent of the total nitrogen excreted but is only partially dependent on total nitrogen metabolism. Absolute values for $\alpha$-amino nitrogen excretion in normal subjects range from 64 to 199 mg/24 hr [71] when the Van Slyke gasometric ninhydrin method is used.[72] Higher values have been reported with the earlier and less specific methods of measurement. Individual amino acids may be identified in the urine by the use of chromatographic techniques. The presence of cystine in the urine may be detected by the nitroprusside test.

NITROPRUSSIDE TEST FOR CYSTINURIA (MODIFIED FROM BRAND *et al.*).[73] *Reagents.* (1) Concentrated ammonium hydroxide; (2) 5-percent sodium cyanide; (3) 5-percent solution of sodium nitroprusside, freshly prepared.

**Method.** To 5 ml of urine, add 1 drop of ammonium hydroxide and 2 ml of sodium cyanide. Mix and allow to stand for 10 min. Add sodium nitroprusside drop by drop and shake. A permanent purplish-red color indicates a positive test. The method measures both cystine and cysteine. A slightly longer but more specific test is that of Sullivan.[73, 74] This may be used to confirm the nitroprusside test.

AMINOACIDURIA IN DISEASE. An increase in urinary exaction of amino acids may occur when the plasma level of amino acids is increased ("overflow aminoaciduria") or when the amino acids of the glomerular filtrate fail to be reabsorbed in the tubules ("renal aminoaciduria"). "Overflow" occurs in severe liver disease when the metabolism of amino acids is impaired. The increased phenylalanine excretion associated with phenylketonuria is also an "overflow" phenomenon. In the common acute and chronic renal disease, significant aminoaciduria does not usually occur.[75] However, in certain diseases, an increased excretion of various amino acids does occur, although plasma levels are normal. These "renal aminoacidurias" are probably the result of specific enzymatic defects.

The congenital diseases associated with generalized aminoaciduria include the deToni-Fanconi syndrome, Wilson's disease, and galactosemia. "Cystinuria" with a tendency to form cystine stones is also congenital. In this disease, lysine, arginine, ornithine, and cystine are all present in increased amounts in the urine. Aminoaciduria may be "acquired" following lead or Lysol poisoning with renal damage. In Wilson's disease, deposition of copper in the renal parenchyma may be responsible for the defect. A number of other rare and poorly understood diseases are also associated with peculiarities of amino acid excretion.[76]

### Abnormal Pigments in the Urine

The exogenous substances that may discolor the urine are listed in Table 59, and discussed on p. 293. These are of no pathologic significance. Endogenous substances giving rise to abnormal color in fresh urine include hemoglobin, myoglobin, bile pigments, certain indoles, porphyrins and related compounds, homogentisic acid, and melanogen. In general, the colored compounds themselves are often lacking in characteristic chemical properties. Their precursors, or chromogens, whose presence may not be apparent to the naked eye, usually have more distinctive properties. Their presence may often be detected by observing the color development under controlled conditions. Fresh urine is usually necessary for these procedures.

#### HEMOGLOBIN

SIGNIFICANCE OF HEMOGLOBINURIA. Following intravascular hemolysis, free hemoglobin enters the glomerular filtrate and probably is partly reabsorbed by the tubules.[11, 77] Recent work indicates that free hemoglobin is bound by a serum mucoprotein (haptoglobin), and appears in the urine only when this is saturated. This may account for the fact that hemoglobin regularly appears in the urine only when the serum level exceeds 100–130 mg/100 ml.[78] In very dilute urine, hemolysis of red cells may release detectable amounts of hemoglobin. Hemoglobinuria without hemoglobinemia has been described in renal infarction.[79] In the urine, hemoglobin undergoes changes that are poorly understood. There is rapid formation of methemoglobin and of a form of hematin.[80] The color of the urine when hemoglobin is present varies from red to brown. Hemoglobin and all its derivatives react with benzidine.

BENZIDINE TEST. *Reagents.* (1) Saturated solution of benzidine dihydrochloride in glacial acetic acid, or benzidine marketed specifically for detection of blood (not benzidine base). This should be fresh and stored only for short periods of time in a brown bottle. (2) Fresh 3-percent hydrogen peroxide made as a 1:10 dilution of stock superoxol.

**Method.** To 3 ml of benzidine solution, add 2 ml of urine and 1 ml of hydrogen peroxide. A blue color indicates the presence of hemoglobin.

TEST FOR DIFFERENTIATION OF HEMOGLOBINURIA FROM MYOGLOBINURIA.[81] **Method.** Dissolve 2.8 gm of ammonium sulfate in 5 ml of urine and then centrifuge or filter. Hemoglobin is rapidly precipitated by this procedure, whereas myoglobin remains in the supernatant.

*Interpretation.* The test differentiates hemoglobin which is insoluble in an 80-percent saturated solution of ammonium sulfate from myoglobin (and other pigments) which are not precipitated.

QUANTITATIVE DETERMINATION OF HEMOGLOBIN IN THE URINE. The concentration of hemoglobin in the urine can be measured quantitatively by the same benzidine methods used in the determination of plasma hemoglobin levels (see Unit 11). Certain salts in urine (for example, sulfates and urates) interfere with the color reaction and cause turbidity by precipitating benzidine. To avoid this, urine should be dialyzed overnight against a 0.9-percent sodium chloride solution prior to the determination.

*Interpretation.* Quantitative study of hemoglobinuria is seldom necessary in clinical medicine. However, the benzidine reaction as well as the hand spectroscope may be utilized simply as a qualitative test to identify urinary pigments as heme proteins (and thus for practical purposes as either hemoglobin or myoglobin).

OTHER TESTS. Oxyhemoglobin can be identified by its absorption spectra. Methemoglobin and hematin are hard to differentiate. On addition of a few drops of concentrated ammonium sulfide at neutral pH, methemoglobin is converted to reduced hemoglobin and hematin is converted to an alkaline hemochromogen with an intense absorption band at 558 $\mu$.

### MYOGLOBIN

Myoglobin appears in the urine after extensive destruction of muscle, as in crush injuries or following occlusion of a main-limb artery,[82, 83] and in the rare disease termed acute paralytic myoglobinuria or acute recurrent rhabdomyolysis.[84, 85]

Myoglobin has only one quarter the molecular weight of hemoglobin; hence it is cleared more rapidly by the kidney. The presence of heme pigments in the urine and not in the serum suggests myoglobinuria.

Separation of myoglobin from hemoglobin depends on fine differences in the absorption maxima. The $\alpha$ band of the oxy compounds is most useful in this respect (see Table 63). A high-grade instrument such as the Hartridge reversion spectroscope or a spectrophotometer is necessary for the differentiation. If the met derivatives are present, these can be reconverted to the oxy compounds with a small amount of sodium hydrosulfite and vigorous shaking.[84]

### INDOLES

PHYSIOLOGY. The urinary and fecal indole derivatives of tryptophane are produced by the action of bacterial flora. Indole and skatole (3-methylindole) represent different metabolic pathways, probably reflecting the actions of different bacterial species.[86, 87] Indole is partially absorbed from the intestine, oxidized to indoxyl, and excreted mainly as a sulfate

ester. Indoxyl sulfate is known as indican because of its similarity to botanical indican (indoxyl glucoside). Urinary derivatives of skatole are not known. However, another urinary indole, indole acetic acid, sometimes parallels the fecal excretion of skatole[88, 89] and may also have a nonenteric origin.[90] Tests for this group of indoles have fallen from popularity because they have no immediate practical significance. Nevertheless, since they give false positive reactions with a variety of tests for substances of greater physiologic significance, the identification of these substances by appropriate tests is still of value.

Recently, there has been a revival of interest in the indoles since the discovery that some of these compounds are of considerable physiologic importance. Among the latter are serotonin and certain characteristic indoles from phenylalanine and tyrosine metabolism which can be detected in the urine of patients with melanotic tumors and in phenylketonuria. An increase of several indoles has also been reported in pellagra.[91] Most indoles give the Ehrlich aldehyde reaction and therefore may be confused with urobilinogen or porphobilinogen.

MELANURIA. Patients with widespread melanotic tumors excrete a colorless precursor of melanin in the urine. Rarely, this spontaneously polymerizes into a melanin-like pigment. The work of Linnell and Raper[92] indicates that the melanogen is a conjugate (glucuronide or sulfate) of 5,6-dihydroxyindole. Unfortunately, no definitive, quantitative method is available. There are reports that the same compound occurs in the urine after the ingestion of large amounts of indole,[93, 94] indicating that the compound may not be specific for melanotic sarcoma.

The following tests for melanuria are helpful but often hard to interpret. Parallel tests must be made on normal urine for comparison.

**Method.** 1. Boil urine with an equal volume of concentrated hydrochloric acid. All urines darken somewhat but urines of high melanogen content turn jet black.

2. Add a few drops of 10-percent ferric chloride to the urine. Filter and expose precipitated ferric phosphate to the air for 30 min. A positive reaction is the *gradual* blackening of the precipitate. Salicylates will obscure this test.

3. Prepare fresh bromine water by adding a few drops of liquid bromine to 100 ml of water. (Discard the solution when the color fades.) Mix equal amounts of bromine water and urine. A yellow precipitate forms which gradually turns black if the reaction is positive.

4. The Thormählen Test. This is alleged to be the most specific test for the condition. However, in practice it is difficult to read and not very sensitive. To 1 ml of urine add several drops of dilute sodium nitroprusside in 10-percent potassium hydroxide. A violet color is produced which changes to blue on the addition of excess acetic acid.

THE CARCINOID SYNDROME. Patients with widespread metastases from carcinoid tumors of the small intestine are subject to attacks of flushing, diarrhea, and asthma, and after a time develop pulmonic stenosis. These changes are related to an overproduction of serotonin (5-hydroxytryptamine).[95] Serotonin itself is difficult to measure,[96] but a metabolic product of serotonin, 5-hydroxyindole acetic acid, is excreted by normal persons in the range of 2 to 8 mg daily and is greatly increased in this condition.[95] A simple test to exclude gross excesses of this compound is that of Sjoerdsma *et al.*[97]

*Reagents.* (1) 1-nitroso-2-naphthol (0.1 gm in 95-percent ethanol); (2) nitrous acid, freshly prepared by mixing 0.2 ml of 2.5-gm/100 ml sodium nitrite solution and 5 ml of 2N sulfuric acid; (3) ethylene dichloride (reagent grade).

**Method.** Pipette into a test tube 0.2 ml of urine, 0.8 ml of water, 0.5 ml of nitrosonaphthol solution, and 0.5 ml of nitrous acid. Mix and leave at room temperature for 10 min, then add 5 ml of ethylene dichloride.

*Interpretation.* A purple color will be visible in the top layer when the concentration of 5-hydroxyindole acetic acid is 4 mg/100 ml or more. Large amounts of keto acids may inhibit the reaction. Nevertheless, the test is usually sensitive enough to detect the increased excretion usually present in the carcinoid syndrome. Where doubt exists, the quantitative method of Udenfriend[98] or paper chromatography[99] should be used.

THE EHRLICH ALDEHYDE REACTION IN MELANURIA AND CARCINOID SYNDROME. Most indoles gives the Ehrlich aldehyde reaction and therefore may be confused with urobilinogen and porphobilinogen. The Watson-Schwartz test was designed to minimize the indole component of this reaction. Another modification of the Ehrlich aldehyde test is useful in distinguishing the physiologically important indoles from other interfering substances and may be used in conjunction with other tests in the diagnosis of melanuria or the carcinoid syndrome.

**Method.** To 5 ml of urine, add several drops of 5-percent Ehrlich's reagent (see Unit 24) in ethanol, 5 ml of ethanol, and 0.5 ml of concentrated hydrochloric acid.

*Interpretation.* Blue colors are produced by the indoles present in melanuria and by 5-hydroxyindole acetic acid. Other compounds give shades ranging from orange to purple.

INDOLE ACETIC ACID AND UROROSEIN. Under a variety of conditions, indole acetic acid condenses into a red pigment, urorosein.[89] This has been repeatedly mistaken for porphyrin.[91] It also masquerades as porphobilinogen in the Watson-Schwartz test.[100] Recently, the excretion of large amounts of this compound has been described in the very rare Hartnup disease.[101]

**Method.** To 10 ml of urine, add 2 ml of concentrated hydrochloric acid and a few drops of 2-percent sodium or potassium nitrate.

*Interpretation.* Formation of large amounts of urorosein results in the instantaneous appearance of a red pigment. Less marked excesses are brought out on heating in a water bath. A faint reaction is seen in normals.[102]

INDOXYL SULFATE OR INDICAN. The identification of this substance is of occasional importance because of its interference in the Ehrlich aldehyde reaction. The Obermayer test [102] is used.

*Reagent.* 2 gm of ferric chloride in 1 L of concentrated hydrochloric acid.

**Method.** If bile is present, remove with ⅛ volume of 10-percent barium chloride and filter. Add 5 ml of reagent to 4 ml of urine or filtrate. Mix, then add 2–3 ml of chloroform. Invert several times. A blue color in the chloroform indicates the presence of indoxyl sulfate.

### PHENOLIC ACIDS

Some 43 different phenolic acids arising largely from the metabolism of tyrosine and phenylalanine have been found in human urine.[103] Certain of these are normal metabolic products of thyroid and adrenal medullary hormones. Gross increases of members of this family occur in four conditions. Three of these, alcaptonuria, phenylketonuria, and tyrosinosis, are examples of inborn errors of metabolism in that they are thought to represent genetic defects in specific enzymes. The other condition, tyrosyluria, occurs in premature infants when fed high-protein diets. This situation is characterized by the appearance of excessive amounts of p-hydroxyphenylpyruvic and p-hydroxyphenyllactic acid.[104] These same compounds, plus increased amounts of 3,4-dihydroxyphen-

ylalanine (DOPA), characterize the single reported case of tyrosinosis.[105]

The urine in both these conditions reduces Benedict's solution and darkens in alkali but to a less striking extent than is seen in alcaptonuria. The iodine titration method of Neuberger will differentiate these from alcaptonuria.[106]

ALCAPTONURIA. This disease is characterized by the excretion of large amounts of homogentisic acid (2,5-dihydroxyphenylacetic acid) in the urine. It is presumed to represent a block in the oxidative pathway of tyrosine metabolism. A high renal clearance of this substance has been reported and suggests that it is actively excreted by renal tubules.[107]

Alcaptonuria is often discovered in infancy because of blackening of the diapers but it remains asymptomatic until later life when an extensive degree of degenerative arthritis sets in. Extensive calcification of the intervertebral disks is a fairly pathognomonic sign.[108] Since the abnormal component is excreted in gram amounts, diagnosis is not difficult. It can be picked up on routine urinalysis because it reduces Benedict's solution, giving a characteristic yellow precipitate and black supernatant fluid in this test.

**Methods.** 1. The urine turns black on the addition of alkali.

2. The urine also has the unique property of developing photographic film. According to Fishberg,[109] a photographic film is exposed to air for 10 min. The urine is alkalinized with 0.5 ml of 2.5N sodium hydroxide to 2 ml of urine. A drop of alkalinized urine is placed on the exposed film. A positive reaction is immediate blackening of the film.

A quantitative method, also easily adaptable for diagnostic use, is the iodine titration method of Neuberger.[106]

*Limitations.* Gentisic acid (2,5-hydroxybenzoic acid), a product of salicylate metabolism, gives all of the reactions of homogentisic acid. It is present at most in milligram amounts and rarely causes confusion.[106]

PHENYLKETONURIA (Phenylpyruvic Oligophrenia). This disease is due to a block in the conversion of phenylalanine to tyrosine. As a consequence, other pathways of phenylalanine metabolism are saturated. A large number of abnormal metabolites accumulate.[110, 111] There is increasing evidence that toxicity of phenylalanine itself is responsible for the idiocy and neurologic symptoms in these patients.[110-112] Early diagnosis is important since it is hoped that dietary phenylalanine restriction, if initiated early enough, will be beneficial.[110, 112] Phenylpyruvic acid is the abnormal metabolite most amenable to screening tests, although estimation of serum phenylalanine levels is considered necessary for proper therapeutic management.[110, 113-115]

A modification of the Penrose and Folling test[115] is used.

*Reagents.* (1) 10-percent ferric chloride, made fresh weekly; (2) 25-percent (by volume) sulfuric acid.

**Method.** Measure 5 ml of urine into each of two test tubes. Add 1 drop of sulfuric acid to the first tube. Then add ferric chloride drop by drop until 5 ml has been added. The tube may cloud or a green color may develop, indicating a positive reaction. If the tube clouds, add 2 drops of acid to a second tube and repeat the test.

## The Porphyrias

### PHYSIOLOGY

A porphyrin is a ring of four pyrrol nuclei connected by methene bridges. The best-known member of this family is ferro-protoporphyrin 9, also known as heme, the prosthetic group of hemoglobin and other respiratory enzymes.

The biochemical processes involved in the synthesis of the porphyrins have been extensively studied.[116] Many of the inconsistencies of earlier studies have been resolved by the recent discovery

Table 63. *Wavelengths (m$\mu$) of spectroscopic absorption bands of important pigments.*

| Pigment | Band | | | |
|---|---|---|---|---|
| | $\alpha$ | $\beta$ | $\gamma$ | |
| Oxyhemoglobin | 577 | 540 | 414 | |
| Oxymyoglobin | 582 | 542 | 418 | |
| CO displaces oxyhemoglobin and oxymyoglobin | | | 4–6 m$\mu$ toward blue | |
| Porphyrins: [a] condensed from Watson and Larson [119] | | | | |
| Coproporphyrin in — | | | | |
| Ether | 624 | 568 | 529 | 498 |
| 7.5$N$ HCl | 594 | 575 | 551 | |
| Uroporphyrin I in — | | | | |
| 0.1$N$ NaOH | 612 | 564 | 539 | 504 |
| 7.5$N$ HCl | 597 | 554 | | |
| Waldenström's porphyrin in | | | | |
| 7.5$N$ HCl | 596 | 553 | | |

[a] Formulas for quantitation from optical density maxima in the near ultraviolet (Soret region), method of Rimington and Sveinsson modified by With;[145] correction in micrograms per milliliter of solution per centimeter light path.

Coproporphyrin: Max 401 in 0.1–0.15$N$ HCl;
$D_{corr} = 2D_{401} - (D_{380} + D_{430}) \times 0.817$
Uroporphyrin: Max 405 in 0.5$N$ HCl;
$D_{corr} = 2D_{405} - (D_{380} + D_{430}) \times 0.831$

that the condensation of porphobilinogen proceeds via uroporphyrinogen and coproporphyrinogen to protoporphyrin.[117, 118] The uro- and coproporphyrins are to be regarded as irreversible oxidation products of the corresponding porphyrinogens. It is possible that porphyrinogens as well as porphyrins occur in the urine and stool.[119]

The pathway of porphyrin biosynthesis is presented in Fig. 33. The porphyrins are derived from the porphyrinogens by dehydrogenation of the connecting methene bridges. Inspection of the structural formula of the porphyrin ring reveals that several isomeric series are possible. The Type III series is the configuration found in heme. The Type I

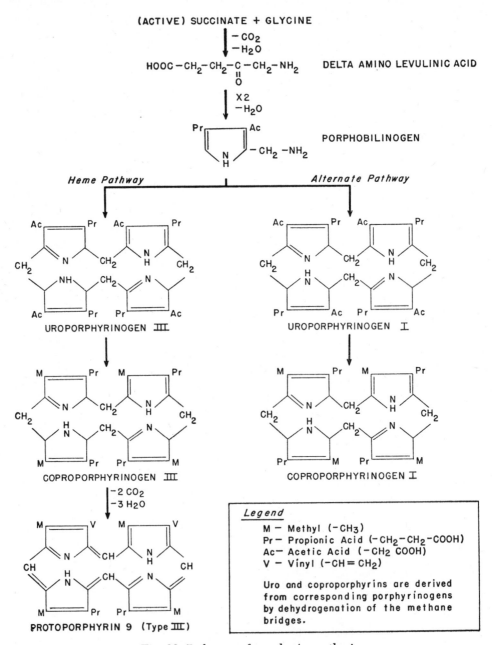

Fig. 33. Pathways of porphyrin synthesis.

porphyrins are also found in biologic materials and are probably by-products of the synthesis of heme. Paradoxically, certain aberrations of the blood-forming organs which are associated with increases in excretion of porphyrins are usually characterized by an excess of the Type I series, whereas in the conditions where nonbiochemical condensation of nonporphyrin precursors into porphyrins may be a factor the Type III series predominates.

The normal red cell contains free protoporphyrin and traces of coproporphyrin. It has been shown that variations in the concentration of these substances have some interesting diagnostic and physiologic implications.[120] Coproporphyrin and to a lesser extent protoporphyrin are normal constituents of the stool.[121] Coproporphyrin is normally found in the urine in amounts varying from 70 to 250 $\mu$g/day. In the majority of normal people, coproporphyrin I is usually in excess of coproporphyrin III.[121]

## Coproporphyrinuria

### SIGNIFICANCE OF COPROPORPHYRINURIA

The biochemical source of normal urinary coproporphyrins is not known. Moderate increases in the excretion of these substances occur in so many conditions that the finding of a moderate increase is of little diagnostic value. The excretion of coproporphyrin I is increased in association with increased erythropoietic activity from any cause, in infectious hepatitis, and in obstructive jaundice. The increased excretion in obstructive jaundice is thought to be related to a rerouting of the coproporphyrins (especially Type I) from feces to urine. Some increase in coproporphyrin III excretion is commonly found in infections, malignant diseases, and alcoholic cirrhosis, and following ingestion of many chemicals. An increase of coproporphyrin III excretion is the only biochemical

derangement produced acutely by ingestion of small amounts of ethanol.[121, 122] Some apparently normal individuals excrete large amounts of coproporphyrin III.[123]

### COPROPORPHYRINURIA IN LEAD POISONING

In lead poisoning, the urinary excretion of coproporphyrin III is markedly increased. Although lead causes some disturbance of heme synthesis, this increase in coproporphyrin excretion may be unrelated to blood formation.[124, 125] In spite of the limitations previously discussed, the measurement of urinary coproporphyrin is a valuable aid in the diagnosis and management of lead poisoning. It is quicker and cheaper than measurement of urinary lead content and avoids the inherent pitfalls of trace-element analysis. Furthermore, it is helpful in distinguishing between patients with clinical lead poisoning and those exposed to lead but not ill because of it. Since the excretion of coproporphyrin III is so large in lead poisoning (up to 10 mg/day), it is usually out of the range seen in the other conditions previously discussed. Moderate increases must always be interpreted with caution. The presence of coproporphyrin does not cause discoloration of the urine.

### METHODS

Coproporphyrin may be measured by the method of Schwartz, Zieve, and Watson,[126] using standards for visual comparison or a photofluorimeter. Quantitative results may also be obtained by measurement of light absorption in the near ultraviolet, using a Beckman DU spectrophotometer (see Table 63). Twenty-four-hour urine collections for coproporphyrin determination should be made with 5 gm of sodium carbonate in the collection flask as a preservative. Urine lead analysis should not be done on the same sample since lead phosphate may precipitate under these conditions.

## THE TRUE PORPHYRIAS

The common denominator of the true porphyrias is the presence of uroporphyrins in the urine and stool. The work of Watson and associates has led to a basic revision in the classification of these diseases.

### PORPHYRIA ERYTHROPOIETICA (CONGENITAL OR PHOTOSENSITIVE PORPHYRIA)

Biochemically, this disease is characterized by an overproduction of uroporphyrin I and coproporphyrin I in the blood-forming organs. The excess porphyrins, especially uroporphyrin, accumulate in the subcutaneous tissues and give rise to photosensitivity. The disease has its onset early in life, and usually manifests itself as a bullous skin eruption (hydroa aestivale), exacerbated by exposure to sunlight. Other unidentified substances may also cause photosensitivity with an identical skin lesion, and only a third of the reported cases of hydroa aestivale are associated with porphyria. Splenomegaly and a hemolytic anemia often develop in porphyria erythropoietica some time after the skin lesion. The teeth and nails may become discolored by deposits of porphyrin. In most cases, the urine is grossly discolored owing to the presence of porphyrin, and varies in color from pink to dark burgundy. Laboratory diagnosis depends on the identification of uroporphyrins in the urine. Porphobilinogen is not present.

### PORPHYRIA HEPATICA

ACUTE INTERMITTENT PORPHYRIA. In this disease, certain compounds that are precursors of porphyrins are produced in excess by the liver and perhaps by other tissues. The disease is characterized clinically by intermittent bouts of abdominal pain, together with variable neurologic and psychiatric disturbances. It differs from congenital porphyria in that the relation between the biochemical disorder and the signs and symptoms is obscure.

A variety of abnormal substances representing porphyrins and their precursors appear in the urine. Most of the porphyrin material in the urine of these patients arises from precursors after the urine has been passed, and as a result the urine may darken visibly on standing. The presence in the urine of porphobilinogen, which gives the Ehrlich aldehyde reaction, is a characteristic of the disease. This substance has recently been identified [127, 128] as one of Shemin's hypothetical intermediates in the metabolic pathway between succinate and glycine and the porphyrins.[116] Delta-amino levulinic acid, another metabolic intermediate, is also excreted in large amounts in the urine.[129] There is some increase in excretion of coproporphyrin III, and a uroporphyrin similar to but not identical with uroporphyrins I and III is also present in the urine. The latter compound, called Waldenström's porphyrin, may be formed to a limited extent in the body, but most of it arises from precursors after the urine has stood. Other uroporphyrins also appear on standing and are apparently derived from porphobilinogen and at least one other precursor.[130] A brown pigment of unknown composition, called porphobilin, also forms on standing.

Diagnostically, the presence of porphobilinogen is characteristic of acute intermittent porphyria in relapse. There are many pitfalls in the identification of this substance. However, if the result of the porphobilinogen test is strongly positive, spectroscopic examination of the red-purple color will show a characteristic strong absorption band at 560 m$\mu$. This gives a reliable means of verifying the diagnosis. Diagnosis may also be ascertained by identification of uroporphyrins after converting the precursors to porphyrins. The conditions for optimum conversion of precursors to uroporphyrins are complex and vary from case to case. The usual procedure is to boil the urine at pH 5.0 for 30 min.[131]

PORPHYRIA CUTANEA TARDA. A disease that clinically resembles porphyria erythropoietica but has its onset later in life has been described.[132, 133] Recent work indicates that the metabolic defect is in the liver, although the relation of this disease to acute intermittent porphyria is not clear.[134] Diagnosis rests on clinical manifestations and the presence of uroporphyrins in the urine. Porphobilinogen is absent.

ACQUIRED PORPHYRIA CUTANEA TARDA. This disease occurs as an occasional complication of alcoholic cirrhosis. Uroporphyrins exceed coproporphyrins in the urine, although both are present in increased quantities.[135] Data on the chemical nature of the excess porphyrins in this disease are fragmentary. The site of condensation appears to be the liver.[134]

CONGENITAL PROTOCOPROPORPHYRIA. This disease usually has its onset in adolescence. Large amounts of coproporphyrins and small amounts of uroporphyrins are found in the urine. Large excesses of coproporphyrins and protoporphyrins are found in the stool. Some patients have episodes of abdominal pain and evidence of neurologic derangements, and porphobilinogen may be found in the urine.

METHODS. 1. *Uroporphyrins.* A simple, satisfactory method of identifying uroporphyrin has not been devised.[136] The method of Brunsting *et al.*, modified by Sunderman,[137] has been widely used. This depends on the extractability at pH 3 of uroporphyrins in a solvent composed of equal parts of normal butanol and ethyl acetate. Small amounts of uroporphyrin may escape detection by this method. A precipitation method[138] has similar limitations but has the advantage of simplicity. The most elegant method is that of Schwartz,[139] by which the por-

phyrins can be eluted in a concentrated form for further study. A great deal of useful information may be obtained by paper chromotography of porphyrins.[140] A simple ascending technique requiring 2 to 3 hr is adequate. Other methods of identification are too laborious for clinical use.[141]

2. *Identification of Porphobilinogen.* Porphobilinogen is usually identified by its reaction with Ehrlich's aldehyde reagent. As emphasized elsewhere, this reaction is far from specific. Porphobilinogen is distinguished from urobilinogen and most other substances giving this reaction by the fact that the colored complex formed is insoluble in chloroform. Nevertheless, false positive reactions are often encountered. These may be due to anticonvulsant drugs,[142] pyridium,[100] or the presence of indoles such as urorosein and indoxyl.[143] False positive reactions may also occur in patients with fecal stasis. Often the interfering chromogen cannot be identified. Many attempts have been made to increase the specificity of this test and to make it quantitative.[129] However, the Watson-Schwartz modification of the Ehrlich aldehyde reaction remains the standard procedure.

WATSON-SCHWARTZ TEST.[144] *Reagents.* (1) Modified Ehrlich's reagent: 3.5 gm of *p*-dimethylamino benzaldehyde, 750 ml of concentrated hydrochloric acid, and 500 ml of water. (2) Saturated sodium acetate, made by adding approximately 1 kg of sodium acetate to 1 L of water at 60°C. A large excess of crystals should remain on cooling. (3) Chloroform.

**Method.** To 2.5 ml of fresh urine in a test tube, add 2.5 ml of Ehrlich's reagent; shake, and after exactly 15 sec add 5 ml of saturated sodium acetate. Then add 5 ml of chloroform, shake, and centrifuge. A positive reaction is a strong red (or red-purple) color, limited to the upper, aqueous phase.

INTERPRETATIONS AND LIMITATIONS. The limitations of the test for porphobilinogen stem from the large number of substances that may give false positive reactions by this test. These are discussed in the preceding paragraphs. False positive reactions due to urorosein and pyridium may be eliminated by repeating the test, substituting hydrochloric acid for Ehrlich's reagent, using acid of the same strength as that used in the reagent. These compounds, but not porphobilinogen, will produce a red color under these conditions. False positive reactions due to indoles may be identified by using the various tests for indoles described elsewhere in this section. The diagnosis of the porphyrias associated with excretion of porphobilinogen cannot be considered firmly established unless uroporphyrins can be identified in the urine following conversion of precursors by boiling for 30 min at pH 5.0.[145]

### Urinary Excretion of Catechol Amines

The presence of a pheochromocytoma may be associated with either paroxysmal or sustained hypertension due to pressor amines liberated into the circulation by the tumor. A variety of pharmacologic tests have been devised to aid in detecting these tumors. These tests are designed to provoke a characteristic paroxysm of hypertension in a nonhypertensive patient or to produce significant lowering of the blood pressure in a hypertensive one. They have been reviewed and evaluated in detail by Chapman and Singh [146] and by von Euler and Ström.[147] Except for the phentolamine (Regitine) test, the pharmacologic tests are not without danger, and they not infrequently give false positive or false negative results. False negative results are especially common where pheochromocytomas give rise to persistent hypertension. Recently, direct chemical determinations have been developed for quantitatively measuring the urinary excretion of catechol amines and their

metabolites. In general, the chemical methods are reliable and specific, and involve no risk to the patient. Where facilities are available for their use, they have largely superseded the pharmacologic tests.

### PRINCIPLES

The pressor amine output of the normal adrenal medulla has an epinephrine content of 75–80 percent, the remainder being chiefly norepinephrine.[148] These are excreted in the urine in a fairly constant proportion of 1–5 percent of circulating catechol amines.[147] Pheochromocytomas contain large amounts of pressor amines, but in contrast to the normal adrenal medulla, norepinephrine usually predominates, together with varying amounts of epinephrine. The norepinephrine/epinephrine ratio in the patient's urine usually parallels that of the tumor.

### METHODS

Determinations are made on 24-hr urine samples, which are more convenient to analyze than blood samples. Since they integrate fluctuations over a 24-hr period, the results are more representative and reproducible. The 24 hr over which a urine sample is collected should ideally include normal activity, sleep, and, if possible, a characteristic hypertensive paroxysm. The urine samples should be acidified to pH 2 with hydrochloric acid during collection, since the catechol amines are unstable at alkaline pH. With acidification, the samples do not deteriorate at room temperature for up to 1 week, and will keep almost indefinitely if refrigerated.

In general, two methods are available. In the trihydroxyindole method,[148, 149] the catechol amines are adsorbed on aluminum oxide and eluted with acid, and the eluate is oxidized with ferricyanide to trihydroxyindoles. These are then tautomerized to the fluorescent compounds adrenolutine and noradrenolutine by alkali, and stabilized with ascorbic acid to prevent further oxidation. Estimations are then performed fluorimetrically. Epinephrine and norepinephrine are differentiated by preferential oxidation at different levels of pH. A recently developed method for simultaneous fluorimetric estimation of epinephrine and norepinephrine following ion-exchange purification is probably the best method currently available for routine clinical use.[150]

The second method makes use of the ethylenediamine condensation reaction.[151] This consists of the formation of a fluorescent substance formed by condensing adrenochrome with ethylenediamine. This test is extremely sensitive, but is less specific, because other catechol derivatives may similarly form fluorescent compounds both in urine and in blood determinations. These derivatives may be especially increased in the presence of renal insufficiency.[152, 153]

INTERPRETATIONS AND LIMITATIONS. The usual 24-hr excretion of pressor amines in the urine of normal subjects is approximately 20–40 $\mu$g of norepinephrine and 4–8 $\mu$g of epinephrine.[147] The total is usually less than 63 $\mu$g/24 hr, of which about 80 percent is norepinephrine.[151] Some fluctuation of these values has been shown to occur in response to stimulation of the carotid-sinus reflex (norepinephrine), during strenuous muscular work, and during exposure to cold and emotional stress.[154] The pressor-amine output at rest is about half that during normal daily activities, and is markedly lowered during the night,[155] but the latter effect may be related to posture and inactivity.

In the vast majority of cases of pheochromocytoma, the 24-hr urine-excretion values for catechol amines are 10–100 times the normal, of which the greater part is usually in the norepinephrine fraction, and present no significant difficulty in evaluation,[147] regardless of the method of determination. Rare cases of pheochromocytoma have been reported with 24-hr values of urinary catechol amines lower than 200 $\mu$g, the lowest being 104 and 109 $\mu$g.[147]

At least three cases have been reported showing normal norepinephrine values.[156–158] Small but significant increases in epinephrine excretion may have been of diagnostic importance in these cases. In all three, catechol amine determinations were made on urine samples collected during paroxysm-free intervals. Although it is generally true that the urinary catechol amines are significantly elevated even between paroxysms,[147, 159] a 24-hr urine collection should include such a paroxysm, if possible. It is preferable to achieve this by repeated determinations rather than by histamine provocation, which may be dangerous.

The current status of false positive results is controversial.[159] Such conditions as hemorrhagic shock, myocardial infarction, severe trauma, insulin hypoglycemia, and others may give significantly elevated values, but in their absence it would appear that false positive results have usually been due to the use of crude techniques. Patients with essential hypertension do not have urinary catechol amine levels exceeding the upper limits of normal.[159]

According to von Euler, when epinephrine constitutes 10–50 percent of urinary catechol amines, the tumor is probably adrenal medullary in location; when it constitutes 0–2 percent, it probably arises in extra-adrenal chromaffin tissues.[160]

METABOLIC DEGRADATION PRODUCTS OF CATECHOL AMINES. Recent work indicates that the metabolic degradation of epinephrine and norepinephrine involves methoxylation and oxidative deamination, with formation of several derivatives, of which the most abundant is 3-methoxy, 4-hydroxy mandelic acid (vanillyl mandelic acid or VMA).[161, 162] The methoxylated derivatives of the pressor amines (metanephrine and normetanephrine) also occur in the urine.[163, 164] Because catabolism of the catechol amines is rapid, these degradation products are much more abundant in the urine than are free epinephrine and norepinephrine. The urinary excretion of VMA is greatly increased in patients with pheochromocytoma,[161, 165] and a constantly increased VMA excretion has been reported in a patient with paroxysmal hypertension in whom catechol amine excretion was normal during the interval between attacks.[166] The clinical use of measurements of VMA, metanephrine, and normetanephrine for diagnosis of pheochromocytoma must await improvements in methodology.

## REFERENCES

1. G. E. Schreiner, "The identification and clinical significance of casts," *A.M.A. Arch. intern. Med.* 99, 356 (1957).
2. T. Addis, *Glomerular Nephritis* (Macmillan, New York, 1949).
3. P. B. Beeson, "The case against the catheter," *Amer. J. Med.* 24, 1 (1958).
4. V. Hawkinson, C. J. Watson, and R. H Turner, "Modification of Harrison's test for bilirubin in urine, especially suited for mass and serial use," *J Amer. med. Ass.* 129, 514 (1945).
5. J. Orloff, "The role of the kidney in the regulation of acid-base balance," *Yale J. Biol. Med.* 29, 211 (1956).
6. G. H. Mudge, "Clinical patterns of tubular dysfunction," *Amer. J. Med.* 24, 785 (1958).
7. A. S. Relman and W. B. Schwartz, "The kidney in potassium depletion," *Amer. J. Med.* 24, 764 (1958).
8. A. F. Muller and C. M. O'Connor, *An Internationl Symposium on Aldosterone* (Little, Brown, Boston, 1958).
9. H. P. Dustan and A. C. Corcoran, "Functional interpretation of renal tests," *Med Clin. N. Amer.* 39, 947 (1955).
10. H. W. Smith, *The Kidney: Structure and Function in Health and Disease* (Oxford University Press, New York, 1951).
11. W. Dock, "Proteinuria and the associated renal changes," *New Engl. J. Med.* 227, 633 (1942).
12. L. J. Rather, "Filtration, resorption, and excretion of protein by the kidney," *Medicine (Baltimore)* 31, 357 (1952).
13. A. L. Sellers, N. Griggs, J. Marmoston, and H. C. Goodman, "Filtration and reabsorption of protein by the kidney," *J. exp. Med.* 100, 1 (1954).
14. J. Hardwicke and J. R. Squire, "The relationship between plasma albumin concentration and protein excretion in patients with proteinuria," *Clin. Sci.* 14, 509 (1955).
15. D. A. Rigas and C. G. Heller, "The amount and nature of urinary proteins in normal human subjects," *J. clin. Invest.* 30, 853 (1951).
16. J. R. Squire, "The nephrotic syndrome," *Advanc. intern. Med.* 7, 201 (1955).
17. J. R. Squire, J. D. Blainey, and J. Hardwicke, "The nephrotic syndrome," *Brit. med. Bull.* 13, 43 (1957).
18. F. P. Chinard, H. D. Lauson, H. A. Eder, R. L. Grief, and A. Hiller, "A study of the mechanism of proteinuria in patients with the nephrotic syndrome," *J. clin. Invest.* 33, 621 (1954).

19. M. Bodansky and O. Bodansky, *Biochemistry of Disease* (ed. 2; Macmillan, New York, 1952).
20. F. B. Kingsbury, C. P. Clark, G. Williams, and A. L. Post, "The rapid determination of albumin in urine," *J. lab. clin. Med. 11*, 981 (1926).
21. E. F. Osserman and D. P. Lawlor, "Abnormal serum and urine proteins in 35 cases of multiple myeloma as studied by filter paper electrophoresis," *Amer. J. Med. 28*, 462 (1955).
22. H. A. Azar, W. T. Hill, and E. F. Osserman, "Malignant lymphoma and lymphatic leukemia with myeloma-type serum proteins," *Amer. J. Med. 23*, 239 (1957).
23. R. J. Cross, ed., "Combined staff clinic. Multiple myeloma," *Amer. J. Med. 23*, 283 (1957).
24. B. M. Jacobson and L. R. Milner, "The detection of urinary Bence-Jones protein," *Amer. J. clin. Path. 14*, 138 (1944).
25. I. Snapper, L. B. Turner, and H. L. Moscovitz, *Multiple Myeloma* (Grune and Stratton, New York, 1953).
26. A. M. Fishberg, *Hypertension and Nephritis* (ed. 5; Lea and Febiger, Philadelphia, 1954).
27. F. Sargent and R. E. Johnson, "Effects of diet on renal function in healthy man," *Amer. J. clin. Nutr. 4*, 166 (1956).
28. S. E. King and D. S. Baldwin, "Production or renal ischemia and proteinuria in man by the adrenal medullary hormones," *Amer. J. Med. 20*, 217 (1956).
29. J. W. Welty, "Febrile albuminuria," *Amer. J. med. Sci. 194*, 70 (1937).
30. G. M. Bull, "Postural proteinuria," *Clin. Sci. 7*, 77 (1948).
31. S. E. King, "Patterns of protein excretion by the kidneys," *Ann. intern. Med. 42*, 296 (1955).
32. M. C. Shevky and D. D. Stafford, "A clinical method for the estimation of protein in urine and other fluids," *Arch. intern. Med. 32*, 222 (1923).
33. R. W. Lippmann, *Urine and the Urinary Sediment* (Thomas, Springfield, Ill., 1952).
34. F. P. Chinard, "Interactions of quarternary ammonium compounds and proteins. A simple method for the rapid esitmation of urinary protein concentrations with alkyldimethylbenzyl ammonium compounds," *J. biol. Chem. 176*, 1439 (1948).
35. J. P. Conner, "Semiquantitative specific test paper for glucose in urine," *Analyt. Chem. 28*, 1748 (1956).
36. W. M. Bell and E. Jumper, "Evaluation of Tes-tape as a quantitative indicator," *J. Amer. med. Ass. 166*, 2145 (1958).
37. J. Leonards, "Evalution of enzyme tests for urinary glucose," *J. Amer. med. Ass. 163*, 260 (1957).
38. J. J. Moran, P. L. Lewis, J. G. Reinhold, and F. D. W. Lukens, "Enzymatic tests for glucosuria," *Diabetes 6*, 358 (1957).
39. P. B. Hawk, B. L. Oser, and W. H. Summerson, *Practical Physiological Chemistry* (ed. 13; Blakiston, Philadelphia, 1954).
40. A. Marble, "The diagnosis of the less common mellitu'ias including pentosuria and fructosuria," *Med. Clin. N. Amer. 31*, 313 (1947).
41. K. J. Isselbacher, "Galactosemia: Clinical staff conference at the National Institutes of Health," *Ann. intern. Med. 46*, 773 (1957).
42. W. G. Exton, "Differential diagnosis of conditions associated with sugar excretion," *N. Y. St. J. Med. 36*, 1545 (1936).

43. F. W. Sunderman *et al.,* "Manual of American Society of Clinical Pathologists: Workshop on glucose," *Amer. J. clin. Path. 26,* 1355 (1956).

44. G. R. Constam, "Paper chromatography, a simple method for the differentiation of sugars in the urine," *Diabetes 7,* 36 (1958).

45. E. R. Froesch and A. E. Renold, "Specific enzymatic determination of glucose in blood and urine using glucose oxidase," *Diabetes 5,* 1 (1956).

46. M. Somogyi, "A rapid method for the estimation of urine sugar," *J. lab. clin. Med. 26,* 1220 (1941).

47. W. T. Wright, unpublished observations.

48. J. Nash, J. Lister, and D. H. Vobes, "Clinical tests for ketonuria," *Lancet 1,* 801 (1954).

49. I. P. Ackerman, unpublished observations.

50. R. Sternheimer and B. Malbin, "Clinical recognition of pyelonephritis with a new stain for urinary sediments," *Amer. J. Med. 11,* 312 (1951).

51. R. C. Larcom and G. H. Carter, "Erythrocytes in urinary sediment; identification and normal limits," *J. lab. clin. Med. 33,* 875 (1948).

52. J. D. Lyttle, "The Addis sediment count in normal children," *J. clin. Invest. 12,* 87 (1933).

53. E. H. Kass, "Chemotherapeutic and antibiotic drugs in the management of infections in the urinary tract," *Amer. J. Med. 18,* 764 (1955).

54. K. P. Poirier and G. G. Jackson, "Characteristics of leucocytes in the urine sediment in pyelonephritis," *Amer. J. Med. 23,* 579 (1957).

55. V. Schilling, "Lebende weisse Blutkörperchen im Dunkenfeld: Beiträge zur normalen und degenerativen Strucktur, besonders der Neutrophilen," *Folia haemat. (Lpz.) 6,* 429 (1908).

56. G. B. Berman, G. E. Schreiner, and J. O. Feys, "Observations on the glitter cell phenomenon," *New Engl. J. Med. 255,* 989 (1956).

57. F. Sargent and R. E. Johnson, "Effects of diet on renal function in healthy men," *Amer. J. clin. Nutr. 4,* 466 (1956).

58. C. A. Stetson, C. H. Rammelkamp, Jr., R. M. Krause, R J. Kohen, and W. D. Perry, "Epidemic acute nephritis: Studies on etiology, natural history, and prevention," *Medicine 34,* 431 (1955).

59. A. C. Allen, *The Kidney: Medical and Surgical Diseases* (Grune and Stratton, New York, 1951).

60. R. W. Berliner, N. G. Levinsky, D. G. Davidson, and M. Eden, "Dilution and concentration of the urine and the action of the antidiuretic hormone," *Amer. J. Med. 24,* 730 (1958).

61. J. Oliver, "New directions in renal morphology: A method, its results, and its future," *Harvey Lect. 40,* 102 (1944–45).

62. R. A. Behrman, "Urinary findings before and after a marathon race," *New Engl. J. Med. 225,* 801 (1941).

63. M. A. Krupp, "Urinary sediment in visceral angiitis," *Arch. intern. Med. 71,* 54 (1943).

64. G. E. Schreiner, "Some observations on telescoped urinary sediments," *Ann. intern. Med. 42,* 826 (1955).

65. R. M. Graham, "Diagnosis of cancer of internal organs by Papanicolaou technique," *Advanc. intern. Med. 6,* 59 (1954).

66. P. A. Herbut, "The value of cytological techniques in the diagnosis of lesions in the genitourinary tract," in *Proceedings, Symposium on Exfoliative Cytology, 1951* (American Cancer Society, New York, 1953).

67. R. Chute and D. Williams, "Experiences with stained smears of cells exfoliated in the urine in the diagnosis of cancer in the genito-urinary tract," *J. Urol. (Baltimore)* 59, 604 (1948).

68. N. C. Foote, G. M. Papanicolaou, N. D. Holmquist, and J. F. Seybolt, "Exfoliative cytology of urinary sediments," *Cancer 11*, 127 (1958).

69. G. M. Papanicolaou, *Atlas of exfoliative cytology* (Harvard University Press, Cambridge, Mass., 1954).

70. R. G. Westall, "The amino acids and other ampholytes of urine. 3. Unidentified substances excreted in normal human urine," *Biochem. J. 60*, 247 (1955).

71. Chemistry Laboratory, Massachusetts General Hospital, unpublished.

72. D. D. Van Slyke, D. A. MacFadgen, and P. B. Hamilton, "The gasometric determination of amino acids in urine by the ninhydrin carbon dioxide method," *J. biol. Chem. 150*, 251–258 (1943).

73. E. Brand, M. M. Harris, and S. Biloon, "Cystinuria: The excretion of a cystine complex which decomposes in the urine with the liberation of free cystine," *J. biol. Chem. 86*, 315–331 (1930).

74. R. J. Block and D. Bolling, *The Amino Acid Composition of Proteins and Foods* (ed. 2; Thomas, Springfield, Ill., 1951), p. 203.

75. W. Latham, K. Baker, and S. E. Bradley, "Urinary amino acid excretion in renal disease, with observations on the Fanconi syndrome," *Amer. J. Med. 18*, 249 (1955).

76. C. E. Dent, "Clinical applications of amino acid chromatography," *Scand. J. clin. lab. Invest. 10*, Suppl. 31, 122–126 (1957).

77. D. R. Gilligan, M. D. Altschule, and E. M. Katersby, "Studies of hemoglobinemia and hemoglobinuria produced in man by intravenous injection of hemoglobin solutions," *J. clin. Invest. 20*, 177 (1941).

78. C. B. Laurel and M. Nyman, "Studies on the serum haptoglobin level in hemoglobinemia and its influence on renal excretion of hemoglobin," *Blood 12*, 493 (1957).

79. E. Libman and A. M. Fishberg, "Unilateral hemoglobinuria: Occurrence in infarction of the kidney," *Ann. intern. Med. 11*, 1344 (1938).

80. L. Heilmeyer, *Spectrophotometry in Medicine* (Hilger, London, 1943).

81. S. H. Blondheim, E. Margoliash, and E. Shafrir, "A simple test for myohemoglobinuria (myoglobinuria)," *J. Amer. med. Ass. 167*, 453 (1958).

82. E. G. L. Bywaters, G. E. Delory, C. Rimington, and J. Smilies, "Myohaemoglobin in the urine of air raid casualties with crushing injuries," *Biochem. J. 35*, 1164 (1941).

83. E. G. L. Bywaters and J. K. Stead, "Thrombosis of the femoral artery with myohaemoglobinuria and low serum potassium concentration," *Clin. Sci. 5*, 195 (1945).

84. D. H. Bowden, D. Fraser, H. Jackson, and N. F. Walker, "Acute recurrent rhabdomyolysis," *Medicine 35*, 335 (1956).

85. H. R. Hipp and H. F. Shrikers, "Spontaneous myoglobinuria with symptoms resembling myotonia," *Ann. intern. Med. 42*, 197 (1955).

86. J. W. Baker and F. C. Happold, "The coli-tryptophane-indole reaction," *Biochem. J. 34*, 657 (1940).

87. C. A. Herter and M. L. Foster, "On the separation of indole from skatole and their quantitative determination," *J. biol. Chem. 2*, 267 (1906).

88. C. A. Herter, "On a relation between skatole and the dimethylaminobenzaldehyde reaction of urine," *J. biol. Chem. 1*, 251 (1905).

89. C. A. Herter, "On indolacetic acid as the chromogen of urorosein of the urine," *J. biol. Chem. 4,* 253 (1908).

90. M. D. Armstrong and K. S. Robinson, "Excretion of indole derivative in phenylketonuria," *Arch. Biochem. 52,* 287 (1954).

91. C. J. Watson and J. A. Layne, "Studies on urinary pigments in pellagra and other pathological states," *Ann. intern. Med. 19,* 183 (1943).

92. L. Linnell and H. S. Raper, "The chromogen of melanuria," *Biochem. J. 29,* 76 (1935).

93. F. Böhm, "Beitrag zur Kenntnis der Thormählenschen Reaktion," *Hoppe-Seylers Z. physiol. Chem. 258,* 108 (1939).

94. S. Rothman, "Studies on melanuria," *J. lab. clin. Med. 27,* 687 (1942).

95. A. Sjoerdsma, H. Weissbach, and S. Udenfriend, "A clinical, physiological, and biochemical study of patients with malignant carcinoid," *Amer. J. Med. 20,* 520 (1956).

96. S. Udenfriend, H. Weissbach, and C. T. Clark, "The estimation of 5-hydroxytryptamine (serotinin) in biological tissues," *J. biol. Chem. 215,* 337 (1955).

97. A. Sjoerdsma, H. Weissbach, and S. Udenfriend, "A simple test for diagnosis of metastatic carcinoid (argentaffinoma)," *J. Amer. med. Ass. 159,* 397 (1955).

98. S. Udenfriend, E. Titus, and H. Weissbach, "The identification of 5-hydroxy-3-indoleacetic acid in normal urine and a method for its assay," *J. biol. Chem. 216,* 499 (1955).

99. G. Curzon, "A rapid chromatographic test for high urinary excretion of 5-hydroxyindoleacetic acid and 5-hydroxytryptamine," *Lancet 2,* 1361 (1955).

100. M. T. Wilson and L. S. P. Davidson, "Ehrlich's aldehyde test for urobilinogen," *Brit. med. J. 1,* 884 (1949).

101. J. B. Jepson, "Indolylacetyl-glutamine and other indole metabolites in Hartnup disease," *Biochem. J. 64,* 14 (1956).

102. P. B. Hank, B. L. Oser, and W. H. Summerson, *Practical Physiological Chemistry* (ed. 13; Blakiston, Philadelphia, 1954).

103. M. D. Armstrong, K. F. Shaw, and P. E. Wall, "The phenolic acids of human urine," *J. biol. Chem. 218,* 293 (1956).

104. S. Z. Levine, E. Marples, and H. H. Gordon, "A defect in the metabolism of tyrosine and phenylalanine in premature infants. I. Identification and assay of intermediary products," *J. clin. Invest. 20,* 199 (1941) and "II. Spontaneous occurrence and eradication by Vitamin C," *ibid.,* 209.

105. G. Medes, "A new error of tyrosine metabolism, tyrosinosis. The intermediary metabolism of tyrosine and phenylalanine," *Biochem. J. 26,* 917 (1932).

106. A. Neuberger, "Studies on alcaptonuria, I. The estimation of homogentisic acid," *Biochem. J. 41,* 431 (1947).

107. A. Neuberger, C. Rimington, and J. M. G. Wilson, "II. Investigation on a case of human alcaptonuria," *Biochem. J. 41,* 438 (1947).

108. M. Goldston, J. M. Steele, and K. Dobriner, "Alcaptonuria and ochronosis," *Amer. J. Med. 13,* 432 (1952).

109. E. H. Fishberg, "The instantaneous diagnosis of alcaptonuria on a single drop of urine," *J. Amer. med. Ass. 119,* 882 (1942).

110. M. D. Armstrong and F. H. Tyler, "Studies on phenylketonuria. I. Reduced phenylalanine intake in phenylketonuria," *J. clin Invest. 34,* 565 (1955).

111. W. E. Knox and D. Y. Y. Hsia, "Pathogenetic problems in phenylketonuria," *Amer. J. Med. 22,* 687 (1957).

112. H. Bickel, "Effects of phenylalanine-free and phenylalanine-poor diets in phenylpyuric oligophrenia," *Exp. Med. Surg. 12,* 114 (1954).

113. R. J. Block and D. Bolling, *Amino Acid Composition of Proteins and Foods— Analytical Methods and Results* (ed. 2; Thomas, Springfield, Ill., 1951, p. 139.

114. A. Fölling, "Ueber Ausscheudung von phenyl-brenzhaubensäure in den Harn als Stoffwechsel anomalie in Verbundung mit Imbezillität," *Hoppe-Seylers Z. physiol. Chem. 227,* 169 (1934).

115. L. S. Penrose, "Two cases of phenylpyruvic amentia," *Lancet 1,* 23 (1935).

116. G. E. W. Wolstenholme and Elaine C. P. Millar, eds., *Porphyrin Biosynthesis and Metabolism* (Ciba Foundation Symposium; Little, Brown, Boston, 1955).

117. L. Bogorad, "The enzymatic synthesis of porphyrins from porphobilinogen. III. Uroporphyrinogens as intermediates," *J. biol. Chem. 233,* 516–519 (1958).

118. D. Mauzerall and S. Granik, "Porphyrin biosynthesis in erythrocytes. III. Uroporphyrinogen and its decarboxylase," *J. biol. Chem. 232,* 1141–1161 (1958).

119. C. J. Watson, R. Pimento-DeMello, S. Schwartz, V. E. Hawkinson, and I. Bossenmaier, "Porphyrin chromogens or precursors in urine, blood, bile, and feces," *J. lab. clin. Med. 37,* 831 (1951).

120. C. J. Watson, "The erythrocyte coproporphyrin," *Arch. intern. Med. 86,* 797 (1950).

121. C. J. Watson, "Porphyrin metabolism," in G. G. Duncan, ed., *Diseases of Metabolism* (ed. 4; Saunders, Philadelphia, 1959).

122. D. A. Sutherland and C. J. Watson, "The effect of alcohol on the per diem excretion and isomer distribution of urinary coproporphyrins," *J. lab. clin. Med. 37,* 29 (1951).

123. C. J. Watson, S. Schwartz, W. Schulze, L. O. Jacobson, and R. Zagaria, "Idiopathic coproporphyrinuria, a hitherto unrecognized form characterized by lack of symptoms in spite of the excretion of large amounts of coproporphyrin," *J. clin. Invest. 28,* 465 (1949).

124. M. Grinstein, H. M. Wikoff, R. Pimento-DeMello, and C. J. Watson, "The biosynthesis of coproporphyrin in experimental lead poisoning," *J. biol. Chem. 182,* 723 (1950).

125. S. F. MacDonald and K.-H. Michl, "The synthesis of the uroporphyrins. II and IV," in Wolstenholme and Millar, *Porphyrin Biosynthesis and Metabolism* (Ciba Foundation Symposium; Little, Brown, Boston, 1955), p. 285.

126. S. Schwartz, L. Zieve, and C. J. Watson, "An improved method for the determination of urinary coproporphyrins and an evaluation of factors influencing the analysis," *J. lab. clin. Med. 37,* 843 (1951).

127. R. G. Westall, "Isolation of porphobilinogen from the urine of a patient with acute porphyria," *Nature 170,* 614 (1952).

128. G. H. Cookson and C. Rimington, "Porphobilinogen," *Biochem. J. 57,* 476 (1954).

129. D. Mauzerall and S. Granick, "The occurrence and determination of delta amino levulinic acid and porphobilinogen in urine," *J. biol. Chem. 219,* 435 (1956).

130. P. Formijne and N. J. Poulie, "Precursors of porphyrin and porphobilinogen,"

in Wolstenholme and Millar, *Porphyrin Biosynthesis and Metabolism* (Ciba Foundation Symposium; Little, Brown, Boston, 1955), p. 246.

131. C. Rimington, S. Krol, and B. Tooth, "Detection and determination of porphobilinogen in urine," *Scand. J. clin. lab. Invest. 8,* 251 (1956).

132. L. A. Brunsting, "Observations on porphyria cutanea tarda," *Arch. Derm. Syph. 70,* 551 (1952).

133. C. Rimington, 'Haems and porphyrins in health and disease II," *Acta med. scand. 143,* 177 (1952).

134. R. Schmid, S. Schwartz, and C. J. Watson, "Porphyrin content of bone marrow and liver in the various forms of porphyria," *Arch. intern. Med. 93,* 167 (1954).

135. J. Waldenström, "Porphyrias as inborn errors of metabolism," *Amer. J. Med. 22,* 758 (1957).

136. L. A. Brunsting, H. L. Mason, and R. A. Aldrich, "Adult form of chronic porphyria with cutaneous manifestations," *J. Amer. med. Ass. 146,* 1207 (1951).

137. F. W. Sunderman, Jr., and F. W. Sunderman, "Practical considerations of porphyrin metabolism," *Amer J. clin. Path. 25,* 1231 (1955).

138. S. L. Sveinsson, C. Rimington, and H. D. Barnes, "Complete porphyrin analysis of pathological urines," *Scand. J. clin. lab. Invest. 1,* 2 (1949).

139. S. Schwartz, M. Kepros, and R. Schmid, "Experimental porphyria. II. Type produced by lead phenylhydrazine and light," *Proc. Soc. exp. Biol.* (N. Y.) 79, 463 (1952).

140. J. E. Falk, "Haem and porphyrin formation from glycine, delta amino levulinic acid, and porphobilinogen," in Wolstenholme and Millar, *Porphyrin Biosynthesis and Metabolism* (Ciba Foundation Symposium; Little, Brown, Boston, 1955), p. 63.

141. S. Schwartz, V. Hawkinson, S. Cohen, and C. J. Watson, "A micromethod for the quantitative determination of the urinary coproporphyrin isomers," *J. biol. Chem. 168,* 133 (1947).

142. M. Markovitz, "Chromogens in the urine of normal individuals and epileptics which react with Ehrlich's aldehyde reagent," *J. lab. clin. Med. 50,* 367 (1957).

143. N. Gössner, "Chemische Untersuchungen zur Ehrlichschen Aldehydereaktion in Normalharn," *Klin. Wschr. 26,* 567 (1948).

144. C. J. Watson and S. Schwartz, "A simple test for urinary porphobilinogen," *Proc. Soc. exp. Biol.* (N. Y.) 47, 393 (1941).

145. T. K. With, "The porphyrin concentration from ultraviolet extinction," *Scand. J. clin. lab. Invest. 7,* 193 (1955).

146. W. P. Chapman and M. Singh, "Evaluation of tests used in the diagnosis of pheochromocytoma," *Modern Concepts of Cardiovascular Disease 23,* 221, 225 (1954).

147. U. S. von Euler and G. Ström, "Present status of diagnosis and treatment of pheochromocytoma," *Circulation 15,* 5 (1957).

148. A. Lund, "Adrenaline and noradrenaline in blood and urine in cases of pheochromocytoma," *Scand. J. clin. lab. Invest. 4,* 263 (1952).

149. U. S. von Euler and I. Floding, "Diagnosis of pheochromocytoma by fluorimetric estimation of adrenaline and noradrenaline in urine," *Scand. J. clin. lab. Invest. 8,* 288 (1956).

150. C. H. DuToit, "A study of chemical methods for quantitative measurements

of catechol amines," *WADC Technical Report* 59–175 (ASTIA, Arlington 12, Virginia, 1959).

151. H. Weil-Malherbe and A. D. Bone, "The chemical estimation of adrenaline-like substances in blood," *Biochem. J. 51*, 311 (1952).
152. C. von Euler, U. S. von Euler, and I. Floding, "Biologically inactive catechol derivatives in urine," *Acta physiol. scand.*, Supp. 118, *33*, 32 (1955).
153. M. S. Zileli, J. T. Hamlin, F. W. Reutter, and D. G. Friend, "Evaluation of catechol amine levels in renal insufficiency," *J. clin. Invest. 37*, 409 (1958).
154. U. S. von Euler, "Adrenaline and noradrenaline. Distribution and action," *Pharmacol. Rev. 6*, 15 (1954).
155. U. S. von Euler, S. H. Björkman, and I. Orwen, "Diurnal variation in the excretion of free and conjugated noradrenalin and adrenalin in urine from healthy subjects," *Acta physiol. scand.*, Supp. 118, *33*, 10 (1955).
156. J. W. Litchfield and W. S. Peart, "Pheochromocytoma with normal excretion of adrenalin and noradrenalin," *Lancet 2*, 1283 (1956).
157. F. W. Reutter, M. S. Zileli, J. T. Hamlin, G. W. Thorn, and D. G. Friend, "Importance of detecting rapid changes in blood catechol amine levels in the diagnosis of pheochromocytoma," *New Engl. J. Med. 257*, 323 (1957).
158. C. H. DuToit, unpublished data.
159. M. Goldenberg, I. Serlin, T. Edward, and M. M. Rapport, "Chemical screening methods for the diagnosis of pheochromocytoma," *Amer. J. Med. 16*, 310 (1954).
160. U. S. von Euler, *Noradrenaline* (Thomas, Springfield, Ill., 1956).
161. M. D. Armstrong and A. McMillan, "Identification of a major urinary metabolite of norepinephrine," *Fed. Proc. 16*, 146 (1957).
162. M. D. Armstrong, A. McMillan, and K. N. F. Shaw, "3-methoxy-4-hydroxy mandelic acid; a urinary metabolite of norepinephrine," *Biochim. biophys. Acta 25*, 422 (1957).
163. J. Axelrod, J. K. Inscoe, S. Senah, and B. Witkop, "O-methylation, the principal pathway for the metabolism of epinephrine and norepinephrine in the rat," *Biochim. biophys, Acta 27*, 210 (1958).
164. A. Sjoerdsma, W. M. King, L. C. Leeper, and S. Udenfriend, "Demonstration of the 3-methoxy analogue of norepinephrine in man," *Science 127*, 876 (1958).
165. "Pheochromocytoma," Leading article, *Lancet 1*, 1080 (1959).
166. O. Kraupp, H. Stormann, H. Bernheimer, and H. Obenaus, "Vorkommen und diagnostische Bedeutung von Phenolsäuren im Harn beim Phaeochromocytom," *Klin. Wschr. 37*, 76 (1959).

# Unit 20

# Tests of Renal Function

### The Use and Interpretation of Renal-Function Tests

In clinical investigation, quantitative methods of measuring renal function have been in use for many years.[1-5] These serve as standards of reference for the less accurate tests used in clinical medicine. The clearance of inulin is well established as a measure of glomerular filtration rate (GFR). The clearance of $p$-aminohippurate measures renal plasma flow. The maximum rate of tubular excretion of $p$-aminohippurate ($Tm_{PAH}$) and the maximum rate of reabsorption of glucose ($Tm_G$) measure the excretory and reabsorptive functions of the renal tubules. These measurements are technically difficult and time-consuming and are rarely used for clinical purposes. The tests that are available for the clinical assessment of renal function are, by comparison, somewhat crude. They provide data that often are influenced by several variables. Nevertheless, they reflect certain discrete functions of the kidney. If the factors that influence them are understood and considered in interpreting the results, the information obtained from these tests can be of considerable value in the evaluation and management of renal disease.

The purpose of renal-function tests is to determine the nature and extent of functional renal impairment. They usually do not give diagnostic information about the nature of the underlying disease, since diffuse damage to all components of the renal architecture is commonly present in renal disease. An exception to this is early acute glomerulonephritis, where filtration rate may be markedly depressed with little evidence of damage to the renal tubules. The combination of azotemia and depressed creatinine or urea clearance with normal phenolsulfonphthalein (PSP) excretion and unimpaired concentrating power is of aid in making this diagnosis.[5] However, in the subacute or chronic stage of glomerulonephritis, tubular damage parallels the depression of GFR. Characteristic functional patterns have been described for other renal diseases, but these are inconstant and unreliable. In general, the most important considerations in the diagnosis of renal disease are the clinical history and careful examination of the urine, rather than the renal-function tests.

Renal-function tests do not distinguish between anatomic and functional impairment of the kidney. Functional impairment without anatomic damage may be present in congestive heart failure, shock, severe dehydration, and other situations where renal circulation is disturbed. Often functional and anatomic impairment coexist. Serial tests of renal function are helpful in determining the extent to which abnormal renal function is reversible and are also useful in following the course of chronic renal disease.

In interpreting renal-function tests it

must be remembered that all measurable renal functions decline with age in apparently normal individuals. The decline becomes apparent after the third decade, and at age 90 there is an average reduction of nearly 50 percent in GFR, renal flow, and $Tm_{PAH}$.[6] Variations due to disease are superimposed on these declining values as age increases.

In addition to the renal-function tests described in this unit, important information about renal function may be obtained from examination of the urine (Unit 19) and from measurement of serum and urine electrolytes (Unit 21).

### Blood Urea Nitrogen (BUN)

PHYSIOLOGY. Urea is the most abundant and most completely oxidized product of protein catabolism. It is distributed throughout the total body water and is in equal concentration in the intracellular and extracellular fluid. Thus its concentration is the same in whole blood as in serum. Although urea itself is virtually nontoxic, its concentration in the blood serves as a convenient index of the kidneys' ability to excrete metabolic wastes and an increase in blood urea nitrogen (BUN) often signals a deterioration in the regulatory functions of the kidney.

In disease as well as in health, the rate of excretion of urea is equal to its rate of production in the body. It is excreted by filtration at the glomerulus, although about half of the amount filtered diffuses back into the blood during passage of the filtrate down the tubule. The relation between BUN and glomerular filtration rate is such that at any given rate of urea production their product remains constant:

$$BUN \times GFR = K.$$

This relation is shown graphically in Fig. 34.[7] When the GFR falls, the BUN rises until constancy of their product is restored. In this way, the rate of urea excretion is kept equal to its rate of production. It is apparent from this relation that the most important factor determining the concentration of urea in blood is the GFR, although it will also be influenced by the rate of urea production. The relation between GFR and BUN is depicted in Curve A of Fig. 34 at a constant rate of urea production. If the rate of protein catabolism is changed, the value of the constant $K$ is changed and the position of the curve is shifted. The dotted line (Curve B) illustrates the relation at a higher rate of protein catabolism. A family of similar curves could be drawn for different rates of urea production.

From inspection of the figure, it can be seen that the BUN rises gradually from the very earliest reduction in the GFR, but the increase is gradual and lies within the arbitrarily defined "normal range" until GFR is reduced to about 40 percent of normal. Further reduction in the GFR below this level then results in a rapid increase in the BUN. Although the BUN is determined by the GFR even within the normal range, interpretation of normal variations is not warranted without precise knowledge of the rate of protein catabolism. For this reason, the upper limit of normal is set at 25 mg/100 ml. Values above this level almost always signify depression of filtration rate.

The relations illustrated in Fig. 34 for urea help to explain the common clinical observation that although patients with renal disease often have very few symptoms despite marked renal impairment, clinical deterioration may occur very abruptly when a critical degree of renal impairment is reached.

INTERPRETATION AND LIMITATIONS. From the preceding discussion, it can be seen that the BUN is not a very precise measure of renal function. Considerable deterioration of renal function must usually be present before the BUN rises above the normal range. At normal rates

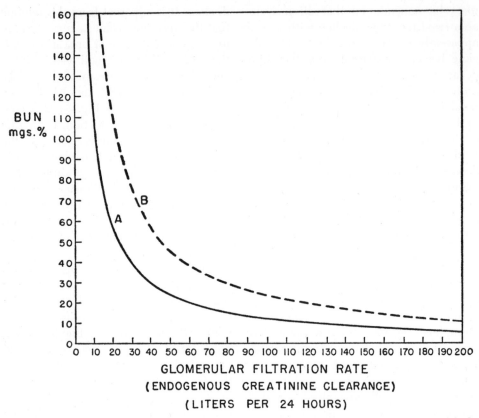

Fig. 34. Relation between blood urea nitrogen and glomerular filtration rate (modified from Leaf and Newburgh,[7] courtesy of Charles C Thomas, Publisher, Springfield, Illinois).

of protein catabolism, an increase of the BUN above the normal range occurs when the GFR is reduced to 30–40 percent of normal. However, the degree of depression of renal function at which the BUN rises may be markedly affected if the rate of protein catabolism changes. If catabolism is rapid, as it is during acute febrile illnesses, following trauma or surgery, or after administration of cytolytic drugs, the BUN may rise above normal limits even when the GFR is diminished by only 50 percent or less. Conversely, when protein catabolism is slow, as it is during protein starvation and in chronic disease, the rise of BUN into the abnormal range may be delayed until the GFR is reduced to as little as 20 percent of normal. In practice, factors influencing the rate of protein catabolism must always

be considered in interpreting the BUN. The high BUN that is often seen following acute gastrointestinal hemorrhage, for example, is a combined effect of low GFR due to blood loss and increased urea production from digestion and absorption of blood from the gastrointestinal tract.

Since urea production depends primarily on the intake of protein, blood urea will exhibit diurnal variations related to ingestion of food. Increase is usually maximal 3 to 4 hr after meals. However, these diurnal variations are small, and for clinical purposes it is usually not necessary to obtain blood in the fasting state.

Technically, analysis of blood for urea is somewhat more difficult than determination of nonprotein nitrogen, and, in inexperienced hands, results are

344

less reliable. Since both these tests are gross measures of renal function, the BUN measurement offers no advantage over the nonprotein nitrogen and the latter is to be preferred for ordinary purposes. If urea clearance is to be measured, however, the BUN must be precisely determined.

### Nonprotein Nitrogen (NPN)

PHYSIOLOGY. The nonprotein nitrogen (NPN) is the nitrogen of whole blood or serum that is not precipitated by the usual protein-precipitating reagents. It is a mixture of compounds including urea, uric acid, creatinine, amino acids, creatine, and small quantities of other nitrogen-containing substances, collectively called the *undetermined nitrogen*. Urea is the most abundant and most variable constituent of the NPN. The concentration of NPN in blood is therefore determined predominantly by the concentration of urea. The factors that determine the NPN level are generally the same as those that determine the BUN, and are discussed in detail in the preceding section.

Urea normally comprises approximately 55 percent of the NPN. When the NPN rises owing to renal insufficiency, the urea fraction is progressively increased and may make up 75–80 percent of the NPN. The other constituents are present in much smaller quantities and are less variable. Amino acids normally comprise approximately 20 percent of NPN, but may represent a larger fraction in severe liver disease if urea synthesis and amino-acid metabolism are impaired. Uric acid, which in health comprises some 20 percent of the NPN, is variably elevated when NPN is increased due to renal insufficiency. Its concentration is also influenced by the factors that govern purine metabolism and it may be elevated in gout and other forms of hyperuricemia despite a normal urea concentration. The undetermined nitrogen is almost entirely confined to cells. It is therefore not available for excretion by the kidney, since the solutes excreted by the kidney are derived from plasma. The factors determining creatinine concentration are discussed elsewhere.

INTERPRETATION AND LIMITATIONS. Since the concentration of NPN is chiefly determined by its urea content, the significance and limitations of the test are the same as those described for the BUN. Technically, the NPN test is somewhat simpler than that for BUN and results may be more reliable in inexperienced hands. For this reason, the test for NPN is preferable for most purposes. Rarely, as in liver failure or severe hyperuricemia, other constituents than urea may become the chief determinant of the NPN concentration. The upper limit of normal for NPN is arbitrarily set at 35 mg/100 ml.

### The Urea Clearance

The clearance of urea measures the volume of plasma necessary to provide the quantity of urea that appears in the urine in 1 min. This volume of plasma is said to be "cleared" of its urea by the kidney each minute. This test, which is the oldest of the quantitative tests of renal function,[8, 9] is still the most widely used renal-function test in clinical medicine. It was observed many years ago that the rate of excretion of urea varies with the urine flow. This led to the development of two urea-clearance tests. One, the clearance at high rates of urine flow, was called the "maximum urea clearance." The other, the clearance measured when the urine flow is less than 2.0 ml/min, was called the "standard urea clearance." Both forms of the test are still in use. However, the "maximum clearance" measured when the urine flow is 2.0 ml/min or greater, is much the more reliable test, and use of the "standard clearance" is seldom necessary. It should be emphasized that the terms "maximum" and "standard" as applied to these tests have no physiologic significance. The effect of urine volume on urea excretion and the differences between the two tests are discussed below.

PHYSIOLOGY OF UREA EXCRETION. Urea is freely filtered at the glomerulus and is present in the glomerular filtrate in the same concentration as in the plasma. As the filtrate passes down the nephron, part of the urea is reabsorbed. As a result, the clearance of urea is always lower than the filtration rate. The reabsorption of urea takes place by passive diffusion. The amount of urea reabsorbed depends on three factors: (i) the concentration gradient for urea between the urine and the plasma, (ii) the rate of flow of fluid down the nephron, and (iii) the permeability of the cells to urea. The reabsorption of urea is therefore closely associated with the reabsorption of water. When urine

volume is small, flow of fluid down the tubule is slow, and urea concentration in the urine is increased. In consequence, more urea is reabsorbed and the clearance of urea is smaller. Conversely, when urine flow is large, a greater fraction of the filtered urea is excreted in the urine and the urea clearance is larger.[10]

The effect of urine volume on urea clearance is greatest when urine flow is low and urea concentration is high. It becomes much less pronounced when urine flow is higher than 2.0 ml/min. In Fig. 35, the urea clearance, expressed as a percentage of the filtration rate, is related to the urine flow, where urine flow is increased from oliguria to 10 ml/min by water diuresis.[2] When urine flow is higher than 2 ml/min, the urea clearance bears a nearly constant relation to the filtration rate, rising only from 59 to 65 percent of the true GFR as urine flow increases from 2 to 6 ml/min.

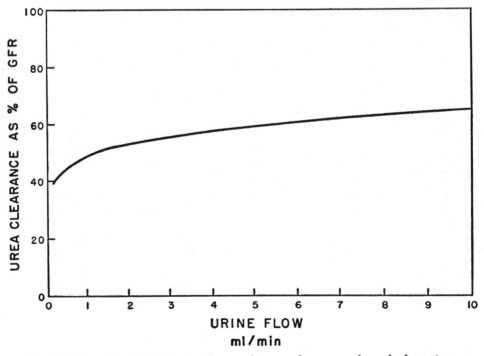

Fig. 35. Effect of variation in urine flow on the urea clearance, where the latter is expressed as a percentage of the true glomerular filtration rate (modified from Smith[2]).

EXCRETION OF UREA BY THE DAMAGED KIDNEY. Since the rate of excretion of urea equals its rate of production, the damaged kidney must excrete just as large a daily load of urea as the normal kidney. As kidney function declines, the remaining functioning nephrons must each handle a larger load of urea.[7, 11] This is done at the expense of an elevated blood urea. If half the nephrons are destroyed, blood urea concentration rises until each remaining nephron receives roughly twice its previous load of urea per unit time. The increased amount of solute, by its osmotic effect, reduces the reabsorption of water, producing an osmotic diuresis in the remaining nephrons. The rate of flow of fluid in the tubules is increased, and urea concentration is relatively low. As a result, a larger fraction of the filtered urea escapes reabsorption in the damaged kidney than in the normal kidney, and the urea clearance becomes a larger fraction of the true glomerular filtration rate. In general, the greater the degree of renal impairment, the more nearly the urea clearance approaches the filtration rate. However, during the recovery phase following acute tubular necrosis,[11] increased permeability to urea can be demonstrated and urea reabsorption is greater than normal, in spite of a large urine volume. This increase is, however, of minor importance in causing the elevated BUN, since the GFR is markedly depressed.

"MAXIMUM" UREA CLEARANCE. When the urea clearance is measured at a urine flow of 2.0 ml/min or more, the test is called the "maximum urea clearance."

The clearance is expressed in milliliters of blood per minute and is calculated as follows:

$$\text{Clearance} = \frac{UV}{B},$$

where $U$ (mg/ml) is the concentration of urea in urine, $V$ (ml/min) is the

urine flow and $B$ (mg/ml) is the concentration of urea in blood.

The concentration of urea in whole blood is usually used rather than the concentration in plasma, although it is only plasma that is cleared by filtration. However, since urea concentration is the same in whole blood as in plasma, this does not affect the result.

The average value in normal subjects is 75 ml/min (57 percent of the filtration rate). By custom, the clearance usually is divided by 75 and multiplied by 100 and is reported as the "percent of normal."

"STANDARD" UREA CLEARANCE. When the urea clearance is measured at a urine flow less than 2.0 ml/min, the test is called the "standard urea clearance." For reasons discussed above, urea clearance varies significantly with the urine flow when the urine volume is small, and it was found [8] that more consistent results could be obtained during oliguria by calculating a "standard" clearance, as follows:

$$\text{Standard clearance} = \frac{U\sqrt{V}}{B}.$$

The calculation is empirical, the use of the square root having the effect of "correcting" the value of $V$ to 1.0 ml/min, thus minimizing the change in clearance due to change in urine value.

The "standard" clearance is not as reliable as the "maximum" clearance. This is chiefly due to two factors: (i) the calculation does not completely correct for change in the clearance with urine flow, and (ii) when urine flow is low, a much greater error is introduced by incomplete emptying of the bladder.

The average value in normal subjects is 54 ml/min (41 percent of the filtration rate). It is usually reported as the "percent of normal."

METHOD OF MEASURING UREA CLEARANCE. Since the "maximum" urea clearance is much to be preferred to the "standard" clearance, the test should always be done with the patient well hydrated to promote urine flow. It should be done in the morning, with the patient in the fasting state to avoid variations in BUN due to food ingestion. The patient drinks 1000 ml of water over a period of ½ hr, and the test is begun one full hour later. If the test is done at a time when urine flow is rising rapidly, falsely high values may be obtained owing to washing out of concentrated urine from the pelvis and ureters. More accurate results are obtained when the urine flow is steady or falling gradually.

Urine is collected during two periods, each 20 or 30 min in duration. Blood is drawn for urea determination during each period. The patient must empty his bladder completely at the beginning of the test and at the end of each period. The beginning and end of each period must be accurately timed to the nearest minute, and the volumes of the urines measured and recorded.

When the test is completed, blood and urine specimens are promptly analyzed for urea content. The clearances are calculated as described previously, and the clearance values for the two periods are averaged.

SOURCES OF ERROR. *Inaccurate timing.* This is probably the commonest source of error. The test requires careful supervision by trained personnel.

*Incomplete bladder emptying.* This is a common source of error, especially in patients with prostatic obstruction. It is partly corrected by averaging several clearance periods.

*Dead-space error.* The washing out of concentrated urea from renal pelvis and ureters may produce a falsely high clearance if the test is done at a time when urine flow is rising rapidly. This can be avoided by making collections when urine flow is steady or falling gradually.[3]

*Infection with urea-splitting organ-* *isms.* This error is increased if urine is not analyzed promptly. Urea-clearance tests often are not feasible in the presence of urinary-tract infections with these organisms.

INTERPRETATION AND LIMITATIONS. The technical limitations of the urea clearance are summarized in the preceding section. Taken together, they combine to make the test much more difficult to perform than the test for 24-hr endogenous creatinine clearance. Furthermore, the custom of relating the urea clearance to an average normal value and reporting it as a "percentage of normal" ignores differences due to age and body size. For these reasons the test for endogenous creatinine clearance is generally preferable to the urea-clearance test for assessment of renal function in adults. Nevertheless, when properly carried out, the urea-clearance test gives highly reproducible results.

The "maximum" urea clearance can generally be interpreted as representing approximately 60 percent of the GFR under conditions where the BUN is normal or only slightly increased. In the late stages of renal disease, it approaches progressively closer to the true filtration rate as the BUN rises, and in terminal uremia it may represent as much as 90 percent of the GFR. Following acute tubular necrosis, urea clearance may be low owing to abnormal back diffusion of urea through damaged nephrons. In this situation, it is not a satisfactory measure of filtration rate, but the comparison of urea clearance with the clearance of creatinine (which diffuses less rapidly) may be a valuable guide to the progress of healing.

## The Serum Creatinine

Creatinine is derived from muscle creatine and phosphocreatine. The quantity produced and excreted depends on skeletal-muscle mass, and is constant in any individual from day to day. It is virtually unaffected by variations in the rate of protein catabolism, and is affected only slightly by variations in the protein content of the diet. Since creatinine is excreted mostly by glomerular filtration, the serum-creatinine concentration rises when filtration rate falls. The relation between these variables is similar to that described for urea in Fig. 34 except that significant variations in the rate of creatinine production do not commonly occur. For this reason, an abnormally elevated serum-creatinine concentration is a reliable indication of depressed renal function. A normal level of serum creatinine, at a time when the NPN is elevated, usually means that much of the NPN elevation is due to increased urea production ("prerenal azotemia") rather than to depression of renal function. This may occur following acute gastrointestinal hemorrhage, or in other situations where protein catabolism is increased. Serum creatinine does not become elevated into the arbitrarily defined abnormal range until the GFR is depressed to some 30 to 40 percent of normal. A normal creatinine concentration therefore cannot be interpreted as an indication of unimpaired renal function. The average value for serum-creatinine concentration varies somewhat with the method of analysis. When a tungstate plasma filtrate is used, it is approximately 1.0 mg/100 ml. The "upper limit of normal" is taken as 1.5 mg/100 ml. Difficulties associated with the measurement and interpretation of creatinine are discussed below.

### Endogenous Creatinine Clearance [12-19]

PHYSIOLOGY. It has been previously emphasized that the daily excretion of creatinine in the urine is remarkably constant. It is unaffected by a wide variety of circumstances, including variations in protein catabolism and in urine volume. This constancy makes it possible to determine the clearance of creatinine over a 24-hr period. Since the serum creatinine is also quite constant, a single blood sample is sufficient for the 24-hr period. The clearance value so obtained measures the total volume of plasma that must have been "cleared" of its creatinine over the period of a day in order to provide the quantity of creatinine found in the urine. The result is expressed in liters per 24 hr, and, with qualifications as discussed below, represents an approximate measure of the glomerular filtration rate.

The creatinine that is formed in the body appears to be excreted by the kidney in a different way from creatinine that is exogenously administered. A distinction is therefore made between the "exogenous" and the "endogenous" creatinine clearances. The clearance of exogenous creatinine is higher than the inulin clearance by 30 or 40 percent,[1] indicating that it is both filtered and excreted by the renal tubular cells. The clearance of endogenous creatinine is very close to the inulin clearance in health, but may diverge from it in disease, behaving in some situations like the clearance of exogenous creatinine. Since the urinary excretion of creatinine does not vary, variations in clearance depend on changes in the serum concentration. The difference between endogenous and exogenous creatinine clearances has been attributed to the presence of noncreatinine substances in the serum which are measured together with true creatinine by the usual colorimetric method of analysis.[1] Of the material that is measured as creatinine by this method, between 80 and 100 percent is true creatinine when measured enzymatically. The remainder consists of noncreatinine "chromogens," the clearances of which may differ from that of creatinine itself.[12] The endogenous-creatinine clearance is therefore a combined clearance of creatinine and several other substances. Its approximate identity with the filtration rate in health is at least partly due to the fact that the relative concentrations of these substances in the serum remain constant. If the proportionate concentrations of creatinine and noncreatinine chromogens change on account of disease, the endogenous creatinine clearance may diverge from the filtration rate. The method of preparing serum for analysis also influences the quantity of chromogens measured. The difference between the "exogenous" and "endogenous" creatinine clearance is not completely explained by the presence of noncreatinine chromogens, since the difference is still apparent when creatinine is measured by a specific enzymatic method.[13]

METHOD OF MEASURING THE 24-HR CREATININE CLEARANCE. The endogenous creatinine clearance may be measured over several short periods in the same manner as the urea clearance. However, since it is not influenced by changes in urine volume, it is possible to measure the clearance over a longer period of time. Six-hour and 24-hr clearance methods have been described. The 24-hr clearance requires only the collection of a 24-hr specimen of urine and a single blood sample. The collection of the urine sample may be started at any time but must be completed at the same time on the following day. At the beginning of the test, the patient voids, the sample is discarded, and the time is recorded. All urine passed subsequent to the beginning of the test is collected in a single container. At the end of 24 hr, the patient voids and adds this urine to the total collection. The blood sample is usually taken near the end of the test, and serum is quickly separated from cells. The volume of the urine is measured, and the creatinine content of serum and urine samples is determined. The clearance is expressed in liters per 24 hr and is calculated as follows:

$$\text{Clearance} = \frac{UV}{P},$$

where $U$ (mg/L) is the urine creatinine concentration, $V$ (L/day) is the urine volume, and $P$ (mg/L) is the serum creatinine concentration.

ANALYTIC METHOD FOR CREATININE. As previously emphasized, the analytic methods for creatinine are not specific, since they measure several chromogenic substances present in the serum in addition to creatinine. The amount of chromogen measured varies somewhat with different methods of precipitating plasma proteins. A satisfactory method, using the Folin-Wu tungstic acid filtrate, is described by Brod and Sirota.[14]

SOURCES OF ERROR. *Incomplete collection of urine.* This is the commonest source of error. However, experience shows that satisfactory 24-hr urine collections are less difficult to obtain than accurately timed short collections. Cooperative patients often can make their own collections with a minimum of supervision. The urinary excretion of creatinine is so constant from day to day that it can be used as a check on the accuracy of collections when more than one 24-hr clearance is measured.

*Creatinine in diet.* Although the constancy of serum creatinine has been emphasized, it may show some diurnal variation in patients on a diet that is high in meat content.[17] In such patients, blood should be drawn in the fasting state.

*Bacterial breakdown of creatinine.* This most commonly occurs when urine is allowed to stand at room temperature. It is preferable to refrigerate the urine during the collection. Samples should be analyzed promptly after completion of the test. Where delay is unavoidable, the 24-hr specimen may be preserved by addition of a few drops of toluol.

LIMITATIONS. In infants and children, the endogenous-creatinine clearance is less satisfactory than in adults, giving values that are generally low in comparison with the inulin clearance.[19] In patients with advanced renal disease, the endogenous-creatinine clearance is higher than the filtration rate by 20–70 percent.[14] In these patients, endogenous creatinine appears to be partly excreted by the renal tubules, its clearance becoming similar to that of exogenous creatinine.[13] Because of this, endogenous-creatinine clearance cannot be interpreted as identical with the filtration rate in these patients. However, creatinine-clearance values that greatly exceed the filtration rate do not occur until extensive damage has taken place, and the error in measurement is not large enough to obscure the presence of severe renal disease. Therefore, in spite of this limitation, the test is sufficiently accurate for use as a clinical measure of renal function even in uremic patients, but the probable error must be borne in mind in interpreting the test.

In patients with congestive heart failure, the endogenous-creatinine clearance is substantially lower than the inulin clearance.[14] The discrepancy is greatest in patients with severe failure and peripheral edema, where creatinine clearance ranges from 56 to 80 percent of the filtration rate. It is less marked in patients who are free of edema or undergoing diuresis where reported values range from 80 to 106 percent of the inulin clearance.

INTERPRETATION AND ADVANTAGES. Despite its limitations, the 24-hr endogenous-creatinine clearance appears to be the best test available at the present time for the clinical assessment of renal function. The simplicity of the 24-hr urine collection and single blood sample make the test feasible for use with out-patients as well as those in the hospital. The inaccuracies of incomplete bladder emptying are largely mitigated by the long duration of the collection period, and the accuracy of collection may be checked by comparison of the 24-hr creatinine excretion, when serial determinations are made. The accuracy of the test may be estimated by its reproducibility in any patient, where variability from day to day is usually no more than $\pm 10$ percent.

In normal subjects and patients with moderate impairment of renal function, the 24-hr clearance may be interpreted as a measure of glomerular filtration rate sufficiently accurate for clinical purposes. The normal value for healthy adults varies in different reported series from 150 to 180 L/24 hr per 1.73 m² of body surface area. It is somewhat lower on a low-protein diet and higher when the meat content of the diet is increased.[17] The average value for normal subjects declines with increasing age. At age 90 the average clearance is approximately 50 percent lower than the normal value at age 20.[6]

### The Phenolsulfonphthalein (PSP) Test [20-23]

PHYSIOLOGY. In the plasma, phenolsulfonphthalein (PSP) is reversibly bound to the albumin fraction of plasma protein. Because of this binding, very little of the dye is excreted by glomerular filtration, and over 90 percent of an administered dose is excreted by the renal tubules.

The PSP test, as it is used clinically, is an empirical measure of the rate of excretion of a standard test dose over a fixed period of time. The rate of excretion depends chiefly on the renal plasma flow, since the test dose produces too low a concentration in the plasma to saturate the tubular excretory mechanism. Since the dye is given as a single injection, it is most rapidly excreted during the first few minutes after injection when the plasma concentration is high. After the plasma concentration is reduced to low levels, the remainder of the dose is excreted more slowly. In the presence of reduced renal blood flow or inactive renal tubules, the blood must be recirculated through the kidney over a longer period of time to excrete the same amount of dye. If allowed sufficient time, the damaged kidney will excrete the same amount of PSP as the normal kidney and abnormally low excretion may be apparent only during the first 15 or 20 min after injection. The cumulative excretion over a period of 2 hr may be the same for normal and damaged kidneys and is usually 70–80 percent of the test dose.

Normally, between 15 and 25 percent of the test dose of PSP is excreted by the liver and is therefore not recovered in the urine.

METHOD OF PERFORMING THE PSP TEST. The patient voids, then drinks 600 to 800 ml of water to promote urine flow, and the test is started 30 min later. It is preferable that the bladder not be emptied after hydration is started, since this may interfere with the patient's ability to void at the end of the first 15-min period. At the beginning of the test, exactly 1.0 ml of phenolsulphonphthalein solution, containing 6 mg of the dye, is injected intravenously. The bladder is emptied exactly 15, 30, 60, and 120 min after the injection. The time of collecting each sample is recorded and its volume is measured.

METHODS OF ANALYSIS. The dye content of the samples may be analyzed either by direct visual colorimetry or, more accurately, with the use of a spectrophotometer. In both instances, the color intensity of PSP in the samples is measured after diluting each sample to the same volume and alkalinizing it to produce the red color of the dye.

*Visual colorimetric method.* Each sample is treated separately. Turbid urine should be centrifuged or filtered before analysis. Add 2 ml of 10-percent sodium hydroxide to each sample to produce full red color development of the dye. Dilute the total sample to 1000 ml in a graduated cylinder and invert several times to insure adequate mixing. Compare the sample with standards containing known amounts of PSP, using a diffuse light source and a cuvette of the same dimensions as that of the standards. The commercially available standards contain dye in amounts expressed as a percentage of 6 mg of PSP diluted to 1000 ml and are sealed to prevent deterioration.

SOURCES OF ERROR. *Inaccurate measurement of test dose.* Since the test depends on the recovery of a known amount of PSP, and is compared with standards prepared from the same test dose, it is essential that the quantity of dye be measured precisely in the syringe. Inaccuracy can also result from loss of a part of the dye into the subcutaneous tissue during injection. A total recovery of more than 90 percent of the test dose at the end of 2 hr suggests liver disease or inaccurate measurement of the dose.

*Interference by bile or blood.* These substances interfere in the colorimetric estimation of PSP. They can be removed by means of a zinc acetate reagent made by adding 50 gm of zinc acetate to 100 ml of absolute methyl alcohol. This should be shaken at intervals and only the supernatant used. To remove bile or blood from urine samples, add a quantity of the reagent equal to the volume of the sample, shake vigorously, let stand 10 min, and filter. The clear filtrate is then analyzed for PSP as described above.

*Interference by BSP dye.* Bromsulfalein, used to measure liver function, gives a purple color in alkaline solution and interferes with PSP determination. At least 24 hr should be allowed to elapse between the performance of these two tests.

*Interference by other pigments.* Since the volume of the urine samples is usually small, dilution to 1000 ml effectively dilutes out normally present urinary pigments. They may interfere when samples are unusually large, but this can usually be avoided by having the patient void at the time hydration is started. Abnormal urinary pigments and pigments due to ingestion of drugs may also interfere in the test.

*Inaccurate timing of urine collections and incomplete bladder emptying.* If excretion of PSP is greater in subsequent samples than in the first sample, it usually signifies an error of this type. Samples smaller than 50 ml in volume frequently are incomplete. Adequate hydration and voiding in the vertical posture help assure complete bladder emptying.

INTERPRETATION AND LIMITATIONS. The significance and inherent limitations of the PSP test have been discussed above. In summary, the test is a crude measure of the integrity of the renal tubules and their rate of perfusion with plasma. The amount of dye excreted during the first 15-min period is the most important information obtained from the test. Collection of the remaining samples serves as a check on the accuracy of urine collection.

When used in conjunction with tests that measure glomerular filtration rate, the PSP test may give information about the relative degree of damage to different parts of the nephron. Early in the course of acute glomerulonephritis, PSP excretion may be normal although creatinine clearance is depressed.[5] PSP excretion may be disproportionately low relative to the GFR in hydronephrosis and pyelonephritis. However, these discrepancies are not sufficiently constant to aid in diagnosis. The normal pattern of PSP excretion is shown in Table 64.[20]

## Concentration Tests

PHYSIOLOGY. The extent to which water is reabsorbed or excreted by the kidney is adjusted to the needs of the organism through variations in the release of antidiuretic hormone (ADH) by the neurohypophysis. Under conditions of de-

Table 64. *Excretion of phenolsulfonphthalein in normal subjects.*[20]

| Time after injection of 6 mg of PSP intravenously (min) | Excretion of PSP (percent) | | |
|---|---|---|---|
| | Minimum | Maximum | Average |
| 15 | 28 | 51 | 35 |
| 30 | 13 | 24 | 17 |
| 60 | 9 | 17 | 12 |
| 120 | 3 | 10 | 6 |
| Total for 2 hr | 63 | 84 | 70 |

hydration, when ADH is maximally activated, water resorption proceeds until a maximum osmotic gradient is established between urine and plasma. At its upper limit, the concentration of the urine may be as great as 1200 mOsm/L—more than four times the concentration of the plasma. A concentration as high as this can be achieved only when a small quantity of osmotically active material is being excreted. If the quantity of solutes being excreted is increased, the concentration of the urine falls in spite of maximum ADH activation. When large quantities of solute are excreted, an "osmotic diuresis" ensues owing to the increased quantity of water that is carried out with the solute, and maximum concentration of the urine may be only slightly greater than that of the serum.[24]

Loss of the ability to form a highly concentrated urine may be due to: (a) a defective neurohypophyseal ADH mechanism (Unit 21); (b) inability of the renal tubular epithelium to sustain a maximum osmotic gradient between urine and plasma, or (c) an increased rate of excretion of solutes, producing an osmotic diuresis. In renal disease, the loss of functioning nephrons requires the remaining nephrons to excrete a larger daily load of solutes. This increased load of solutes produces an osmotic diuresis which is probably the principal cause of the loss of concentrating power that occurs in renal disease. In addition, nephrons that are damaged are unable to sustain a maximum osmotic gradient.

353

METHOD OF MEASURING THE URINE-CONCENTRATING ABILITY. A large number of different test schedules have been described for testing urine-concentrating ability.[25] As previously emphasized, maximum concentration will be achieved only when ADH is fully activated by adequate dehydration and when the excretion of solutes is at a minimum. Concentrating ability can also be measured by administering Pitressin (see Unit 21). Concentration tests are contraindicated in patients with manifest renal insufficiency, since they may result in severe dehydration and exacerbation of uremic symptoms.

The following test usually causes little discomfort and is applicable to ambulatory as well as hospitalized patients.

*Procedure.* All fluids are restricted after breakfast until the following morning. The usual diet is allowed, omitting foods containing free fluids. On retiring, the patient voids and discards the urine. The following morning, the bladder is emptied on awakening and the sample is saved. Two additional samples are collected at hourly intervals. Each of the three samples is examined for volume, specific gravity, and protein. The first (night) sample is examined for sediment. Where facilities are available, measurement of urine osmolality (by freezing-point depression) is preferable to specific-gravity determination.

INTERPRETATION AND LIMITATIONS. Normally, the specific gravity in at least one of the samples will reach 1.025 or higher, corresponding to a concentration of approximately 800 mOsm/L. Failure to achieve this concentration is a generally reliable indication of renal damage. In severe renal disease, the specific gravity becomes fixed in the vicinity of 1.008 to 1.012, indicating severe impairment of concentrating ability. In addition to patients with structural kidney disease, inability to concentrate the urine has been reported in patients with sickle-cell anemia and sickle-cell trait and with panhypopituitarism. Reversible loss of concentrating ability may be seen in severe anemia from any cause, and in the nephropathy associated with potassium deficiency.

Concentration tests are not reliable in edematous patients who are undergoing diuresis, and are of questionable value in any edematous patient because of the likelihood of spontaneous diuresis. Failure to concentrate the urine may be the result of a defective mechanism for formation and release of ADH. Characteristically, this is associated with a urine more dilute than the plasma (specific gravity below 1.010). Methods of testing this mechanism are discussed in Unit 21.

### Special Diagnostic Procedures in Renal Disease

Despite the development of many new radiologic techniques and urologic procedures, the diagnosis of parenchymal renal disease still depends to a large extent on clinical findings and, especially, on careful examination of the urine (Unit 19). Bacteriologic studies of the urine (Unit 26) should also be made whenever renal disease is suspected. Biopsy of the kidney is of considerable value and has been employed with increasing frequency in recent years, especially where conventional diagnostic methods fail to give adequate information.

RADIOLOGIC STUDIES. A discussion of diagnostic radiology is beyond the scope of this book. Standard radiologic procedures, such as intravenous pyelography, are of considerable diagnostic value, not only in visualizing disease within the renal collecting system and lower urinary tract, but also in the diagnosis of parenchymal renal diseases such as pyelonephritis and tuberculosis. It should be emphasized that estimation of the concentration of radiopaque dye as judged by x-ray visualization is not a satisfactory measure of the adequacy of renal function, since a "normal" concentration is frequently seen, in spite of considerable depression of function as measured by creatinine clearance. Measurement of the length of the renal shadows may give important diagnostic clues. In normal adults, length of the renal outline is from 10 to 14.5 cm, and varies with body size. Abnormally large kidneys suggest hydronephrosis, polycystic disease, amyloidosis, acromegaly, or lymphoma with involvement of the renal parenchyma. Small kidneys may be seen in many kinds of advanced renal disease. Normally, the difference in length between the two kidneys does not exceed 1.0 cm, and larger discrepancies suggest disease of one kidney (see below).

SPECIAL TESTS FOR DETECTION OF RENAL VASCULAR DISEASE. The detection of abnormalities of renal blood flow is of considerable importance in patients with hypertension, since surgical correction of the abnormality may restore blood pressure to normal. Several tests have recently been developed for the purpose of detecting and defining this type of renal lesion. It has been emphasized that minor differences in the relative size of the kidneys and in the rate of excretion of radioactive dye in the intravenous pyelogram provide important clues to the presence of renal vascular lesions and help in selecting patients for the specialized studies described below.[26, 27]

A test described by Howard[28] (the "Howard test") involves bilateral ureteral catheterization and collection of timed urine samples from each kidney. The urine volume and sodium concentration are measured and compared. Reduction in urine volume by 50 percent and of sodium concentration by 15 percent on one side as compared to the other suggests ischemia of the kidney with the lower urine volume. The test is technically cumbersome, and, except where unilateral disease of the main renal artery is present, has not given consistent results.[26]

A test utilizing the intravenous injection of a small amount of radioactive Iodopyracet has been described by Winter.[29] In this test, two crystal scintillation counters are positioned over the skin of the back, and the radioactivity is recorded for a 15-min period following the injection. The curves representing the two kidneys are analyzed and compared. Experience with the test is still limited, but suggests that it may prove to be of value as a screening test for the detection of renal vascular disease.[30] Difficulties in interpretation are frequently encountered, owing chiefly to imperfections in the geometry of surface counting. The proximity of the right kidney to the liver also causes difficulty, since the liver takes up some of the radioactive dye.

The only procedure that provides definitive anatomic information about the renal vasculation is renal angiography. Recently, modifications in the technique of performing angiography[31] have greatly reduced the morbidity of this procedure.

BIOPSY OF THE KIDNEY. When the ordinary diagnostic techniques fail to give adequate information, a histologic diagnosis can often be made in parenchymal renal disease by needle biopsy of the kidney.[31] In pyelonephritis, organisms can sometimes be recovered from culture of biopsy material, although urine cultures are sterile.[32] Improvements in the technique of renal biopsy have recently been described.[33] The procedure is reasonably safe, if proper precautions are taken, but should not be used where adequate information can be obtained by the usual tests. Biopsy can be done only on cooperative patients, and is contraindicated in the presence of bleeding tendencies, hydronephrosis, pyonephrosis, perinephric abscess, renal tuberculosis, renal tumors, and cysts, and when only one kidney is present. Uremia is not a contraindication unless it is associated with a bleeding tendency. The test is usually followed by transient microscopic or gross hematuria. Complications include back pain, renal colic, severe hematuria, and retroperitoneal hematoma.

## REFERENCES

1. H. W. Smith, *The Kidney, Structure and Function in Health and Disease* (Oxford University Press, New York, 1951).
2. H. W. Smith, *Principles of Renal Physiology* (Oxford University Press, New York, 1956).
3. W. Goldring and H. Chasis, *Hypertension and Hypertensive Disease* (The Commonwealth Fund, New York, 1944).
4. A. M. Fishberg, *Hypertension and Nephritis* (ed. 5; Lea and Febiger, Philadelphia, 1954).
5. D. P. Earle, "Renal function tests in the diagnosis of glomerular and tubular disease," *Bull. N. Y. Acad. Med. 26,* 47 (1950).
6. D. F. Davies and N. W. Shock, "Age changes in glomerular filtration rate, effective renal plasma flow, and tubular excretory capacity in adult males," *J. clin. Invest. 29,* 496 (1950).
7. A. Leaf and L. H. Newburgh, *Significance of the Body Fluids in Clinical Medicine* (ed. 2; Thomas, Springfield, Ill., 1955).
8. J. H. Austin, E. Stillman, and D. D. Van Slyke, "Factors governing the rate of excretion of urea," *J. biol. Chem. 46,* 91 (1921).
9. D. D. Van Slyke, "The effect of urine volume on urea excretion," *J. clin. Invest. 26,* 1159 (1947).
10. J. A. Shannon, "The renal reabsorption and excretion of urea under conditions of extreme diuresis," *Amer. J. Physiol. 123,* 182 (1938).
11. F. H. Epstein, "Reversible uremic states," *J. Amer. med. Ass. 161,* 494 (1956).
12. B. F. Miller and A. W. Winkler, "The renal excretion of endogenous creatinine in man in comparison with exogenous creatinine and inulin," *J. clin. Invest. 17,* 31 (1938).
13. B. F. Miller, A. Leaf, A. R. Mamby, and Z. Miller, "Validity of the endogenous creatinine clearance as a measure of glomerular filtration rate in the diseased human kidney," *J. clin. Invest. 31,* 309 (1952).
14. J. Brod and J. H. Sirota, "The renal clearance of endogenous creatinine in man," *J. clin. Invest. 27,* 645 (1948).
15. J. H. Sirota, D. S. Baldwin, and H. Villareal, "Diurnal variations of renal function in man," *J. clin. Invest. 29,* 187 (1950).
16. D. S. Baldwin, J. H. Sirota, and H. Villareal, "Diurnal variations of renal function in congestive heart failure," *Proc. Soc. exp. Biol. (N. Y.) 74,* 578 (1950).
17. T. Addis, E. Barrett, L. J. Poo, H. J. Ureen, and R. W. Lippman, "The relation between protein consumption and diurnal variations of the endogenous creatinine clearance in normal individuals," *J. clin. Invest. 30,* 206 (1951).
18. A. A. Camara, K. D. Arn, A. Reiner, and L. H. Newburgh, "The 24 hourly endogenous creatinine clearance as a measure of the functional state of the kidneys," *J. lab. clin. Med. 37,* 743 (1951).
19. R. S. Hare, "Endogenous creatinine in serum and urine," *Proc. Soc. exp. Biol. (N. Y.) 74,* 148 (1950).
20. E. M. Chapman and J. A. Halstead, "The fractional phenolsulfonphthalein test in Bright's Disease," *Amer. J. med. Sci. 186,* 233 (1933).

21. E. M. Chapman, "Further experience with the fractional 'phthalein test," *New Engl. J. Med. 214,* 16 (1936).

22. W. Goldring, R. W. Clarke, and H. W. Smith, "The phenol red clearance in normal man," *J. clin. Invest. 15,* 221 (1936).

23. W. W. Smith and H. W. Smith, "Protein binding of phenol red, Diodrast, and other substances in plasma," *J. biol. Chem. 124,* 107 (1938).

24. S. Rapaport, W. A. Brodsky, C. D. West, and B. Mackler, "Urinary flow and excretion of solutes during osmotic diuresis in hydropenic man," *Amer. J. Physiol. 156,* 433 (1949).

25. F. H. Lashmet and L. H. Newburgh, "An improved concentration test of renal function," *J. Amer. med. Ass. 99,* 1396 (1932).

26. I. H. Page, "Mechanisms, diagnosis, and treatment of hypertension of renal vascular origin," *Ann. intern. Med. 15,* 196 (1959).

27. H. P. Dustan, I. H. Page, and E. F. Poutasse, "Renal hypertension," *New Engl. J. Med. 261,* 647 (1959).

28. J. E. Howard, "A functional test for detection of hypertension produced by one kidney," *Trans. Ass. Amer. Phycns 69,* 291 (1956).

29. C. C. Winter, "Unilateral renal disease and hypertension: Use of the radioactive Diodrast renogram as a screening test," *J. Urol. (Baltimore) 78,* 107 (1957).

30. M. Serratto, J. T. Grayhack, and D. P. Earle, "A clinical evaluation of the Iodopyracet (Diodrast) renogram," *Arch. intern. Med. 103,* 851 (1959).

31. E. Poutasse and H. P. Dustan, "Arteriosclerosis and renal hypertension: Indications for aortography in hypertensive patients and results of surgical treatment of obstructive lesions of renal artery," *J. Amer. med. Ass. 165,* 1521 (1957).

32. R. M. Kark, R. C. Muehrcke, C. L. Pirani, and D. E. Pollak, "The clinical value of renal biopsy," *Ann. intern. Med. 43,* 807 (1955).

33. R. C. Muehrcke, R. M. Kark, and C. L. Pirani, "Techniques of percutaneous renal biopsy in the prone position," *J. Urol. 74,* 267 (1955).

# Unit 21

## Disorders of Water Excretion and the Electrolyte Composition of Body Fluids

### DISORDERS OF WATER EXCRETION

PHYSIOLOGIC REGULATION OF
WATER EXCRETION

Regulation of the osmolality of the extracellular fluid is normally achieved through variations in rate of release of the antidiuretic hormone (ADH) by the neurohypophysis. This hormone acts on the cells of the renal tubules to promote the reabsorption of water. In its absence, the urine is dilute and copious, amounting in volume to as much as 10–15 percent of the glomerular filtration rate. The structural formula of ADH, based on analyses of beef and hog pituitaries, is that of an octapeptide amide.[1,2] Recent work indicates that it is formed in the supraoptic and paraventricular nuclei of the hypothalamus and is then transported distally along the axones of the supraoptico-hypophyseal tract and stored in the posterior pituitary gland in axonal end plates adjacent to vascular channels.[3,4] Its rate of release into the blood stream is under neural control and is governed by "osmoreceptors" in the hypothalamus (Verney)[5] which are sensitive to changes of as little as 2 percent in the osmolality of the extracellular fluid. The mechanism by which ADH promotes the reabsorption of water is incompletely understood. The site of action appears to be in the medullary area of the kidney and involves the loops of Henle and collecting ducts.[6]

The normal stimulus to the osmoreceptor-neurohypophyseal mechanism is an increase in the osmolality of extracellular fluid induced by a deficit of water or an excess of solute. Certain drugs also stimulate the release of ADH. Nicotine and acetyl choline are powerful stimulants [7–9] which are thought to act directly on cells of the hypothalamic nuclei rather than through the osmoreceptors.[10] Morphine is a potent stimulant to release of ADH in animals,[11] but this action is less consistent in man. Pain, fright, and strenuous exercise also stimulate ADH release, although epinephrine alone does not.[7] Marked antidiuresis may follow contraction of extracellular-fluid volume, with no rise, or even with a fall, in plasma osmolality.[12,13]

While ADH governs the rate of water excretion, the intake of water is governed by the sensation of thirst. There is evidence that a "thirst center" located in the hypothalamus and sensitive to changes in osmolality [14] and volume [15] of extracellular fluid gives rise to this sensation and insures that fluid losses are replaced.

358

## DISORDERS OF WATER EXCRETION

Abnormal water excretion with polyuria and polydipsia may result from diseases affecting the formation and release of ADH, the thirst mechanism, or the site of action of ADH in the renal tubules. In all three types of defect the urine is more dilute than the plasma (specific gravity less than 1.010), distinguishing this type of polyuria from osmotic diuresis which may result from glycosuria or advanced renal disease.

*Diabetes insipidus* is the result of absent or inadequate production or release of ADH and may result from any lesion involving the hypothalamic nuclei, supraoptico-hypophyseal tract, or posterior lobe of the pituitary. Diagnosis depends on the demonstration that: (i) the neurohypophyseal mechanism does not respond normally to stimulation by releasing adequate amounts of ADH, and (ii) the kidneys are capable of responding normally to exogenously administered antidiuretic hormone (Pitressin).

*Disorders of the thirst mechanism* resulting in primary polydipsia are usually of psychogenic origin. These disorders are distinguished from diabetes insipidus by demonstrating that the neurohypophyseal mechanism responds normally to stimulation.

*Nephrogenic diabetes insipidus* is a rare, sex-linked familial disorder transmitted by females and appearing in males during infancy.[16] ADH is apparently released normally by the neurohypophysis, but the kidney does not respond to the hormone. Diagnosis depends on the demonstration of an absent response to exogenously administered ADH (Pitressin).

*Hypercalcemia* from any cause may cause polyuria and polydipsia, with failure to respond to neurohypophyseal stimulation or exogenously administered Pitressin.[17–19] When the serum calcium concentration returns to normal, the ability of the kidney to respond to ADH is rapidly restored.[17] The mechanism by which hypercalcemia inhibits renal water reabsorption is not understood. It has been suggested that deposition of calcium in the renal tubules may be responsible. However, histologic studies on animals in which hypercalcemic polyuria has been induced in acute and short-term experiments show only minor changes in the collecting ducts, and significant intrarenal calcium deposition is not found.[20]

*Hypokalemia.* In subjects depleted of potassium as a result of gastrointestinal or renal losses or primary aldosteronism, there may be marked polyuria and polydipsia with defective ability to concentrate the urine.[21, 22] In most instances, the urine is only moderately dilute (180–210 mOsm/L) and becomes isosmotic or slightly hypertonic in response to water deprivation or Pitressin.[23] The defect in concentrating ability is partially or completely restored to normal when the potassium deficit is replaced. Histologically, potassium depletion is associated with vacuolar and degenerative changes in the renal tubular epithelium.[22]

### CLINICAL TESTS IN DISORDERS OF WATER EXCRETION

No reliable method for direct measurement of ADH is available for clinical use. The clinical evaluation of the antidiuretic mechanism depends instead on observing the changes in urine flow and urine concentration after stimulating the neurohypophysis to release ADH by increasing serum osmolality or by giving nicotine. Since the released ADH is "assayed" on the patient's own kidneys, it is essential to determine also whether or not the patient responds normally to exogenously administered Pitressin whenever an abnormal response to neurohypophyseal stimulation occurs.

In these tests, the osmotic concentration of the urine is usually measured as its specific gravity. However, more reliable and quantitative information is obtained if the urine osmolality is measured directly by determination of the freezing-point depression (Unit 19).

FLUID-DEPRIVATION TEST. In diabetes insipidus, prolonged deprivation of fluid can lead to a dangerous degree of dehydration. It is therefore not possible to standardize a fluid-deprivation test that will be applicable to all cases. The standard concentration tests (Unit 20) are too strenuous.

Fluid deprivation should be embarked upon only in alert and cooperative patients. When the urine volume is large and rapid losses are anticipated, it is preferable that the test be carried out during the daytime, to permit close observation. The patient should be weighed at the beginning of the test and every 2–3 hr thereafter. Fluid is withheld for as long a period as the patient can tolerate without extreme discomfort.[24] Urine is collected at hourly intervals and its volume, specific gravity, and osmolality are determined. Osmolality of the serum determined at the beginning and end of the test gives useful additional information.

*Interpretation.* In normal subjects there is a progressive reduction in urine volume with a rise in specific gravity of the urine to 1.016 or above, usually within 6–8 hr (if food is also withheld). There is little or no discomfort for up to 12 hr, weight loss is usually no greater than 1 lb, and there is no significant change in serum osmolality after 12 hr. In diabetes insipidus (or nephrogenic diabetes insipidus), urine volume remains high and specific gravity usually does not exceed 1.010 at any time. There are a steady loss of weight and progressive thirst and discomfort as the test progresses. Patients with psychogenic polydipsia respond like normal subjects but complain of extreme thirst. In patients with diabetes insipidus who are severely dehydrated as a result of fluid deprivation, glomerular filtration rate (GFR) falls somewhat and urine concentration may increase, although the urine remains

more dilute than the plasma. With an extreme reduction in GFR in animals, an osmotically concentrated urine may be formed even in the absence of ADH.[25] This is theoretically possible in man, but it is doubtful whether this phenomenon ever results from the moderate reduction in GFR that results from even severe water deprivation.

RESPONSE TO HYPERTONIC SODIUM CHLORIDE (Hickey-Hare Test). The following test is a modification of the procedure described by Hickey and Hare.[26] Water diuresis is induced by hydration and control observations are made on urine flow and osmolality. Hypertonic sodium chloride solution is then rapidly infused by vein in amounts sufficient to significantly elevate the serum osmolality and stimulate the osmoreceptors. Additional observations are made on urine flow and concentration during and following the infusion. Measurement of serum osmolality during the control period and at the completion of the infusion provides useful additional information.

*Procedure.* During the hour preceding the test the patient drinks 20 ml of water per kilogram of body weight. Urine is collected by voiding at 15-min intervals and the test is started when the urine flow exceeds 5 ml/min. The urine is first collected for two 15-min control periods. An intravenous infusion of 3-percent sodium chloride solution is then begun and administered at a rate of 0.25 ml/min per kilogram of body weight for a period of 45 min (approximately 800 ml of fluid). Urine collections are continued for 30 min after completion of the infusion. The appropriately labeled urine samples are examined for volume, specific gravity, and osmolality.

*Interpretations and limitations.* A normal response to the infusion of hypertonic sodium chloride solution is a marked reduction in urine volume with a rise in urine concentration to well above that of the plasma (specific gravity 1.016 or more). These changes usually are evident within less than 30 min after starting the infusion. Patients with psychogenic polydipsia respond like normal subjects. In diabetes insipidus, the urine volume remains unchanged or may increase.[26, 27] The specific gravity may rise somewhat but usually not above 1.010. Measurement of urine osmolality gives more precise information and shows that the urine remains more dilute than the plasma. Similar responses occur in nephrogenic diabetes insipidus and hypercalcemic polyuria. Occasional patients who respond in a normal or near-normal fashion to nicotine stimulation will fail to respond to hypertonic saline or fluid deprivation. It has been suggested that the defect in these patients is in the osmoreceptor itself, rather than in the neurohypophysis.[10]

The infusion of a large volume of saline may be dangerous or undesirable in patients with cardiac or liver disease, and certain other situations. Clinical judgment should determine when the test ought to be omitted. Modifications may be devised in some cases, using smaller volumes of saline, but if this is done measurements of serum osmolality should be made to determine whether a significant increase in osmolality has been induced.

NICOTINE STIMULATION. Tests using nicotine stimulation are difficult to standardize, owing to the wide variability in the dose required to produce a response in smokers.[8, 9] The drug may be given as pure nicotine alkaloid, or as nicotine tartrate or salicylate. Alternatively, nicotine stimulation may be achieved by smoking from 1 to 4 cigarettes in rapid succession with deep inhalation. In general, it may be assumed that stimulation is adequate when side effects of nicotine such as dizziness, nausea, vomiting, or palpitation are induced. The following test is based on the use of the pure alkaloid.

*Procedure.* The patient is hydrated and urine collections are made as described in the hypertonic sodium chloride test. Two 15-min control collections are obtained when the urine flow exceeds 5 ml/min. Nicotine is given intravenously, 1 mg at a time at 3-min intervals, using a total of 1–2 mg for nonsmokers and 3 or 4 mg for smokers. Injection is discontinued sooner if side effects of nicotine occur. Urine collections are continued at 15-min intervals for 1 hr. Measurements are made of the volume, specific gravity, and osmolality of each sample.

*Interpretations and limitations.* If nicotine stimulation has been adequate, normal subjects respond with a prompt decrease in urine flow and an increase in the concentration of the urine (specific gravity 1.016 or higher), which is usually evident within 15–30 min. Patients with complete diabetes insipidus and patients with nephrogenic diabetes insipidus show no response. Patients with diabetes insipidus of mild or moderate degree, as evidenced by other tests, may respond in a normal or near-normal fashion to nicotine. It has been suggested that the defect in these patients is in the osmoreceptor rather than in the neurohypophysis or hypothalamus.

The nicotine test is of use when large infusions of hypertonic saline are contraindicated. Its value is limited by the fact that patients with clinically important diabetes insipidus may respond to the drug like normal subjects. In subjects who do not respond normally to nicotine, there is no assurance that an adequate amount has been given unless toxic side effects occur. These are usually transient but occasionally are severe and prolonged. The test is contraindicated in patients with severe coronary disease, Buerger's disease, and other forms of arterial insufficiency, and in patients with tobacco amblyopia.

PITRESSIN TEST. Pitressin is a purified preparation of vasopressin closely resembling the endogenous antidiuretic hormone. It is available in aqueous solution and as Pitressin tannate in oil. Tests using both preparations have been described. In general, the antidiuretic response is more consistent and sustained and more nearly maximal when Pitressin tannate in oil is used, as described below. However, Hickey and Hare [26] and others [27] have combined the Pitressin test with the hypertonic-saline test by giving 0.1 unit of aqueous Pitressin in 1 ml of isotonic sodium chloride solution intravenously at the end of the procedure and collecting the urine for two additional periods. If negative or equivocal results are obtained with the use of aqueous Pitressin, a second Pitressin test should be made using Pitressin tannate in oil.

*Procedure.* Pitressin tannate in oil is given by deep intramuscular injection at the time of the evening meal. The patient voids at bedtime and again on arising in the morning. The overnight specimen is examined for specific gravity and osmolality. *Whenever Pitressin tannate in oil is used, it is essential that the vial be placed in warm water for several minutes, then agitated thoroughly and carefully inspected* at the time the syringe is filled, since Pitressin tannate precipi-

tates at room temperature and settles to the bottom of the vial. The dose for healthy young adults is 5 units (1 ml), which usually results in an antidiuresis lasting from 24–48 hr. In thin or aged persons, half the usual dose is used. It is contraindicated in coronary disease.

*Interpretations and limitations.* In normal subjects and patients with diabetes insipidus whose renal concentrating mechanisms are normal, the overnight urine specimen following stimulation with Pitressin tannate in oil is highly concentrated. The specific gravity is 1.025 or higher and osmolality often greater than 800 mOsm/L. In elderly patients or those with renal disease, lesser degrees of concentration are achieved, but an increase in osmolality above that of the plasma occurs in all except those with nephrogenic diabetes insipidus or hypercalcemic polyuria.

The test is reliable, simple, and, except in patients with coronary disease, safe. It may be used in place of the usual concentrating test (Unit 20) as a measure of renal function. The most common source of error in the Pitressin test is failure to suspend the precipitated vasopressin in the oil prior to injection.

## DISORDERS OF SERUM ELECTROLYTE COMPOSITION

An enormous amount of experimental data has been accumulated in recent years bearing on the regulation of the volume and ionic composition of body fluids. This has been well summarized in several recent monographs [28-30] and reviews [31, 32] and will not be reviewed in detail here.

Representative normal values for the principle serum electrolytes are shown in Table 65, which illustrates the fact that the total quantities of cations and of anions must be equal. Although each species of ion is subject to different physiologic influences, their serum concentrations normally remain constant within

Table 65. *Representative normal values for the principal electrolytes of serum.*[28]

| Cations | mEq/L | Anions | mEq/L |
|---|---|---|---|
| $Na^+$ | 138 | $Cl^-$ | 102 |
| $K^+$ | 4 | $HCO_3^-$ | 26 |
| $Ca^{++}$ and $Mg^{++}$ | 7 | $PO_4^{---}$ and | |
| | | $SO_4^{--}$ | 3 |
| | | Undetermined | 3 |
| | | Protein | 15 |
| Total | 149 | Total | 149 |

narrow limits. Separate mechanisms exist in the kidney that govern the rate of excretion of each of the electrolytes. Evaluation of abnormalities in serum concentration is often helped by measurement of the rate of urinary excretion.

The intracellular ions are not accessible for direct measurement, and knowledge of the factors that govern their distribution is very incomplete. In the case of potassium, which is chiefly intracellular in distribution, marked changes in the quantity present in the body may occur with no change in the serum concentration. Knowledge of the physiologic role of magnesium [33, 34] is in its infancy.

### METHODS OF MEASURING ELECTROLYTE CONCENTRATIONS

SODIUM AND POTASSIUM. Determination of sodium and potassium done with a lithium internal-standard flame photometer are accurate to $\pm 2$ percent. The method is applicable to either serum or urine. Blood for determination of potassium must be carefully drawn to prevent mechanical hemolysis, and the serum must be separated promptly from the cells, since potassium diffuses out of red cells on standing, giving falsely high serum values.

CHLORIDE. A variety of acceptable methods are available for quantitative determination of serum chloride. The method of Schales and Schales [35] is applicable to urine as well as serum, provided the urine pH is adjusted.[36] A semiquantitative method for urine chloride adaptable to office or bedside use is that of Fantus.[37]

*Semiquantitative urine chloride test* (*Fantus test*). Titration of a chloride-containing solution with silver nitrate results in precipitation of silver chloride. In the presence of potassium chromate, formation of rust-colored silver chromate becomes apparent when all the chloride is combined.

*Reagents.* (1) Twenty-percent potassium chromate; (2) $N/10$ silver nitrate (1.7 percent); (3) 1-percent phenolphthalein in 95-percent alcohol; (4) 10-percent acetic acid.

*Procedure.* Ten drops of urine is carefully measured into a test tube and 1 drop of phenolphthalein is added. If the urine is alkaline, 10-percent acetic acid is added drop by drop to the end point of phenolphthalein. One drop of potassium chromate is then added. The dropper with which the urine was measured is then rinsed twice with distilled water and twice with silver nitrate, and silver nitrate is added drop by drop until the color of the solution changes from yellow to rust. The dropper should be held at the same angle when measuring urine and silver nitrate to assure that drop size is the same.

*Calculation.* (No. of drops Ag $No_3$ − 1) × 10 = chloride (mEq/L).

BICARBONATE. Methods for determination of serum bicarbonate are discussed below (p. 370).

SERUM OSMOLALITY. The osmolality of the serum may be calculated from its freezing-point depression. This can be determined quickly and accurately with a Fiske osmometer or similar device. The serum osmolality gives a measure of the total concentration of osmotically active material, both electrolyte and nonelectrolyte. It has recently been in use as a means of assessing clinical states of dehydration and overhydration. However, since sodium and its attendant anions represent the chief osmotic constituents of extracellular fluid, measurements of osmolality generally parallel the serum sodium concentration.[38] Since both methods are quick and accurate, measurement of osmolality offers no definite advantage over serum sodium. There are also pitfalls in the interpretation of serum osmolality which stem from the fact that it measures nonelectrolytes as well as electrolytes. If blood urea is elevated, osmolality will be increased, thus falsely signifying "dehydration." Physiologically, the elevated urea concentration does not exert an osmotic effect, since the urea is equally distributed between cells and extracellular fluid. Osmolality may be corrected for the contribution of elevated NPN as follows: [38]

Corrected osmolality

$$= \text{measured osmolality} - \frac{\text{NPN (mg/100 ml)}}{2.8}.$$

Measurement of urine osmolality is discussed elsewhere (p. 359 and Unit 19).

INTERPRETATION OF CHANGES IN SERUM ELECTROLYTE CONCENTRATION AND LIMITATIONS RELATED TO METHODOLOGY. *Accuracy of methods.* In general, the methods used for measuring serum electrolytes have a high degree of precision, provided that they are performed by an analyst skilled in quantitative chemical techniques and provided that the instruments are frequently standardized. The necessity for care in handling blood samples for potassium determinations has been mentioned.

*Serum water correction.* Electrolyte concentrations are usually expressed in milliequivalents per liter of serum, although it would be more accurate to express their concentrations in serum water, since they are confined to the aqueous phase. Normally, serum is approximately 93 percent water. When lipids and lipoproteins are elevated, this figure may be significantly decreased and falsely low values for electrolytes are recorded. Determinations of serum water content are usually made gravimetrically by evaporating weighed aliquots of serum to dryness and determining the difference in weight. A rapid method for determining serum water has recently been described, based on measurement of freezing-point depression before and after addition of a known amount of sodium chloride.[39]

ABNORMALITIES IN SERUM SODIUM CONCENTRATION AND EXTRACELLULAR-FLUID (ECF) VOLUME

PHYSIOLOGIC REGULATION OF SODIUM EXCRETION. Normally the osmolality of body fluids is kept constant by regulation of water excretion as detailed above. Since sodium and its anions represent the chief osmotic constituents of extracellular fluid, gains and losses of sodium salts are accompanied by isosmotically equivalent gains and losses of water. The total quantity of sodium in the body therefore determines the volume of the extracellular fluid (ECF). Normally the excretion of sodium in the urine is regulated primarily by the action of the adrenal cortical hormone aldosterone,[30] which promotes renal tubular reabsorption of sodium. Considerable evidence indicates that the release of aldosterone is governed by a "volume receptor," [32] which probably lies within the vascular system. Through this mechanism, sodium excretion is increased whenever fluid volume is expanded, even when the expansion is due to retention of water and serum sodium concentration is decreased.[40] Similarly, sodium is retained when fluid volume is contracted, even if there is an associated increase in serum sodium concentration. In general, changes in plasma volume have a greater effect on sodium excretion than do equivalent changes in the volume of ECF or total body water.[41] Many other factors in addition to aldosterone influence the excretion of sodium. These include hemodynamic alterations which influence glomerular filtration rate and other hormones of adrenal cortical and gonadal origin, or their synthetic analogues.[30] Osmotic diuresis from increased excretion of solutes such as glucose and urea also promotes increased sodium excretion.

ABNORMALITIES OF URINARY SODIUM EXCRETION. Through the action of aldosterone, the daily urinary excretion of sodium in normal subjects approximates the dietary intake. Whenever changes occur in sodium intake, similar changes in output follow, but several days are required before balance is achieved. In normal subjects depleted of sodium, the urinary excretion of sodium diminishes to 2 or

3 mEq/24 hr. If sodium is abruptly withdrawn from the diet, 3 or 4 days are required before this level of output is reached.[42] An inability to conserve sodium in the urine may result from renal disease or adrenal insufficiency. Administration of desoxycorticosterone or other preparations that simulate the action of aldosterone may be necessary to distinguish between these possibilities.[43]

A marked increase in urine sodium excretion occurs in certain patients with diffuse brain damage ("cerebral salt losers") and advanced pulmonary disease ("pulmonary salt wasters"). Abnormal sodium loss has also been described in patients with carcinoma of the lung and mediastinal metastases.[44] In these patients the urine is highly concentrated in spite of marked reduction in serum sodium concentration and an expanded ECF volume. The pathogenesis appears to be continuous and inappropriate ADH release. Sodium excretion diminishes when ECF volume is restored to normal by fluid deprivation.

ABNORMALITIES OF SODIUM CONCENTRATION AND EXTRACELLULAR-FLUID VOLUME. As indicated in the preceding paragraphs, two homeostatic systems act together to maintain constancy of the extracellular fluid. The regulation of water excretion by ADH governs the *concentration* of body fluids and regulation of sodium excretion under the predominant influence of aldosterone governs ECF *volume*. As long as these two systems operate harmoniously, sodium and water are gained and lost in isosmotic proportions and the concentration of serum sodium remains normal.

Deviations from the normal in serum sodium concentration imply that sodium and water have been gained or lost in other than isosmotic proportions. The possible deviations from normal in volume and sodium concentration have been classified by Welt[28] as *isosmotic, hypertonic,* and *hypotonic* expansions and con-

Table 66. *Expansions and contractions of body-fluid compartments with associated sodium concentration.*[28]

| Type | Change in volume | | Change in sodium concentration |
|---|---|---|---|
| | ECF | ICF | |
| Isotonic contraction | Decrease | None | None |
| Isotonic expansion | Increase | None | None |
| Hypertonic contraction | Decrease | Decrease | Increase |
| Hypertonic expansion | Increase | Decrease | Increase |
| Hypotonic contraction | Decrease | Increase | Decrease |
| Hypotonic expansion | Increase | Increase | Decrease |

tractions of ECF volume (Table 66). Since there is no barrier to diffusion of water between cells and ECF, associated changes in the volume of intracellular fluid also occur as indicated in the table. It is apparent that no conclusion concerning changes in ECF volume can be drawn from changes in sodium concentration. A variety of techniques are used experimentally for measurement of body-fluid "compartments," but there are none that can be considered practical for routine clinical use. Appraisal of body-fluid volumes depends on measurements of total body weight and clinical judgment.

*Expanded ECF volume.* Expansion of ECF volume is most commonly *isosmotic.* Examples are edematous states such as congestive heart failure and nephrotic syndrome. *Hypotonic expansion* may occur in severe congestive failure when both sodium and water are retained, and in postoperative patients receiving large volumes of hypotonic fluids by vein. Abnormal antidiuresis leading to hypotonic expansion has also been reported in patients with mediastinal metastases.[44] These patients respond to the hypervolemia by excreting large quantities of sodium in the urine, even though serum sodium concentration is low. *Hypertonic expansion* is usually iatrogenic and may result from administration of hypertonic sodium chloride solutions.

*Contracted ECF volume.* Moderate losses of sodium from any cause may result in an *isotonic contraction.* More severe losses produce a *hypotonic contraction,* since a marked contraction of fluid volume stimulates ADH release. Antidiuresis continues as long as volume remains contracted, even though serum osmolality falls. Sodium may be lost through the gastrointestinal tract from diarrhea or vomiting, or in the urine as a result of renal disease or adrenal insufficiency. *Hypertonic contraction* results from loss of water alone, or of water in excess of sodium.

#### ABNORMALITIES IN SERUM POTASSIUM CONCENTRATION AND BODY STORES OF POTASSIUM

FACTORS INFLUENCING SERUM POTASSIUM CONCENTRATION. The bulk of the body potassium is distributed within cells, where its concentration is roughly 15 times greater than in the serum. The serum potassium concentration often fails to reflect abnormalities in intracellular potassium.[45] A marked deficiency of potassium may exist at a time when serum potassium is normal or even high.

During acidosis, serum potassium rises, apparently as the result of a shift in potassium from the intracellular to the extracellular site. This increase in serum potassium may occur even when total body potassium is low. A common example is diabetic acidosis.

In either metabolic or respiratory alkalosis, serum potassium concentration falls somewhat,[46] but remains within the normal range unless potassium deficiency is present. When the patient with diabetic acidosis is treated with alkalinizing salts and insulin, correction of acidosis may be accompanied by a marked drop in serum potassium, "unmasking" the presence of potassium deficiency.

Regulation of potassium excretion is governed largely by adrenal steroids, which promote potassium excretion as well as sodium retention. Hyperadrenalism, as in Cushing's disease and primary aldosteronism, is often associated with a decrease in serum potassium level, while adrenal insufficiency is characterized by an increase.

HYPOKALEMIC ALKALOSIS. When potassium is lost from the body, the resulting deficiency of intracellular cation is replaced by sodium and hydrogen ion derived from extracellular fluid. Balance studies suggest that for each 3 mM of potassium lost, 2 mM of sodium and 1 mM of hydrogen ion are gained by the cells.[47] The loss of hydrogen ion from extracellular fluids results in extracellular alkalosis, while the gain of hydrogen ion by the cells results in intracellular acidosis. Deficiency of potassium sufficient to cause alkalosis is usually, although not always, associated with an abnormally low serum potassium concentration.

ABNORMALITIES OF URINARY POTASSIUM EXCRETION. Experimentally, a wide variability can be demonstrated in the renal excretion of potassium, indicating that it is filtered at the glomerulus, partly or wholly reabsorbed by the tubule, and also actively excreted by the tubular cells [48] in exchange for sodium, which is reabsorbed. There is also evidence that sodium and hydrogen ions share or compete for some component of a common secretory mechanism. Potassium excretion is increased when the urine is made alkaline by inhibiting hydrogen-ion excretion. Conversely, in potassium depletion with alkalosis, the urine pH may be inappropriately low ("paradoxical aciduria"), presumably because of preferential excretion of hydrogen ion.

Unlike sodium, potassium is not efficiently conserved by the kidney. A daily urinary excretion of 10–15 mEq or more may continue in spite of potassium deficiency.[49] Measurement of urinary potassium excretion is therefore not an accurate index of body potassium stores. However, in severe and prolonged deficiency, urinary excretion may drop to less than 10 mEq/day,[50] and this measurement may be helpful in gauging the severity of the depletion. Urinary potassium excretion is increased in primary aldosteronism in spite of coexisting hypokalemia. However, an increased excretion may not be apparent in patients on low-sodium diets. Renal losses of potassium also occur in Cushing's disease, renal tubular acidosis, and Fanconi syndrome. Osmotic diuresis from glycosuria or other solutes also promotes urinary potassium loss. In chronic renal failure, excretion of potassium frequently remains high in spite of marked reduction in renal function.[51]

CLINICAL EVALUATION OF ABNORMALITIES IN BODY POTASSIUM STORES. It has been emphasized that total body stores of potassium are poorly reflected by serum values, and measurement of urinary potassium excretion is also unreliable as a guide to potassium deficiency. For practical purposes, an abnormally *low* serum potassium concentration almost always means that potassium deficiency exists, although a normal or even high value does not exclude this possibility.[49] However, potassium depletion may be suspected from the clinical history, from characteristic electrocardiogram changes or from the presence of alkalosis, with or without "paradoxical aciduria." Potassium deficiency is most commonly the result of losses of secretions from the gastrointestinal tract through vomiting, diarrhea, or gastric suction. The causes of renal potassium loss are listed above.

Moderate elevations of serum potassium occur in adrenal insufficiency and in acidosis. In chronic renal failure, moderate elevation of serum potassium associated with acidosis is common.

Marked increases are associated with characteristic electrocardiogram abnormalities, cardiac arrythmias, and death. Serum potassium seldom rises into the lethal range except in renal failure with oliguria.

ABNORMALITIES IN SERUM CHLORIDE CONCENTRATION AND CHLORIDE EXCRETION

PHYSIOLOGIC REGULATION OF CHLORIDE CONCENTRATION. Chloride has been less completely studied than any of the other serum electrolytes. Its physiologic behavior suggests that it assumes a passive role, increasing or decreasing in concentration in the serum in response to changes in the concentrations of other anions and thus preserving the electroneutrality of extracellular fluid.

The sum of chloride and bicarbonate is usually about 10 mEq/L less than the concentration of serum sodium, the difference being due to phosphate, sulfate, and the other "unmeasured anions." When bicarbonate increases or decreases, a reciprocal change occurs in the chloride concentration. Similarly, when "unmeasured anions" increase, a corresponding decrease in serum chloride occurs. In subjects receiving sodium or ammonium chloride, the serum chloride concentration rises, and bicarbonate falls. However, since both these salts are acidifying, the decrease in bicarbonate probably results chiefly from the effect of the acid load on the bicarbonate buffer system.

ABNORMALITIES IN URINARY EXCRETION OF CHLORIDE. Excretion of chloride in the urine closely parallels that of sodium in health and in many disease states. When sodium chloride is withdrawn from the diet, chloride excretion diminishes to a few milliequivalents per day. In diseases characterized by a high sodium excretion, chloride is usually increased as well. When measurement of urine sodium excretion is available, the measurement of chloride provides no additional information and is, of course, a less accurate measure of sodium excretion than is sodium itself. The semiquantitative determination of urine chloride provides a rapid means of obtaining approximate information about sodium chloride excretion.

ABNORMALITIES IN SERUM CHLORIDE CONCENTRATION. As indicated above, chloride appears to "fill the gap" between the total cation concentration and the concentration of other anions. When serum bicarbonate rises, as in metabolic alkalosis, there is a reciprocal drop in serum chloride. Conversely, in acidosis due to renal tubular disease, chloride concentration is high, while bicarbonate is low. These states have been designated as "hypochloremic alkalosis" and "hyperchloremic acidosis" respectively, although the changes in chloride concentration are in themselves of dubious physiologic significance. It has been pointed out [52] that in acidosis with reduced renal function the rise in "unmeasured anion" usually offsets the decrease in bicarbonate and chloride does not increase.

"Hypochloremic alkalosis" may occur following prolonged vomiting, after vigorous diuresis induced by mercurial diuresis, and in association with potassium depletion.

"Hyperchloremic acidosis" occurs in renal tubular acidosis, and as a result of therapy with ammonium chloride or carbonic anhydrase inhibitors.

## Abnormalities of Acid-Base Equilibrium

### INTRODUCTION

A full discussion of the physiologic regulation of acid-base equilibrium is outside the scope of this book. A majority of the discussions of this subject have, until recently, used an archaic terminology in which sodium, potassium, and other cations have been called "bases,"

and chloride, phosphate, and other inorganic anions have been called "acids." A more satisfactory terminology is used in several recent monographs.[28, 29] The renal mechanisms of acid-base regulation have been reviewed by Orloff.[53]

### PHYSIOLOGIC CONSIDERATIONS

An acid may be defined as "any substance that donates or yields hydrogen ions" and a base as "any substance that accepts hydrogen ions,"[52] of which the prototype is hydroxyl ($OH^-$) ion. The hydrogen-ion concentration of serum and extracellular fluid, expressed as pH, normally varies between 7.35 and 7.45. Deviation from these limits is combatted by buffer systems and by respiratory and renal homeostatic mechanisms. The limits of pH compatible with life are 6.9 and 7.8.

*Buffer systems* represent the first defense of body-fluid neutrality. They consist of weak acids and their salts which react with strong acids to form a neutral salt and a weakly dissociated acid, and react with strongly alkaline salts to form a neutral and a weakly alkaline salt. The principal buffer systems in the body consist of bicarbonate, phosphate, and protein. They are distributed in heterogeneous phases of the body fluids, including the intracellular fluid. Recent studies [54–56] indicate that the activity of these systems in combatting administered loads of acid or alkali involves exchanges of sodium and potassium for hydrogen ions between the intracellular and extracellular fluids. By means of these exchanges over half of an administered load of acid or alkali is neutralized by intracellular buffers.

Since the principal buffer of blood is bicarbonate, the pH of the serum and extracellular fluid can be defined by the relation between bicarbonate and carbonic acid. According to the Henderson-Hasselbach equation:

$$pH = pK_{(HCO_3)} + \log \frac{NaHCO_3}{H_2CO_3}.$$

The buffer ratio of bicarbonate at pH 7.4 is approximately 20:1. Thus of the 27 mM/L of bicarbonate normally present in serum, the carbonic acid normally represents only 1.2 mM.

*The respiratory defense* of body-fluid pH is based on the fact that carbonic acid readily dissociates to carbon dioxide and water, and the rate of loss of $CO_2$ can be controlled by varying the rate and depth of respiration. The carbonic acid that is generated by the reaction of the bicarbonate system with a strong acid can thus be "blown off" as $CO_2$, thereby diminishing the total bicarbonate content but at the same time elevating the buffer ratio toward normal. Similarly, carbonic acid may be generated when the buffer ratio rises by reducing the rate of respiratory loss and increasing the partial pressure of $CO_2$ [$P(CO_2)$] in the serum. This elevates the total bicarbonate while reducing the buffer ratio toward normal.

*The renal defense* of body-fluid pH consists of tubular transport systems by which the daily dietary load of nonvolatile acids comprising 50 to 100 mEq of hydrogen ion is excreted, principally in the form of phosphate and ammonium salts, at an average pH above 5.0. In the process of excreting hydrogen ion, bicarbonate is generated and returned to the blood. In response to an increase in the acid load, ammonia excretion is increased, enabling a larger amount of acid to be excreted and returning a larger amount of bicarbonate to the circulation. During alkalosis, the urine rapidly becomes alkaline in response to the decrease in $P(CO_2)$,[57] and bicarbonate is excreted.

### CLASSIFICATION OF ACID-BASE DISTURBANCES

As a result of the respiratory and renal responses that have been briefly described, deviations from the normal in serum pH are accompanied by changes in bicarbonate concentration. Much of the time the nature and severity of the disorder can be surmised from the bicarbonate concentration together with clinical findings. However, complete and accurate definition requires measurement of the serum pH (Unit 34) as well. Clinical disorders of acid-base balance usually represent one of the four types of disturbance described below, although confusing combinations of these disturbances are occasionally encountered.

METABOLIC ACIDOSIS. This condition results from a gain in nonvolatile acids. The *serum pH* and *total bicarbonate are reduced.* The latter change is a result of respiratory compensation. Examples are *diabetic ketoacidosis,* where the load of ketoacids exceeds the capacity of the kidney to excrete acid, and *uremic acidosis,* in which the renal capacity to excrete acid is impaired. Specific impairment of the renal mechanisms for hydrogen-ion excretion without reduction in filtration rate may result in *renal tubular acidosis.*[58, 59]

RESPIRATORY ACIDOSIS. This condition results from an increase in carbonic acid due to abnormal retention of $CO_2$. *Serum pH is reduced* and *total bicarbonate is increased.* The latter change is due largely to increased renal reabsorption of bicarbonate and partly to the increased concentration of carbonic acid. Respiratory acidosis usually results from pulmonary insufficiency.

METABOLIC ALKALOSIS. This condition results from loss of acid or gain of alkali. *Serum pH* and *total bicarbonate are increased.* The latter change is due chiefly to reduced respiratory loss of $CO_2$. Metabolic alkalosis may result from ingestion of alkali, or loss of acid due to prolonged vomiting. It is often associated with, and may be caused by, potassium depletion (see p. 366).

RESPIRATORY ALKALOSIS. This condition results from hyperventilation with increased loss of $CO_2$. *Serum pH is elevated* and *total bicarbonate is decreased.* The reduction in bicarbonate results chiefly from renal loss of bicarbonate in response to alkalosis and lowered $P(CO_2)$. Hyperventilation may be of psychogenic origin or may result from disease of the central nervous system.

METHODS OF MEASURING BICARBONATE

CARBON DIOXIDE CONTENT OF SERUM. The bicarbonate content of serum is measured by the method of Van Slyke and Neill,[60] in which serum obtained under anaerobic conditions is transferred to a Van Slyke apparatus and shaken with acid under negative pressure. The volume of released gas is measured and results are expressed as milliequivalents per liter of bicarbonate.

*Sources of error.* The method is highly accurate, having an error of less than 2 percent. However, sources of sizable error are involved in obtaining and handling the blood sample. Most accurate results are obtained when arterial blood is used, or when venous blood is "arterialized" by soaking the subject's arm for 10 min in water at a temperature of 46–47°C. For most clinical purposes, venous blood is adequate, but it should be drawn without stasis, the tourniquet being released after the vein is entered, and care must be exercised to prevent air from entering the syringe.

After the blood is drawn, it is transferred to a test tube under mineral oil. Mineral oil does not completely prevent the escape of $CO_2$, especially when the interface between the blood and oil is disturbed. Considerable skill is also required to prevent loss of $CO_2$ during centrifugation and transfer to the Van Slyke apparatus. With care, most of these sources of error can be controlled. However, more accurate results may be obtained by retaining the blood in the syringe throughout the procedure, as described by Davenport.[61]

CARBON DIOXIDE COMBINING POWER.[60] In this method, the bicarbonate content of serum is measured after the blood is equilibrated with a gas mixture containing carbon dioxide at a partial pressure of 40 mm Hg.

*Interpretations and limitations.* Since the dissolved $CO_2$ of the plasma is constant at 1.2 mM/L when $P(CO_2)$ is 40 mm Hg, the carbon dioxide combining power gives a measure of the serum bicarbonate which is bound to cation plus 1.2 mM. The measurement is inaccurate by the extent to which the subject's true $P(CO_2)$ is higher or lower than 40 mm Hg (as in respiratory acidosis and alkalosis). Measurement of carbon dioxide combining power offers the advantage of not requiring anaerobic handling of blood samples. However, results are considerably less accurate than measurement of total $CO_2$ and may be misleading.

# REFERENCES

1. V. DuVigneaud, C. Ressler, J. M. Swan, C. W. Roberts, P. G. Katsoyannis, and S. Gordon, "Synthesis of octapeptide amide with hormonal activity of oxytocin," *J. Amer. chem. Soc.* 75, 4879 (1953).
2. V. DuVigneaud, H. C. Lawlor, and E. A. Popenoe, "Enzymatic cleavage of glycinamide and proposed structure of this pressor-antidiuretic hormone of posterior pituitary," *J. Amer. chem. Soc.* 75, 4880 (1953).
3. E. Scharrer and B. Scharrer, "Hormones produced by neurosecretory cells," *Recent Progr. Hormone Res. 10*, 183 (1954).
4. W. Bargmann and E. Scharrer, "The site of origin of the hormones of the posterior pituitary," *Amer. Scientist* 39, 255 (1951).

5. E. B. Verney, "The antidiuretic hormone and the factors which determine its release," *Proc. roy. Soc. B 135*, 25 (1947).
6. R. W. Berliner, N. G. Levinsky, D. G. Davidson, and M. Eden, "Dilution and concentration of the urine and the action of antidiuretic hormone," *Amer. J. Med. 24*, 730 (1958).
7. T. M. Chalmers and A. A. G. Lewis, "Stimulation of the supraopticohypophyseal system in man," *Clin. Sci. 10*, 137 (1951).
8. A. A. G. Lewis and T. M. Chalmers, "A nicotine test for the investigation of diabetes insipidus," *Clin. Sci. 10*, 137 (1951).
9. J. D. Cates and O. Garrod, "The effect of nicotine on urinary flow in diabetes insipidus," *Clin. Sci. 10*, 144 (1951).
10. J. K. Dingman, K. Benirschke, and G. W. Thorn, "Studies of neurohypophyseal function in man; diabetes insipidus and psychogenic polydipsia," *Amer. J. Med. 23*, 226 (1957).
11. W. C. Thomas, "Diabetes insipidus," *J. clin. Endocr. 17*, 565 (1957).
12. A. Leaf and A. R. Mamby, "An antidiuretic mechanism not regulated by extracellular fluid tonicity," *J. clin. Invest. 31*, 60 (1952).
13. H. P. Wolff, K. R. Koczorek, and E. Buchborn, "Aldosterone and ADH in liver disease," *Acta endocr. (Kbh.) 27*, 45 (1958).
14. B. Andersson, "Polydipsia caused by intra-hypothalamic injections of hypertonic sodium chloride solutions," *Experientia (Basel) 8*, 157 (1952).
15. P. Fourman and P. M. Leeson, "Thirst and polyuria," *Lancet 1*, 268 (1959).
16. R. H. Williams and H. Cole, "Nephrogenic diabetes insipidus: transmitted by females and appearing during infancy in males," *Ann. intern. Med. 27*, 84 (1947).
17. S. I. Cohen, M. G. Fitzgerald, P. Fourman, W. J. Griffiths, and H. E. deWardener, "Polyuria in hyperparathyroidism," *Quart. J. Med. 26*, 423 (1957).
18. G. Klatskin and M. Gordon, "Renal complications of sarcoidosis and their relation to hypercalcemia," *Amer. J. Med. 15*, 484 (1953).
19. F. H. Epstein, L. R. Freedman, and H. Levitin, "Hypercalcemia, nephrocalcinosis and reversible renal insufficiency associated with hyperthyroidism," *New Engl. J. Med. 258*, 782 (1958).
20. F. H. Epstein, M. J. Rivera, and F. A. Carone, "The effect of hypercalcemia induced by calciferol upon renal concentrating ability," *J. clin. Invest. 37*, 1702 (1958).
21. W. B. Schwartz and A. S. Relman, "Metabolic and renal studies in chronic potassium depletion resulting from overuse of laxatives," *J. clin. Invest. 32*, 258 (1953).
22. A. S. Relman and W. B. Schwartz, "Nephropathy of potassium depletion; clinico-pathologic entity," *J. clin. Invest. 34*, 959 (1955).
23. S. W. Stanbury, "Some aspects of disordered renal tubular function," *Advanc. intern. Med. 9*, 231 (1958).
24. W. E. Brown and E. H. Rynearsen, "A procedure for the diagnosis of diabetes insipidus," *Proc. Mayo Clin. 19*, 67 (1944).
25. R. W. Berliner and D. G. Davidson, "Production of hypertonic urine in the absence of antidiuretic hormone," *J. clin. Invest. 36*, 1416 (1957).
26. R. C. Hickey and K. Hare, "The renal excretion of chloride and water in diabetes insipidus," *J. clin. Invest. 23*, 768 (1944).
27. A. C. Carter and J. Robbins, "The use of hypertonic saline infusions in the

differential diagnosis of diabetes insipidus and psychogenic polydipsia," *J. clin. Endocr.* 7, 753 (1947).

28. L. G. Welt, *Clinical Disorders of Hydration and Acid-Base Equilibrium* (Little, Brown, Boston, 1955).

29. J. E. Elkinton and T. S. Danowski, *The Body Fluids* (Williams & Wilkins, Baltimore, 1955).

30. M. B. Strauss, *Body Water in Man* (Little, Brown, Boston, 1957).

31. H. W. Smith, "Salt and water volume receptors," *Amer. J. Med.* 23, 623 (1957).

32. F. H. Epstein, "Renal excretion of sodium and the concept of a volume receptor," *Yale J. Biol. Med.* 29, 282 (1957).

33. J. R. Elkinton, "The role of magnesium in the body fluids," *Clin. Chem.* 3, 319 (1957).

34. R. E. Randall, E. C. Rossmeisl, and K. H. Bleifer, "Magnesium depletion in man," *Ann. intern. Med.* 50, 257 (1959).

35. O. Schales and S. S. Schales, "Simple and accurate method for determination of chloride in biological fluids," *J. biol. Chem.* 140, 879 (1941).

36. S. P. Asper, Jr., and O. Schales, "Importance of controlling pH in the Schales and Schales method of chloride determination," *J. biol. Chem.* 168, 779 (1947).

37. B. Fantus, "Fluid postoperatively; a statistical study," *J. Amer. med. Ass.* 107, 14 (1936).

38. I. S. Edelman, J. Liebman, M. P. O'Meara, and L. W. Birkenfeld, "Interrelations between serum sodium concentration, serum osmolarity and total exchangeable sodium, total exchangeable potassium, and total body water," *J. clin. Invest.* 37, 1236 (1958).

39. M. J. Albrink, P. M. Hald, E. B. Man, and J. P. Peters, "The displacement of serum water by hyperlipemic serum. A new method for the rapid determination of serum water," *J. clin. Invest.* 34, 1483 (1955).

40. A. Leaf, F. C. Bartter, R. F. Santos, and O. Wrong, "Evidence that urinary electrolyte loss induced by Pitressin is a function of water retention," *J. clin. Invest.* 32, 868 (1953).

41. F. C. Bartter, G. W. Liddle, L. E. Duncan, and C. Delea, "The role of extracellular fluid volume in the control of aldosterone excretion in man," *J. clin. Invest.* 35, 688 (1956).

42. A. Leaf and W. T. Couter, "Evidence that renal sodium excretion in normal human subjects is regulated by adrenal cortical activity," *J. clin. Invest.* 28, 1067 (1949).

43. G. W. Thorn, G. F. Koepf, and M. Clinton, Jr., "Renal failure simulating adrenocortical insufficiency," *New Engl. J. Med.* 231, 74 (1944).

44. W. B. Schwartz, W. Bennett, S. Curelop, and F. C. Bartter, "A syndrome of renal sodium loss and hyponatremia probably resulting from inappropriate secretion of ADH," *Amer. J. Med.* 23, 529 (1957).

45. D. C. Darrow, "Body fluid physiology: the role of potassium in clinical disturbances of body water and electrolytes," *New Engl. J. Med.* 242, 978, 1014 (1950).

46. R. E. Keating, T. E. Weichselbaum, M. Alanis, H. W. Margraf, and R. Elman, "The movement of potassium during experimental acidosis and alkalosis in the nephrectomized dog," *Surg. Gynec. Obstet.* 96, 323 (1953).

47. D. C. Darrow, R. Schwartz, J. F. Ianucci, and F. Coville, "The relation of

serum bicarbonate concentration to muscle composition," *J. clin. Invest. 27*, 198 (1948).

48. R. W. Berliner, T. J. Kennedy, and J. Orloff, "Relationship between acidification of the urine and potassium metabolism: effect of carbonic anhydrase inhibition of potassium excretion," *Amer. J. Med. 11*, 274 (1951).

49. D. A. K. Black, "Body fluid depletion," *Lancet 1*, 353 (1953).

50. W. B. Schwartz, "Potassium and the kidney," *New Engl. J. Med. 253*, 601 (1955).

51. A. Leaf and A. A. Camara, "Renal tubular secretion of potassium in man," *J. clin. Invest. 28*, 1526 (1949).

52. W. B. Schwartz and A. S. Relman, "Acidosis in renal disease," *New Engl. J. Med. 256*, 1184 (1957).

53. J. Orloff, "The role of the kidney in the regulation of acid-base balance," *Yale J. Biol. Med. 29*, 211 (1956).

54. R. F. Pitts, "Mechanisms for stabilizing alkaline reserves of the body," *Harvey Lectures*, No. 172 (Academic Press, New York, 1954), vol. 48.

55. W. B. Schwartz, K. J. Ørning, and R. Porter, "The internal distribution of hydrogen ions with varying degrees of metabolic acidosis," *J. clin. Invest. 36*, 373 (1957).

56. J. R. Elkinton, "Whole body buffers in the regulation of acid-base equilibrium," *Yale J. Biol. Med. 29*, 191 (1957).

57. P. Brazeau and A. Gilman, "Effect of plasma carbon dioxide tension on renal tubular reabsorption of bicarbonate," *Amer. J. Physiol. 175*, 33 (1953).

58. G. H. Mudge, "Clinical patterns of tubular dysfunction," *Amer. J. Med. 24*, 785 (1958).

59. H. E. F. Davies and O. Wrong, "Acidity of urine and excretion of ammonium in renal disease," *Lancet 2*, 625 (1957).

60. J. P. Peters and D. D. Van Slyke, *Quantitative Clinical Chemistry*, vol. 2, *Methods* (Williams and Wilkins, Baltimore, 1931).

61. H. W. Davenport, *The ABC of Acid-Base Chemistry* (ed. 3; University of Chicago Press, Chicago, 1950).

# Unit 22

## Examination of the Stool

Examination of the stool is one of the basic procedures that should be part of every physical examination. A routine stool examination includes inspection and a test for occult blood. In special cases, there may be indications for a microscopic examination for red and white blood cells and for fat and undigested muscle fibers. Investigation for ova and parasites is beyond the scope of this chapter. If disorders of digestion and absorption are suspected, a quantitative determination of fat and nitrogen in the stool may be desired. The stool can be collected in a paper or glass container and should be uncontaminated with urine. If the stool is liquid, a glass jar with screw top is preferred. At the time of the rectal examination, a film of stool may be made from the gloved finger directly onto a piece of filter paper. This sample can be inspected and tested immediately for occult blood. Study of the stool provides information about motility and digestive capacity of the intestinal tract, and the demonstration of occult blood indicates the need for a careful search for the cause of the bleeding.

### Physiology

After ingested foodstuffs have undergone digestion and absorption during transit through the small intestine, the residue is passed on into the large bowel where there is absorption of additional water. The solid fecal material is stored in the descending colon and sigmoid until evacuation occurs. The normal frequency of bowel movements may vary from two or three per day to one every 2 or 3 days. Transit time through the small bowel is from 2 to 6 hr, but there is a marked variation in the normal period of time required for the feces to traverse the colon. This may range from less than 12 to more than 48 hr. Moreover, material does not move along the small and large bowel in an orderly fashion like cars on a train. Rather, there is a streaming effect. For example, after the ingestion of a single dose of a stool marker such as carmine, the color may appear in several successive stool specimens.

The normal stool consists of undigested and unabsorbed remnants of food, water, products of the digestive tract such as bile pigments, enzymes, and mucus, products of decomposition such as indole and skatole, epithelial-cell debris from the intestinal-tract mucosa, and large numbers of bacteria, which may constitute one-third to one-half of the total dry stool weight. The quantity of stool is usually from 100 to 200 gm/day, depending upon the amount of water present.

### Laboratory Tests Related to the Stool

#### INSPECTION

Inspection should be conducted personally by the physician on freshly

374

passed specimens. The characteristics to be observed are listed in Table 67.

Table 67. *Stool characteristics observed on inspection.*

| Quantity and Frequency |
| Form and Consistency |
| Color |
| Odor |
| Mucus |
| Blood and Pus |
| Undigested Food |

### QUANTITY AND FREQUENCY

The normal quantity and frequency have already been described. In diseases of the gastrointestinal tract, the number of stools may be greatly increased. Watery discharges containing mere flecks of feces may be passed frequently in severe diarrhea. Sprue and other forms of steatorrhea often result in copious, mushy, foul-smelling stools. Small hard balls of feces, known as scybala, are associated with constipation. Alternating scybalous stools and diarrhea are frequently associated with a spastic or irritable colon. A diet high in meat and protein will usually result in much smaller amounts of stool than that from a person who consumes large amounts of vegetables.

### FORM AND CONSISTENCY

The normal stool is soft and formed or semiformed. The hard, dry scybala of constipation reflect excessive absorption of water or inadequate fluid intake. Mushy and liquid stools may be the result of laxatives, excessive fruit juice or roughage in the diet, a hyperirritable colon, or organic diseases of the gastrointestinal tract. Gassy, foamy stools indicate fermentation which suggests impaired intestinal absorption of foodstuffs. Small, flattened, or pencillike stools are due to stricture, cancer, or ulceration of the rectum, or to spasm of the anal canal secondary to fissure or hemorrhoids. Massive stools of large caliber, especially

in children, may suggest a diagnosis of megacolon.

### COLOR

The color of stool varies normally from light to dark brown. The normal stool darkens on standing, owing in part to oxidation of bile pigments. Food, drugs, and disease may modify the color from white to black. Some causes of color change are as follows:

(*a*) A white color is seen after ingestion of barium for x-ray study.

(*b*) A gray or putty-colored stool may be due to absence of bile pigments and is called acholic (see Unit 24). Excess fat in the stool will cause a similar gray color, even when bile pigments are present. These are pseudo-acholic stools.

(*c*) A silvery or aluminum-paint appearance to the stool suggests a diagnosis of cancer of the pancreas.[1]

(*d*) A golden yellow color is due to unchanged bilirubin. This is normal for the breast-fed infant and may be seen in adults who are having diarrhea.

(*e*) A green stool most frequently means the presence of biliverdin, which is a regular feature of oral antibiotic therapy since the drugs eliminate colon bacteria which reduce biliverdin to urobilinogen. Diarrhea in children is often associated with green stools, also due to biliverdin. Spinach and calomel produce a green color in feces.

(*f*) A red color, often mistaken for blood in the stool, may appear after eating beets or carrots. If the stool is alkaline, it will have a red-purple color after administration of bromsulfalein dye, whose presence can be established by disappearance of the red-purple color when the stool is acidified.

(*g*) A dark brown color may indicate ingestion of large amounts of meat or chocolate.

(*h*) A black stool can result from oral intake of bismuth, iron, or charcoal.

Observation of color variation in the stool is thus most often indicative of what has been ingested. The color changes associated with steatorrhea and disturbances of bile pigment metabolism have clinical diagnostic significance.

The most important reason for observing stool color is for the detection of blood. This is therefore discussed separately. There may be considerable amounts of blood in the stool, representing up to as much as 75 to 200 ml of bleeding in the upper gastrointestinal tract, without any change in color or appearance of the stool.[2] On the other hand, very slight bleeding from hemorrhoids, anal fissures, polyps, cancer, and ulceration of the rectum may appear as streaks of red blood on the outside of the stool or on the toilet paper. Massive bleeding of more than 200 ml will produce either a dark red or black, tarry stool, depending upon the site of bleeding and transit time through the intestinal tract.[3] In general, a tarry stool indicates hemorrhage from the upper gastrointestinal tract, above the ileocaecal valve. The exact nature of the black color of tarry stools is not known, but it is due to digested blood. Consequently, if the transit time through the small and large bowel is sufficiently short, namely 5–8 hr, the blood will appear undigested and give the stool a dark or bright red color. Massive bleeding in the esophagus, stomach, and duodenum often causes intestinal hurry and results in red, bloody stools. Bleeding at any level in the colon causes dark red or bright red bloody stools. In evaluating the clinical significance of tarry stools, it should be emphasized that they may be passed for as long as 5 days after bleeding has stopped.[2] Consequently, the appearance of tarry stools does not indicate continued bleeding. Moreover, tarry stools can result from eating spleen, liver, or blood pudding. Finally, the presence of blood in any tarry or red stool should be confirmed by a chemical test for occult blood.

### ODOR

The odor of the normal stool is due chiefly to indole and skatole, and is not unduly offensive. The strength of this odor is greater with a high meat diet and less if the patient eats primarily fruit and vegetables. Pathologic odors include the sour, acrid quality of fatty acids passed in cases of steatorrhea and the putrid stench of ulcerating lesions, either benign or malignant.

### MUCUS

There are normally small amounts of mucus in and on the stool. Visible traces to large amounts of mucus, varying from gelatinous globs of different colors to shreds or mucus casts resembling worms, are most often seen in patients who have a spastic or irritable colon. These manifestations of mucus, while frightening to the patient, do not signify organic lesions of the colon. Inflammatory infections, ulcerations, and neoplasms of the colon may also cause increased mucus in the stool, but in these cases the mucus is usually mixed with flecks of blood and pus.

### BLOOD AND PUS

The gross appearance of pus and flecks or small quantities of red blood in the feces is indicative of inflammatory ulcerating lesions of the lower colon and rectum. These may include ulcerative colitis, diverticulitis, specific dysenteric infections, and ulcerating cancers. The microscopic study of stool for blood and pus cells is described below.

### UNDIGESTED FOOD

The presence of undigested and readily identifiable pieces of corn and other vegetables and fruit skins and fibers is normal and of no clinical significance. Observation of their transit time may give an estimate of intestinal motility, and the nature of the food remnants in the stool can be used as a check on the dietary history. In rare instances, the appearance within an hour or two after eating of large amounts of poorly digested food in the stool is suggestive of a fistula that short-circuits the normal pathway for food through the intestinal tract, such as a gastrocolic fistula.

### CHEMICAL DETERMINATION OF OCCULT BLOOD

The detection of occult blood in the stool has been carried out by many modifications of procedures that employ phenolic compounds like gum guaiac, orthotolidine, benzidine, phenolphthalein, and others.[4-6] Many methods appear to be too sensitive, demand meat-free diets, or are too complex. The filter-paper–guaiac test seems to have the required simplicity and sensitivity and is recommended as a routine screening test for occult blood.

#### PRINCIPLE

Gum guaiac contains the oxidizable phenol guaiacetic acid, which when oxidized to an unknown quinone type of compound yields a blue-colored product by intermolecular reaction.[7] Oxidation is brought about by oxygen liberated from hydrogen peroxide. The reaction is catalyzed by peroxidases, some of the most effective of which are found in the heme moiety of hemaglobin.

#### METHOD

REAGENTS. (1) Filter paper that has been tested with the reagents and proved to be free of positive color reaction. (2) Glacial acetic acid. (3) Saturated alcoholic solution of gum guaiac which is made by dissolving 1 gm of powdered gum guaiac in 5 ml of 95-percent ethyl alcohol; this reagent is stable for at least 1 month.[4] (4) Three-percent hydrogen peroxide, which must be fresh so that it bubbles when added to a drop of blood; this reagent should be stored under refrigeration.

PROCEDURE. A small quantity of stool is smeared on a piece of filter paper with an applicator stick. Two drops of glacial acetic acid is added and mixed with the stool. Two drops of guaiac solution and 2 drops of hydrogen peroxide is then added and mixed. The appearance and intensity of any blue or blue-green color is looked for at the end of 1 and 5 min; the presence of color is considered a positive reaction. An arbitrary system of grading the reaction is used and this varies from laboratory to laboratory. In general, a deep blue color appearing within 1 min is considered 4+, and no color or only a slight trace of green at any time during the 5-min period is graded negative. Lesser degrees of color development occurring between 1 and 5 min can be graded from 1+ to 3+ according to the physician's experience.

#### INDICATION AND INTERPRETATION

The guaiac test should be part of every physical examination and should be performed frequently in the study of gastrointestinal diseases. Any degree of positivity of the test above 1+ usually indicates significant bleeding in the gastrointestinal tract and suggests that there be a thorough investigation for the source of bleeding, since Barnet found that the test was 96.5-percent positive when there were lesions that were expected to bleed.[8]

#### LIMITATIONS AND SOURCES OF ERROR

The guaiac test, as well as all other tests for occult blood in the stool, is qualitative and not even semiquantitative. The sensitivity of the guaiac reaction is illustrated by the fact that it is negative when normal diets are ingested and, contrary to some earlier opinions[4] is not positive after ingestion of medicinal iron.[5-7, 9] On a normal diet, the guaiac reaction may become positive when 2 to 12 ml of blood is introduced into the stomach,[5, 6, 9] although one investigator[10] reported that as much as 25 to 50 ml of bleeding in the gastrointestinal tract might be missed with the guaiac test. A positive guaiac-test result does not indicate the presence of active bleeding. A positive reaction may persist for as long as 7 days [11] to 12 days [2] after massive bleeding has ceased.

There are sources of error with the guaiac test. Lots of gum guaiac may have varying sensitivities. The stability of hydrogen peroxide and gum guaiac should be checked by performing the test regularly with known positive and negative stool specimens. The moistened filter paper should not be placed on laboratory benches or other surfaces that might be contaminated with blood.

### MICROSCOPIC EXAMINATION OF THE STOOL

Microscopic examination of the stool for white blood cells, red blood cells, and fat of muscle fibers is not a routine procedure but is a simple test which should be employed if there are clinical indications.

#### EXAMINATION FOR PUS AND BLOOD

When inflammatory lesions of the colon or infectious diarrhea are suspected, a drop of liquid stool, a fleck of mucus or pus, or, less frequently, a watery emulsion of solid stool may be studied under the microscope. The presence of large numbers of white blood cells and red blood cells suggests infection or inflamed ulcerating lesions in the large bowel. This observation is of assistance in differentiating diarrhea of organic origin from the watery stools associated with an irritable colon. In the latter, there would be very few white blood cells or red blood cells in the stool.

#### EXAMINATION FOR FAT

PRINCIPLE. Globules of neutral fat are stained directly with a fat stain, sudan III; fatty acids are similarly stained after hydrolysis from calcium soaps and other fatty-acid combinations.[12]

REAGENTS. (1) Ninety-five-percent ethanol. (2) Saturated solution of sudan III in 95-percent ethanol. (3) Thirty-six-percent acetic acid.

**Method.** A specimen of stool is mixed thoroughly with an applicator stick and small aliquots about 3 to 5 mm in diameter are placed on each of two glass microscope slides. Unless the stool is liquid, it is emulsified on the first glass slide with 2 drops of water. Then 2 drops of 95-percent ethanol is added and mixed, followed by 2 or 3 drops of saturated alcoholic solution of sudan III. After mixing, a coverslip is applied and the specimen examined under high dry magnification. Yellow- or orange-stained globules of fat are looked for, with special attention to the edges of the coverslip since neutral fat tends to collect there. This is the examination for neutral fat.

To study for fatty acids, the aliquot of stool on the second glass slide is mixed with 2 to 3 drops of 36-percent acetic acid. Then 2 to 3 drops of saturated alcoholic solution of sudan III is added and mixed, after which a coverslip is applied. Hydrolysis is carried out by gently heating the slide over a low flame until there is boiling under the coverslip. This heating should be repeated two or three times to assure complete hydrolysis. The specimen should be examined while still warm under high dry magnification. The stained fatty-acid globules will appear as deep orange globules scattered throughout the preparation. A standardized micrometer eyepiece is used to determine the size of the fat globule. If the preparation is permitted to cool, the fatty acids may crystallize out into colorless sheaves of needlelike crystals.

INDICATIONS AND INTERPRETATIONS. The microscopic examination of stool for fat should be used as a screening test to confirm the gross appearance of a fatty, bulky stool and also should be used to study any patient with symptoms suggesting intestinal malabsorption. Very few, if any, neutral fat globules are found in a normal stool. The presence of large amounts of neutral fat should make one suspicious that the patient has been taking an oily laxative. Some patients with pancreatic insufficiency may have an increase in neutral fat content of stools, but all other forms of steatorrhea are associated with no increase in neutral fat.

In the microscopic evaluation of fatty acids, classification is on an arbitrary basis, depending upon the examiner's experience. Normal and 1+ amounts of fatty acids in the stool may appear as many tiny globules, up to 1 to 4 $\mu$ in size, and as frequent as 100 per high-power field, scattered throughout the preparation. At the other end of the scale, a 4+ screening-test result for fat, indicating clinical steatorrhea, will show every high-power field loaded with large orange-stained globules ranging in size from 10 to 75 $\mu$. Gradations of fat content between these two limits depends upon the number and size of fat globules present. Experience in correlating microscopic screening examination of the stool with quantitative measurements of fecal fat loss have shown that all patients with 4+ screening results have excessive fecal fat losses, and most patients with more than a 1+ screening result have some degree of steatorrhea. On the other hand, 86 percent of the stool specimens with a normal or 1+ microscopic examination for fatty acids showed normal quantities of fat when measured chemically.[12]

LIMITATIONS AND SOURCES OF ERROR. A screening test for fat in the stool is of no value unless the patient eats more than 60 gm of fat a day. Since most stools, even in the absence of pancreatic enzymes, contain large amounts of split fats, the use of microscopic screening tests for neutral and fatty acids in the stool will not differentiate steatorrhea of pancreatic insufficiency from other causes.

EXAMINATION FOR MUSCLE FIBERS

The study of stools for the presence of undigested, striated muscle fibers is an aid in establishing the diagnosis of pancreatic insufficiency.

A small piece of stool is emulsified on a glass microscope slide with 2 drops of water. Next, it is stirred with an applicator stick that has been moistened with a 2-percent aqueous solution of eosin and the preparation is covered with a coverslip. Examination with high dry magnification is carried on for precisely 5 min. A count is made of the number of square-ended, reddish-stained muscle fibers with well-preserved striations. Normally, very few undigested muscle fibers are found in a 5-min search, but in pancreatic insufficiency from 10 to 100 undigested muscle fibers may be counted in 5 min. There may be an increased number if the patient has complete biliary-tract obstruction or a gastrocolic fistula. This screening procedure requires the patient to eat adequate amounts of red meat if the test is to have any significance.

## REFERENCES

1. H. Ogilvie, "Thomas's sign, or the silver stool in cancer of the ampulla of Vater," *Brit. med. J. 1*, 208 (1955).
2. L. Schiff, R. J. Stevens, N. Shapiro, and S. Goodman, "Observations on the oral administration of citrated blood in man. II. The effect on the stool," *Amer. J. med. Sci. 203*, 409 (1942).
3. J. H. Hilsman, "The color of blood-containing feces following the instillation of citrated blood at various levels of the small intestine," *Gastroenterology 15*, 131 (1950).

4. S. O. Hoerr, W. R. Bliss, and J. Kaufman, "Clinical evaluation of various tests for occult blood in feces," *J. Amer. med. Ass. 141*, 1213 (1949).

5. A. Peranio and M. Bruger, "The detection of occult blood in feces including observations on the ingestion of iron and whole blood," *J. lab. clin. Med. 38*, 433 (1951).

6. T. E. Morgan and R. J. Roantree, "Evaluation of tests for occult blood in the feces. Significance of guaiac and orthotolidine tests after ingestion of iron," *J. Amer. med. Ass. 164*, 1665 (1957).

7. J. C. Harvey, "The lack of effect of ingested ferrous sulfate on the guaiac test for occult blood in the stool," *Amer. J. med. Sci. 232*, 17 (1956).

8. R. N. Barnett, "The guaiac test. Correlation with clinical findings," *Gastroenterology 21*, 540 (1952).

9. J. W. B. Forshaw and G. W. Mason, "Evaluation of occult-blood tests on faeces," *Lancet 2*, 470 (1954).

10. A. I. Mendeloff, "Selection of a screening procedure for detecting occult blood in feces," *J. Amer. med. Ass. 152*, 798 (1953).

11. W. C. Breidenbach and G. R. Priddy, "The duration of chemically demonstrable blood in the feces following ingestion of whole blood," *Gastroenterology 26*, 469 (1954).

12. G. D. Drummey, J. A. Benson, Jr., and C. M. Jones, "The microscopic examination of the stool for malabsorption," to be published.

# Unit 23

## Tests of Gastric Secretory Function

Gastric juice is a complex of substances actively secreted by the mucosal cells of the stomach. Quantitative study of the components of human gastric juice has been hampered by technical difficulties in complete collection of pure secretion uncontaminated by saliva or duodenal contents. Although the techniques are rather crude, and in spite of many gaps in the knowledge of basic mechanisms of secretory function, there is sufficient information to permit the application of the results of gastric secretory studies to an evaluation of pathologic physiology of the stomach.[1-3] Correlation between alterations in the components of gastric secretion and histologic changes in the specimens of gastric mucosa obtained by biopsy has resulted in the concept of a "chemical gastric biopsy."[4] Study of the rate, quantity, and qualitative changes of gastric secretory products has become a diagnostic aid in such diseases as peptic ulcer and pernicious anemia, as well as in providing a rational basis for medical and surgical management of diseases of the stomach.

### Physiology

The chief function of the gastric juice is to promote the gastric phase of digestion by liquefying ingested food and modifying the chyme so it can be tolerated by the duodenum.[1] Partial hydrolysis of protein is initiated by the pepsin of the gastric juice if the pH of the gastric contents is lower than 3.5. The mucus fraction provides protection for the gastric mucosal cells and prevents autodigestion. Biologically active materials such as intrinsic factor, blood-group substances, and possibly many other as yet unidentified factors are elaborated with the mucin fraction.[5] Each component of the gastric juice seems to be secreted by a particular type of cell in the mucosa of the stomach.[1, 3, 4]

#### HYDROCHLORIC ACID

Hydrochloric acid is secreted by the parietal cells located in the neck and body of the gastric glands which are in the mucosa of the fundus and upper half of the body of the stomach. The quantity of hydrochloric acid is proportional to the density of the parietal cells.[1, 2] The secretion of hydrochloric acid is an "active" process requiring the expenditure of metabolic energy by the cells. The mechanism of the transport process remains controversial.

Stimulation of hydrochloric acid production by the parietal cells can be effected in several ways:

In the cephalic phase, vagal-nerve stimulation acts upon the parietal cell as a specific end organ with an outpouring of water and hydrochloric acid. Maximal stimulation via this route can be produced by insulin-induced hypoglycemia, the so-called Hollander test for demonstrating the integrity of the vagus nerves.

A second type of stimulation is hormonal. This is the gastric phase of hydrochloric acid secretion. A hormone, gastrin, is formed in the stomach wall of the pyloric region in response to mechanical distension of the pyloric antrum or by contact of the antral mucosa with chemical substances derived from partial hydrolysis of proteins. The gastrin thus formed circulates in the blood stream and acts directly on the parietal cell to stimulate hydrochloric acid production. Histamine given parenterally also acts directly on the parietal cell in a manner similar to gastrin. Histamine can provoke a maximal secretory response of both volume and acidity.

The intestinal phase of gastric secretion is brought about by a variety of substances that are absorbed into the circulation by the small bowel. Among such are nitrogenous meat and liver extracts, amino acids, alcohol, and histamine. These exogenous, humoral stimulants act directly upon the parietal cell to increase production of hydrochloric acid and water. Their action may be augmented by vagal stimulation. Of the three phases of acid production, the intestinal phase is of minor importance.

In contrast to the digestive phases of secretion described above, there is the interdigestive, or basal, secretion which occurs in the absence of all intentional or avoidable stimulation.[2] It has not yet been established whether parietal cells are capable of some degree of spontaneous activity or whether even in the basal state there are some phasic vagal impulses.[1, 2] Basal secretion can be measured by continuous overnight aspiration of the stomach contents or during a "fasting" period of 1 to 2 hr in the morning.[6-8] Basal secretion varies greatly among individuals and in the same person from day to day, but each person has a general pattern of high, medium, or low secretion.[6] The volume of secretion and hydrochloric acid concentration can fluctuate independently.[6] The normal level of 1-hr basal and also maximal se-

Table 68. *Basal gastric secretion and histamine response in normal persons (1-hr continuous aspiration).*[a]

| Sex | No. | Basal secretion | | Histamine response | |
|---|---|---|---|---|---|
| | | Volume (ml) | Free HCl conc. (c.u.) | Volume (ml) | Free HCl conc. (c.u.) |
| Male | 319 | 79.4 | 25.8 | 133.1 | 69.9 |
| Female | 241 | 65.2 | 20.5 | 101.2 | 55.9 |

[a] Modified from E. Levin, J. B. Kirsner, and W. L. Palmer.[7]

cretion are shown in Table 68. With age, an increasing number of normal people fail to secrete acid even after histamine.[7] This is illustrated in Table 69. Anacidity

Table 69. *Incidence of anacidity in basal secretion and after histamine in normal persons (percent of studies).*[a]

| Sex | Age group (years) | Basal | After histamine |
|---|---|---|---|
| Male | 20–29 | 20.0 | 6.0 |
| | 30–39 | 19.0 | 3.0 |
| | 40–49 | 20.0 | 6.0 |
| | 50–59 | 24.0 | 19.0 |
| | 60+ | 50.0 | 33.0 |
| Female | 20–29 | 24.0 | 5.0 |
| | 30–39 | 28.0 | 3.0 |
| | 40–49 | 33.0 | 11.0 |
| | 50–59 | 45.0 | 20.0 |
| | 60+ | 42.0 | 24.0 |

[a] Modified from E. Levin, J. B. Kirsner, and W. L. Palmer.[7]

with low volume after maximal stimulation is observed in virtually all patients who have gastric atrophy or pernicious anemia, as well as in many cases of carcinoma of the stomach. Gastric ulcers and some cancers of the stomach are associated with a low level of acid production. On the other hand, duodenal-ulcer patients have continuous basal secretion with greatly increased volume and acid concentration.[7, 8]

The functions of hydrochloric acid are to promote peptic activity, as described below, and to effect sterilization of the stomach chyme by destroying bacteria.[1]

### NONPARIETAL SECRETIONS

Gastric juice as obtained from the stomach is a mixture of hydrochloric acid and the alkaline, nonparietal components—enzymes, mucin, and inorganic ions of the interstitial fluid. The concentration of free hydrochloric acid in a specimen of gastric juice is a function of the relative proportion of the two components. The chief buffering capacity of the nonparietal secretions resides in the alkaline mineral bases adsorbed on gastric mucin.[9] The acid-binding capacity of gastric mucin and pepsin is very limited.[3] The neutralizing capacity of the nonparietal components does not mean that they have a single specific cell of origin or result from a particular stimulus. There is an independent mechanism of formation for each of the various components.[9]

ENZYMES. Pepsin is the principal enzyme of gastric juice. It is synthesized as zymogen granules, pepsinogen, in the peptic chief cells of the body of gastric glands in the fundus, the body, and possibly the pyloric areas of the stomach.[1, 3] Inactive pepsinogen granules are secreted into the lumen of gastric glands. There, hydrochloric acid initiates an autocatalytic reaction converting the zymogen to active pepsin.[1] Although pepsinogen is primarily an exocrine secretion, approximately 1 percent is extruded from the peptic chief cells into the surrounding interstitial fluid and thence into the blood stream. It is excreted in the urine as uropepsinogen.[1, 10–12] The level of pepsinogen in the blood or urine varies directly with the rate of gastric pepsin secretion.

Stimulation of pepsin secretion is mediated primarily by the vagus nerve.[3] Both the cephalic phase of gastric digestion and insulin-induced hypoglycemia produce a gastric juice high in pepsin as well as hydrochloric acid. Gastrin does not appear to stimulate pepsin secretion. There are conflicting reports about the effect of histamine on pepsin secretion. Many have attributed the increase in gastric pepsin after histamine administration to the washing out of pepsin from the gastric glands by increased production of hydrochloric acid and water.[3] There is, however, fairly convincing evidence that continuous administration of histamine causes a prolonged elevation of the secretion of pepsin in the gastric juice.[13]

The function of pepsin is proteolytic. It hydrolyzes dietary proteins to polypeptides by hydrolysis of peptide bonds. The rate of peptic hydrolysis varies with the pH of the reaction mixture, being optimum at pH 2 and ceasing above pH 4.5.[1] This peptic activity depends directly upon the quantity of hydrochloric acid secretion.

Normal values for gastric pepsin and blood and urinary pepsinogen vary from laboratory to laboratory, depending upon the precise conditions of the analytic method, so each laboratory must establish its own normal range. There is general agreement, however, that pepsin production is increased in patients with duodenal ulcer, normal or slightly decreased in gastric ulcer and cancer of the stomach, and low to absent in cases of pernicious anemia and gastric atrophy.[11, 12, 14, 15] Anacidity together with a high blood-pepsinogen level suggests inflammatory lesions of the gastric mucosa.[4]

Little is known of the origin or mechanisms of secretion or clinical significance of other enzymes of the gastric juice. These include among others cathepsin, urease, lipase, and lysozyme.[1, 16]

MUCIN. The three main components of human gastric mucin are dissolved mucoproteose, dissolved glandular muco-protein, and mucoid of the visible gastric mucus.[17, 18] They are a heterogeneous mixture of mucoproteins—a complex of protein and mucopolysaccharide moie-ties—each with a specific cell of origin. Identification depends on separation and characterization by chemical means [17, 18] or by resin-column fractionation.[5] Knowl-edge in this area is still very rudimen-tary.

Mucoid of the visible gastric mucus is secreted by the surface epithelial cells of the gastric mucosa. In the presence of hydrochloric acid, the mucoid is pre-cipitated as a visible, viscous, adherent gel, whose chief function is to form a protective coating over the mucosal lin-ing of the stomach.[18] Its production is strongly stimulated by substances that irritate the gastric mucosa locally.[3]

Dissolved mucoproteose is a complex of intermediate products of digestion of gastric mucus. This digestion does not seem to be caused by pepsin or lysozyme but by a postulated, but as yet unidenti-fied, specific proteolytic enzyme, "muci-nase." [18] Some of the mucoproteose may be secreted directly by the surface epi-thelial cells of the gastric mucosa.[17] Mu-coproteose is constantly present in all gastric juice, normal and pathologic, basal and stimulated. Its constancy re-flects the continuous secretory activity of the surface epithelial cells. The con-centration of mucoproteose in the gastric juice is roughly inverse to the secretion of hydrochloric acid.[18] The highest levels of mucoproteose concentration are found in the gastric juice of patients with per-nicious anemia, gastric atrophy, and car-cinoma of the body of the stomach. Va-gal stimulation has little effect on muco-proteose secretion.[18]

The function of mucoproteose may be inhibitory to gastric secretion. It appears to absorb histamine and pepsin.[18]

Dissolved mucoprotein is secreted by the mucoid or neck chief cells of the gastric glands. Its secretion is intermit-tent and roughly parallel to hydrochloric acid secretion. Both histamine and vagal stimulation increase the output of glan-dular mucoprotein.[17, 18] As might be an-ticipated, glandular mucoprotein of the gastric juice is increased in patients with duodenal ulcer, and greatly diminished or absent when there is pernicious ane-mia and gastric atrophy.[18]

The function of glandular mucopro-tein has not been determined, but the intrinsic factor of Castle appears to be elaborated in this fraction of gastric se-cretion.[18]

ELECTROLYTES. Electrolytes of the gastric juice include sodium, potassium, mag-nesium, calcium, chloride, phosphate, and, in the absence of hydrochloric acid secretion, bicarbonate.[1] The electrolytes provide the major buffering capacity of the nonparietal component of gastric se-cretion. Phosphates are present in very small amounts, and the concentration of calcium and magnesium never exceeds that of blood.[1] Consequently, these elec-trolytes may get into the gastric juice by simple diffusion from the interstitial fluid.

The sodium concentration of the fast-ing gastric juice of both normal and an-acid individuals averages 57 to 61 mEq/L. With increased hydrochloric acid secretion following insulin stimu-lation, there is a corresponding decrease of gastric-juice sodium by as much as 37 percent; but if there is no acid secre-tory response, the sodium level remains the same as in a fasting specimen.[9]

Total chlorides of fasting gastric con-tents average 120 mEq/L and after in-sulin stimulation they increase to as high as 149 mEq/L. This increase occurs ir-respective of acid secretion. Neutral chlorides are determined by the differ-ence between total chlorides and the chloride contained in the hydrochloric acid. In acid producers, the neutral chlorides are greatly reduced after stimulation. In anacid individuals, the neutral chloride fraction is increased after insulin stimulation.[9]

Potassium content of fasting gastric juice of both normal and anacid individuals averages 17–18 mEq/L—several times its concentration in serum.[9] After insulin stimulation, the potassium concentration remains unchanged in both groups,[9] but following histamine stimulation there is a considerable increase of gastric-juice potassium in acid secretors but not in achlorhydric subjects.[19] This is thought to indicate that potassium secretion is a function of parietal-cell activity,[19] but other investigators believe that potassium is secreted mainly by the mucoid cells of the gastric glands and by surface epithelial cells.[3]

In summary, it must be emphasized that each component of gastric juice has its particular cell of origin and mechanism of secretion. To acquire a complete picture of the physiology of gastric secretory activity in health and disease would necessitate quantitative analysis of each component. Such study is impractical here. For clinical purposes, a few quantitative and semiquantitative procedures have proved valuable.

## Methods of Studying Gastric Secretory Function

An outline of methods commonly used in clinical practice is presented below. Most require specialized techniques beyond the scope of the ordinary clinical laboratory. Only the tests for parietal-cell function will be described in detail in a subsequent section.[1, 2, 4]

### TESTS OF PARIETAL-CELL FUNCTION

(1) Direct measurement of hydrochloric acid concentration of gastric juice obtained by aspiration through a stomach tube.

(2) Indirect measurement of hydrochloric acid by "tubeless gastric analysis."

### TESTS OF PEPTIC-CELL ACTIVITY

(1) Measurement of gastric-juice pepsin.[20, 21]

(2) Measurement of blood pepsinogen.[11]

(3) Measurement of urinary excretion of uropepsinogen.[12]

Although all three methods reflect peptic-cell activity in general, both blood and urine pepsinogen levels may be used only as approximate indices of peptic-cell activity.[15] Inaccurate and incomplete collection of gastric-juice and urine samples may introduce errors. Urinary pepsinogen can vary considerably among consecutive 24-hr urine samples from the same person and the diurnal level of uropepsin tends to be greater than the nocturnal.[15] Blood levels in any given individual are more constant. Renal disease, diabetes mellitus, and hyperparathyroidism, all associated with diminished renal blood flow, may result in abnormally elevated blood pepsinogen levels and decreased uropepsinogen excretion without any correlation with gastric-juice pepsin.[22]

### TEST FOR SOLUBLE MUCOPROTEIN SECRETION: MEASUREMENT OF INTRINSIC FACTOR ACTIVITY [23]

The determination of intrinsic-factor activity by measuring the absorption of orally administered radioactive vitamin $B_{12}$ is the only practical test in this area. Uptake of the labeled $B_{12}$ may be determined by counting radioactivity over the liver or in the stool; but the Schilling test [22] is most convenient (see Unit 14). Normal 24-hr urinary excretion of radioactive $B_{12}$ is 7 percent or more of the oral dose. Greatly diminished urinary excretion in the range of 2 percent suggests absence of intrinsic-factor production, especially when a normal range of labeled $B_{12}$ excretion is restored by giving exogenous intrinsic factor along with the radioactive $B_{12}$. Such findings are evidence of absent intrinsic-factor production in patients with pernicious anemia and gastric atrophy.

## Cytologic Examination for Malignant Cells

### STUDY OF EXFOLIATIVE GASTRIC CYTOLOGY

Papanicolaou observed that malignant growths desquamate cells that can be identified after suitable fixation and staining.[24] From this there developed the cytologic method as an aid in the diagnosis of gastric carcinoma.[25] Success depends upon obtaining a fasting sample of gastric juice free of food contamination by aspiration through a stomach tube. Immediate centrifugation and fixation of the sedimented cells on a glass microscope slide is essential if digestion of the cells is to be prevented. Newer methods such as the Ayre brush,[26] antral abrasive balloon, and chymotrypsin lavage [27] have been developed in an attempt to increase the yield of well-preserved cells in the aspirated gastric contents. In experienced hands, there is still a 10–15-percent error of false negatives in patients who are found to have cancer, while in patients without cancer there may be 6–8 percent of false positive cytologic examinations reported.[28, 29] Cytologic diagnosis of gastric carcinoma is performed accurately only by individuals who have had a long experience in the identification of malignant cells.

### HISTOLOGY OF GASTRIC MUCOSA OBTAINED BY SUCTION BIOPSY

The development of a satisfactory tube for suction biopsy of the gastric mucosa [30] has made it possible to begin a correlation between histologic changes of the mucosal cells and the various studies of gastric secretory activity described above.[4]

### MISCELLANEOUS USES OF THE STOMACH TUBE

(1) Examination of gastric contents for tubercle bacilli recovered from swallowed sputum.

(2) Treatment of dilatation of the stomach associated with pyloric obstruction or diabetic coma.

(3) Removal of poisons, drugs, and other toxic substances that may have been ingested.

## Basic Examination of Contents of the Stomach—"Gastric Analysis"

### DIRECT MEASUREMENT OF PARIETAL-CELL FUNCTION

#### PRINCIPLE

Samples of gastric juice are obtained from the stomach in a fasting or basal state and after stimulation of parietal-cell secretion. Contamination of gastric secretions by saliva and duodenal contents must be avoided.[2, 31] Quantitative results will depend upon completeness of recovery of the gastric contents. This can be more nearly assured by accurate placement under fluoroscopic control of the tip of the tube in the dependent portion of the stomach with the patient sitting upright and by continuous aspiration of gastric contents with a hand syringe throughout the period of collection.[31]

Examination of the gastric juice consists of a description of its physical appearance and volume and analysis for acidity by determination of pH and titration with sodium hydroxide. Any suitable indicator paper (pHydrion, for example) or a glass electrode may be used to measure pH. Chemical analysis for free acid and combined acid is carried out by titration with $0.1N$ sodium hydroxide, using either a chemical indicator or a glass electrode to determine the end point. The accepted end point for determination of free hydrochloric acid in a gastric sample is pH 3.5. The indicator of choice is dimethylaminoazobenzene (Töpfer's reagent). It is red below pH 3.0, orange at pH 3.5, and yellow above pH 4.0.[32] In measuring combined acid or total acidity, a titration end point of pH 8.3 to pH 8.5 is probably best.[32] Phenolphthalein is the indicator of choice for this determination and the end point is described as when the first tinge of red color appears and persists for at least 5 sec.[32] Total acidity is an expression of the sum of units of free acid and combined acid.

The measurement of acidity is frequently expressed in clinical units or degrees. This is the number of milliliters of $0.1N$ sodium hydroxide required for the titration of hydrochloric acid in 100 ml of gastric juice. Since a clinical unit is equivalent to 1 mEq/L, it is perhaps more desirable to express gastric acidity in milliequivalents per liter and bring it into line with measurement of concentration of solutes in other body fluids.[2]

The type of stomach tube used for aspirating gastric contents is optional. Most frequently used is the Levin tube of smooth rubber or plastic with a catheter tip. It is available in sizes from 12 to 18 French scale. It can be introduced through the nose or mouth. The nasal route is preferred because there is less gagging when the tube does not touch the soft palate.

### METHOD

The patient receives neither food nor water after the evening meal and gastric analysis is performed in the morning while the patient is in a fasting state.

TECHNIQUE OF INTRODUCING THE LEVIN TUBE. Just before use, the first 5 to 10 cm of the Levin tube is lubricated with surgical (water-soluble) lubricant. The patient is placed in a comfortable sitting position, draped with suitable towels, and reassured by a brief explanation of what is to occur. The tip of the tube is inserted gently into a patent nostril and passed backward along the floor of the nasal cavity until the tip impinges upon the posterior nasopharynx. Then the patient is asked to swallow and the tube is advanced along the posterior pharynx and beyond the epiglottis. When the tube is in the esophagus, the operator will be aware of a tug upon the tube with each swallow. If the patient experiences difficulty in getting the tip of the tube past the epiglottis, he may take a few sips of water through a drinking tube. Any water he drinks will dilute the fasting gastric contents. Once the tube has entered the esophagus, the operator may advance the tube rapidly until the tip of the tube should be in the stomach, a distance of approximately 55 cm from the nose.

Passage of the Levin tube may be complicated by having the tube coil up in the nasopharynx. In such cases, the tube should be withdrawn slowly and reinserted with repeated swallowing. If the tube enters the trachea instead of the esophagus, the patient will cough vigorously and the respiratory movement of air will be felt at the open end of the Levin tube. Again, the tube should be withdrawn and reinserted. The introduction of a stomach tube should be attended with caution or omitted in patients with esophageal varice, aortic aneurysms, or severe hypertension. If the tube cannot be passed through the nose, it may be passed through the mouth, but this usually induces considerable gagging because of contact with the soft palate.

Once the tube is in place, it may be secured to the side of the patient's face with a small strip of adhesive tape. Gagging can be reduced by instructing the patient to breathe in and out gently (to "pant") with his mouth held wide open. This procedure reduces the contact between the tube and the soft palate.

Once the tube is in place, the patient is asked to expectorate all saliva into a basin in order to minimize contamination of pure gastric juice.[2] Likewise, any specimen of juice that is bile-stained must be discarded because the yellow color indicates admixture with alkaline duodenal contents that have refluxed into the stomach.

Samples of gastric juice are collected with a syringe of at least 30-ml capacity attached to the open end of the tube. Gentle, continuous suction is advised. Vigorous suction may cause bleeding or obstruction of the fenestrated opening at the tip of the tube by indrawn gastric mucosa. If no gastric juice is obtained, the tube may be advanced or withdrawn a few centimeters.

STIMULATION OF GASTRIC SECRETION. Since the most frequent use of gastric analysis is to establish the qualitative presence of free acid as a screening test, it would be sufficient to demonstrate free hydrochloric acid in the fasting specimen by adding 3 drops of Töpfer's reagent. If, however, there is no free acid, or if it is desired to study parietal-cell secretory activity in its various phases, stimuli will have to be employed. Test meals and 7-percent alcohol have been much used but these cause only mild stimulation via the gastric phase and may modify the concentration of hydrochloric acid by dilution. Maximal stimulation by insulin-induced hypoglycemia or parenteral administration of histamine is essential if true achlorhydria is to be established or the completeness of vagotomy is to be tested.

For insulin stimulation,[33] the patient is given an intravenous injection of regular insulin in a sufficient dose (10 to 20 units) to produce a blood-sugar level of less than 50 mg/100 ml. Blood-sugar levels are taken at 30-min intervals to ensure an adequate degree of hypoglycemia for vagal stimulation. Gastric-juice samples are collected fractionally over a 3-4-hr period after injection. The production of hypoglycemia is unwise in patients with hypertension or coronary-artery disease.

Histamine stimulation acts directly upon the parietal cell. A subcutaneous injection of 0.01 mg of histamine base per kilogram of body weight is an adequate and tolerated dose.[2] The use of histamine in patients who have a history of asthma or paroxysmal hypertension is contraindicated. The injection of histamine may also produce unpleasant but transitory side effects such as headache, flushing, sweating, hypotension, tachycardia, and a burning pain at the site of injection. An isomeric analog of histamine,[34] Histalog, has proved to be a satisfactory maximal stimulus of parietal-cell activity with few unpleasant side effects.

A second sample of gastric juice, aspirated 30 to 40 min after histamine injection, is sufficient for the diagnosis of presence or absence of free acid. Fractional gastric analysis with continuous aspiration of samples divided into 10-min periods for an hour or longer is of value in studying the physiology of gastric secretion.

REAGENTS. (1) Töpfer's reagent : 0.5 gm of dimethylaminoazobenzene dissolved in 100 ml of 95-percent ethyl alcohol. (2) Phenolphthalein : 1 gm dissolved in 100 ml of 95-percent alcohol. (3) One-tenth normal sodium hydroxide.

EXAMINATION OF GASTRIC JUICE. Each sample of gastric juice should be measured, described, and analyzed for free and combined acid soon after aspiration. The free-acid content of the gastric juice will not change appreciably if the gastric juice is permitted to remain at room temperature for several hours.

*Description.* The following items are noted: volume; color; odor; mucus—quantity and quality; presence of bile, blood, food particles; salivary contamination, indicated by stringy material floating on the surface.

*Determination of Acidity.* Measurement of pH by indicator paper or glass electrode is a simple, direct method for determining the acid-producing capacity of the stomach. *Titration:* Titration of acidity is performed as follows. The liquid phase of gastric juice may be obtained free of food particles or salivary contamination by filtration through three or four layers of gauze, but if the patient has been fasting, unfiltered gastric juice is usually satisfactory for titration. A sample of 10 ml of gastric juice is measured into a white dish. Addition of 10 to 20 ml of distilled water will make the titration easier if much mucus is present. *Free hydrochloric acid:* For measurement of free hydrochloric acid, add 2 or 3 drops of Töpfer's reagent. A red color indicates the presence of free acid. To titrate, 0.1N sodium hydroxide is added drop by drop from a pipette or burette with constant stirring. The appearance of a faint pink color indicates that the end point of titration is near; and a few more drops of sodium hydroxide are added cautiously until an orange color results. This is the "end point" of approximately pH 3.5. The volume (ml) of sodium hydroxide used is recorded. Calculation:

$$\frac{\text{Vol. (ml) of 0.1N sodium hydroxide} \times 100}{\text{Vol. (ml) of gastric-juice sample}}$$
$$= \frac{\text{Units of free hydrochloric}}{\text{acid per 100 ml of gastric juice.}}$$

*Combined acid:* After completion of titration for free hydrochloric acid, 2 or 3 drops of phenolphthalein solution is added to the same sample. The 0.1N sodium hydroxide is again added drop by drop with constant stirring until a faint pink color appears and persists for at least 5 sec. The quantity of sodium hydroxide used for this second titration is noted. Calculation of the units of combined acid is accomplished by the same formula as for free acid. If no free acid was demonstrated originally, only the titration for combined acid is carried out.

*Test for Blood.* Occult blood in the gastric juice may be proved by the guaiac test described in Unit 22. It is more satisfactory to pick out red- or brown-colored mucus particles from the gastric juice, smear the particles on filter paper, and apply the guaiac test.

INDICATIONS AND INTERPRETATION. A gastric analysis is indicated whenever knowledge of gastric secretory function will aid in diagnosis or add to the rationale of medical or surgical measures for treatment. The normal range of variation in acid secretion and volume is shown in Table 70 both for basal secre-

Table 70. *Usual range of variation of hydrochloric acid and volume of gastric juice in normal adults.*[a]

| Function | Response per 1-hr sample | |
|---|---|---|
| | Basal | After histamine |
| Free acid (clinical units per 100 ml) | 10–40 | 35–90 |
| Volume (ml) | 40–95 | 75–155 |

[a] The values in this table are somewhat arbitrary, being based on results reported in the literature, but it is expected that they may represent the normal range of variation in most subjects.

tion and after maximal stimulation. Use of 7-percent alcohol or other test meals, which produce submaximal stimulation, will result in values of an intermediate range. Normal individuals may have a transient achlorhydria due to emotional tension and such findings indicate the need for a repetition of gastric analysis with maximal stimulation.

*Achlorhydria and Hypochlorhydria.* Proved achlorhydria is a criterion for differentiating Addisonian pernicious anemia from the other macrocytic anemias of sprue, pregnancy, malnutrition, and tapeworm infestation. Atrophy of the gastric mucosa is associated with a failure to produce hydrochloric acid. Gastric analysis with demonstration of achlorhydria or hypochlorhydria is a valuable screening test for cancer of the stomach.[35, 36, 37] A gastric ulcer associated with achlorhydria should be considered malignant until proved otherwise. In patients who have achlorhydria, cancer of the stomach develops 3.2 times as often as the national incidence.[35] Although normal acid production by the stomach does not rule out cancer, it makes a malignant ulceration much less probable.

If no free acid is demonstrable, even after maximal stimulation, a decrease in pH from 6 or 7 to 4 or 5 is evidence of some acid-secreting activity of the stomach glands, but probably not enough to be of diagnostic significance.

*Hypersecretion.* An increased volume and concentration of hydrochloric acid above the normal is found usually in both the basal and the stimulated specimens from patients with duodenal ulcer. Gastric analysis, however, is no substitute for the barium-meal x-ray examination as the method of choice for the diagnosis of duodenal ulcer. Extremely large volumes of gastric juice are associated with the Zollinger-Ellison syndrome.[38] After subtotal gastrectomy, gastric analysis may show evidence of continued excessive secretory activity and confirm a suspicion of a stomal ulcer. The use of insulin stimulation and gastric analysis is indicated to test the completeness of vagus-nerve resection.

*Achylia.* In an occasional older person with atrophy of the gastric mucosa, there will be complete absence of gastric juice, acid, and enzymes, even after maximal stimulation. This is termed achylia.

*Physical Characteristics of the Gastric Juice.* Attention to the physical characteristics of the gastric juice is of value in cases where there may be pyloric obstruction, bleeding lesions, small-bowel obstruction, or fistulae between the stomach and intestines. A volume in excess of 100 ml obtained from the fasting stomach is presumptive evidence for pyloric obstruction. If, in addition, particles of food ingested the day before are recognized, obstruction is almost a certainty. Normal gastric juice has a pearly opalescent color, and a slightly sour odor. The juice from an obstructed stomach may be cloudy and much more sour or putrid in odor if a necrotic lesion is in the stomach. Small-bowel obstruction or a gastrojejunocolic fistula gives the aspirated contents of the stomach a fecal color and odor. Bile, regurgitated from the duodenum, will cause the gastric juice to have a yellow or greenish color, and bile in the gastric juice is an indication that there is little or no pyloric obstruction. Flecks of bright-red blood in the juice are usually from trauma due to passage of the tube through the nose or produced by too vigorous aspiration which has sucked the gastric mucosa into openings at the end of the tube. Bleeding lesions of the stomach or duodenum, such as ulcer, cancer, gastritis, or varices, are associated with brown lumps in the gastric contents. These so-called "coffee grounds" are the result of the action of hydrochloric acid on the blood to form acid hematin. If no acid is present or the bleeding is brisk, then red blood may be aspirated. Excessive amounts of thick, glary mucus in the gastric juice may indicate excessive psychic stimulation or the swallowing of mucus from the irritation of the tube in the nose and throat.

In summary, the single most important use of gastric analysis is the qualitative demonstration of the presence or absence of free hydrochloric acid. To this end, advantage should be taken of random specimens of gastric contents produced by vomiting. Evidence of free acid by the addition of 2 or 3 drops of Töpfer's reagent to the vomitus may be of as much value as a gastric analysis.

LIMITATIONS AND SOURCES OF ERROR. Gastric analysis at best is a semiquantitative procedure. Complete recovery of gastric contents is difficult because the fenestrated openings of the tube may not be in the most dependent portion of the stomach. Even continuous aspiration with a hand syringe does not prevent the loss of some gastric juice via gastric emptying through the pylorus. If a subtotal gastric resection has been performed, even more difficulty in quantitative recovery of juice will be experienced.

In evaluating the quantity of free acid, the neutralizing effects of saliva, gastric mucus, and bile must all be taken into account. If these contaminants are present to any degree, the amount of combined acid may be considerably increased while the free acid is reduced.

Since there is an increased incidence of achlorhydria normally in the older age groups, the absence of free acid in these patients loses some of its diagnostic significance. The use of a stomach tube and histamine stimulation is contraindicated in certain patients, as mentioned above.

### Tubeless Gastric Analysis

Carboxylic cation-exchange resin (Amberlite XE–96) has been combined with substances such as quinine [39] or Azure A [40] which replace the hydrogen ions of the carboxylic acid groups of the resin. When ingested, the gastric hydrochloric acid displaces the indicators quinine or Azure A with hydrogen ion. Maximum displacement occurs at pH 1.5 and is negligible above pH 3.2.[41] The indicators thus displaced are absorbed from the small bowel and excreted in the urine. Identification of quinine in the urine depends on a tedious process of extraction and fluorescent measurement. The quinine compound has given way to the Azure A compound which imparts a blue color directly to the urine that can be compared semiquantitatively with standards. At times, the Azure A is excreted in the urine as a conjugated colorless compound. By acidification of the urine and boiling, free blue-colored Azure A is released for comparison with the standards.

Prior to ingestion of the Azure A resin compound, stimulation of hydrochloric acid secretion by the stomach is brought about by the oral administration of caffeine sodium benzoate or parenteral injection of Histalog or histamine.

REAGENTS. (1) Azure A–resin compound : Hydrogen ions of each gram of carboxylic cation-exchange resin are displaced with 45 mg of Azure A [40] (commercially available as Diagnex Blue, Squibb).

(2) Caffeine sodium benzoate : Available as two 250-mg tablets with the Diagnex Blue kit; or Histalog (Lilly) in 1-ml sterile ampules.

(3) Eighteen-percent ($6N$) hydrochloric acid.

(4) Azure A : Standards in concentrations of 0.6 and 0.3 mg/300 ml are made from a 0.01-percent stock solution. (The commercially available Diagnex Blue kits are provided with a comparator block that has built-in blue color standards.)

METHOD.[40] The patient fasts after midnight of the day before the test. In the morning, all urine is voided and discarded. The patient then ingests 500 mg of caffein sodium benzoate with 1 glass of water or receives a subcutaneous injection of 1 ml of Histalog and drinks 1 glass of water. One hour later, he voids completely, saves all of the sample of urine, and labels it "control urine." The packet of Azure A–resin compound or Diagnex Blue, already measured in a dosage of 2 gm, is then emptied into ¼ glass of water, stirred well, and drunk. The granules remaining in the glass are rinsed out with a little more water and swallowed. The granules are not to be chewed. All urine produced during the next 2 hr after taking the Diagnex Blue is collected and marked "test urine." The control urine and test urine are both diluted to a volume of 300 ml. Aliquots of approximately 10 ml of control urine are measured into each of two test tubes and 10 ml of the test urine into a third tube. The two control tubes are placed in a comparator block in the two lateral holes. The test urine sample is placed in the central hole. Comparison of color is made against a natural light source. Measurement may also be made with the use of a photoelectric colorimeter. If blue color is not present in the test-urine sample, both of the control aliquots and the test-urine aliquot should be acidified with 1 drop of 18-percent hydrochloric acid. All three tubes are boiled in a water bath for 10–15 min and then allowed to cool to room temperature for 2 hr. Any blue color present in the test sample may disappear during boiling, but will reappear during cooling. At the end of the cooling period, the samples are read in the comparator block.

INDICATION AND INTERPRETATION. Tubeless gastric analysis with Diagnex Blue is a simple procedure, well adapted to mass surveys of populations for the presence or absence of achlorhydria. Since direct gastric analysis with a stomach tube is unwise in patients with esophageal lesions, esophageal varices, severe heart disease, or debilitating illness, tubeless gastric analysis is of value for qualitative assay of gastric secretory activity of such patients.[41] After subtotal gastrectomy, both rapid emptying of the gastric remnant and reflux of small-bowel contents into the stomach may result in a finding of achlorhydria by direct gastric analysis. Tubeless gastric analysis will therefore permit a more accurate appraisal of gastric secretory function after subtotal gastrectomy.[42]

If the test urine sample shows more than 0.6 mg of Azure A per 300 ml, the test is positive for hydrochloric acid secretion by the stomach. Less than 0.3 mg of Azure A per 300 ml in the test sample indicates no free hydrochloric acid in the gastric juice. Values between 0.3 and 0.6 mg of Azure A per 300 ml are borderline, but in general are consistent with hypochlorhydria or intermittent acid secretion.[40, 43]

Tubeless gastric analysis is qualitative. If acid secretion is present by direct gastric analysis, the tubeless method has been positive in 95–97 percent of cases.[40, 44] Achlorhydria by direct analysis has been confirmed in every case by the tubeless method.[40, 44] False positive results by tubeless gastric analysis must be very unusual.

LIMITATIONS AND SOURCES OF ERROR. Tubeless gastric analysis must never be considered a quantitative test.[40] It merely establishes the presence or absence of free hydrochloric acid in the gastric juice. The major source of error in the use of tubeless gastric analysis occurs in the cases of false negative results. Pyloric obstruction, severe hepatic disease, renal impairment, malabsorption from the intestine, and urinary-bladder retention may cause absence of excretion of Azure A dye in the urine even when there is secretion of hydrochloric acid.[40] Inadequate stimulation of secretory function of the stomach by caffeine may be another cause of false negatives. The use of histamine or Histalog will overcome this defect.[45]

REFERENCES

1. F. Hollander, "Current views on the physiology of the gastric secretions," *Amer. J. Med. 13*, 453 (1952).
2. H. D. Janowitz, "Quantitative tests of gastrointestinal function," *Amer. J. Med. 13*, 465 (1952).
3. G. B. Jerzy Glass and L. J. Boyd, "Studies on the non-parietal component of gastric secretion in humans, Part II. Present concept of the 'alkaline constituent' of the gastric juice," *Gastroenterology 20*, 442 (1952).

4. I. J. Poliner and H. M. Spiro, "The independent secretion of acid, pepsin, and 'Intrinsic Factor' by the human stomach," _Gastroenterology 34,_ 196 (1958).

5. V. Richmond, R. Caputto, and S. Wolf, "Biochemical study of the large molecular constituents of gastric juice," _Gastroenterology 29,_ 1017 (1955).

6. J. B. Kirsner, D. Bock, W. L. Palmer, E. Levin, and H. Ford, "Variation in basal gastric secretion in man and the evaluation of gastric secretory stimulants," _Gastroenterology 30,_ 779 (1956).

7. E. Levin, J. B. Kirsner, and W. L. Palmer, "A simple measure of gastric secretion in man. Comparison of one hour basal secretion, histamine-secretion and twelve hour nocturnal gastric secretion," _Gastroenterology 19,_ 88 (1951).

8. E. Levin, J. B. Kirsner, W. L. Palmer, and C. Butler, "The fasting nocturnal gastric secretion in normal individuals and in patients with duodenal ulcer, gastric ulcer, and gastric carcinoma," _Arch. Surg. 56,_ 345 (1948).

9. G. B. Jerzy Glass, L. J. Boyd, I. Drekter, and A. Heisler, "Studies on the nonparietal component of gastric secretion in humans, Part I. Variations in electrolytes and dissolved mucin of the gastric juice following insulin stimulation," _Gastroenterology 20,_ 430 (1952).

10. H. D. Janowitz and F. Hollander, "Relation of uropepsinogen excretion to gastric pepsin secretion in man," _J. appl. Physiol. 4,_ 53 (1951).

11. H. M. Spiro, A. R. Ryan, and C. M. Jones, "The utility of the blood pepsin assay in clinical medicine," _New Engl. J. Med. 253,_ 26 (1955).

12. S. J. Gray, C. G. Ramsey, and R. W. Reifenstein, "Clinical use of the urinary uropepsin determination in medicine and surgery," _New Engl. J. Med. 251,_ 835 (1954).

13. B. I. Hirschowitz, J. L. London, and H. M. Pollard, "Histamine stimulation of gastric pepsin secretion in man," _Gastroenterology 32,_ 85 (1957).

14. D. A. Cubberley, A. E. Dagradi, H. O. Carne, and S. J. Stempien, "Uropepsin parallels gastric acid secretion in gastric atrophy and hypertrophic gastritis," _Gastroenterology 28,_ 80 (1955).

15. G. Van Goidsenhoven, L. Wilkoff, and J. B. Kirsner, "Serum and urine pepsinogen and gastric pepsin; simultaneous analyses for 24 hour periods in normal persons and in patients with duodenal ulcer, gastric ulcer, and achlorhydria," _Gastroenterology 34,_ 421 (1958).

16. L. L. Miller, H. L. Segal, and E. J. Plumb, "Proteolytic enzyme activity. II. Gastric and urinary proteolytic activities of pH 1.5 and 3.5," _Gastroenterology 33,_ 566 (1957) .

17. G. B. Jerzy Glass and L. J. Boyd, "The three main components of the human gastric mucin: Dissolved mucoproteose, dissolved mucoprotein, and mucoid of the gastric visible mucus," _Gastroenterology 12,_ 821 (1949).

18. G. B. Jerzy Glass, "Gastric mucin and its constituents: Physicochemical characteristics, cellular origin, and physiological significance," _Gastroenterology 23,_ 636 (1953).

19. L. Martin, "The relationship of potassium to the electrolytes and to the proteins of the gastric juice of man," _Gastroenterology 15,_ 326 (1950).

20. G. R. Bucher, M. I. Grossman, and A. C. Ivy, "A pepsin method: The role of dilution in the determination of peptic activity," _Gastroenterology 5,_ 501 (1945).

21. M. L. Anson, "The estimation of pepsin, trypsin, papain, and cathepsin with hemoglobin," _J. gen. Physiol. 22,_ 79 (1938).

22. H. M. Spiro, A. E. Ryan, and C. M. Jones, "The relation of blood pepsin to

gastric secretion, with particular reference to anacidity and achylia," *Gastroenterology 30*, 563 (1956).

23. R. F. Schilling, "Intrinsic factor studies, II. Effect of gastric juice on urinary excretion of radioactivity after oral administration of radioactive vitamin B$_{12}$," *J. lab. clin. Med. 42*, 860 (1953).
24. G. N. Papanicolaou, "A new procedure for staining vaginal smears," *Science 95*, 438 (1942).
25. R. M. Graham, H. Ulfelder, and T. H. Green, Jr., "The cytologic method as an aid in the diagnosis of gastric carcinoma," *Surg. Gynec. Obstet. 86*, 257 (1948).
26. J. E. Ayre and B. G. Oren, "New rapid method for stomach cancer diagnosis: Gastric brush," *Cancer 6*, 1177 (1953).
27. C. E. Rubin, B. W. Massey, J. B. Kirsner, W. L. Palmer, and D. D. Stonecypher, "The clinical value of gastrointestinal cytology," *Gastroenterology 25*, 119 (1953).
28. J. F. Seybolt and G. N. Papanicolaou, "The value of cytology in the diagnosis of gastric cancer," *Gastroenterology 33*, 369 (1957).
29. W. O. Umiker, R. J. Bolt, A. D. Hoekzema, and H. M. Pollard, "Cytology in the diagnosis of gastric cancer. The significance of location and pathologic type," *Gastroenterology 34*, 859 (1958).
30. I. J. Wood, R. K. Doig, R. Motteram, S. Weiden, and A. Moore, "The relationship between the secretions of the gastric mucosa and its morphology as shown by biopsy specimens," *Gastroenterology 12*, 949 (1949).
31. D. H. Johnson and B. H. McCrew, "Gastric analysis—evaluation of collection techniques," *Gastroenterology 35*, 512 (1958).
32. H. Shay, S. A. Komarov, and J. E. Beth, "Some fallacies in the clinical measurement of gastric acidity with special reference to the histamine test," *Gastroenterology 15*, 110 (1950).
33. F. Hollander, "The insulin test for the presence of intact nerve fibers after vagal operations for peptic ulcer," *Gastroenterology 7*, 607 (1945).
34. C. E. Rosiere and M. I. Grossman, "An analog of histamine that stimulates gastric acid secretion without other actions of histamine," *Science 113*, 657 (1951).
35. M. W. Comfort, M. P. Kelsey, and J. Berkson, "Gastric acidity before and after the development of carcinoma of the stomach," *Proc. Mayo Clin. 23*, 135 (1948).
36. C. R. Hitchcock, W. A. Sullivan, and O. H. Wangensteen, "The value of achlorhydria as a screening test for gastric cancer. A ten-year report," *Gastroenterology 29*, 621 (1955).
37. C. W. Wirts, J. Groves, and L. Calderon, "Gastric analysis as a screening method in gastric cancer detection," *Amer. J. med. Sci. 229*, 1 (1955).
38. R. M. Zollinger and E. H. Ellison, "Primary peptic ulcerations of the jejunum associaated with islet cell tumors of the pancreas," *Surgery 142*, 709 (1955).
39. H. L. Segal, L. L. Miller, and J. J. Morton, "Determination of gastric acidity without intubation by use of cation exchange indicator compounds," *Proc. Soc. exp. Biol. (N. Y.) 74*, 218 (1950).
40. H. L. Segal, L. L. Miller, and E. T. Plumb, "Tubeless gastric analysis with an Azure A ion-exchange compound," *Gastroenterology 28*, 402 (1955).
41. C. A. Flood, B. Jones, W. M. Rotton, and H. Schwarz, "Tubeless gastric analysis: A study of 100 cases," *Gastroenterology 23*, 607 (1953).

42. H. Shay, R. Ostrove, and H. Siplet, "Study of tubeless method for determining gastric acidity and pH value," *J. Amer. med. Ass. 156*, 224 (1954).

43. M. L. Sieverg and R. V. Gieselman, "Tubeless gastric analysis. Evaluation of a technic using a dye-resin compound," *Amer. J. dig. Dis. 1*, 241 (1956).

44. R. J. Bott, T. G. Ossius, and H. M. Pollard, "A clinical evaluation of tubeless gastric analysis," *Gastroenterology 32*, 34 (1957).

45. I. J. Poliner, M. A. Hayes, and H. M. Spiro, "Detection of achlorhydria by indirect gastric analysis," *New. Engl. J. Med. 256*, 1051 (1957).

# Unit 24

## Tests Related to the Liver and Biliary System

The establishment of an accurate diagnosis in diseases of the liver and biliary system is frequently difficult, yet it is often of great importance for determining proper treatment. For example, surgery in the presence of medical jaundice, such as hepatitis and cirrhosis, is associated with increased mortality and morbidity and should be avoided if possible. On the other hand, failure to operate and relieve an extrahepatic obstruction of the biliary tree may lead to the development of an irreversible biliary cirrhosis. Even among the diseases classified under medical jaundice, there are some that are benign, have an excellent prognosis, and require no therapy other than reassurance. Included in this group are neonatal jaundice, Gilbert's constitutional hepatic dysfunction, chronic idiopathic jaundice with liver pigment (Dubin-Johnson syndrome), and chronic idiopathic jaundice without liver pigment.[1-3] It would be unfortunate in such cases to institute a rigorous course of therapy and give the more serious prognosis indicated in cases of viral hepatitis and nutritional cirrhosis. The diagnosis and management of obstructive jaundice also are complicated by the need to differentiate extrahepatic biliary-tract obstruction from intrahepatic obstruction or cholestasis caused either by certain drugs such as chlorpromazine, methyl testosterone, and so on, or by hepatitis viruses.[4]

In approaching the problem of diagnosis of diseases of the liver and biliary tract, it should be emphasized that interpretation of a careful history and complete physical examination is all-important. The so-called liver-function tests are supplementary and serve to confirm or refute the clinical impression. These tests should be considered as yielding a measure of pathologic physiologic alterations, rather than being specifically diagnostic for a particular liver disease.[5] "Diverse pathologic processes often give rise to similar types of derangements, and function tests are but indices to be incorporated in the general clinical appraisal."[6] All attempts to correlate alterations in function with histologic change in the liver have met with failure.[5, 6] Moreover, most liver-function tests not only reflect the total metabolic and excretory activity of the liver as a functioning unit, but, in addition, are modified by other bodily processes outside of the liver. Over the years, countless tests have been developed with respect to the many functions of the liver. Most have been discarded as being too cumbersome or unreliable. Those tests which have survived are more generally accepted as being the most practical, simple, and reliable, although their principle is not often completely understood and they may be in part empirical.[5-7] Only the tests that have achieved increasing acceptance for clinical application will be discussed in this chapter.

Liver-function tests may be used as an adjunct to the history and physical examination for one or more of the following four reasons:[7]

1. Screening to detect the presence of minimal or latent hepatobiliary-tract disease;

2. The differential diagnosis of jaundice—hemolytic, medical, and surgical;

3. Measurement of the severity of liver disease;

4. To follow the course of hepatic disease and help to establish a prognosis.

### Physiology

Some basic concepts of liver physiology have been described by Bollman,[8] Hanger,[6] and Seligson.[9] In summary, the function of the liver is to help regulate the addition, removal, and alteration of the individual constituents of the blood by means of metabolic and excretory processes. From the anatomic viewpoint, the liver parenchyma should be considered as a barrier of cells between the vascular bed and the biliary tree, with a functioning surface in direct contact with each. Biochemically, each specific function of the liver reflects the activity of integrated enzyme systems which may be modified by the availability of metabolites, oxygen supply, factors that enhance or depress individual enzyme activities, and the function of other organs in the body as well as the mass and health of the liver cells. From these general statements, it is obvious that there are countless functions of the liver that can be subjected to investigation and measurement; but in this section on physiology, discussion will be limited to those liver functions which pertain to the tests that have been most widely accepted as of clinical value. Such essential metabolic functions as regulation of blood sugar, deamination of amino acids, and phosphorylation of fatty acids will scarcely be mentioned because there are no practical tests for measuring these functions of the liver.

#### BILIRUBIN METABOLISM

Jaundice is the manifestation of yellow color in the sclerae of the eyes, the mucous membranes, and the skin. It is a dramatic symptom which frequently directs the attention of the patient and physician to disorders of the liver and red blood cells. Jaundice is due to an abnormal accumulation of bilirubin in the tissues of the body. Knowledge of bilirubin metabolism is fundamental to understanding the clinical significance of jaundice. Bilirubin metabolism has been well summarized in reviews by Billing and Lathe,[10] Schmid,[11] Watson,[12] and in a panel discussion by Butt, Schmid, Arias, Bollman, and Isselbacher.[13]

NORMAL BILIRUBIN METABOLISM. At the end of their life span, normally 100 to 120 days, the erythrocytes are destroyed and the red pigment, hemoglobin, is liberated. The hemoglobin molecule is broken down in the reticuloendothelial system by a mechanism that is not yet understood. Globin is returned to the body's protein pool for further metabolic uses. The iron molecule is removed from the heme portion and is stored for new synthesis of hemoglobin or other iron-containing compounds. The protoporphyrin ring splits out the alpha-methene bridge with loss of carbon monoxide to form a chained molecule of four pyrrole nuclei which is the basic structure for the bile pigments. The chemical relation between the protoporphyrin ring and bilirubin is shown in Fig. 36.[13]

The first bile pigment released from the reticuloendothelial system into the blood stream may be biliverdin, which, if present, is rapidly reduced to free bilirubin, a yellow, water-insoluble pigment transported in the blood, linked to protein, mostly albumin.[14] Free bilirubin is taken up or removed by the parenchymal cells of the liver where the bilirubin is made water-soluble by conjugation. Most of the bilirubin is conjugated with glucuronic acid supplied in an activated form by uridine diphosphate glucuronic acid. The enzymatic transfer of glucuronide to bilirubin is carried out by glucuronyl

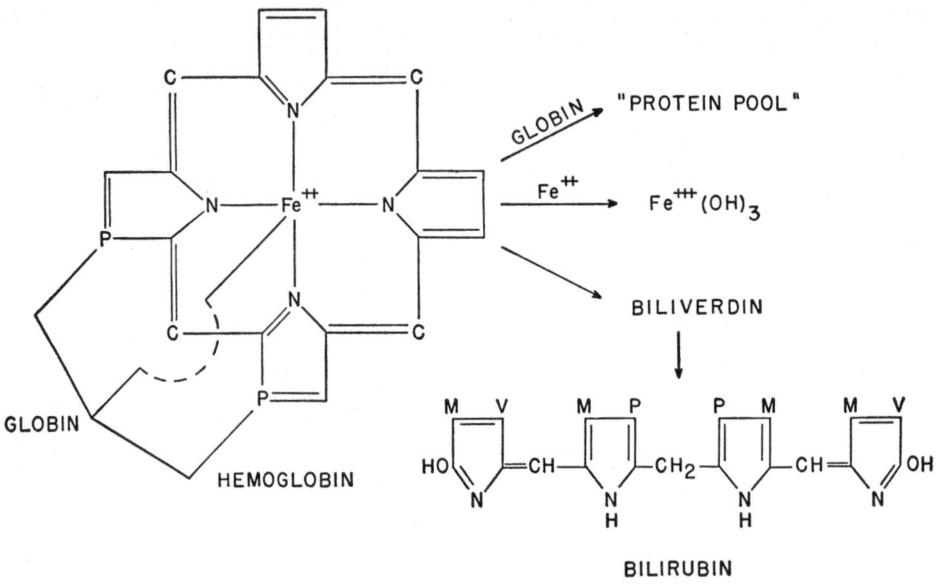

Fig. 36. Breakdown of hemoglobin.[13]

transferase that is present in the microsomes of liver cells. The scheme of this reaction is shown in Fig. 37.[10] Chemical studies have confirmed the theory that glucuronic acid is attached to the bilirubin molecule by an ester linkage at the carboxyl group of the propionic acid side chains of bilirubin. This is depicted in Fig. 38.[13] From chromatographic separation of conjugated bilirubin and from enzymatic hydrolysis with β-glucuronidase, both a di- and a mono-glucuronide pigment appear to be present. Although glucuronide conjugation accounts for the major portion of conjugated bilirubin, up to 20 percent of the water-soluble bilirubin in bile is conjugated with other hydrophilic substances. One of these is sulfate, which is believed to be linked with the bilirubin molecule at the hydroxyl groups.[15]

The contrast in water solubility of free and conjugated bilirubin not only accounts for the differences in physiologic behavior of the two pigments as summarized in Table 71,[10] but also makes possible the chemical differentiation of the two types of pigment by means of the van den Bergh reaction. Water-soluble, conjugated bilirubin after splitting

Table 71. *Differences between the two types of bile pigment (modified from Billing and Lathe* [10]*).*

| Property | Bilirubin | Conjugated bilirubin |
|---|---|---|
| Van den Bergh reaction | Indirect | Direct |
| Solubility in aqueous solution at acid or neutral pH | − | + |
| Solubility in chloroform and lipid solvents | + | − |
| Occurrence in icteric urine | − | + |
| Affinity for brain tissue | + | − |
| Attachment to plasma albumin | + | + |
| Ease of oxidation | + | 2+ |
| Association with hemolytic jaundice | 2+ | (+) |
| Association with obstructive jaundice and hepatitis | + | 3+ |

into two dipyrrole molecules couples immediately with Ehrlich's diazo reagent to produce a red color in neutral or weakly acid solutions. This is the direct van den Bergh reaction. Reaction between the diazo reagent and free bilirubin does not take place until the latter is rendered soluble by the addition of alcohol or other nonpolar solvents to the mixture, and is called the indirect van den Bergh reaction.

Conjugated bilirubin, but not the free,

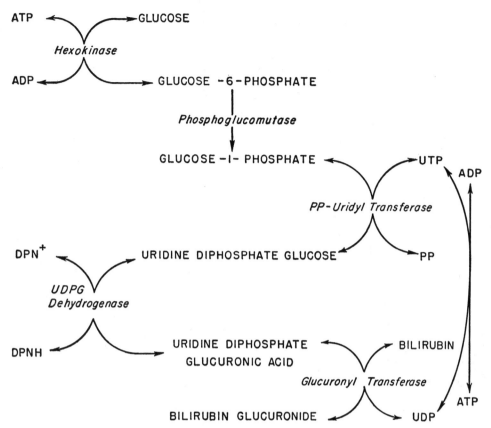

Fig. 37. A possible mechanism for the conjugation of bilirubin with glucuronic acid.[10]

is excreted by an unknown mechanism from the liver cells into the bile canaliculi, and makes up a component of the bile which flows into the intestinal tract. A small fraction of the conjugated bilirubin may be hydrolyzed to the free form in the bile or in the gut, but most remains as conjugated bilirubin which is reduced in the gut by bacteria to a group of colorless chromagens collectively called urobilinogen. The urobilinogens all have the same basic chemical structure of a chain of four pyrrole nuclei and differ only in the number of hydrogen atoms, as shown in Fig. 39.[12] The red color that results from the reaction of urobilinogen with Ehrlich's benzaldehyde reagent makes possible the identification and quantitation of urobilinogen.

An unknown portion of the urobilinogen is absorbed from the intestinal tract into the portal circulation and returns to the liver, where most of it is cleared by the liver cells and reexcreted into the bile as urobilinogen.[16] This circuit of urobilinogen is known as an enterohepatic circulation. A small amount of urobilinogen escapes clearance by the liver cells, passes into the general circulation, and is excreted by the kidneys as urine urobilinogen. Normally, urine urobilinogen amounts to about 1 percent of the daily production of bilirubin.

Eventually, approximately 99 percent of the urobilinogen is excreted in the feces, but some of it is oxidized to orange-colored urobilin (see Fig. 39) by bacteria in the colon and additional urobilinogen is converted to urobilin after the feces are exposed to the air. Thus the stool contains a mixture of urobilinogens, urobilins, and possibly a trace of bilirubin. The brown color of stool may be in part due to urobilin. Most of the

## CONJUGATED BILIRUBIN

## "DIRECT-REACTING"

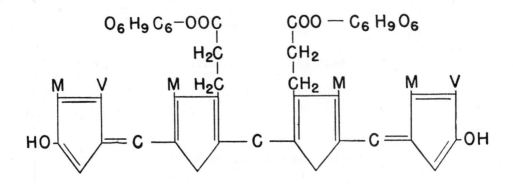

## FREE BILIRUBIN

## "INDIRECT-REACTING"

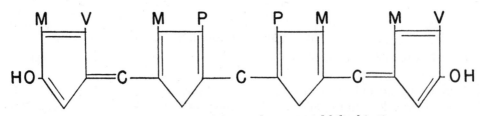

Fig. 38. Structures of free and conjugated bilirubin.[13]

hemoglobin heme released from hemoglobin breakdown can be accounted for usually in these catabolic end products of bilirubin metabolism. A summary of normal bilirubin metabolism is shown diagrammatically in Fig. 40.

A quantitative estimation of daily bilirubin metabolism can be arrived at by the following calculations. Assume a normal adult with a circulating blood volume of 5000 ml, and a hemoglobin concentration of 15 gm/100 ml. This makes 750 gm of circulating hemoglobin. Since the normal life span of the erythrocyte is 100 to 120 days, approximately 1 percent, or 7.5 gm, of hemoglobin will be liberated each day. Each gram of hemoglobin destroyed results in approxi-

mately 35 mg of bilirubin or its derivatives. Therefore, the theoretical calculated daily bilirubin production would be about 260 mg. Although there may be occasional discrepancies between erythrocyte life span and quantity of daily fecal urobilinogen,[12] the theoretical daily output of 260 mg is in harmony with the observed normal range of 100 to 250 mg/day.[17]

ABNORMALITIES OF BILIRUBIN METABOLISM. Jaundice or an increase in the concentration of bilirubin in the blood may result from: (*a*) overproduction (hemolysis), (*b*) failure of removal of free bilirubin by the liver cells, (*c*) failure of conjugation of bilirubin by the liver cells,

400

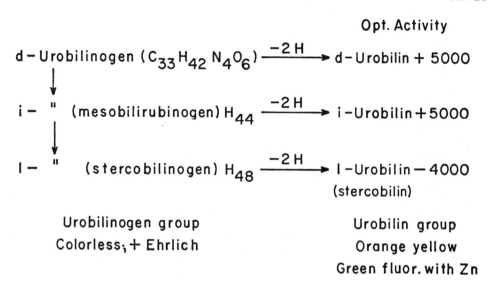

Fig. 39. Interrelations and characteristics of members of the urobilinogen and urobilin group.[12] Although the three members are designated conveniently as *d-*, *i-*, and *l*-forms, it is recognized that they are not isomers.

(*d*) failure of the liver cells to excrete conjugated bilirubin, (*e*) reentry of conjugated bilirubin into the blood due to either hepatocellular damage or biliary-tract obstructions.

The first three of these abnormalities will cause an elevation of free bilirubin in the plasma but no bile in the urine, since free bilirubin, which is water-insoluble, cannot be excreted by the kidneys. There is no increase in the plasma level of conjugated bilirubin. These abnormalities of bilirubin metabolism may be classed together in a group called "retention jaundice."

The last two result in an increase of water-soluble, conjugated bilirubin in the plasma and the appearance of bile in the urine. There may also be an elevation of free bilirubin in the plasma under these conditions. A possible explanation for this is that the accumulation of conjugated bilirubin in the liver cells, due to interference with excretion, slows down the forward progress of the conjugation reaction. The type of jaundice resulting from the mechanisms listed under (*d*) and (*e*) has been called in the past "regurgitation jaundice."

(*a*) *Overproduction or hemolysis.* He-

molytic states may result in a five- or tenfold increase in the rate of destruction of red blood cells. Such conditions include hemolytic anemias, transfusion reactions, large collections of extravasated blood as in hematomas, and massive infarcts of lungs, heart, or other organs. There may also be overproduction in disturbances of porphyrin metabolism. In these situations, the production of free bilirubin exceeds the capacity of the liver to handle the load. The resulting jaundice, due solely to an increase in the plasma concentration of free bilirubin and without any bile in the urine, is called acholuric jaundice. In these hemolytic states, with a normal liver function, there is an increased excretion of conjugated bilirubin in the bile. Urobilinogen output in the stools may then rise to levels of 1000 to 2000 mg/day or even more. The greater-than-normal amount of urobilinogen in the intestine causes more to be absorbed into the enterohepatic circulation. In spite of normal liver function in hemolytic states, more than the usual amount of urobilinogen may escape reexcretion by the liver and appear as an increase in urine urobilinogen. The pattern of bilirubin metabolism asso-

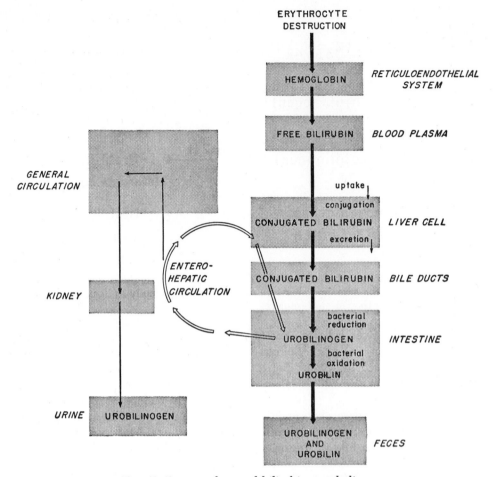

Fig. 40. Pattern of normal bilirubin metabolism.

ciated with overproduction is shown in Fig. 41. Note that the principal clinical abnormalities are increased plasma concentration of free bilirubin, greatly elevated fecal urobilinogen and urobilin, and a slightly larger amount of urine urobilinogen. Of greatest significance is the absence of conjugated bilirubin in the urine.

(*b*) *Decreased uptake by the liver cell.* A number of patients with a benign form of jaundice due to a mild elevation of the plasma concentration of free bilirubin have been studied. This type of jaundice is called constitutional hepatic dysfunction or Gilbert's disease. The rate of erythrocyte destruction is normal in this group. Histologic study of the liver has shown no abnormalities. Investiga-

tion of the conjugating mechanism in these patients has suggested that there is no defect in the glucuronyl transferase enzyme system,[2, 18] although there is some difference of opinion about this.[19] The output of urine and fecal urobilinogen is normal. To explain the mild plasma retention of free bilirubin in these patients, there is speculation about a possible impairment of uptake or transfer of free bilirubin from the plasma to the hepatic cell.[18]

(*c*) *Decreased conjugation of bilirubin.* There are several types of nonhemolytic, acholuric jaundice that have been associated with marked impairment of the glucuronyl transferase enzyme activity of the hepatic cell. One of these is a severe, and usually fatal, congenital, non-

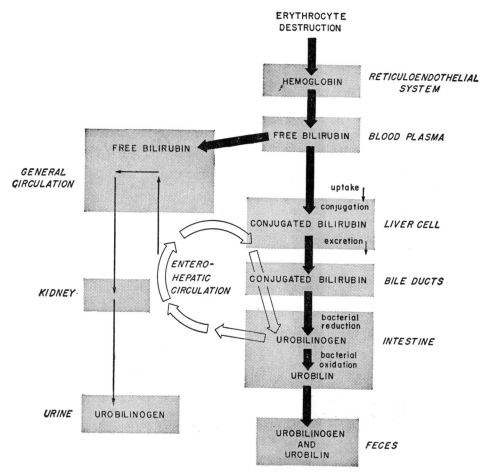

Fig. 41. Pattern of bilirubin metabolism associated with overproduction.

hemolytic jaundice of children called the Crigler-Najjar syndrome.[20, 21] The jaundice of premature and newborn infants is probably due to impaired glucuronide conjugation, since the enzyme systems of fetal and neonatal livers do not approach adult levels of activity until 10 days or so after birth.[22, 23] In both of the above classifications, the plasma concentration of free bilirubin may reach quite high levels. Since there is a defect of conjugation, a marked decrease in the excretion of conjugated bilirubin into the bile will cause a reduction of urobilinogen and urobilinogen production. The mild jaundice of Gilbert's disease has also been attributed to a conjugating enzyme defect, but, as mentioned above, this is debatable. The pattern of bilirubin metabo-

lism associated with defective conjugation is shown in Fig. 42.

It should be noted that the salient clinical features in this group of jaundiced patients is the normal rate of production of free bilirubin, almost complete absence of conjugated bilirubin in the bile, and little or no fecal and urine urobilinogen. The marked retention of free bilirubin in the plasma leads to jaundice without bile in the urine.

(d) Decreased excretion by the liver cell. The next type of abnormality that might disrupt the orderly progress of bilirubin metabolism is impaired transfer of conjugated bilirubin across the hepatic-cell membrane from cell to bile canaliculi. Such a defect of excretion has been postulated for two types of benign

403

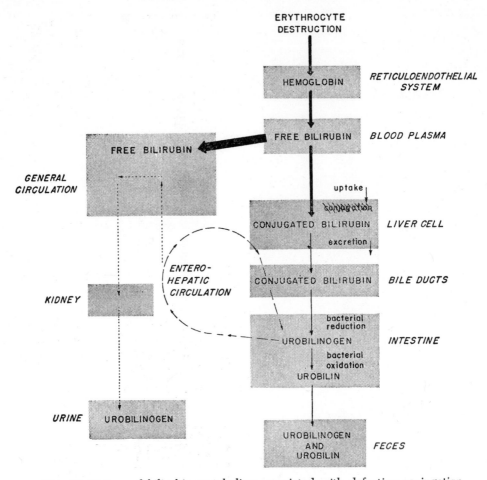

Fig. 42. Pattern of bilirubin metabolism associated with defective conjugation.

jaundice with bile in the urine (choluric jaundice). One of these is chronic idiopathic jaundice with unidentified pigment in liver cells or Dubin-Johnson syndrome. The other is familial, nonhemolytic jaundice, or chronic idiopathic jaundice without pigment in liver cells.[3] Both types are relatively rare, the latter more so. Since in these conditions there is increased plasma concentration of conjugated bilirubin and bile in the urine, it is assumed that enzymatic conjugation of bilirubin is normal. It is not understood why the conjugated bilirubin gets back into the blood stream. An increase in plasma free bilirubin is also found in these patients, explained either by a superimposed impairment in uptake by the hepatic cells or, more likely, by satu-

ration and slowing down of forward progress of the bilirubin-glucuronide-conjugating system.

Although there is an impairment of cellular excretion of conjugated bilirubin into the bile, the block is not complete. Consequently, urobilinogen is formed and reabsorbed into the enterohepatic circulation. Apparently the hepatic-cell excretory defect also applies to reexcretion of urobilinogen because the urinary excretion of urobilinogen is increased in these patients.

(e) *Hepatocellular and obstructive jaundice.* Although the previously described types of jaundice have contributed greatly to our knowledge of the pathophysiology of bilirubin metabolism, hepatocellular and obstructive jaundice have by far the higher incidence and are of greater clinical importance with respect to differential diagnosis. Hepatocellular or medical jaundice implies diseases associated with necrosis or lesser damage to the hepatic parenchymal cells and includes hepatitis in its broad sense, both viral and toxic, as well as cirrhosis. The classification of obstructive jaundice comprises both extrahepatic biliary-tract obstruction or surgical jaundice and intrahepatic obstruction, called cholestasis.

The rate of hemoglobin breakdown and production of free bilirubin is generally normal in these patients. An exception occurs in cirrhosis, where the life span of erythrocytes may be reduced and an element of hemolysis may be present.[24] Enzymatic conjugation of bilirubin

is also active in this group, but, with much hepatocellular damage, the overall conjugating capacity in the liver may be somewhat reduced. The term "regurgitation jaundice" suggests the passage of conjugated bilirubin into the blood stream. The mechanism of regurgitation is not understood. Among the theories to explain regurgitation of conjugated bilirubin is a break in the hepatic-cell barrier between blood in the sinusoid and bile canaliculi because of focal necrosis of hepatic cells in hepatitis. Another explanation is that increased hydrostatic pressure due to extra- or intrahepatic obstruction may rupture the smaller bile canaliculi and permit the entry of conjugated bilirubin into the blood stream. According to the current concept, the

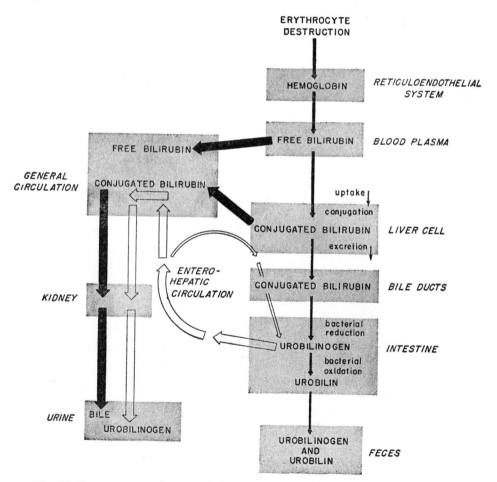

Fig. 43. Pattern of bilirubin metabolism associated with hepatocellular jaundice.

most probable basis for an increase in the blood level of conjugated bilirubin for both hepatocellular and obstructive jaundice is failure of excretion by the liver cells.[25] Because of the reentry of conjugated bilirubin into the blood stream, both hepatocellular and obstructive jaundice are associated with bile in the urine.

The striking difference between hepatocellular and obstructive jaundice is in the metabolism of urobilinogen which is demonstrated by comparing the pattern of bilirubin metabolism in hepatocellular jaundice, as shown in Fig. 43, with the pattern of obstructive jaundice as shown in Fig. 44 which summarizes bilirubin metabolism in the obstructive type. In hepatocellular jaundice, conju-

gated bilirubin continues to be excreted into the intestinal tract. The urobilinogen thus formed is not so efficiently reexcreted by the sick liver, passes into the general circulation, and causes a striking increase in the urinary output of urobilinogen. In obstructive jaundice, on the other hand, little or no conjugated bilirubin reaches the intestine, so there is not much urobilinogen formed. A marked decrease or absence of urine urobilinogen is a characteristic of obstructive jaundice.

Frequently, however, this distinction between hepatocellular and obstructive jaundice is not so clear-cut. The differential may be confused by obstruction appearing in hepatocellular disease due to edema and inspissation of bile in the bile

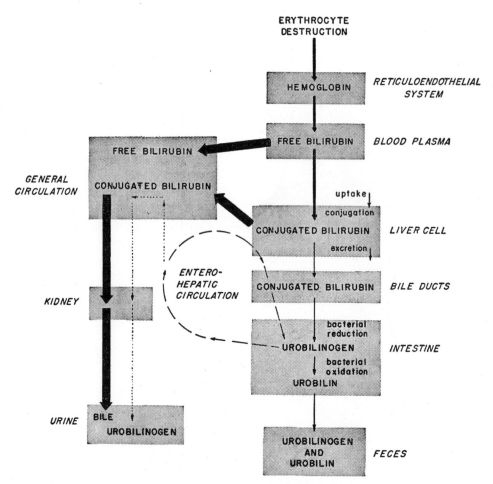

Fig. 44. Pattern of bilirubin metabolism associated with obstructive jaundice.

canaliculi. Then the urinary urobilinogen will become reduced or absent. On the other hand, infection in the biliary tree behind an obstruction may cause bacterial reduction of the conjugated bilirubin present. The urobilinogen so formed can then be absorbed into the general circulation and cause an increase of urine urobilinogen in obstructive jaundice.

The chief differences in bilirubin me-tabolism for the various types of jaundice are summarized in Table 72.

In conclusion, it should be pointed out that the preceding discussion of bilirubin metabolism is somewhat dogmatic and arbitrary, for the sake of simplicity. Intermediate steps have been skipped, and controversial aspects such as the clinical significance of mono- and diglucuronide esters of bilirubin [10, 13] have been omitted.

Table 72. *Classification of disorders of the liver and biliary tract, with notes on pathologic physiology and changes observed in liver-function tests.*

| Anatomic abnormality in liver or biliary system | Clinical entity | Alterations in bilirubin metabolism | Tests for disease of parenchymal cells (exclusive of bilirubin metabolism) | Tests for obstruction to biliary tract (exclusive of bilirubin excretion) |
|---|---|---|---|---|
| None | Hemolytic jaundice | Overproduction; increased free bilirubin in plasma; increased stool urobilin; some increase in urine urobilinogen | Normal | Normal |
| None | Gilbert's disease (constitutional hepatic dysfunction) | Impaired uptake; increased free bilirubin in plasma | Normal | Normal |
| None | Neonatal jaundice (Crigler-Najjar syndrome) | Impaired conjugation; increased free bilirubin in plasma | Normal | Normal |
| Normal hepatic cells; pigment deposition | Dubin-Johnson syndrome | Impaired excretion; bile in urine; increased conjugated bilirubin in plasma | Normal | Normal |
| Hepatocellular necrosis or damage; if cirrhosis, there may also be fibrosis and inflammation of portal areas | Medical jaundice | Reentry of conjugated bilirubin into plasma; bile in urine; increased urine urobilinogen | Abnormal | Essentially normal, except for some elevation of alkaline phosphatase |
| + Bile plugs in bile canaliculi | + Cholangiolitic obstruction | Changes to: Decreased or absent stool urobilin and decreased urine urobilinogen | Abnormal | Abnormal |
| Normal hepatic parenchymal cells; obstruction in biliary tree either extra- or intrahepatic | Obstructive jaundice | Reentry of conjugated bilirubin into plasma; bile in urine; decreased to absent stool urobilin and urine urobilinogen | Normal | Abnormal |
| + Pericholangiolar inflammation | + Cholangitis | Changes to: Increased urine urobilinogen | Somewhat abnormal, depending on duration of disease | Abnormal |

## OTHER EXCRETORY FUNCTIONS

In discussing the metabolism of a single substance, bilirubin, it was shown that several functions of the liver were involved. These were uptake, conjugation by enzyme activity within the liver cell, and excretion. A similar complexity of function must be kept in mind when considering the physiology of other tests related to the liver. Nevertheless, there are several which, along with bilirubin, are considered to be tests of excretory function. These include the excretion of dyes such as bromsulfalein (BSP) and radioactive rose bengal, as well as alkaline phosphatase, and are discussed below under liver-function tests.[26-29]

## PROTEIN METABOLISM

The metabolism of protein is one of the vital functions of the liver. This includes deamination and transamination of amino acids, urea formation, and the synthesis of serum proteins, prothrombin, and enzymes. All of the plasma protein fractions except gamma globulin are synthesized entirely by the liver.[30] Even minor abnormalities of liver function may be associated with abnormal protein synthesis.[31, 32]

Prothrombin and fibrinogen are considered separately because they are essential to blood coagulation (Unit 14). Prothrombin is formed from an unknown precursor in the liver through the influence of vitamin K. A deficiency of prothrombin in the plasma will result when there is decreased synthesis due either to hepatocellular dysfunction or to an inadequate supply of vitamin K. Since the intestinal absorption of vitamin K depends upon the presence of bile salts in the gut, obstructive jaundice is associated with prothrombin deficiency. The parenteral administration of vitamin K will soon restore prothrombin synthesis to normal. If there is sufficient damage to the liver cells, however, no amount of parenteral vitamin K will bring about an improvement in the plasma prothrombin concentration.[33]

## AMMONIA METABOLISM

Ammonia is produced both by deamination of amino acids in the liver and by the action of bacteria on urea in the intestine. It is rapidly removed by synthesis of urea in the liver through glutamic acid and the Krebs-Henseleit ornithine cycle. In the failing liver, urea synthesis is impaired and the accumulation of ammonia in the blood and body tissues may contribute to the clinical picture of hepatic coma.[34-36] Ammonia intoxication may occur even when hepatic parenchymal function is satisfactory, if the products of intestinal bacterial action gain access to the general circulation via the shunts, either natural or iatrogenic, associated with portal hypertension. Methods for measuring the volatile-base content of alkalinized plasma,[37, 38] which is interpreted as the blood ammonia level, have been employed with increasing frequency in clinical laboratories, although the techniques are somewhat nonspecific and are difficult to control without considerable experience. A screening test, employing a semiquantitative estimate of blood ammonia, has been suggested for differentiating the bleeding of esophageal varices from other types of upper-gastrointestinal-tract hemorrhage.[39]

## CARBOHYDRATE METABOLISM

One of the basic, life-preserving functions of the liver is the stabilization of the blood sugar level. This is accomplished by the uptake of ingested carbohydrates, conversion to glucose, and storage in the liver in the form of glycogen for future release as glucose into the general circulation when needed. The liver further maintains the blood sugar level by changing amino acids and other precursors such as glycerol to glucose. The details of carbohydrate metabolism in the liver are beyond the scope of this discussion and may be studied by reference to reviews elsewhere.[9, 31] In liver disease, the storage of glycogen and the metabolism of glucose precursors are reduced. As might be anticipated, there is also a delay in the uptake of ingested glucose, and in the rate of conversion of fructose and galactose to glucose. These pathophysiologic alterations have formed the basis for using tolerance tests for glucose, fructose, and galactose as measures of carbohydrate metabolism by the liver. Glucose and fructose tolerance tests have proved unsatisfactory for this purpose because so many other factors such as metabolism by other tissues may modify the results. The galactose tolerance test,[40] although it is more specific for carbohydrate metabolism in the liver, and can be used as a sensitive index of severe liver damage, has not been generally accepted for clinical use as a liver-function test because it is time-consuming in administration and analysis.

### FAT METABOLISM

The metabolism of fat in the liver appears to be more complex and less well understood than the metabolism of protein and carbohydrate. Such details of fat metabolism as are known are beyond the scope of this discussion and the reader is referred to reviews for further information.[9, 31, 41] In summary, the liver both oxidizes and synthesizes fatty acids. It may convert the latter to triglycerides and phospholipids and make cholesterol from the two carbon residues of fatty-acid oxidation. The liver is also responsible for esterifying cholesterol with fatty acids and for promoting the transport of triglycerides in the blood stream via the fat- and water-solubilizing properties of phospholipids and cholesterol esters. In addition, fat transport is promoted by the coupling of fatty acids, phospholipids, and cholesterol with albumin as alpha lipoprotein and with beta globulin as beta lipoprotein.[41] These complexes, as well as the proteins, are probably synthesized in the liver. The liver makes bile acids from cholesterol, conjugates them with taurine and glycine, and excretes them into the intestine with the bile where they play an important role in the emulsification, digestion, and absorption of dietary fats.

### LIVER ENZYMES

The liver is extremely rich in enzymes.[9] In recent years, there have been rapid advances in the discovery and characterization of the liver enzymes in the serum. Experience with only a few of these enzymes has been sufficiently great, however, to warrant the use of alterations in their serum concentration as tests of liver function. Determinations of serum cholinesterase, of glutamic-oxalacetic transaminase, and of glutamic-pyruvic transaminase fall into this category.

### DETOXIFYING MECHANISMS OF THE LIVER

Conjugation, a function essential to the excretion of bilirubin, bile acids, steroids, and other substances normally metabolized by the liver, is also utilized to rid the body of noxious agents when they have been ingested. This mechanism is employed for such tests of liver function as hippuric acid synthesis,[42] which has been pointed out by Hanger to be much more complex than a simple coupling of benzoic acid with glycine.[6] An ample supply of glycine, high-energy phosphate bonds, plus coenzyme-A, various enzymes, and adequate renal function are all essential to a normal hippuric acid test. This procedure has lost popularity as a liver-function test because of these modifying factors. Other detoxifying mechanisms of the liver such as degradation, phagocytosis, and excretion in the bile have not been used as liver-function tests.

## Methods for Studying Liver Function

Although there are many functions of the liver that might be investigated, "the experience of the last decade has led to the obsolescence of many of the more cumbersome procedures, and has given increasing prominence to those that can be performed rapidly, inexpensively, and accurately, with minimal hardship to the patient and with economy of time and effort to the investigator." [6] Only those tests which are widely used will be described.

MEASUREMENT OF BILIRUBIN IN THE<br>BLOOD

PRINCIPLE. Ehrlich described in 1883 the diazotizing reaction of bilirubin with a mixture of sulfanilic acid, hydrochloric acid, and sodium nitrite, resulting in a red-violet colored pigment called azobilirubin. The quantitative measurement of bilirubin by means of this chemical reaction was reported in 1913 by van den Bergh and Snapper. Since then, this determination of blood bilirubin has been known as the van den Bergh reaction, and the reagent, as Ehrlich's diazo reagent. The technique for quantitative measurement of azobilirubin has been adapted to the photoelectric-cell colorimeter by dilution of the serum with water.[43] If color develops immediately when serum and the diazo reagent are mixed, it is due to the conjugated bilirubin present. This is known as the direct van den Bergh reaction. The free bilirubin in serum will not be diazotized for the most part until it has been made soluble by the addition of methyl alcohol. This is called the indirect van den Bergh reaction. The kinetics of the diazotizing reaction with bilirubin are not completely understood. If serum containing both conjugated and free bilirubin is mixed with the diazo reagent, there will be an immediate development of color, followed by a slow, gradual increase over the following minutes, even without the addition of alcohol. There has been some difference of opinion as to the optimum time to allow for reaction in order to estimate more accurately the

true concentration of conjugated bilirubin. The 1-min reaction time for direct bilirubin as suggested by Ducci and Watson [44] appears to be the most desirable.[45]

METHOD. Fresh Ehrlich's diazo reagent is mixed with diluted serum in a photoelectric colorimeter tube and the amount of color developed is measured exactly 1 min after mixing. Methyl alcohol is then added to the tube and the total color present at the end of 15 min is determined. The quantities of conjugated (direct) and total (15 min) bilirubin are established by reference to calibration curves for the colorimeter. The amount of free (indirect) bilirubin is determined by the following calculation:

Total bilirubin — direct bilirubin
= indirect bilirubin.

INDICATION AND INTERPRETATION. Measurement of serum bilirubin is one of the basic tests related to diseases of the liver. The level of total bilirubin provides a quantitative record of the degree of jaundice, and is used serially in following such cases. The van den Bergh reaction is preferred to the nonspecific icteric index for this purpose.[6, 45] Since the determination of direct-reacting bilirubin, especially by the 1-min direct method, gives an approximate qualitative and quantitative estimate of the concentration of conjugated bilirubin in the blood, there is probably no indication for performing the direct van den Bergh reaction when the urine contains bile (choluria). The direct reaction should be carried out, however, whenever there is jaundice without bile in the urine (acholuric jaundice).

Normal values for the serum concentration of conjugated bilirubin vary somewhat, depending on the arbitrary time interval chosen for duration of the direct van den Bergh reaction. By the 1-min method, the direct-reacting bilirubin ranges from 0 to 0.26 mg/100 ml.

410

The total bilirubin is normally less than 1.0 mg/100 ml.[45] The diagnostic significance of increases in conjugated and free bilirubin is evident from the discussion on physiology and by reference to Table 72. In general, there is an increase in free bilirubin in the serum without an appreciable elevation of conjugated bilirubin when there is overproduction or hemolysis, decreased uptake or Gilbert's disease, and decreased conjugation as in neonatal jaundice and the Crigler-Najjar syndrome. Decreased excretion and reentry of conjugated bilirubin, due to hepatocellular disease or biliary-tract obstruction, are associated with an increase in the serum concentration of both free and conjugated bilirubin. The ratio of direct to total van den Bergh reaction is of little value in the differential diagnosis of medical from surgical types of reentry jaundice.[6] On the other hand, Watson[45] has demonstrated that increases of the 1-min fraction above 0.26 mg/100 ml of serum when the total bilirubin level is still normal may have diagnostic value in preicteric and anicteric hepatitis, portal cirrhosis, carcinoma of the liver, and partial obstruction of the bile duct. Prognostically, there is no correlation between the level of serum bilirubin and the severity of hepatocellular disease.

LIMITATIONS AND SOURCES OF ERROR. The diazo reaction between bilirubin and the van den Bergh reagent is quite specific. Biliverdin is not measured by the diazo test. When free bilirubin has been made water-soluble by addition of methyl alcohol, the quantitative measurement of total serum bilirubin is accurate, provided the serum is diluted to prevent precipitation of protein with adsorbed bilirubin.[43] The measurement of the direct-reacting fraction is less well defined. Theoretically, the direct fraction should be equivalent to the serum concentration of conjugated bilirubin. But at the lower levels of the direct van den Bergh reaction, there are sources of error which may give evidence of conjugated bilirubin when none is present. The technical limitations of the photoelectric colorimeter at low dilutions are one factor.[6, 24, 46] Another is the fact that some free bilirubin may be made water-soluble by urea or protein linkages and thus give a false direct reaction. Then, as has been emphasized, the color due to direct reaction of reagent with bilirubin increases with time, so the levels of direct-reacting bilirubin may be inconsistent with the quantity of conjugated bilirubin present.[45] These difficulties with the accurate determination of low levels of conjugated bilirubin have led to confusion in differentiating mild hepatocellular jaundice (hepatitis) from the mild forms of hemolytic jaundice and constitutional hepatic dysfunction. The significance of small amounts of direct-reacting bilirubin found in the serum of patients with hemolytic jaundice has been reexamined by Tisdale *et al.*,[24] who suggest that there is some reentry of conjugated bilirubin into the blood stream from normal liver cells. Moreover, the fraction of direct-reacting pigment found in the serum under these circumstances is more closely correlated with the amount of bilirubin excreted in the bile than with the total bilirubin concentration of the serum.

DETERMINATION OF BILE IN THE
URINE

The presence of conjugated bilirubin in the urine (choluria) or its absence (acholuria) may be determined by a number of tests which vary from the qualitative and presumptive to the semi-quantitative and specific (see Unit 19). Fortunately, the most reliable tests are inexpensive and simple to perform.

A test for bilirubin in the urine should be used as a routine screening test on every urine specimen. A positive result indicates the presence of liver disease which requires further investigation and has the same significance as an increase of the direct-reacting bilirubin in blood. The lowering of the renal threshold for conjugated bilirubin early in the course of hepatitis makes a screening test for urine bilirubin especially valuable in case detection.

### DETERMINATION OF UROBILINOGEN
### IN THE URINE

A number of methods are available for measuring the group of urobilinogen and urobilin pigments excreted in the urine. An absolutely quantitative measurement of urine urobilinogen requires careful 24-hr collection of urine in specially prepared bottles, reduction of all urobilin to urobilinogen, and extraction of the pigments.[47] This method is not employed as a routine clinical procedure because of the demanding nature of the technique and will not be discussed further. Semiquantitative determination of urine urobilinogen is possible by either the Watson [48] or the Wallace and Diamond method.[49]

WATSON'S METHOD FOR UROBILINOGEN IN THE URINE. *Principle*. Urobilinogen, along with other aldehyde reacting substances found in the urine, reacts with Ehrlich's aldehyde reagent to produce a red color whose intensity is proportional to the amount of pigment present. Since the color continues to deepen over a period of time, the reaction is stopped after 15 sec by the addition of sodium acetate. The amount of urobilinogen is quantitated against pontacyl dye standards in a comparator block or with a colorimeter that has been calibrated.[50] Since other aldehyde reacting substances besides urobilinogen are found in urine, the results are expressed in terms of Ehrlich units. One Ehrlich unit is the color equivalent of 1 mg of pure urobilinogen per 100 ml of solution. There is a greater quantity of urobilinogen excreted in the urine during the afternoon and evening than during the morning. In order to make the test more quantitative, the total urine excreted during a 2-hr period in the afternoon is used. The analysis should be performed soon after collecting the urine in order to avoid the oxidation of urobilinogen to urobilin. Urobilin will not react with Ehrlich's aldehyde reagent.

METHOD. *Reagents*. Saturated aqueous solution of sodium acetate is made as follows. Approximately 1000 gm of sodium acetate containing 3 molecules of water of crystallization is added to 1 L of distilled water in a flask. The mixture is heated to approximately 60°C. When the solution has cooled, it should show a large excess of crystals. The solution must be fully saturated when used or it will fail to stop the color reaction. Ehrlich's aldehyde reagent (Watson's modification) is made as follows: 0.7 gm of paradimethylaminobenzaldehyde is dissolved in a mixture of 150 ml of concentrated hydrochloric acid and 100 ml of distilled water. This reagent is stable if stored in a brown glass bottle.

*Procedure*. At approximately 1 p.m. the patient drinks a large glass of water, empties the bladder, discarding the urine, and records the time of voiding. At 3 p.m., the patient voids again, collecting all of the specimen. The volume and the total time of excretion are recorded. Analysis for urobilinogen is carried out promptly on the fresh urine specimen. If bile is present in considerable amount, it is removed by mixing an aliquot of urine with an equal amount of 10-percent aqueous solution of barium chloride and filtering. The color reaction for urobilinogen is then carried out by measuring 2.5 ml of urine into each of two test tubes. Next, 2.5 ml of Ehrlich's aldehyde reagent is added to the first tube and the contents are thoroughly mixed. At the end of 15 sec, the color reaction is stopped by the addition of 5 ml of saturated sodium acetate solution with careful mixing. This is the unknown tube. The urine sample in the second tube is prepared for a "blank" by first adding 5 ml of sodium acetate solution with thorough mixing, and then adding 2.5 ml of aldehyde reagent. The quantity of urobilinogen equivalent to the color developed can be determined by comparing the color in the unknown tube with pontacyl dye standards in a comparator block, but this is not as satisfactory as the use of a photoelectric colorimeter with a calibration curve.[50]

*Calculation.* The concentration of urobilinogen in the unknown tube is recorded in Ehrlich units per 100 ml. This is multiplied by 4 because the urine has been diluted 4 times in conducting the test. The volume of urine excreted in 2 hr is divided by 100 to convert this volume to the number of 100-ml amounts excreted. If the period of urine excretion is not exactly 2 hr, the volume is corrected to the equivalent of a 2-hr excretion at the rate observed. If bile is removed from the urine, there is a further dilution of the urine by a factor of 2 and this also is put into the equation for calculating the output of urobilinogen. Thus the formula becomes:

$$\text{Ehrlich units in unknown} \times 4 \times \frac{\text{2-hr urine vol. (ml)}}{100 \text{ ml}}$$
$$\times \text{ dilution factor if bile removed} = \text{Ehrlich units/2 hr.}$$

INDICATIONS AND INTERPRETATIONS. Determination of urine urobilinogen excretion is one of the most sensitive tests for the detection of hepatic dysfunction. Its use is indicated in the discovery and in following the progress of various types of hepatocellular disease. It is also of value in differentiating medical from surgical jaundice. The range of normal values for urine urobilinogen excretion by this method is from 0.3 to 1.0 Ehrlich unit/ 2 hr.[51] Values greater than 1.5 Ehrlich units are usually associated with abnormal liver function. If less than 0.3 Ehrlich units are excreted, it usually indicates an impairment of bilirubin excretion in the bile. An increase of urine urobilinogen is characteristic of the pre-

icteric phase of hepatitis and frequently continues after the jaundice has disappeared. Then it may serve as a sensitive index of residual liver damage during the recovery phase.[52] Elevation of urine urobilinogen is frequently found in patients with cirrhosis even though there is only mild icterus. Infection in the bile ducts (cholangitis) associated with partial obstruction may cause an increased output of urobilinogen in the urine. This finding can lead to confusion in the differential diagnosis of obstructive jaundice. The increase of urobilinogen production due to hemolysis may lead to abnormal amounts of urine urobilinogen, especially if there is some associated liver-cell dysfunction.

Small to negligible amounts of urine urobilinogen will be observed when there is either intra- or extrahepatic obstruction, the reduction being proportional to the degree of obstruction. A similar situation occurs during the obstructive (cholangiolitic) phase of hepatitis and again may cause difficulty in the differential diagnosis of medical and surgical jaundice. A reduction in urine urobilinogen may also be caused by reduced rate of red-cell destruction, as in severe hypoplastic anemias.

LIMITATIONS AND SOURCES OF ERROR. The determination of urobilinogen with the aldehyde reagent is not specific for urobilinogen. Other aldehyde reacting chromagens, notably indoles, are excreted in the urine (see Unit 19). In general, their increase or decrease parallels that of urobilinogen so that their presence does not vitiate the diagnostic value of the urine urobilinogen test. Abnormalities of porphyrin metabolism in cases of porphyria and pernicious anemia may also add to the color development during the reaction with Ehrlich's aldehyde reagent.[12] The presence of these other chromagens as well as the diurnal variation in urine urobilinogen excretion makes it impossible to use the simplified

Watson method as a quantitative measure of urobilinogen. Correlation between the urine Ehrlich test and the 24-hr quantitative urinary urobilinogen is satisfactory in about 75 percent of cases.[53]

Sources of error in the use of the semiquantitative test for urobilinogen may be either technical or physiologic. Technically, the greatest errors may be caused by inadequate mixing of the urine and reagents during each step of the procedure. Experience with large groups of students has demonstrated difficulties with the procedure because of contamination of reagents by the careless use of dirty pipettes. Physiologic errors may be introduced by acute febrile illnesses, circulatory disturbances, or severe anemias which impair liver function and result in an increase of urobilinogen. Diarrhea and other states of intestinal malabsorption may decrease the interohepatic circulation of urobilinogen and reduce urine urobilinogen. A special note of caution is indicated concerning the use of urine urobilinogen determinations when antibiotics are administered because they interrupt the formation of urobilinogen in the intestine by inhibiting the growth of intestinal bacteria.

### WALLACE AND DIAMOND METHOD FOR UROBILINOGEN IN THE URINE

PRINCIPLE. In general, the same principle holds for this method as for the Watson method. Urobilinogen and other chromagens react with paradimethylaminobenzaldehyde to produce a red color. The concentration of chromagens in the urine is determined semiquantitatively by serial dilutions of the urine.[49]

METHOD. *Reagents.* Ehrlich's aldehyde reagent is made by dissolving 2 gm of paradimethylaminobenzaldehyde in 100 ml of a 20-percent aqueous solution of concentrated hydrochloric acid.

*Procedure.* From 6 to 10 clean test tubes of the same internal diameter are placed in a test-tube rack for the serial dilution of a fresh random urine sample. Cool tap water, in 5-ml aliquots, is placed in all but the first test tube Then 5-ml aliquots of urine are pipetted into each of the first two tubes. If the urine contains much bilirubin, it should be removed with barium chloride as previously described. The urine and water in the second tube are mixed and 5 ml of the mixture is transferred to the third tube. Serial dilutions are thus carried out until the last tube, from which 5 ml of mixture is removed and kept for further dilution, if required. After the dilutions—1 : 1, 1 : 2, 1 : 4, 1 : 8, 1 : 16, . . . —have been made, 0.5 ml of Ehrlich's aldehyde reagent is added to each tube and thoroughly mixed. The tubes are allowed to stand for 5 min for color development, which is then read by looking vertically through the solution at a white background placed in bright daylight. The last dilution in which a faint pink color appears is recorded as the end point. If the end point is not reached by the dilutions made, the series is extended.

INDICATIONS AND INTERPRETATIONS. The same indications and interpretations hold for the use of the Wallace and Diamond method as for the Watson method, but the latter, more quantitative procedure is preferred, if available. The normal range for urine urobilinogen with the Wallace and Diamond technique is an end point in the 1 : 8 or 1 : 16 dilution. A pink color in dilutions of 1 : 64 or higher is indicative of an increased urine urobilinogen excretion, while a faint pink color found only in the undiluted or 1 : 2 dilution is evidence for a decrease in urobilinogen excretion. If bile has been removed from the urine, it must be remembered that the dilution in the first tube is 1 : 2 and the rest of the dilutions are increased correspondingly.

LIMITATIONS AND SOURCES OF ERROR. The Wallace and Diamond procedure will detect one part of urobilinogen in 640,000 parts of water, but it is not as specific or quantitative as the Watson method. The former does not take into account the variations in urinary volume output per hour, nor is the time for color development controlled. Consequently, the chromagens other than urobilinogen may play a larger role in color development. The same physiologic sources of error apply here as for the Watson technique.

#### QUALITATIVE DETECTION OF UROBILIN AND UROBILINOGEN IN THE STOOL

The quantitative measurement of the end products of bilirubin metabolism in the stool involves such demanding technical procedures that it is used primarily for clinical investigation.[47] A qualitative method devised by Watson [51] has proved to be a rapid and simple screening procedure of considerable value.

PRINCIPLE. Urobilin and urobilinogen are extracted from the stool with an alcoholic solution of zinc acetate. Urobilin reacts with zinc to produce a green fluorescence that is roughly proportional to the amount of urobilin. The reaction with Ehrlich's aldehyde reagent is used to demonstrate the presence of urobilinogen.[51]

METHOD. *Reagents.* A saturated alcoholic solution of zinc acetate is prepared as follows. Approximately 50 gm of zinc acetate, with 2 molecules of water of crystallization, is added to a flask containing 1 L of 95-percent ethyl alcohol. The mixture is heated to 50°C in a water bath, with frequent stirring, until dissolved. On cooling, the solution should show some recrystallization and should be used only when saturated. The Ehrlich's aldehyde reagent (Watson modification) and saturated aqueous solution of sodium acetate are made as already described (p. 412) for the urine urobilinogen method of Watson.

*Procedure.* Fresh stool is required for the estimation of urobilinogen, but any stool may be used for detection of urobilin. A sample of stool, approximately 2 gm in amount, is emulsified with an applicator stick in 10 ml of saturated alcoholic solution of zinc acetate. The mixture is filtered and 2.5 ml of clear filtrate is mixed thoroughly in a test tube with 2.5 ml of Ehrlich's aldehyde reagent. Fifteen seconds later, 5 ml of the saturated aqueous solution of sodium acetate is added with complete mixing. The final product may be slightly cloudy, but a pink color development is due primarily to urobilinogen. The presence of urobilin may be demonstrated in a sample of untreated zinc acetate filtrate from the stool by the production of green fluorescence when a narrow beam of light, as from a pencil flashlight, is transmitted through the solution.

INDICATIONS AND INTERPRETATIONS. Although the brown color of feces usually indicates the presence of adequate amounts of urobilin, the physician cannot be sure whether urobilin and urobilinogen are absent, decreased, or normally present in gray, clay-colored, or putty-colored stools where the major factor contributing to the change in stool color is an excess amount of fat (see Unit 22). The qualitative screening test for urobilin and urobilinogen should be applied to light-colored stools. Absence of both a green fluorescence in the clear filtrate and pink color after reacting with the aldehyde reagent indicates that conjugated bilirubin has been excluded from the intestinal tract and the stool is acholic. This has all of the diagnostic implications that have been previously described. Marked reduction of both green fluorescence and pink color, as compared with that obtained from a normal stool, suggests partial obstruction in the biliary tract. If the screening test shows either a normal range of green fluorescence or pink color, the stool content of bile pigments should be within normal limits.

415

An excessive amount of urobilinogen production in association with hemolysis may result in a very deep-red color and a bright-green fluorescence when this screening test for urobilinogen and urobilin is applied to such stools.

LIMITATIONS AND SOURCES OF ERROR. As already indicated, this procedure is qualitative, but may be interpreted in a semiquantitative manner. The major source of error results from the oral administration of antibiotics which disrupt the bacterial production of urobilinogen.

BROMSULFALEIN (BSP) EXCRETION TEST

"This test appears to approach nearer than any to the perfect function test, although it must be remembered that only one function is being tested." [6]

PRINCIPLE. When the dye bromsulfalein (phenoltetrabromphthalein sodium sulfonate; BSP) is injected intravenously, it circulates in the blood in combination with serum proteins. It is taken up by the hepatic cells at a rate of 10–16 percent per minute of the concentration of dye remaining in the blood.[54] Transfer of BSP from blood to bile is a rate-limited mechanism depending in part upon the conjugation of BSP with glycine and glutamic acid.[55] The volume of liver blood flow and the health and mass of liver parenchymal cells affects the rate of clearance of the dye. Obstruction in the biliary tract interferes with excretion of the dye into the bile. Shock, anemia, fever, and advanced age may cause increased retention of BSP in the plasma.[56] An enterohepatic circulation of the dye has been suggested.[57] When made alkaline, BSP becomes red-purple in color, which makes it possible to determine the concentration of the dye in serum. When given intravenously in a dose proportional to body weight, the amount of dye remaining in the blood at the end of a measured period of time can be corre-

lated with the degree of impairment of liver function.[29, 48]

METHOD. The patient is weighed, but no allowance is made for obesity or ascites. Bromsulfalein, available in ampules as a sterile 5-percent solution, is drawn into a sterile 10-ml syringe. The quantity of the dye used is calculated at the rate of 5 mg/kg body weight or 1 ml of solution for 10 kg of weight. It is injected slowly into an antecubital vein. Note the time when the injection is completed. Caution must be exercised to see that none of the dye escapes outside the vein, or a painful slough may result. Forty-five minutes later, a 10-ml sample is withdrawn from a vein in the other arm, and a clear syringe is used in order to avoid any contamination of the sample with dye. The blood is permitted to clot and the serum is separated. A 2.5-ml aliquot of serum is pipetted into each of two colorimeter tubes. Two drops of a 10-percent aqueous solution of sodium hydroxide is added to one tube. This converts any dye present in the serum to its colored form. One drop of 5-percent hydrochloric acid is mixed with the serum in the other tube to maintain the dye in a colorless state. This second tube serves as a "blank" in the colorimeter or comparator block. Although comparator blocks with standards are available, it is preferable to use a photoelectric colorimeter to measure the concentration of BSP in the serum, which is reported as percentage of BSP retained. When a 5 mg/kg dose of dye and a time interval of 45 min have been used for the test, the standard reference curve for the colorimeter is based upon a concentration of 10 mg of BSP per 100 ml of serum as being equivalent to 100-percent retention.

INDICATIONS AND INTERPRETATION. Normal values are less than 5-percent retention of the dye. The BSP test is indicated as a sensitive detector of early or latent hepatocellular disease and is of value in following the progress of hepatitis or cirrhosis. There is some correlation between the severity of liver damage and the amount of BSP remaining in the serum. The test has also been of help in differentiating bleeding of esophageal varices from that associated with ulcer or gastritis, because the former is usually secondary to portal cirrhosis which favors a higher and more persistent retention of dye in the serum.[56] Finally, the BSP test is an adjunct to the diagnosis of partial obstruction to the outflow of bile, even without significant retention of bilirubin, a condition that may prevail with either extrahepatic obstruction [58] or intrahepatic space-occupying lesions.[59] Thus, the BSP test may provide an early indication of metastatic cancer in the liver.

LIMITATIONS AND SOURCES OF ERROR. Although the BSP test is perhaps the most sensitive of all liver-function tests, elevation of BSP level in the serum does not indicate the type of dysfunction in the liver. Hepatocellular damage, decreased circulation, as in portal cirrhosis, or impairment of bile outflow, will all result in BSP retention. If performed with care, there is little chance of technical error in the test. There are, however, physiologic causes for a "false positive" BSP test, such as fever, shock, anemia, and old age.[56] A note of caution is indicated regarding the slight hazard associated with giving BSP. The danger of tissue necrosis and thrombosis at the site of injection from extravasated dye has been mentioned previously. Occasional toxic reactions, headache, weakness, chills, and fever, have been reported. These can be prevented by injecting the dye slowly over a period of 5 min. There have also been rare allergic manifestations [60] and at least one death [61] associated with repeated use of the dye in sensitive individuals. In these cases, BSP appears to act as a hapten.

## DETERMINATION OF ALKALINE PHOSPHATASE OF SERUM

PRINCIPLE AND METHOD. Alkaline phosphatase comprises one or more enzymes of the blood capable of hydrolyzing organic phosphates such as glycerol and phenyl phosphates in the alkaline pH range with a maximum activity at pH 9.5.[62] Origin and more specific identity of blood alkaline phosphatase is obscure, but zone electrophoresis suggests a method for separating alkaline phosphatases.[63] Some of it arises in osteoblastic activity of the bones. Small amounts have been demonstrated by histochemical techniques in the normal liver, but regenerating liver tissue is rich in the enzyme and the epithelial cells of bile ducts show increased staining for alkaline phosphatase when there is obstruction in the biliary tract. The relation of these histochemical observations to the level of blood alkaline phosphatase is not known. Alkaline phosphatase is excreted into the bile presumably by a different mechanism than bilirubin.[6, 7] The excretory mechanism of alkaline phosphatase appears to be more readily impaired by even slight degrees of obstruction to the biliary tree than is the excretion of bilirubin.[6, 58] The marked increase in concentration of serum alkaline phosphatase with infiltrative diseases of the liver suggests that production by the liver cells as well as impaired excretion may play a role in elevating the blood alkaline phosphatase.[64] Although the pathophysiology of alkaline phosphatase is poorly understood, experience has shown that the demonstration of an elevated serum alkaline phosphatase is a valuable adjunct to the diagnosis of obstructive jaundice.[6, 7, 62, 64] Alkaline phosphatase of the serum is determined by its activity in liberating inorganic phosphorus from an organic phosphate ester, glycerophos-

417

phate. The substrate is made up in a barbiturate buffer at pH 8.6 in such a concentration that 10 ml of buffered organic phosphate solution will yield 5 mg of inorganic phosphorus. One milliliter of serum is incubated at 37°C for 1 hr with 10 ml of buffered substrate. The inorganic-phosphorus concentration resulting from this reaction is measured, and the concentration present in the serum prior to incubation is also determined. The difference between these two values is the result of alkaline phosphatase activity, which is expressed in Bodansky units. A Bodansky unit is the activity needed to liberate 1 mg of inorganic phosphorus under the conditions of the reaction as stated.[65] Other substrates and units of activity have also been used to determine alkaline phosphatase activity. In the King-Armstrong method, the amount of phenol hydrolyzed from phenyl phosphate is measured.[66]

INDICATIONS AND INTERPRETATION. The normal range of alkaline phosphatase activity is 0.5 to 4.0 Bodansky units [65] or 3 to 13 King-Armstrong units.[66] Determination of serum alkaline phosphatase is very useful in differentiating the jaundice due to hepatocellular dysfunction from that caused by obstruction. Gutman *et al.*[67] observed that 90 percent of patients with common-duct obstruction had serum alkaline phosphatase levels above 10 Bodansky units, while a similar percentage of hepatitis patients had less than 10 Bodansky units. Although there is some overlap, our experience has shown that most cases of obstructive jaundice are associated with an alkaline phosphatase level of more than 15 Bodansky units and medical jaundice with less than 15 units. When using King-Armstrong units, the dividing line is set at 30. The differential diagnostic value of alkaline phosphatase determination is increased when it is combined with the cephalin flocculation test.[68] There is usually an element of obstruction, cholangio-

litis, or fibrosis in those patients with medical jaundice who show greater elevations of serum alkaline phosphatase.

There is frequently a very marked increase in serum alkaline phosphatase activity without jaundice in patients with cancer in the liver or liver abscesses,[59] as well as in some cases of cirrhosis. An enlarged liver and increasing serum alkaline phosphatase should make the physician very suspicious of metastatic cancer of the liver, lymphoma, or a granulomatous disease like sarcoid or tuberculosis.

LIMITATIONS AND SOURCES OF ERROR. Determination of serum alkaline phosphatase activity is considered an empirical test of liver function because it measures no known function and the source of the alkaline phosphatase has not been completely established. Nevertheless, this test has been proved to be of considerable clinical value in spite of its lack of specificity. Bone disease, such as rickets, Paget's disease, or osteogenic sarcoma, as well as hyperparathyroidism, will cause an elevation of alkaline phosphatase. These must be considered when interpreting the significance of this test (see Unit 32).

MEASUREMENT OF SERUM PROTEINS

Alterations in the concentration of various fractions of serum proteins in liver disease can be measured by chemical or electrophoretic methods,[69-72] and are of value both in differentiating hepatocellular jaundice from obstructive jaundice and in estimating the severity of liver disease (see Unit 16). Of even greater importance from the diagnostic standpoint in hepatocellular disease, quantitative and qualitative alterations in serum protein fractions are the basis for a series of flocculation tests which determine the stability of serum proteins.[73-76] Since albumin is synthesized in the liver parenchymal cells and gamma globulin, the major component of the globulin fraction, originates in the reticuloendothelial system, there is little relation between these two components. Consequently, there is no real meaning to the so-called A/G (albumin/globulin) ratio which has been used for many years in clinical medicine. In diseases of the liver, there is a lowering of the albumin fraction somewhat in proportion to the degree of damage to the hepatic cells. It takes a number of days for decreased synthesis of albumin in the liver to be reflected by a measurable chemical change in serum proteins. Therefore there is no appreciable alteration in acute hepatitis. Decreased serum albumin and elevations of serum globulin are characteristic of chronic liver disease, either hepatitis or cirrhosis. An increasing serum albumin level associated with treatment is a hopeful prognostic sign in these cases. No changes are to be found in obstructive jaundice unless there is liver damage secondary to prolonged obstruction.

Paper electrophoresis is discussed in Unit 16. When serum proteins are analyzed by this technique in acute hepatitis, the albumin fraction may be decreased with some elevation of alpha$_2$ globulin and no change in beta globulin. At first, the gamma globulin fraction is unchanged, but with duration of the disease and for weeks or months after clinical recovery, gamma globulin is elevated. With advanced parenchymal liver disease, chronic hepatitis, or cirrhosis of all etiologies, there is a marked reduction of albumin, variable changes in alpha$_1$, alpha$_2$, and beta globulins, and an increase in gamma globulin, often to a marked degree.[72] As far as the lipoproteins are concerned, there is elevation of the beta lipoproteins in obstructive jaundice and in hepatitis,[77] while the beta lipoproteins may be decreased to virtually absent in advanced cirrhosis.[72]

None of the changes in serum proteins described above are specific for diseases of the liver. Low serum albumin levels may be found also in nephrotic syndrome and in malnutrition states such as inadequate intake, impaired intestinal absorption, or excessive protein loss from ulcerating surfaces. Hyperglobulinemia is by no means restricted to chronic liver disease (see Table 52, Unit 16). Therefore the changes in serum protein patterns must be interpreted in the light of the total clinical picture.

### STABILITY REACTIONS OF SERUM

Included under this heading is a group of empirical tests, developed as a result of chance observations, that have proved to be helpful in the diagnosis of liver disease.

PRINCIPLE. The mechanisms responsible for positive turbidity and flocculation reactions are not understood completely. In a general way, they all reflect an absolute or relative increase in gamma globulin, and pathologic globulin may also have a more intense flocculating power than normal globulin. Normal albumin acts as an inhibitor to positive stability reactions, but this inhibitory effect is decreased in hepatocellular diseases which cause both a reduction in quantity and a qualitative change in albumin. An increase in beta lipoproteins contributes to abnormal thymol turbidity reaction.[62, 73, 76]

The physicochemical basis for flocculation and turbidity reactions has been reviewed by Saifer[76] and by Maclagan.[78] Details are beyond the scope of this chapter. In summary, proteins are stabilized in solution by an electric double layer at their surface, and by solvation. Instability is introduced by a change of pH to the isoelectric point of the proteins, which reduces the potential difference across the electric double layer, and by dilution, which decreases the ionic strength of the solution. In developing flocculation and turbidity tests, the physicochemical details of the procedure are established in such a way that the proteins in pathologic serums become unstable and precipitate, while normal serum proteins remain stabilized under the same conditions.

The many tests for stability reaction of the serum can be divided into three general categories, each somewhat different in principle.[76] The tests chosen as examples of these categories are the three tests most commonly used in clinical medicine.

(*a*) In the cephalin-cholesterol flocculation reaction, the reagent is a charged colloidal suspension which is flocculated out of solution by a change in charge distribution of the proteins in the fluid tested.[76]

(*b*) The thymol turbidity test is an example of the category in which certain protein fractions of pathologic serums are precipitated out either by organic compounds containing phenolic linkages or by strongly polar compounds like water and alcohol, which neutralize the charged field around the protein molecules.[76]

(*c*) The third classification is represented by the zinc sulfate turbidity test, which depends primarily upon an interaction between protein and a divalent metal ion.[76]

METHODS. (*a*) *Cephalin-cholesterol flocculation.*[79] The reagent is a cephalin-cholesterol emulsion prepared from sheep brain and now available commercially. One milliliter of a fresh dilution of this emulsion, prepared from the stock solution according to directions, is added to 4 ml of a 1 : 20 dilution of fresh serum with 0.85-percent sodium chloride solution. After mixing in a stoppered test tube, it is left undisturbed in a dark cabinet at room temperature for 24 and 48 hr. A saline blank, a known normal serum, and a known positive serum are set up at the same time to check on the stability of the reagent. The degree of flocculation is read at the end of 24 and 48 hr. It is graded and reported as follows:

| Report | Grade of Flocculation |
|---|---|
| 0 | No precipitation, fluid opalescent as in original set-up |
| 1+ | Slight precipitation, slight clearing of fluid |
| 2+ | Moderate precipitation, moderate clearing of fluid |
| 3+ | Heavy precipitation, almost complete clearing of fluid |
| 4+ | Heavy precipitation, complete clearing of fluid |

Flocculations of 0 and 1+ are normal, 2+ is borderline, and 3+ and 4+ are evidence of an abnormal protein pattern in the serum.

(*b*) *Thymol turbidity.* The reagent is a saturated solution of thymol in barbiturate buffer at pH 7.8 made according to the directions of Maclagan.[80] Six milliliters of reagent is added to 0.1 ml of serum, mixed, and observed for turbidity at the end of 30 min. Originally, the degree of turbidity was determined by comparing the test mixture with the Kingsbury standards for urine protein (see Unit 19). Quantitation of the turbidity has been improved by measuring it in a photoelectric colorimeter, using a filter for 650 m$\mu$, and comparing with a standard curve prepared from barium sulfate suspensions.[81] The colorimeter modification eliminates the difficulties caused by bilirubin or hemoglobin when the visual-comparison technique is employed. If the pH of the reagent is changed from 7.8 to 7.55, the thymol turbidity test appears to become more sensitive for hepatocellular dysfunction without introducing false positive results.[82] Normal values by the colorimeter method are 0 to 4 Shank-Hoagland units.[81]

The thymol flocculation test is not a necessary part of the thymol turbidity reaction, but may be used as an adjunct. If the reaction mixture for the turbidity test is set aside in a dark cabinet, it may be observed after 24 and 48 hr for turbidity which is graded and reported according to the same criteria as for the cephalin-cholesterol test.

(*c*) *Zinc sulfate turbidity.* The reagent for this procedure consists of 24 mg of zinc sulfate, with seven molecules of water of crystallization dissolved in 1 L of barbiturate buffer at pH 7.5. Six milliliters of reagent is mixed with 0.1 ml of serum in a colorimeter tube. After 30 min, the degree of turbidity is read in a photoelectric colorimeter at 650 m$\mu$. The units of turbidity are determined by comparison with a standard curve derived from barium sulfate suspensions similar to that for thymol turbidity. The normal range is from 2 to 12 units.[83]

INDICATIONS AND INTERPRETATION. The use of protein-flocculation tests is indicated for the detection of acute and chronic diseases of the hepatic parenchymal cells. These procedures are also of value in the differential diagnosis of medical and surgical jaundice. The choice of which tests of stability reaction of serum to use depends in part upon the simplicity and reliability of the method and in part on the personal experiences of the physician with the various tests. All three protein-flocculation tests might well be employed because they vary in selectivity and sensitivity,[62] since each test measures different changes in the serum protein pattern.

As a general rule, the protein-flocculation test results are usually positive in parenchymal diseases of the liver and most often negative when there is uncomplicated biliary-tract obstruction. When flocculation tests are combined with alkaline phosphatase determinations, the accuracy of differentiating between medical and surgical jaundice is improved over the results of either test by itself.[68, 84] In the diagnosis and follow-up study of acute hepatitis, the cephalin flocculation becomes positive early in the course of the disease, but the thymol turbidity is elevated later be-

cause of the delayed rise of serum lipids in hepatitis[85] and persists for many months after clinical recovery. The thymol turbidity is also markedly elevated in active post-necrotic cirrhosis and chronic hepatitis, while the cephalin flocculation is more often positive in other forms of cirrhosis if the process is active. The zinc sulfate turbidity, which is primarily a measure of gamma globulin, is the most sensitive test for the study of long-standing hepatocellular degeneration.[86] Although the flocculation tests are usually negative in obstructive jaundice, the increase of serum lipoproteins caused by prolonged obstruction may result in a positive thymol turbidity.

LIMITATIONS AND SOURCES OF ERROR. The limitation of these tests lies in their lack of specificity, since the change in serum-protein pattern responsible for a positive reaction is common to a number of diseases.[78] Included in this list of diseases are malaria, infectious mononucleosis, pneumonia, kala-azar, chronic lung infections, endocarditis, brucellosis, rheumatic fever, rheumatoid arthritis, disseminated lupus, tuberculosis, and multiple myeloma.[76] The lipemic serum associated with nephrosis may cause a nonspecific elevation of thymol turbidity. The specificity of these tests is further limited by the fact that they may remain negative in 10 to 20 percent of patients with hepatitis,[68, 78] and positive flocculations may occur in up to 16 percent of patients with obstructive jaundice.[79] Technical factors may play a role in reducing the reliability of protein-flocculation tests. This is particularly true for the cephalin-cholesterol flocculation. The preparation and stability of the reagent presents difficulties. Exposure to light, increase in temperature of the reaction, age of the serum, and contamination of glassware with traces of acid may cause false positive cephalin flocculations. Purity of the barbiturates and pH of the buffer must be carefully controlled to avoid lowered pH which makes the thymol-turbidity test positive even with normal serum. Variations in the normal range for thymol turbidity and zinc sulfate turbidity may result from a lack of uniformity in the preparation of barium sulfate suspension standards.[87] The results of stability reactions of serum must be interpreted with an understanding of the role of nonhepatic diseases in causing positive test results and the causes of technical errors must be considered also.

### DETERMINATION OF TOTAL CHOLESTEROL AND CHOLESTEROL ESTERS IN THE SERUM

The measurement of cholesterol and cholesterol esters of the serum is a technically exacting procedure.

PRINCIPLE AND METHOD. Cholesterol is extracted from serum with a mixture of three parts absolute ethyl alcohol and one part anhydrous ethyl ether. The extracted mixture is carefully evaporated to dryness and the cholesterol is taken up in chloroform. The concentration of cholesterol is determined by the development of a blue color resulting when concentrated sulfuric acid in acetic anhydride is added. This is the Liebermann-Burchard reaction. The amount of cholesterol is measured in a photoelectric colorimeter and quantitated by comparison with a standard curve made with known cholesterol solutions.[88]

Cholesterol esters are determined in a somewhat similar fashion after the free cholesterol of the alcohol-ether extract has been precipitated by digitonin. The alcohol-ether mixture is evaporated and the cholesterol esters are selectively extracted with petroleum ether, leaving the precipitated cholesterol-digitonide behind. After the petroleum ether has been evaporated from the cholesterol esters, the latter are dissolved in chloroform and the Liebermann-Burchard reaction is carried out. The amount of cholesterol esters is quantitated in a photoelectric colorimeter with a standard curve of reference.[89]

INDICATIONS AND INTERPRETATION. The normal values for total cholesterol range from 150 to 280 mg/100 ml and the esters comprise 50 to 65 percent of the total. Determination of total cholesterol and cholesterol esters is an adjunct to the study of both obstructive jaundice and parenchymal liver disease. In patients with obstructive lesions of the biliary tract there may be a significant rise in both total cholesterol and esters so that the percentage of esters remains within normal limits. The increase in serum cholesterol is somewhat proportional to the duration of biliary-tract obstruction. In both acute and chronic parenchymal disease of the liver, the total cholesterol concentration in the serum may be normal or reduced, but esterification is markedly depressed. Both the total cholesterol and esters are greatly reduced in liver failure. Consequently, serial determinations of cholesterol and esters are of prognostic value in patients with medical jaundice.

LIMITATIONS AND SOURCES OF ERROR. There are significant limitations to this test as a measure of liver function, since changes may occur in other diseases that do not affect the liver or biliary tree. Total cholesterol may be greatly elevated in nephrotic syndrome, diabetes mellitus, and hypothyroidism, while severe malnutrition in association with malignant obstruction of the bile duct may result in a marked decrease of total cholesterol. The determination of cholesterol esters is a time-consuming procedure, hence its routine use is limited.

### DETERMINATION OF LIVER ENZYMES IN THE SERUM

Among the many enzymes of hepatic origin which have been investigated in the serum, three have become useful as clinical tools. These are the serum cholinesterase, serum oxalacetic-glutamic transaminase (SGOT), and serum pyruvic-glutamic transaminase (SGPT).

SERUM CHOLINESTERASE. *Principle and method.* The cholinesterase activity of the serum may be measured electrometrically or colorimetrically. The first method depends upon the measurement of the amount of acetic acid resulting from the action of cholinesterase on acetyl choline over a 2-hr period, at standard temperature and pH of the reaction medium. The quantity of acetic acid liberated is determined by the change in pH, which is measured with a glass electrode.[90] In the colorimetric method, the enzyme hydrolyzes carbonaphthoxycholine, a choline ester, and liberates $\beta$-naphthol, which combines with a diazonium salt, tetrazotized diorthoanisidine, to form a colored dye. The dye is extracted with ethyl acetate and measured in a colorimeter. The readings are converted to milligrams of $\beta$-naphthol and the enzyme activity is expressed in units, one unit being equivalent to the amount of enzyme activity needed to liberate 10 mg of $\beta$-naphthol in 1 hr.[91]

*Indication and interpretation.* The normal range of values may vary from one laboratory to another, according to the method or modification.[91, 92] Each laboratory should establish its own norm. The determination of serum cholinesterase may be of value when used serially to follow the course of subacute or chronic parenchymal liver disease. The serum level is depressed in compensated cirrhosis and even more so in decompensated cirrhosis.[93] Very low levels in hepatitis or cirrhosis presage a fatal outcome.

*Limitations and sources of error.* The cholinesterase determined in the serum is nonspecific. The range of normals overlaps widely the range in disease states. Consequently, the test is of little diagnostic value.[94] It is of no help in differentiating medical from surgical jaundice. Malnutrition will decrease the se-

rum cholinesterase.[95] This test is not recommended for routine clinical use.

SERUM TRANSAMINASES. *Principle and method* (see also Unit 17). Transaminases are enzymes that promote the transfer of an amino group from an $\alpha$ amino acid to a keto acid with formation of a new amine and $\beta$ acid. The following equations describe the chemical reactions which concern SGOT and SGPT:

$$\text{Aspartate} + \text{ketoglutarate} \underset{}{\overset{\text{SGOT}}{\rightleftharpoons}} \text{glutamate} + \text{oxalacetate,}$$

$$\text{Alanine} + \text{ketoglutarate} \underset{}{\overset{\text{SGPT}}{\rightleftharpoons}} \text{glutamate} + \text{pyruvate.}$$

The transaminase activity can be measured by quantitating the amount of glutamate with the aid of paper chromatography,[96] but this is less practical than the spectrophotometric determination of the change from reduced DPNH to oxidized DPN brought about by the formation of oxalacetate or pyruvate. These reactions are depicted in the following two equations.[96, 97]

$$\text{Oxalacetate} + \text{DPNH} \underset{\text{dehydrogenase}}{\overset{\text{malic}}{\rightleftharpoons}} \text{l-malate} + \text{DPN,}$$

$$\text{Pyruvate} + \text{DPNH} \underset{\text{dehydrogenase}}{\overset{\text{lactic}}{\rightleftharpoons}} \text{lactate} + \text{DPN.}$$

The oxidation of DPNH to DPN is followed by the change in light absorption at 340 m$\mu$ which is decreased as oxidation proceeds. A transaminase unit is defined as the decrease of optical density by 0.001 in 1 min.[96]

*Indication and interpretation.* The normal values for SGOT are 5 to 40 units/ml min [98] and for SGPT are 7 to 25 units/ml min.[99] Since transaminase is released from the cell, these tests are of value in the diagnosis of diseases that cause hepatic necrosis, especially acute hepatitis, where the serum levels of transaminases are frequently elevated early in the course of the disease before jaundice appears. The serum transaminases are also greatly increased in cases of toxic hepatitis and metastatic involvement of the liver. Elevation of transaminases may occur with extra- or intrahepatic obstruction as well as with hepatocellular disease; but in the former, the values may increase up to 300 or 400 units/ml min, whereas in the latter, there are often elevations above 2500 or 3000 units/ml min.[98–100]

*Limitations and sources of error.* There are large quantities of oxalacetic-glutamic transaminase in heart, kidney, and muscle. Diseases that cause cellular damage to these organs may result in elevations of SGOT in a range similar to that in biliary-tract obstruction. SGPT is more specific for hepatic parenchymal damage than SGOT. The final evaluation of transaminase determinations in the study of liver function awaits further experience.

### DUODENAL DRAINAGE AND X-RAY

Drainage of duodenal juice with examination of the bile is an adjunct to the study of patients with disease of the biliary system.[101, 102] Careful placement of the fenestrated tip of a duodenal tube at the ampulla of Vater under fluoroscopic control and the meticulous collection of clear, bile-colored juice with siphonage makes it a tedious and time-consuming procedure. This test is indicated in patients who are suspected of having stones or obstructing lesions in the biliary system when oral and intravenous cholecystograms and cholangiograms fail to show a satisfactory filling of the gall bladder and bile ducts. Demonstration of bilirubin crystals and cholesterol plates in the spun sediment of duodenal juice is presumptive evidence for stones or gravel in 70 to 85 percent of the cases when found. The presence of bile-stained white cells is suggestive of infection in the biliary tree.

The importance of cholecystography and intravenous cholangiography is well known, but with jaundice, and sometimes in the presence of serious hepatocellular disease without jaundice, the excretion of the dye may be so decreased as to make visualization of the gall bladder and bile ducts impossible. Barium-meal x-rays of the esophagus, stomach, and duodenum may permit the observation of esophageal varices and the extrinsic pressure of gall bladder or pancreatic lesions upon the stomach or duodenum.

### LIVER BIOPSY

Histologic examination of a biopsy specimen of the liver may provide information of value in diagnosis and in making therapeutic decisions. A biopsy specimen of the liver may be obtained under direct vision at laparotomy or by peritoneoscopy, but in most instances a percutaneous needle biopsy of the liver with any of several types of needles available is the method of choice, since it is simple and produces satisfactory material for study at minimal discomfort and risk to the patient. A needle biopsy is not necessary for a correct diagnosis in most cases of liver disease.[103] It does not supplant other liver-function tests. Biopsy is indicated in a small group of cases where other tests have not resolved the differential diagnosis between medical and surgical jaundice. In most instances, biopsy does not distinguish extrahepatic obstruction from intrahepatic cholestasis. Metastatic cancer of the liver is frequently detected by needle biopsy, thus avoiding a needless abdominal operation. A biopsy may be helpful in treatment and prognosis by defining the stage of known liver disease, as in cirrhosis.

A review of large series of liver-biopsy experiences [103] has shown a 2- to 4.8-percent failure to get a satisfactory specimen of tissue. Significant complications such as hemorrhage, perforation of the gall bladder or bile ducts, collapse of the right lower lobe of the lung, and severe right upper quadrant pain have been reported in 0.23 percent of cases. Contraindications to a needle biopsy of the liver are a prothrombin concentration of less than 50 percent, hemorrhagic diathesis, chronic passive congestion of the liver, cholangitis, infection in the right pleural cavity if the transthoracic approach is used, and an actively uncooperative patient. Although it is a relatively safe procedure, the over-all mortality from liver biopsy is between 0.085 and 0.19 percent. Consequently, liver biopsy should be employed with due regard for indications and in anticipation of the benefits to be derived. It should be performed by a physician who is well trained in its technique and who is aware of the contraindications.

### Choice of Liver-Function Tests

Not all of the liver-function tests described above should be performed on any individual patient. Moreover, the indiscriminate use of a routine battery of liver-function tests is to be discouraged. Such tests should be chosen as will serve the particular purpose of liver-function tests as outlined in the introduction of this chapter, with due regard for simplicity, reliability, and lack of expense for the patient. The following groups of tests are the author's suggestion for each purpose.

#### SCREENING TESTS

These tests should be of the more sensitive type to detect subclinical or latent hepatocellular disease. A suggested group is the following:

> Urine bile,
> Van den Bergh (1-min direct and total),
> Urine urobilinogen,
> Flocculation tests (thymol and cephalin),
> Bromsulfalein excretion,
> Serum transaminases.

#### TESTS TO DIFFERENTIATE MEDICAL AND SURGICAL JAUNDICE

The tests chosen for this purpose should be those which reflect excretory processes of the liver on one hand and, on the other, tests which are affected primarily by disturbances of hepatocellular function. These tests are listed in Table 73, together with the changes to be observed in medical and surgical jaundice. It should be noted that tests for urine bile, the direct and total van den Bergh reactions of the serum, and BSP excretion are of no differential diagnostic value because they are affected to more or less the same degree by both medical and surgical jaundice.

#### TESTS FOR SEVERITY OF LIVER DISEASE

Included in this group are the following less sensitive tests of hepatocellular function whose degree of abnormality is

Table 73. *Tests to differentiate medical and surgical jaundice.*

| Test | Medical jaundice | | Surgical jaundice | |
|---|---|---|---|---|
| | Uncomplicated | Obstructive phase | Uncomplicated | With cholangitis |
| Urine urobilinogen | ↑ | ↓ | ↓ | ↑ |
| Alkaline phosphatase | <15 B.U. | <15 B.U. | >15 B.U. | >15 B.U. |
| Flocculation | 4+ | 4+ | Negative | Negative |
| Cholesterol | Normal or decreased | Normal or decreased | Increased | Increased |
| Percentage of cholesterol esters | Greatly decreased | Greatly decreased | Normal | Normal |
| Transaminases | Greatly increased | Greatly increased | Mildly increased | Mildly increased |
| Prothrombin after vitamin K | Depressed | Depressed | Normal | Normal |
| Stool urobilin (color) | Brown | Clay | Clay | Clay |
| Liver biopsy | Parenchymal disease | Parenchymal disease; bile stasis | Bile stasis | Bile stasis; cholangiolitis |

to some extent proportional to the severity of liver damage:

Serum albumin,
Serum globulin,
Bromsulfalein,
Prothrombin after vitamin K,
Cholesterol esters (percentage),
Cholinesterase,
Transaminase.

### TESTS FOR FOLLOWING THE COURSE OF LIVER DISEASE

When choosing tests for this group, the physician desires either sensitive tests that permit him to decide when the liver has recovered completely from a hepatocellular disease, or else tests that reflect the relentless progression of parenchymal damage to the point where it will become incapacitating or fatal. In other words, these tests are used for prognosis. They will be performed periodically at the discretion of the physician. Rather than using all of the tests listed below, only those tests that are most sensitive or that give the most abnormal results should be repeated:

Van den Bergh (total),
Urine urobilinogen,
Serum albumin,
Serum globulin,
Prothrombin after vitamin K,
Cholesterol and cholesterol esters,
Cholinesterase,
Transaminases,
Bromsulfalein,
Liver biopsy.

In this group, the omission of flocculation tests is notable because they may give positive results for months after clinical recovery from hepatitis since they are possibly a reflection of an immune state with elevated serum gamma globulin.

In conclusion, it should be reemphasized that there is no one test of liver function appropriate to all cases, and that there may be considerable difference of opinion as to which tests to use for any particular purpose.

## REFERENCES

1. I. Dubin, "Chronic idiopathic jaundice. A review of fifty cases," *Amer. J. Med. 24,* 268 (1958).
2. W. T. Foulk, H. R. Butt, C. A. Owen, F. F. Whitcomb, Jr., and H L. Mason, "Constitutional hepatic dysfunction (Gilbert's Disease): Its natural history and related syndromes," *Medicine 38,* 25 (1959).
3. L. Schiff, B. H. Billing, and Y. Oikawa, "Familial nonhemolytic jaundice with conjugated bilirubin in the serum. A case study," *New Eng. J. Med.* 260 1315 (1959).
4. H. C. Johnson and J. P. Doenges, "Intrahepatic obstructive jaundice (primary cholestasis), a clinicopathologic syndrome of varied etiology: A review with observations of the use of cortocotropin as a diagnostic tool," *Ann. intern. Med. 44,* 589 (1956).
5. W. E. Rickets, "An analysis of tests widely used in the differential diagnosis of jaundice," *Gastroenterology 23,* 391 (1953).
6. F. M. Hanger, "The meaning of liver function tests," *Amer. J. Med. 16,* 565 (1954).
7. A. M. Snell, "Liver function tests and their interpretation," *Gastroenterology 34,* 675 (1958).
8. J. L. Bollman, "Physiology of the liver," in L. Schiff, ed., *Diseases of the Liver* (Lippincott, Philadelphia, 1956).
9. D. Seligson, "Biochemical considerations of the liver," in L. Schiff, ed., *Diseases of the Liver* (Lippincott, Philadelphia, 1956).

10. B. H. Billing and G. H. Lathe, "Bilirubin metabolism in jaundice," *Amer. J. Med.* 24, 111 (1958).

11. R. Schmid, "Jaundice and bilirubin metabolism," *Arch. intern. Med.* 101, 669 (1958).

12. C. J. Watson, "Some challenging aspects of hemoglobin metabolism," *Ann. intern. Med.* 47, 611 (1957).

13. H. R. Butt, R. Schmid, I. M. Arias, J. L. Bollman, and K. Isselbacher, "Panel: Bilirubin metabolism," *Gastroenterology 36*, 161 (1959).

14. G. Klatskin and L. Bungards, "Bilirubin-protein linkages in serum and their relationship to the van den Bergh reaction," *J. clin. Invest.* 35, 537 (1956).

15. K. J. Isselbacher and E. A. McCarthy, "Studies on bilirubin sulfate and other nonglucuronide conjugates of bilirubin," *J. clin. Invest.* 38, 645 (1959).

16. J. D. Mann and R. D. Koler, "The excretion in the bile of urobilinogen administered orally and parenterally," *Gastroenterology 17*, 400 (1951).

17. C. J. Watson, "Studies of urobilinogen. III. The per diem excretion of uro-bilinogen in the common forms of jaundice and disease of the liver," *Arch. intern. Med.* 59, 206 (1937).

18. R. Schmid and L. Hammaker, "Glucuronide formation in patients with con-stitutional hepatic dysfunction (Gilbert's disease)," *New Engl. J. Med. 260*, 1310 (1959).

19. I. M. Arias and I. M. London, "Bilirubin glucuronide formation in vitro: demonstration of defect in Gilbert's disease," *Science 126*, 563 (1957).

20. J. Axelrod, R. Schmid, and L. Hammaker, "Biochemical lesion in congeni-tal, non-obstructive, non-hemolytic jaundice," *Nature 180*, 1426 (1957).

21. R. Schmid, J. Axelrod, L. Hammaker, and I. Rosenthal, "Congenital defects in bilirubin metabolism," *J. clin. Invest. 36*, 927 (1957).

22. A. K. Brown and W. W. Zuelzer, "Studies on the neonatal development of the glucuronide conjugating system," *J. clin. Invest. 37*, 332 (1958).

23. G. H. Lathe and M. Walker, "The synthesis of bilirubin glucuronide in ani-mal and human liver," *Biochem. J. 70*, 705 (1958).

24. F. A. Allen, M. H. Carr, and A. P. Klotz, "Decreased red blood cell survival time in patients with portal cirrhosis," *J. Amer. med. Ass. 164*, 955 (1957).

25. W. A. Tisdale, G. Klatskin, and E. D. Kinsella, "The significance of the direct-reacting fraction of serum bilirubin in hemolytic jaundice," *Amer. J. Med. 26*, 214 (1959).

26. E. S. Cohen, T. L. Althausen, and J. E. Giansiracusa, "Studies on brom-sulfalein excretion. IV. Variations in the mechanism of hepatic excretory function when challenged with different dyes," *Gastroenterology 30*, 232 (1956).

27. G. U. Taplin, O. M. Meredith, Jr., and H. Kade, "The radioactive ($I^{131}$-tagged) rose bengal uptake-excretion test for liver function using external gamma-ray scintillation counting techniques," *J. lab. clin. Med. 45*, 665 (1955).

28. A. B. Gutman, K. B. Olson, E. B. Gutman, and C. A. Flood, "Effect of disease of the liver and biliary tract upon the phosphatase activity of the serum," *J. clin. Invest. 19*, 129 (1940).

29. J. G. Mateer, J. I. Baltz, P. D. Comanduras, H. H. Steele, and S. W. Brouwer, "Further advances in liver function tests and the value of a therapeutic test in facilitating the earlier diagnosis and treatment of liver impairment," *Gas-troenterology 8*, 52 (1947).

30. L. L. Miller and W. F. Bale, "Synthesis of all plasma protein fractions except gamma globulins by the liver," *J. exp. Med. 99*, 125 (1954).

31. P. K. Bondy, "Some metabolic abnormalities in liver disease," *Amer. J. Med. 24*, 428 (1958).

32. W. Volwiler, P. D. Goldsworthy, M. P. MacMartin, P. A. Wood, I. R. MacKay, and K. Freemont-Smith, "Biosynthetic determinations with radioactive sulfur of the turnover of various plasma proteins in normal and cirrhotic man," *J. clin. Invest. 34*, 1126 (1955).

33. G. Mindrum and H. I. Glueck, "Plasma prothrombin in liver disease: Its clinical and prognostic significance," *Ann. intern. Med. 50*, 1370 (1959).

34. S. P. Bessman and A. N. Bessman, "The cerebral and peripheral uptake of ammonia in liver disease with an hypothesis for the mechanism of hepatic coma," *J. clin. Invest. 34*, 622 (1955).

35. W. V. McDermott, Jr., "Metabolism and toxicity of ammonia," *New Engl. J. Med. 257*, 1076 (1957).

36. S. Sherlock, "Pathogenesis and management of hepatic coma," *Amer. J. Med. 24*, 805 (1958).

37. E. J. Conway, *Micro-Duffusion Analysis and Volumetric Error* (ed. 4; Crosby Lockwood, London, 1957).

38. D. Seligson and K. Hirahari, "The measurement of ammonia in whole blood, erythrocytes and plasma," *J. lab. clin. Med. 49*, 962 (1957).

39. W. V. McDermott, Jr., "Simple discriminatory test for upper gastrointestinal hemorrhage," *New Engl. J. Med. 257*, 1161 (1957).

40. A. M. Bassett, T. L. Althausen, and G. C. Coltrin, "New galactose test for differentiation of obstructive from parenchymatous jaundice," *Amer. J. dig. Dis. 8*, 432 (1941).

41. W. E. King, "Liver Function," in F. A. Jones, ed., *Modern Trends in Gastro-enterology* (series 2; Hoeber, New York, 1958).

42. A. J. Quick, "Clinical value of the test for hippuric acid in cases of disease of the liver," *Arch. intern. Med. 57*, 544 (1936).

43. H. T. Malloy and K. A. Evelyn, "Determination of bilirubin with the photo-electric colorimeter," *J. biol. Chem. 119*, 481 (1937).

44. H. Ducci and C. J. Watson, "The quantitative determination of serum bilirubin with special reference to prompt reacting and the chloroform-soluble types," *J. lab. clin. Med. 30*, 293 (1945).

45. C. J. Watson, "The importance of fractional serum bilirubin determination in clinical medicine," *Ann. intern. Med. 45*, 351 (1956).

46. L. Zieve, E. Hill, M. Hanson, A. B. Falcome, and C. J. Watson, "Normal and abnormal variations and clinical significance of the one-minute and total serum bilirubin determinations," *J. lab. clin. Med. 38*, 446 (1951).

47. C. Schwartz, V. Sborov, and C. J. Watson, "Studies of urobilinogen. IV. The quantitative determination of urobilinogen by means of the Evelyn photo-electric colorimeter," *Amer. J. clin. Path. 14*, 598 (1944).

48. O. H. Gaebler, "Determination of bromsulfalein in normal, turbid, hemo-lyzed or icteric serums," *Amer. J. clin. Path. 15*, 452 (1945).

49. G. B. Wallace and J. S. Diamond, "The significance of urobilinogen in the urine as a test for liver function. With a description of a simple quantitative method for its estimation," *Arch. intern. Med. 35*, 698 (1925).

50. C. J. Watson and V. Hawkinson, "Studies of urobilinogen. VI. Further experience with the simple quantitative Ehrlich reaction. Corrected calibra-

tion of the Evelyn colorimeter with a pontacyl dye mixture in terms of uro-bilinogen," *Amer. J. clin. Path. 17,* 108 (1947).

51. C. J. Watson, S. Schwartz, V. Sborov, and E. Bertie, "Studies of urobilinogen. V. A simple method for the quantitative recording of the Ehrlich reaction as carried out with tissue and feces," *Amer. J. clin. Path. 14,* 605 (1944).

52. H. A. Lindberg and G. V. LeRoy, "Excretion of urobilinogen in urine in infectious hepatitis," *Arch. intern. Med. 80,* 175 (1947).

53. W. L. Voegtlin, M. H. Moss, and E. March, "A comparison of the quantitative urinary urobilinogen determination (Watson) with the urine Ehrlich test," *Gastroenterology 14,* 538 (1950).

54. F. J. Inglefinger, S. E. Bradley, A. I. Mendeloff, and P. Kramer, "Studies with bromsulphalein. I. Its disappearance from the blood after a single intravenous injection," *Gastroenterology 11,* 646 (1948).

55. G. J. Gabuzda, Jr., R. D. Eckhardt, and C. S. Davidson, "Urinary excretion of amino-acids in patients with cirrhosis of the liver and in normal adults," *J. clin. Invest. 31,* 1015 (1952).

56. N. Zamchek, T. C. Chalmers, F. W. White, and C. S. Davidson, "The bromsulphalein test in the early diagnosis of liver disease in gross upper gastrointestinal hemorrhage," *Gastroenterology 14,* 343 (1950).

57. S. H. Lorber, M. J. Oppenheimer, H. Shay, P. Lynch, and H. Siplet, "Enterohepatic circulation of bromsulphalein: intraduodenal, intraportal, and intravenous dye administration in dogs," *Amer. J. Physiol. 173,* 259 (1953).

58. P. J. Culver, W. V. McDermott, and C. M. Jones, "Diagnostic value of selective interference with certain excretory processes of the liver," *Gastroenterology 33,* 163 (1957).

59. T. H. Brem, "Recognition of biliary tract obstruction without jaundice," *J. Amer. med. Ass. 159,* 1624 (1955).

60. G. Morey, G. J. Gabazda, and H. H. Scudamore, "Sensitization to bromsulfalein (Phenol tetrabromphthalein–disodium sulfonate)," *Gastroenterology 13,* 246 (1949).

61. H. C. Walker, Jr., "Fatal bromsulphalein reaction," *Ann. intern. Med. 47,* 362 (1957).

62. N. F. Maclagan, "Liver function tests," in L. Schiff, ed., *Diseases of the Liver* (Lippincott, Philadelphia, 1956).

63. J. M. Walshe, "Disturbances of amino-acid metabolism following liver injury," *Quart. J. Med. 22,* 483 (1953).

64. R. S. Ross, F. L. Iber, and A. M. Harvey, "The serum alkaline phosphatase in chronic infiltrative disease of the liver," *Amer. J. Med. 21,* 850 (1956).

65. A. Bodansky, "Phosphatase studies. II. Determination of serum phosphatase. Factors influencing accuracy of determination," *J. biol. Chem. 101,* 93 (1933).

66. E. J. King and A. R. Armstrong, "A convenient method for determining serum and bile phosphatase activity," *Canad. med. Ass. J. 31,* 376 (1934).

67. A. B. Gutman, K. B. Olson, E. B. Gutman, and C. A. Flood, "Effect of disease of the liver and biliary tract upon the phosphatase activity of the serum," *J. clin. Invest. 19,* 129 (1940).

68. A. B. Gutman and F. M. Hanger, Jr., "Differential diagnosis of jaundice by combined serum phosphatase determination and cephalin flocculation test," *Med. Clin. N. Amer. 25,* 845 (1941).

69. P. E. Howe, "The use of sodium sulfate as the globulin precipitant in the determination of proteins in blood," *J. biol. Chem. 49*, 93 (1921).

70. H. Popper, W. B. Bean, J. de la Huerga, M. Franklin, Y. Tsumageri, J. I. Rouch, and F. Steigmann, "Electrophoretic serum protein fractions in hepatobiliary disease," *Gastroenterology 17*, 138 (1951).

71. I. R. MacKay, W. Volwiler, and P. D. Goldworthy, "Paper electrophoresis of serum proteins: Photometric quantitation and comparison with free electrophoresis," *J. clin. Invest. 33*, 855 (1954).

72. R. L. Wall, "The use of serum protein electrophoresis in clinical medicine. Principle and method of paper electrophoresis described," *Arch. intern. Med. 102*, 618 (1958).

73. R. Armas-Cruz, G. Lobo-Parga, M. Madrid, and C. Velasco, "Normal and pathologic proteins and flocculation tests. A contribution to the study of the mechanism of flocculation tests," *Gastroenterology 35*, 298 (1958).

74. E. A. Kabat, F. M. Hanger, D. H. Morre, and H. Landow, "The relation of cephalin flocculation and colloidal gold reactions to the serum proteins," *J. clin. Invest. 22*, 563 (1943).

75. D. B. Moore, P. S. Pierson, F. M. Hanger, and D. H. Moore, "Mechanism of the positive cephalin-cholesterol flocculation reaction in hepatitis," *J. clin. Invest. 24*, 292 (1945).

76. A. Saifer, "Protein flocculation reactions. A physicochemical approach," *Amer. J. Med. 13*, 730 (1952).

77. H. A. Eder, E. M. Russ, R. A. Rees Pritchett, A. M. Wilber, and D. P. Barr, "Protein-lipid relationships in human plasma: In biliary cirrhosis, obstructive jaundice, and acute hepatitis," *J. clin. Invest. 34*, 1147 (1955).

78. N. F. Maclagan, "Flocculation tests: Chemical and clinical significance," *Brit. med. J. 2*, 892 (1948).

79. F. M. Hanger, "Serological differentiation of obstructive from hepatogenous jaundice by flocculation of cephalin-cholesterol emulsions," *J. clin. Invest. 18*, 261 (1939).

80. N. F. Maclagan, "Thymol turbidity test as indicator of liver dysfunction," *Brit. J. exp. Pathol. 25*, 234 (1944).

81. R. E. Shank and C. L. Hoagland, "A modified method for the quantitative determination of the thymol turbidity reaction of the serum," *J. biol. Chem. 162*, 133 (1946).

82. L. M. Hershenson, H. M. Rawnsley, and J. G. Reinhold, "Factors influencing the reliability of hepatic turbidity and flocculation tests in the differential diagnosis of obstructive jaundice," *Gastroenterology 34*, 1146 (1958).

83. H. G. Kunkel, "Estimations of alterations of serum gamma globulin by a turbidimetric technique," *Proc. Soc. exp. Biol. (N. Y.) 66*, 217 (1947).

84. H. Ducci, "The flocculation tests in the differential diagnosis of jaundice," *Gastroenterology 15*, 628 (1950).

85. H. G. Kunkel and C. L. Hoagland, "Mechanism and significance of the thymol turbidity test for liver disease," *J. clin. Invest. 26*, 1060 (1947).

86. T. E. Wilson, C. H. Brown, and A. Hainline, Jr., "The zinc sulfate turbidity test," *Gastroenterology 32*, 483 (1957).

87. M. H. Friedman, "Technical factors affecting the estimation of serum gamma globulin by the zinc turbidimetric method of Kunkel," *Gastroenterology 17*, 57 (1951).

88. W. R. Bloor, "The determination of cholesterol in the blood," *J. biol. Chem.* 24, 227 (1916).
89. W. R. Bloor and A. Knudson, "The separate determination of cholesterol and cholesterol esters in small amounts of blood," *J. biol. Chem.* 27, 107 (1916).
90. H. O. Michel, "An electrometric method for the determination of red blood cell and plasma cholinesterase activity," *J. lab. clin. Med.* 34, 1564 (1949).
91. H. A. Ravin, K. C. Tsou, and A. M. Seligman, "Colorimetric estimation and histochemical demonstration of serum cholinesterase," *J. biol. Chem.* 191, 843 (1951).
92. M. H. Sleisenger, T. P. Almy, H. Gilder, and G. Perle, "Colorimetric determination of serum cholinesterase; its value in hepatic and biliary tract disease," *J. clin. Invest.* 32, 466 (1953).
93. H. J. Wetstone, R. Tennant, and B. V. White, "Studies of cholinesterase activity. I. Serum cholinesterase, methods and normal values," *Gastroenterology* 33, 41 (1957).
94. J. D. Mann, W. I. Mandell, P. L. Eichman, M. A. Knowlton, and V. M. Sborov, "Serum cholinesterase activity in liver disease," *J. lab. clin. Med.* 39, 543 (1952).
95. H. M. Williams, R. V. La Motta, and H. J. Wetstone, "Studies of cholinesterase activity. III. Serum cholinesterase in obstructive jaundice and neoplastic disease," *Gastroenterology* 33, 55 (1957).
96. A. Karmen, F. Wroblewski, and J. S. LaDue, "Transaminase activity in human blood," *J. clin. Invest.* 34, 126 (1955).
97. F. Wroblewski and J. S. LaDue, "Serum glutamic pyruvic transaminase in cardiac and hepatic disease," *Proc. Soc. exp. Biol.* (N. Y.) 91, 569 (1956).
98. F. Wroblewski, G. Jervis, and J. S. LaDue, "The diagnostic, prognostic, and epidemiologic significance of serum glutamic oxaloacetic transaminase (SGO–T) alterations in acute hepatitis," *Ann. intern. Med.* 45, 782 (1956).
99. F. Wroblewski and J. S. LaDue, "Serum glutamic pyruvic transaminase (SGP–T) in hepatic disease: A preliminary report," *Ann. intern. Med.* 45, 801 (1956).
100. F. Wroblewski, "The significance of alterations in serum enzymes in the differential diagnosis of jaundice," *Arch. intern. Med.* 100, 635 (1957).
101. C. M. Jones, "The rational use of duodenal drainage. An attempt to establish a conservative estimate of the value of this procedure in the diagnosis of biliary tract pathology," *Arch. intern. Med.* 34, 60 (1924).
102. K. Juniper, Jr. and E. N. Burson, Jr., "Biliary tract studies. II. The significance of biliary crystals," *Gastroenterology* 32, 175 (1957).
103. N. Zamcheck and R. L. Sidman, "Needle biopsy of the liver. I. Its use in clinical and investigative medicine. II. Risk of needle biopsy," *New Engl. J. Med.* 249, 1020, 1062 (1953).

# Unit 25

# Tests Related to the Exocrine Function of the Pancreas

Accurate diagnosis of diseases of the pancreas is one of the most difficult areas in medicine. Symptoms of the various types of pancreatic disease are often non-specific and may range from complaints of disturbed digestion or vague headaches to such severe abdominal pain that it resembles an acute surgical emergency. The anatomic location of the gland makes it almost inaccessible to physical examination. As yet, no direct method of x-ray examination of the pancreas has been developed to the point where it can be used in the same way as gallbladder x-rays or barium studies of the gastrointestinal tract. X-ray studies can aid, however, in the study of pancreatic disease if there is calcification in the gland or if pathologic processes of the pancreas enlarge it sufficiently to displace and alter the contour of adjacent organs, such as the stomach and duodenal loop.

On the other hand, laboratory study of the exocrine secretions of the pancreas in duodenal contents, blood serum, and urine has increased our knowledge of the pathologic physiology of pancreatic disease and has provided some tests of diagnostic value. Additional indirect evidence of disturbances in pancreatic function can be gained from determinations of altered digestive capacity secondary to pancreatic insufficiency.

## Physiology

Thomas,[1] Grossman,[2] and Dreiling and Janowitz [3] have written excellent re-

views of the exocrine secretion of the pancreas. The exocrine secretion, or pancreatic juice, is produced by the acinar cells, centroacinar cells, and epithelial cells of the intralobular ducts, in contrast to the purely endocrine products of the islet cells of the pancreas. Only the exocrine secretion will be considered in this unit.

### PANCREATIC JUICE

Pure pancreatic juice is a colorless fluid of low viscosity, with a pH of 8. It consists of water, electrolytes, and a protein moiety of mucus, mucoproteins, and digestive enzymes.[3] Its osmolality is equivalent to that of blood.[1] Electrolytes include sodium, potassium, calcium, chloride, and bicarbonate. There are also small amounts of zinc, phosphate, and sulfate. In the fasting state, the concentrations of sodium, potassium, calcium, chloride, and bicarbonate in the pancreatic juice approximate the concentrations of these diffusible ions in the interstitial fluid.[4] With stimulation to secretion, the sum of concentrations of chloride and bicarbonate remains constant, but there is an inverse ratio of the two: as the bicarbonate concentration rises with increased rate of fluid secretion, the chloride concentration drops. The maximum concentration of electrolytes in pancreatic juice after stimulation is given in Table 74.

The digestive enzymes of the pancreatic juice fall into three categories: amylase, lipase, and trypsin. There are

432

Table 74. *Maximum concentration of electrolytes in pancreatic juice after stimulation.*[1, 4]

| Electrolyte | Concentration |
| --- | --- |
| Sodium | 138–143 mEq/L |
| Potassium | 5–9 mEq/L |
| Calcium | 3–4 mgm/100 ml |
| Bicarbonate [a] | 90–103 mEq/L |
| Chloride [a] | 51–64 mEq/L (minimum) |

[a] Total of bicarbonate and chloride concentration constant at 154–161 mEq/L.

two amylases, alpha and beta, and one lipase. These are all secreted in an active state. At least four proteolytic enzymes have been identified, including trypsin, chymotrypsin, carboxypeptidase, and a collagenase.[1, 3] Trypsin and chymotrypsin are secreted in an inactive form, trypsinogen and chymotrypsinogen. They are activated in the intestinal tract by enterokinase. Once some trypsin is formed, it continues the autocatalytic activation of trypsinogen.[1] There is also a trypsin inhibitor secreted by the pancreas. This inhibitor prevents digestion of the normal pancreas by any active trypsin in the gland and the inhibitor is inactivated by some substance similar to enterokinase in the intestinal tract.[5] In addition to its digestive properties in the intestinal tract, trypsin, when it gets into the blood stream, causes changes in blood coagulability.[3]

MECHANISM OF EXOCRINE SECRETION

In man, the secretion of pancreatic juice appears to be continuous, but it is augmented by stimulation through humoral and neurogenic factors.[1] Although the vascular supply, if insufficient, may limit or influence the rate of secretion, the quantity of blood flowing through the pancreas does not control secretion.[6] Secretion in response to stimulation is an active process requiring energy derived from utilization of carbohydrate and oxygen.[1] Both experimental studies employing selective destruction of acinar cells and clinical observations on the composition of pancreatic juice in various disease states suggest a differentiation of cellular function of the pancreatic glands.[3, 7] Water and bicarbonate are probably secreted by the centroacinar cells and epithelial cells of the intralobular ducts.[2] The digestive enzymes are produced by the acinar cells.[1]

The mechanism of active secretion of water and bicarbonate has not been established definitely. An attractive theory is based on the demonstration of carbonic anhydrase in pancreatic tissue and the suppression of stimulated secretion of total volume and total bicarbonate by the pancreas to below basal secretory levels with the administration of a potent carbonic anhydrase inhibitor, acetozolamide.[8] Some (perhaps 20 percent) of the bicarbonate of pancreatic juice is derived from the plasma; but the majority is probably derived from intracellular oxidation in the pancreas with production of carbon dioxide. The availability of bicarbonate ions from this source would be increased by carbonic anhydrase, which accelerates the hydration of carbon dioxide to carbonic acid. Therefore at higher rates of secretion the pancreas seems to be more dependent upon carbonic anhydrase activity for its supply of bicarbonate ions.[8] Since the concentrations of sodium and potassium in the pancreatic juice remain unaffected by stimulation, acetozolamide, or pancreatic disease,[8] it is assumed that these ions are passively diffused into the juice in equilibrium with the interstitial fluid.

The digestive enzymes of the pancreas are continuously synthesized in the acinar cells and appear as zymogen granules, which migrate during maturation to the apex of the cell. After stimulation to secretion, which causes the acinar cell to contract, the zymogen granules are extruded into the gland lumen where they dissolve in the fluid.[1] In addition to this exocrine secretion of pancreatic enzymes, there is an "endocrine" component to the secretion of pancreatic enzymes.[9] Thus pancreatic amylase, lipase, and possibly trypsinogen are always normally present in the blood. It is not known how the pancreatic ferments get into the blood stream but it is postulated that there is a physiologic secretion or diffusion from the base of the acinar cells via the interstitial spaces.[9] If obstruction to outflow from the pancreatic ducts exists, then there appears to be a pathologic diffusion due to hydrostatic pressure of greatly increased quantities of enzymes into the tissue spaces and blood.[10] The production of pancreatic enzymes is believed to occur in a parallel fashion for each individual enzyme both in the normal pancreas and in diseased states,[3] but there is experimental evidence in animals to suggest that pancreatic-enzyme secretion may be adapted to the type of food in the diet when fed for a long period of time.[11] For example, a high-carbohydrate diet resulted in an increased production of amylase and decrease in trypsin, while a high-protein diet was associated with elevation of trypsin in the pancreatic secretion.[11]

REGULATION OF PANCREATIC SECRETION

The relative importance of neural and humoral regulation of pancreatic secretion is still unsettled.[3] Secretin, a hormone produced by the mucosa of the upper small intestine in response to hydrochloric acid, amino acids, and products of fat digestion, is the major stimulus to active outpouring of fluid and bicarbonate.[2] Secretin appears to act directly on the secretory cells,[2] but its mode of action has not been discovered.[8] By stimulating the outpouring of alkaline pancreatic juice to neutralize the acid chyme from the stomach, secretin is credited with providing the optimal pH for activity of the pancreatic digestive enzymes in the intestinal lumen.[1] Secretin has no effect on enzyme release.[2] Consequently, pancreatic juice produced in response to an injection of secretin is voluminous, rich in bicarbonate, and poor

in enzymes. Anticholinergic drugs tend to inhibit the response to secretin.

Pancreazymin is a second hormone released by the mucosa of the upper small intestine in response to fats, peptone, casein, starch, maltose, lactose, saline and even water. Hydrochloric acid does not stimulate the elaboration of pancreazymin. This hormone acts in some fashion on the acinar cells and augments the secretion of pancreatic enzymes, but has little effect on the secretion of water or bicarbonate.[2]

Neural stimulation via the vagus nerve or cholinergic drugs cause increased elaboration of enzymes.[1] In animals, vagal-nerve stimulation may potentiate the effect of secretin,[1] but there is no evidence that the vagus modifies water and electrolyte secretion in response to secretin in man.[12, 13] On the other hand, vagal activity augments and may condition the pancreatic enzyme output in response to pancreazymin stimulation.[12, 13] The role of the splanchnic nerves in the control of pancreatic secretion is not clearly defined,[3] but there seems to be no demonstrable effect in man.[12] Finally, in addition to the major regulatory mechanisms, namely the secretin-water-bicarbonate and the pancreozymin-vagus-enzymes relations, there are postulated intestino-pancreatic reflexes in the sympathetic ganglia that may respond to the mechanical and chemical stimulation of foodstuffs.

## Tests of Pancreatic Function

Diseases that disturb pancreatic function may cause obstruction to outflow of pancreatic juice or destruction of acinar-gland cells or both. Such alterations should be reflected in: (i) measurable change of enzyme levels in blood and urine; (ii) abnormalities of pancreatic juice obtained via duodenal intubation; and (iii) disturbances in the intestinal phase of digestion. A list of pancreatic-function tests is shown in Table 75.

Table 75. *Pancreatic-function tests.*[a]

| Determination of blood or serum constituents |
| --- |
|   Serum amylase |
|   Serum lipase |
|   Serum trypsin |
|   Plasma antithrombin titer |
|   Provocative pancreatic enzyme tests |
|   Glucose-tolerance test |
|   Serum calcium |
|   Serum carotene |
| Determination of urine constituents |
|   Urinary amylase |
|   Urinary lipase |
| Determination of stool constituents |
|   Microscopic examination |
|   Quantitative fecal fat content |
|   Fecal nitrogen content |
|   Fecal trypsin activity |
| Detection of alteration in digestive capacity |
|   Vitamin A tolerance |
|   Starch tolerance |
|   Gelatin tolerance |
|   $I^{131}$-labeled fat meals |
|   $I^{131}$-labeled protein meals |
|   Estimation of phospholipid synthesis with radioactive phosphorus |
| Detection of abnormalities of pancreatic secretion via duodenal intubation |
|   Volume of secretion |
|   Bicarbonate concentration |
|   Enzyme concentration |
|   Concentration of biliary pigment |
|   Cytology of duodenal aspiration |

[a] Modified from Sterkel and Kirsner.[14]

The clinical application of pancreatic-function tests for the diagnosis of specific diseases of the pancreas is limited by a number of factors.[14–16] The reserve capacity of the gland is so great that more than ⅘ may be destroyed before there is evidence of insufficiency of pancreatic enzymes. Since alterations in blood, urine, and pancreatic-juice enzyme levels depend on obstruction and destruction, interpretation of laboratory-test results may be difficult and confusing. Many of the tests lack specificity for disturbances of pancreatic function, so these tests must be used with caution and with an understanding of the nonpancreatic causes for abnormal laboratory results. Inasmuch as many tests of pancreatic function are currently in the stage of investigation and development, there is often a lack of reproducibility and standardization. Finally, some of the tests present technical difficulties that have restricted widespread utilization. Therefore, only those tests which have proved helpful frequently in the diagnosis of pancreatic disease will be discussed in some detail.

### DETERMINATION OF SERUM AMYLASE

The serum amylase determination is the most generally useful procedure in the diagnosis of acute pancreatitis or of acute recurrences of chronic pancreatitis.[3, 16]

PRINCIPLE. Of several methods described, the saccharogenic method of Somogyi [17] is the one most frequently used and the most accurate.[14, 16] The method involves the determination by copper reduction of the amount of glucose formed when starch is hydrolyzed by amylase. The values are expressed as Somogyi units, defined as the amount of amylase required to digest 1.5 gm of starch in 8 min at 37°C. The normal range for serum amylase by this method is 60–200 units/100 ml.[14, 16] Since modifications of the method with different ranges of normal values have been established by various clinical laboratories, it behooves the physician to ascertain the range for his particular laboratory.

INDICATION AND INTERPRETATION. Serum amylase determinations should be made routinely in all patients with acute abdominal pain.[18] Serial measurements of serum amylase are of value in establishing the cessation of an inflammatory process of the pancreas.[18]

The amylase normally present in the blood serum is derived from the pancreas, salivary glands, liver, muscle, and adipose tissue.[3, 14] Any pathologic process that restricts the outflow of pancreatic juice will result in elevation of serum amylase. This rise takes place within a

435

matter of very few hours after the onset of acute pancreatitis, generally reaches a maximum in 24 hr, and usually returns to a normal range within 3 to 6 days.[14, 18] The magnitude of elevation usually exceeds four to six times the normal value.[14] Although increases of lesser degree may occur in very mild cases, any value less than four times the normal range is not diagnostic of acute pancreatitis. There is no correlation between the concentration of serum amylase and the severity of the inflammation of the pancreas.[3, 18]

In cases of chronic recurrent pancreatitis, acute exacerbations are associated with a similar elevation of serum amylase; but in these cases, there is often a slower return to normal values which may be interpreted as indicating a continuation of the inflammatory process or obstruction.[18] With repeated attacks of pancreatitis, there may be so much destruction of pancreatic tissue that subsequent bouts of pain are associated with no increase of serum amylase.[18] Similar massive destruction in acute pancreatitis may be heralded by an abrupt fall of serum amylase to low levels.[3]

Demonstration of a significant rise in serum amylase may be of diagnostic value in cancer of the ampulla or head of the pancreas, but this test has been useless in the diagnosis of cancer of the body or tail.[18]

LIMITATIONS AND SOURCES OF ERROR. Although elevation of serum amylase is relatively specific, increases may occur in the absence of pancreatic disease. Such conditions include duodenal ulcers, either penetrating into the pancreas or acutely perforating, mumps and other diseases of the salivary glands, diseases of the biliary tract, peritonitis, intestinal obstruction, abdominal operations, and mesenteric thrombosis.[3, 14, 16, 18–20] In general, the elevation of serum amylase noted in these conditions was not as high as in acute pancreatitis.[16]

Since amylase is excreted in the urine, false positive elevations of serum amylase are associated with renal failure and uremia.[3, 14, 16, 20] Another cause of confusion in the interpretation of serum amylase determination is the varying reports of the effect of morphine, other opiate derivatives, and demerol on elevations of pancreatic enzymes in the blood.[21–24] Although many subjects showed no increase in serum amylase after parenteral administration of the narcotics, there were some without any evidence of pancreatic disease who had a significant rise of serum amylase for as long as 24 hr after injection of morphine. The number of false positive results was greater when the secretion of the pancreas had been stimulated.[21, 22] Such variations in response to narcotic injection seem related to differing sensitivities of the sphincter of Oddi and to anatomic arrangements of the pancreatic and biliary duct system.[24] Therefore, antecedent morphine injection must be taken into account when evaluating serum amylase levels.

Finally, since the serum amylase may return to normal within 48 hr after the onset of acute pancreatitis, the test loses its diagnostic value unless performed early in the course of the disease.

DETERMINATION OF SERUM LIPASE

Serum lipase elevations tend to parallel rises of amylase, but may persist longer.[14, 16]

PRINCIPLE. The lipase activity of the serum is determined by titrating with a standard solution of sodium hydroxide the fatty acid liberated as a result of hydrolysis of an olive-oil emulsion by the lipase.[25] Results are expressed in milliliters of $N/20$ sodium hydroxide used for titration. The normal range is less than 1.2 ml. Since there are other esterases normally found in blood serum, the choice of a specific substrate for pancreatic lipase activity is important. Olive oil satisfies this requirement. Attempts to shorten the time required for the analytic method by the use of other substrates have raised a question of the specificity of such modifications.

INDICATION AND INTERPRETATION. The measurement of serum lipase activity is of complementary value in the diagnosis of pancreatitis, since elevation of lipase may persist after the transient rise of serum amylase has disappeared.[26, 27] Greater organ specificity for origin of lipase in the serum makes lipase determinations useful for differentiating the elevation of serum amylase due to pancreatitis from the hyperamylasemia of inflammatory diseases of the salivary glands.[18] Elevation of serum lipase has been reported to occur early in the course of cancer of the head of the pancreas.[27] Serial determinations of serum lipase will show elevations in 40 to 67 percent of cancers. The normal range of values for serum lipase is up to 1.0 to 1.2 ml of $N/20$ sodium hydroxide. Larger amounts indicate elevation of serum lipase activity with diagnostic significance as indicated.

LIMITATIONS AND SOURCES OF ERROR. The 24-hr period of incubation of substrate and serum required before titration limits the usefulness of this procedure in the diagnosis of acute pancreatitis.[14] Modifications of substrate have been proposed in an effort to shorten the time needed for incubation, but such changes in substrate may alter the specificity of the test for pancreatic lipase.[28] Elevations of serum lipase have been associated with a number of nonpancreatic causes. Such "false positive" results may be due to renal insufficiency, hepatic and biliary-tract disease, intestinal obstruction, or peritonitis, or may follow the use of opiates.[14, 16]

DETERMINATION OF SERUM TRYPSIN

Until recently, trypsin levels of the blood serum have not been measured directly because of the presence of antitryptic activity of the blood [3, 16] and because of lack of a specific substrate. Tryptic activity has been related to the plasma antithrombin titer, but this test has many pitfalls.[16] Alpha-benzoyl-1-arginine amide hydrochloride appears to be a specific substrate for enzymes with tryptic-like activity. It is hydrolyzed rapidly by trypsin to yield benzoyl-1-arginine and ammonia. The amount of ammonia liberated is believed to be proportional to the "tryptic activity" of the serum. In a small series of cases so far reported, the serum "trypsin" was a more sensitive and reliable index of pancreatic disease than the serum amylase or lipase.[29] The value of this test awaits confirmation by other investigators.

PROVOCATIVE ENZYME TESTS

In theory, if organic obstruction of the pancreatic ducts exists or if functional obstruction is created by the use of opiates, stimulation to secretion of pancreatic juice or to elaboration of pancreatic enzyme should result in an increase in blood enzyme levels unless there has been much destruction of pancreatic glandular tissue. Although there are occasional reports of various combinations of provocative enzyme tests that appear to have some diagnostic value in chronic pancreatitis and cancer of the pancreas,[30, 31] careful evaluations have shown inconsistencies in results and lack of correlation with observed pathologic changes in the pancreas. Therefore, provocative enzyme tests offer little promise of diagnostic significance.[30, 32, 33]

DETERMINATION OF AMYLASE IN URINE

Amylase is readily excreted by the kidneys and can be measured in the urine by methods similar to those used for serum. There are differences of opinion about the relation between blood and urinary amylase. On one side, a close parallelism between blood and urine amylase levels in acute pancreatitis seems to have been demonstrated.[34] On the other, a serial, quantitative study of serum and urinary amylase values showed increases of urinary amylase output in every case where the serum level was elevated, but there were also many instances of pancreatitis where the urinary output was elevated and persisted above the normal range for 7 to 10 days after the serum level had become normal.[15, 35] Both sides agree that the measurement of amylase concentration in a random specimen of urine is of no diagnostic value because of great variability. Hence the use of random urine amylase determinations has been replaced by serum amylase tests in the diagnosis of acute pancreatitis. Nevertheless, timed 1- or 2-hr urine collections, with amylase determined as a quantitative rate of excretion in terms of units excreted per hour, would seem to give the urinary amylase measurements diagnostic value.[34, 35] If the increased reliability and sensitivity of the quantitative rate of urinary excretion of amylase is confirmed by other investigators, then the routine use of such urine amylase tests may be recommended in preference to serum amylase determinations.[15, 35] When renal insufficiency complicates an episode of acute pancreatitis, even transiently, neither the serum nor the urinary amylase gives reliable information.[34, 35]

### DETERMINATION OF LIPASE IN URINE

A fat-splitting enzyme of pancreatic origin has been demonstrated to be regularly present in the urine.[36] By the same method as for serum lipase determinations,[25] the average concentration of urinary lipase in 100 normal subjects was found to be 0.35 ml of $N/20$ sodium hydroxide per milliliter of urine, with a range of 0.1 to 0.75 ml. This concentration range was relatively constant and showed no significant variation with fasting, after fat-rich meals, or from day to day. The 24-hr urinary lipase output varied from 180 to 780 units in these 100 normal subjects. The excretion rate was unrelated to urine volume.[37] Use of urinary lipase measurements in the study of diseases of the pancreas has not been reported as yet.

### DETERMINATION OF VOLUME, BICARBONATE CONCENTRATION, AND ENZYME CONTENT OF STIMULATED PANCREATIC JUICE— THE SECRETIN TEST

With the advent of purified preparations of secretin, a direct test of the quantity and composition of uncontaminated pancreatic juice has been developed.[38, 39]

PRINCIPLE. Semiquantitative recovery of pancreatic juice uncontaminated by gastric contents is accomplished via a double-lumen tube whose fenestrated openings are accurately positioned near the ampulla of Vater and at the stomach outlet. Constant suction is maintained on both lumens for the period of the test. A standard dose of secretin is given intravenously to produce a submaximal stimulation of pancreatic juice. The volume of juice recovered is measured in milliliters per kilogram of body weight per time of collection. The bicarbonate concentration is determined in milliequivalents per liter and the quantity of amylase is expressed as units per kilogram of body weight per time of collection. For simplicity, other enzymes are not measured, since there is a parallelism of secretion of amylase, lipase, and trypsin. Values characteristic of normal exocrine pancreatic secretion have been established and alterations due to disease of the pancreas have been described.[38, 40, 41]

METHOD. The patient is tested in the fasting state. A double-lumen gastroduodenal tube is positioned under fluoroscopic control and constant suction is applied to both outlets. After the duodenal aspirate has become crystal clear and alkaline, the fluid is collected for a control period of 20 min. Then 1 unit of secretin per kilogram of body weight is given intravenously. Following this, duodenal specimens are collected during four successive 20-min periods. The volume of single and combined specimens is measured. Bicarbonate concentration is determined by the Van Slyke volumetric method, and amylase by the Somogyi method.[38]

INDICATION AND INTERPRETATION. The secretin test is indicated in the study and diagnosis of suspected chronic diseases of the pancreas such as chronic pancreatitis, pancreatic fibrosis, cancer of the pancreas, and obstruction of the pancreatic ducts. The test is unwarranted in cases of acute pancreatitis because the patient is too ill to withstand the rigors of such a test [3] and the diagnosis can be made more readily from serum or urinary enzyme studies. The minimum normal values of the stimulated juice are: [38]

Total volume, 2.0 ml/kg body weight per 80 min (mean 3.2 ml/kg);
Maximum bicarbonate concentration, 90 mEq/L (mean 108 mEq/L);
Total amylase secretion, 6.0 units/kg body weight (mean 14.2 units/kg).

Since hypersecretion of pancreatic juice is unknown, only values less than the lower limits of normal are of clinical significance.[40] If the secretin test is performed in cases of acute pancreatitis, alterations of volume, bicarbonate concentration, and amylase secretion may be observed, but such changes are seldom below the lower level of the normal range and there is no characteristic diagnostic pattern.[41] After subsidence of clinical signs and symptoms, any abnormality in secretion is suggestive of persistent disease.[41]

In chronic pancreatitis, there is a persistent and marked lowering of bicarbonate concentration in 97 percent of the cases. The volume and amylase secretion are affected much less, with about half of the cases falling within the normal range.[41]

With obstruction of the pancreatic duct by stone or tumor of the ampulla or head of the pancreas, the volume will be considerably reduced, but bicarbonate concentration and amylase will be altered very little.[41, 42] Diffuse cancers of the pancreas cause a marked reduction of all three components of the pancreatic juice, while a cancer in the tail has little or no effect on any.[42]

Fibrocystic disease of the pancreas or advanced fibrosis will likewise result in a marked decrease of volume, bicarbonate concentration, and amylase.[3] In this respect, fibrosis of the pancreas cannot be differentiated from diffuse carcinoma.

LIMITATIONS AND SOURCES OF ERROR. The time-consuming nature of the secretin test and the elaborate set-up required for it have limited widespread clinical application.[16] Since secretion of amylase is not stimulated by secretin, but the enzyme is only washed out by the increase in volume of pancreatic juice, there is great variability of enzyme content in normal subjects. Hence amylase determinations are of less clinical significance than volume and bicarbonate concentration.[39]

Care must be exercised in avoiding contamination of pancreatic juice with gastric contents which will lower bicarbonate concentration by neutralization and enzyme content by inactivation.[38] To avoid such errors, any specimen of duodenal aspirate with a pH of less than 7.0 should be discarded. The recovery of duodenal contents is semiquantitative at best, so any 20-min collection whose volume is much less than other consecutive specimens should arouse suspicion of inadequate recovery.

DETERMINATION OF INSUFFICIENCY
OF PANCREATIC ENZYMES

The pancreas has such a tremendous reserve that most of the gland may be replaced by cancer or fibrosis before there is clinical evidence of enzyme deficiency.[41, 42] Changes in volume and bicarbonate concentration of the pancreatic juice become apparent long before enzyme deficiency is demonstrable.[42] Marked obstruction of the pancreatic ducts will also result in a deficiency of pancreatic enzymes in the intestinal tract. Determination of enzymes can be made directly on duodenal contents or stool. Tests of alteration in digestive capacity may give an indirect estimate of the secretion of pancreatic enzymes.

### DIRECT MEASUREMENT OF ENZYMES IN PANCREATIC JUICE AND IN FECES

The content of amylase, lipase, or trypsin in duodenal aspirate may be measured. It is usually sufficient to determine just one of these. Since there is normally much variability of enzyme content in pancreatic juice, only an almost complete absence will be clinically significant.[39] Qualitative demonstration of proteolytic (tryptic) activity in the stool is another method for direct measurement. The gelatin-film test [43] is a simple screening technique for establishing the presence or absence of trypsin in the stools of infants and children under the age of 4 years. To avoid false positive results due to proteolytic enzymes of intestinal bacterial origin (gelatinases), a special dilution technique may be used.[44] The use of the gelatin-film test in adults is of no value because trypsin is generally inactivated during the slow passage of feces through the colon.[43]

### DETERMINATION OF ALTERED DIGESTIVE CAPACITY

A gross deficiency of pancreatic enzymes is associated with diarrhea, steatorrhea, and creatorrhea. Examination of the stool for fat, muscle fibers, and nitrogen, as well as various oral tolerance tests, may indicate pancreatic insufficiency, but such procedures are frequently nonspecific for pancreatic ferments and do not distinguish between

the various causes of intestinal malabsorption.

Tests for the study of intestinal absorption are still in the process of development, and their value and limitations are still to be determined. The most helpful screening tests include serum carotene level, oral D-xylose absorption tests, and microscopic examination of stool for fat and muscle fiber.[45] Vitamin A tolerance tests are of limited value in the differential diagnosis of intestinal malabsorption.[3] The oral glucose-tolerance test as a measure of intestinal absorption is subject to such variation both in normal patients and in disease that it cannot be used.[45] Intake and output balance studies for fat and nitrogen are the most reliable way of measuring the degree of malabsorption but are tedious and time-consuming. Moreover, such balance studies do not differentiate between the various causes of disturbed absorption. There is a possibility that the differential absorption between radioactive-iodine-labeled fatty acids and radioactive-iodine-labeled neutral triglycerides may distinguish the malabsorption due to pancreatic insufficiency from that caused by other conditions. The Schilling test with cobalt [60]-labeled vitamin $B_{12}$ with and without intrinsic factor has proven effective in differentiating the malabsorption secondary to intrinsic factor deficiency, as in pernicious anemia, from that due to primary or secondary sprue.[45]

STOOL EXAMINATION. Inspection of the stool often gives the first suggestion of pancreatic insufficiency. Such stools are bulky and light-colored, or have a silvery sheen, and have a rancid odor due to increased content of fat. They usually float on the water in the toilet bowl.[15, 16] Microscopic examination of a bit of stool stained with sudan III (see Unit 22) will show increased neutral fat and total fatty acids when there is a deficiency of pancreatic enzymes.[15] The demonstration of a large number of undigested muscle fibers with well-preserved longitudinal and transverse striations indicates inadequate digestion of protein.[15] There must be an adequate intake of fat and red meat if stool examinations for fat and muscle fiber are to be valid. Delayed transit through the intestinal tract may permit digestion by enzymes of intestinal and bacterial origin.[15] Consequently, absence of neutral fat or undigested muscle fibers in the stool does not eliminate the possibility of pancreatic insufficiency.

Quantitative determination of the solids, fat, and nitrogen in stools of patients who have a measured oral intake may show fecal losses that are roughly in proportion to pancreatic damage.[46] Increased fecal fat loss is more often present than an increase in solids or nitrogen. Quantitative study of stool fat, nitrogen, and solids does not differentiate pancreatic insufficiency from other forms of malabsorption.

ORAL TOLERANCE TESTS WITH RADIOACTIVE ISOTOPES. Alterations in the digestive capacity for protein and fat have been studied by the use of I[131]-labeled albumin[47] and glycerol trioleate[48] respectively. Increased fecal radioactivity has been demonstrated in patients with advanced pancreatic insufficiency, but these methods are not specific for a decrease of pancreatic enzymes. A combined test using tagged neutral fat (I[131]-triolein) and fatty acid (I[131]-oleic acid) at different times offers promise of being a more specific measurement for the digestive capacity of pancreatic lipase.[49] Impaired absorption in both parts of the test suggests some cause of malabsorption other than pancreatic insufficiency. A decrease of pancreatic lipase will impair hydrolysis of the triolein, and hence its absorption, but the tagged oleic acid is absorbed normally in pancreatic insufficiency.

OTHER TESTS OF VALUE IN PANCREATIC DISEASE

DETERMINATION OF SERUM CALCIUM. Measurement of serum calcium (see Unit 32) may be of prognostic value in acute pancreatitis. It is believed that the degree of hypocalcemia may be somewhat related to the severity of the disease and may be looked upon as a quantitative equivalent of the amount of fat necrosis.[50] The loss of calcium is attributed mainly to its incorporation with fatty acids liberated in fat necrosis to form calcium soaps. Additional calcium deficiency may be caused by increased excretion of calcium into the bowel and impaired absorption.[50]

ORAL GLUCOSE-TOLERANCE TEST. Destruction of a sufficient number of islet cells may occur in chronic pancreatitis or carcinoma of the pancreas to produce a deficiency of insulin. Then a diabetic type of oral glucose-tolerance test will result. Although there is no way to differentiate the glucose-tolerance curve of diabetes mellitus from that of chronic pancreatitis or cancer, application of this test is warranted in every case of suspected pancreatic disorder.[14] If positive, the results should increase suspicion of a diagnosis of cancer of the pancreas or chronic pancreatitis. If negative, these diseases are not ruled out.

SERUM LEUCINE AMINOPEPTIDASE DETERMINATION. Leucine aminopeptidase is a proteolytic enzyme found in liver, pancreas, intestinal mucosa, and many other body tissues. The nature of its entry into blood plasma is not known, but it may be identified in both serum and urine by its hydrolytic action on the substrate *l*-leucyl-β-naphthylamide hydrochloride. This reaction liberates β-naphthylamine which is then diazotized and converted to an azo dye that can be measured quantitatively.[51] The urinary excretion of the enzyme may be increased in pregnancy and in many malignant and other diseases, so the urinary determination is not a specific diagnostic test. Preliminary reports of experiences with measurements of leucine aminopeptidase in the serum, however, suggest that a persistent and greatly elevated level is quite suggestive of cancer of the pancreas.[52] Pancreatitis and stones in the common bile duct may be associated with fluctuating serum levels of a lesser degree of increase. The eventual value of this test will be established with greater experience.

## REFERENCES

1. J. E. Thomas, *The External Secretion of the Pancreas* (Thomas, Springfield, 1950).
2. M. I. Grossman, "Gastrointestinal hormones," *Physiol. Rev. 30*, 33 (1950).
3. D. A. Dreiling and H. D. Janowitz, "Exocrine pancreatic secretion: Effects of pancreatic disease," *Amer. J. Med. 21*, 98 (1956).
4. D. A. Dreiling and H. D. Janowitz, "The secretion of electrolytes by the human pancreas," *Gastroenterology 30*, 382 (1956).
5. M. H. Kalser and M. I. Grossman, "Secretion of trypsin inhibitor in pancreatic juice," *Gastroenterology 29*, 35 (1955).
6. H. I. Tankel and F. Hollander, "The relation between pancreatic secretion and local blood flow: A review," *Gastroenterology 32*, 633 (1957).
7. M. H. F. Friedman and W. J. Snape, "Dissociation of secretion of pancreatic enzymes and bicarbonate in patients with chronic pancreatitis," *Gastroenterology 15*, 296 (1950).
8. D. A. Dreiling, H. D. Janowitz, and M. Halpern, "The effect of a carbonic anhydrase inhibitor, Diamox, on human pancreatic secretion," *Gastroenterology 29*, 262 (1955).
9. H. D. Janowitz and F. Hollander, "The exocrine-endocrine partition of enzymes in the digestive tract," *Gastroenterology 17*, 591 (1951).
10. M. I. Grossman, "Experimental pancreatitis," *Arch. intern. Med. 96*, 298 (1955).
11. M. I. Grossman, H. Greengard, and A. C. Ivy, "The effect of diatary composition on pancreatic enzymes," *Amer. J. Physiol. 138*, 676 (1942).
12. R. B. Pfeffer, H. E. Stephenson, and J. W. Hinton, "The effect of thoracolumbar sympathectomy and vagus resection on pancreatic function in man," *Ann. Surg. 136*, 585 (1952).
13. D. A. Dreiling, L. J. Druckerman, and F. Hollander, "The effect of complete vagisection and vagal stimulation on pancreatic secretion in man," *Gastroenterology 20*, 578 (1952).
14. R. L. Sterkel and J. B. Kirsner, "The laboratory diagnosis of pancreatic disease," *Arch. intern. Med. 101*, 114 (1958).
15. M. N. Nothman, "The value of functional tests for the diagnosis of diseases of the pancreas," *Ann. intern. Med. 34*, 1358 (1951).
16. T. E. Machella, "Useful diagnostic laboratory procedures in pancreatitis," *Arch. intern. Med. 96*, 322 (1955).
17. M. Somogyi, "Micromethods for estimation of diastase," *J. biol. Chem. 125*, 399 (1938).
18. T. S. Malinowski, "Clinical value of serum amylase determination," *J. Amer. med. Ass. 149*, 1380 (1952).
19. T. W. Challis, L. C. Reid, and J. W. Hinton, "Study of some factors which in-

fluence the level of serum amylase in dogs and humans," *Gastroenterology 33*, 818 (1957).

20. E. C. Raffensperger, "Elevated serum pancreatic enzyme values without primary intrinsic pancreatic disease," *Ann. intern. Med. 35*, 342 (1951).

21. R. B. Pfeffer, H. E. Stephenson, Jr., and J. W. Hinton, "The effect of morphine, demerol, and codeine on serum amylase values in man," *Gastroenterology 23*, 482 (1953).

22. H. Wapshaw, "The pancreatic side-effects of morphine," *Brit. med. J.*, No. 4806, 373 (1953).

23. A. Bogoch, J. L. A. Roth, and H. L. Bockus, "The effects of morphine on serum amylase and lipase," *Gastroenterology 26*, 697 (1954).

24. H. L. Nossel, "The effect of morphine on the serum and urinary amylase and the sphincter of Oddi: With some preliminary observations on the effect of alcohol on the serum amylase and the sphincter of Oddi," *Gastroenterology 29*, 409 (1955).

25. I. S. Cherry and L. A. Crandall, "The specificity of pancreatic lipase: Its appearance in the blood after pancreatic injury," *Amer. J. Physiol. 100*, 266 (1932).

26. H. O. Lagerlöf, "Normal serum esterase and pancreatic lipase in diseases of the biliary ducts and pancreas," *Acta med. scand.*, Supp. 196, *128*, 399 (1947).

27. T. A. Johnson and H. L. Bockus, "Diagnostic significance of determinations of serum lipase," *Arch. intern. Med. 66*, 62 (1940).

28. H. A. Ravin and A. M. Seligman, "Determinants for the specificity of action of pancreatic lipase," *Arch. Biochem. 42*, 337 (1953).

29. G. L. Nardi and C. W. Lees, "Serum trypsin: A new diagnostic test for pancreatic disease," *New Engl. J. Med. 258*, 797 (1958).

30. D. A. Dreiling and A. Richman, "Evaluation of provocative blood enzyme tests employed in diagnosis of pancreatic disease," *Arch. intern. Med. 94*, 197 (1954).

31. T. S. Malinowski, "Serum amylase response to pancreatic stimulation as a test of pancreatic disease," *Amer. J. Med. Sci. 222*, 440 (1951).

32. J. O. Burke, K. Plummer, and S. Bradford, "Serum amylase response to morphine, mecholyl, and secretin as a test of pancreatic function," *Gastroenterology 15*, 699 (1950).

33. L. A. Sachar, J. G. Probstein, and J. M. Whittico, "The effect of pancreatic stimulants on blood diastase," *Gastroenterology 18*, 104 (1951).

34. A. Danker and C. J. Heifetz, "The interrelationship of blood and urinary diastase during transient acute pancreatitis," *Gastroenterology 18*, 207 (1951).

35. B. I. Saxon, W. C. Hinkley, W. C. Vogel, and L. Zieve, "Comparative value of serum and urinary amylase in the diagnosis of acute pancreatitis," *Arch. intern. Med. 99*, 607 (1957).

36. M. M. Nothman, J. H. Pratt, and A. D. Callow, "Studies on urinary lipase. I. On a fat-splitting enzyme in urine and its relations to pancreas," *Arch. intern. Med. 95*, 224 (1955).

37. M. M. Nothman, J. H. Pratt, and A. D. Callow, "Studies on urinary lipase. II. Urinary lipase in man," *Arch. intern. Med. 96*, 188 (1955).

38. D. A. Dreiling and F. Hollander, "Studies in pancreatic function. I. Preliminary series of clinical studies with the secretin test," *Gastroenterology 11*, 714 (1945).

39. D. A. Dreiling and F. Hollander, "Studies in pancreatic function. II. A statistical study of pancreatic secretion following secretin in patients without pancreatic disease," *Gastroenterology 15*, 620 (1950).

40. G. R. Dornberger, M. W. Comfort, E. E. Wollaeger, and M. H. Power, "Pancreatic function as measured by analysis of duodenal contents before and after stimulation with secretin," *Gastroenterology 11*, 701 (1948).

41. D. A. Dreiling, Sr., "Studies in pancreatic function. V. The use of the secretin test in the diagnosis of pancreatitis and in the demonstration of pancreatic insufficiencies in gastrointestinal disorders," *Gastroenterology 24*, 540 (1953).

42. D. A. Dreiling, "Studies in pancreatic function. IV. The use of the secretin test in diagnosis of tumors in and about the pancreas," *Gastroenterology 18*, 184 (1951).

43. H. Shwachman, P. R. Patterson, and J. Laguna, "Studies in pancreatic fibrosis: A simple diagnostic gelatin film test for stool trypsin," *Pediatrics 4*, 222 (1949).

44. D. E. Johnstone, "Studies in cystic fibrosis of the pancreas. Role of various diluents and the dilution factor in the interpretation of the X-ray film test for fecal trypsin," *Amer. J. Dis. Child. 84*, 191 (1951).

45. P. J. Culver, "Survey of methods for study of intestinal absorption," *Amer. J. dig. Dis. 2*, 620 (1957).

46. G. R. Dornberger, M. W. Comfort, E. E. Wollaeger, and M. H. Power, "Total fecal solids, fat and nitrogen. IV. A study of patients with chronic relapsing pancreatitis," *Gastroenterology 11*, 691 (1948).

47. A. B. Chinn, P. S. Lavik, R. M. Stitt, and G. W. Buckaloo, "Use of I[131]-labelled protein in the diagnosis of pancreatic insufficiency," *New Engl. J. Med. 247*, 877 (1952).

48. W. W. Shingleton, G. J. Baylin, J. K. Isley, A. P. Sandos, and J. M. Ruffin, "The evaluation of pancreatic function by use of I[131]-labelled fat," *Gastroenterology 32*, 28 (1957).

49. B. J. Duffy and D. A. Turner, "The differential diagnosis of intestinal malabsorption with I[131]-fat and fatty acid," *Ann. intern. Med. 48*, 1 (1958).

50. H. A. Edmondson, C. J. Berne, J. Homann, and M. Wertman, "Calcium, potassium, magnesium, and amylase disturbances in acute pancreatitis," *Amer. J. Med. 12*, 34 (1952).

51. J. A. Goldbarg and A. M. Rutenburg: "The colorimetric determination of leucine aminopeptidase in urine and serum of normal subjects and patients with cancer and other diseases," *Cancer 11*, 283 (1958).

52. A. M. Rutenburg, J. A. Goldbarg, and E. P. Pineda, "Leucine aminopeptidase activity. Observations in patients with cancer of the pancreas and other diseases," *New Engl. J. Med. 259*, 469 (1958).

# Unit 26

# Infectious Diseases

The diagnosis of infectious disease is made either by direct isolation and identification of the causative agent or by obtaining indirect but specific evidence of the presence of an offending pathogen by serologic tests on the blood serum or by skin tests. The physician is referred to textbooks of bacteriology for the details of classification and identification of bacteria, rickettsiae, protozoa, fungi, and viruses.[1-5] The purpose of this unit is to indicate the methods for diagnosis of causative agents in blood, urine, cerebrospinal fluid, pleural, pericardial, peritoneal, and synovial fluids, and exudates from the throat and other sites. The techniques for the Gram stain and the Ziehl-Neelsen acid-fast stain are described in Unit 27.

## Diagnostic Bacteriology of Exudates and Body Fluids

### NOSE AND THROAT CULTURES

INTRODUCTION. The nasopharynx and the oropharynx are easily accessible for culture, and the bacteriologic diagnosis of many infectious diseases can be made by examination of secretions obtained from these sites. Meningococcal carrier states are established by culture of nasopharyngeal secretions, and such isolations have particular epidemiologic significance. The finding of group A *Streptococcus hemolyticus* in the nasopharynx usually correlates with a similar isolation from the throat and provides sound rationale for prompt chemotherapy. Isolation of *Staphylococcus aureus hemolyticus* or *Hemophilus influenzae* by nasopharyngeal swab may reflect acute sinusitis caused by these bacteria or may be indicative of more benign clinical carrier states. Culture of the oropharynx is also a useful laboratory procedure in the problem of pharyngitis where a specific bacteriologic agent such as beta hemolytic *Streptococcus, Corynebacterium diphtheriae* and, rarely, *Staph. aureus* may produce disease. In infants, *H. influenzae* should be sought as a cause for sore throats. Pharyngitis associated with normal pharyngeal flora is caused by a viral infection. Furthermore, there is still the rare situation in which the appearance of the oropharynx suggests diphtheria, and throat culture provides the only certain means by which this disease may be excluded. In these, as in all bacteriologic determinations, the cultural data should be evaluated in conjunction with the rest of the clinical protocol.

METHODS OF OBTAINING SPECIMENS. *Nose culture.* Secretions from the nose may be obtained by passing swabs through a nasal speculum and gently wiping the posterior aspect of the nasal passages. In children, and especially when meningococcal organisms are suspected, cultures are best obtained by inserting a bent swab through the mouth and behind the uvula. Care should be taken to prevent the swab from coming in contact with

445

the tonsils, tongue, or saliva, since the mouth organisms and secretions in the mouth may inhibit growth of the meningococcus. In the case of meningococci, culture swabs should be streaked onto media at once. For other organisms, if culture media are not close at hand, the swab may be placed in a sterile cotton-plugged test tube and taken to the bacteriology laboratory before the material on the swab becomes dry or contaminated.

*Throat culture.* The swabbing of the oropharynx should be done with proper illumination and a tongue depressor should be used. Care should be exercised not to touch the base of the tongue. A quick maneuver allows the passage of the swab from one tonsil or tonsillar fossa across the posterior oropharyngeal wall to the opposite tonsillar area without disturbing the patient and with minimal stimulation of the gag reflex. As with nose cultures, prompt plating of the swab is indicated.

CULTURE MEDIA. Five-percent defibrinated horse-blood agar is a good nutrient medium for the cultivation of most nose and throat pathogens. Incubation of agar plates at 37°C should not exceed 24 hr and gross examination for colony morphology and presence of hemolysis is then made.

Pneumococci may be differentiated from alpha hemolytic streptococci by inspection of colonial morphology under a hand lens, and by testing for bile solubility.

Staphylococci may be further classified by means of the coagulase test or mannitol fermentation. Whenever gross colony identification is doubtful, microscopic appearance with Gram stain should be used for confirmation.

The identification of group A beta hemolytic streptococci in nose and throat cultures is especially important because of the possibility of nonsuppurative sequelae such as rheumatic fever and glomerulonephritis. When horse-blood agar is used, there may be false positive instances of beta hemolysis due to *H. influenzae.* A Gram stain of hemolytic colonies is used to identify streptococci. Sheep-blood agar is a better medium for the accurate identification of beta hemolytic streptococci, since the latter medium does not support the growth of *H. influenzae.* Since primarily group A beta hemolytic streptococci are pathogenic for man, the serologic identification of streptococci showing beta hemolysis on sheep-blood agar has practical implications. Group specific antiserums against many of the subgroups of beta hemolytic streptococci are available and the precipitin reaction between an acid extract of the bacteria and the various antiserums allows for precise characterization of group A organisms. Among group A streptococci, there may be further classification into subtypes, but such typing is usually done in special study laboratories as a research project. Approximately 10 to 15 percent of beta hemolytic streptococci isolated from the nose and throat during clinical infections are found to be other than group A and are therefore of no importance etiologically.

*Diphtheria.* In cases of acute exudative pharyngitis, especially in the presence of membranous lesions, diphtheria should be suspected and inoculation of specialized media should be made in addition to the usual blood-agar plate. Corynebacteria grow most readily on Löffler's medium, which contains coagulated serum, and the characteristic growth on a potassium tellurite plate enables differentiation between the three types of *C. diphtheriae.* In addition to such cultural methods, smears of the membrane with methylene-blue stain may show the typical beaded rods with "club-shaped" irregular swellings at either end. If the patient has received penicillin, the cultures should be kept for at least 7 days, since penicillin inhibits the growth of the organism without killing it.

*Meningococci.* Nasopharyngeal swabs suspected of containing *Neisseria intracellularis* should be plated immediately. Chocolate-agar inoculation and growth in an atmosphere containing 5–10 percent of $CO_2$ (candle jar) provides optimal conditions for isolation of these organisms, but final differentiation of the meningococcus from other benign *Neisseria* requires the use of differential sugar fermentation.

*Cough plate for Hemophilus pertussis* (whooping cough). Primary isolation of *H. pertussis* requires complex enriched media. A plate containing Bordet-Gengou's medium may be held about 6 in. from the patient's mouth and the patient instructed to cough at it. A spontaneous cough during a paroxysm yields a higher chance of positive culture. An alternative method is the use of a nasal swab which is then streaked through a drop of penicillin solution (10–100 $\mu g/ml$) and placed on the Bordet medium. Growth of *H. pertussis* is sluggish and will appear in 48 to 72 hr, particularly in the zone where penicillin has inhibited the growth of other organisms. Cells from typical colonies may then be finally identified by agglutination with specific antiserum.

*Monilia,* which may be found in thrush or during long-term therapy with antibiotics, grow readily on blood agar and are easily identified.

*Vincent's organisms* are of importance in the differential diagnosis of membranous pharyngitis. These organisms are not easily cultured but may be demonstrated in a direct Gram stain of a smear from the membrane or from the gingivae.

BLOOD CULTURES

INTRODUCTION. Bacterial invasion of the blood stream occurs during the course of many infectious diseases, and the isolation of such specific etiologic organisms is of crucial importance in directing proper antimicrobial therapy. The possibility of bacteremia should be considered in all febrile illnesses and should particularly be suspected when chills accompany spiking fever. Intermittent bacteremia is characteristic of cholangitis, pyelonephritis, septic thrombophlebitis, undrained abscess, brucellosis, and many other infections. In these situations, repeated blood cultures may be necessary to isolate the organism, and cultures are best obtained just prior to a predictable chill or on the ascending limb of a fever spike. In certain other infections, such as subacute bacterial endocarditis and typhoid fever during the first four or five febrile days, bacteremia is relatively constant and isolation of the organism can be reasonably assured if four or five cultures are obtained over a 24–48-hr span. In such instances, when antimicrobial therapy is urgently indicated, it may be initiated after the requisite four or five cultures have been obtained, with the knowledge that in a large majority of instances positive cultures will be found. Antimicrobial therapy administered to the patient prior to hospitalization or otherwise prematurely may partially or wholly suppress bacteremia and render isolation of the etiologic organism from the blood difficult or impossible. In some instances, addition of penicillinase to the blood culture medium will overcome the inhibitory effect of penicillin and allow recovery of organisms; but often it is necessary to withhold further therapy and await recrudescence of the suppressed infection in order to make a precise diagnosis.

The interpretation of positive blood cultures must always be viewed with the possibility of contamination in mind. The skin of the patient, and the hospital milieu, offer fertile soil for bacterial growth, and therefore extreme care to avoid contamination must be taken in obtaining blood cultures. In general, the recovery of identical organisms from several blood cultures indicates that true bacteremia is present. Recovery in blood cultures of common skin or environmental contaminants such as *Staph. albus,* diphtheroids, and yeasts, generally indicates contamination; but recovery of *Staph. aureus* often presents a difficult problem, as this organism is a common and serious pathogen, as well as a widespread contaminant of the hospital environment.

METHODS. *Technique of blood culture.* Venous blood is the most satisfactory to obtain for culture. The operator should wear a surgical mask. A wide area of skin over the antecubital vein should be carefully cleaned with an aqueous solution of zephiran or other detergent antiseptic. The antiseptic area should then be cleaned with tincture of iodine and a final cleansing carried out with 70-percent alcohol. At least 10 ml of blood should be withdrawn via needle into a sterile syringe. The needle should then be removed from the syringe and the syringe tip flamed in a bedside burner prior to introducing the blood into the liquid culture flask. Paired 5–10-ml aliquots of sterile blood should be added to approximately 100 ml of aerobic and thioglycollate media. It is also advisable to incubate cultures under increased carbon dioxide pressure. In addition, it is often desirable to incorporate 1 ml of blood into an agar pour plate as a means of quantitating the degree of bacteremia.

*Reading and interpretation of blood cultures.* Blood-culture flasks should be inspected daily during incubation. Evidence of bacterial growth may be manifested either by diffuse turbidity or by colony growth on the surface of the sedimented cells. Early growth may often be suspected if the color of the sedimented cell turns from crimson to a more purple hue. If growth is suspected, the flask should be entered under aseptic conditions with a sterile pipette and a sample removed for subculture and Gram stain. Although growth in a positive culture is usually apparent after 48

hr, in many instances growth may take much longer to appear, and certain organisms such as *Brucella* and *Pasteurella tularensis* may require weeks. If inhibitory antibiotics have been taken by the patient prior to blood culture, growth may also be delayed, so cultures should be kept under observation for 3 weeks before a final negative report is issued. The addition of para-aminobenzoic acid will serve to neutralize sulfonamides in blood cultures obtained following such therapy. Penicillinase will neutralize penicillinemia that exists at the time of blood culture. There are at present no suitable antagonists for the many other antibiotics.

*Special problems in blood culture.* Some organisms require specialized media or cultural conditions and for their isolation the laboratory must be informed that the clinician suspects their presence. Most bacteriology laboratories do not routinely culture blood under strictly anaerobic conditions, so if bacteremia with strict anaerobes such as *Bacteroides* is suspected the laboratory should be so notified.

The isolation of the *Brucella* group of organisms is best accomplished with specialized mediums, now commercially available. The Castaneda double-medium technique is an excellent one and employs both trypticase soy agar and broth in a single flask containing 10 percent of $CO_2$.

One of the most fastidious organisms encountered in clinical infectious disease is *Past. tularensis.* Its isolation from the tularemic patient requires a complex blood-glucose-cystine agar as well as serum-enriched broth. Guinea pig inoculation and subsequent recovery of the organism from blood, lymph nodes, and spleen may be useful.

URINE CULTURES

INTRODUCTION. Infections of the urinary tract may be caused by almost any microorganism, but more than half of such infections are due to *Escherichia coli.* Culture of the urine is indicated whenever chronic pyelonephritis is suspected (see Unit 19). The presence of leukocytes or white-blood-cell casts in the urine is an indication for bacteriologic study of the urine. Urine cultures may be of value in the diagnosis of chills and fever.

METHOD AND INTERPRETATION. Urine is best collected by the "clean-catch" method, making certain that the external genitalia have been scrupulously cleansed, and collecting only the terminal portion of urine voided. A sterile container should be used. Gram staining should be carried out on the fresh, uncentrifuged urine. If organisms are detected on such a smear, there are usually $10^5$ or more bacteria per milliliter of urine; this is usually indicative of urinary-tract infection. Cultures of fresh urine should be planted on blood agar and Endo's or other inhibitory media.

Often when cultures are positive but no organisms are seen by smear, a colony count may be helpful in differentiating between bacterial contamination and infection. If fewer than 10,000 organisms per milliliter are present, the organisms usually represent contamination. Colony counts should be made immediately after voiding, since bacteria multiply rapidly in warm specimens. Refrigeration allows reasonably accurate counts within 4 hr. Two plates are usually made for a colony count. The first consists of 0.5 ml of undiluted urine mixed with 10 ml of melted agar. Twice the number of observed colonies represents the number of bacteria per milliliter of urine. If the colonies are too numerous to count, a second dilution, in which the urine has been diluted to 1:100 and from which 0.1 ml has been mixed with 10 ml of melted agar, will be helpful. The number of observed colonies mutiplied by 1000 represents the number of organisms per milliliter of urine.

Acid-fast bacilli may be demonstrated in the sediment of a centrifuged urine sample by staining a smear by the Ziehl-Neelsen method. Tubercle bacilli, however, cannot be differentiated by their appearance in the smear from acid-fast saprophytes which may easily find access to the urine from the genitalia. If renal tuberculosis is suspected, the urine should be cultured on appropriate mediums and inoculated into a guinea pig.

### BACTERIOLOGIC EXAMINATION OF FECES

INTRODUCTION. The etiologic agents of infectious gastrointestinal disease can be demonstrated frequently by appropriate bacteriologic examination of the feces. Since carrier states of enteric pathogens may exist without overt symptomatology, the finding of a potentially pathogenic organism in the stool is not always conclusive evidence that this agent is responsible for an active disease state. In addition to primary diarrheal states caused by known enteric pathogens, the use of antibiotics has introduced an important group of secondary diarrheas, presumably due to the inhibition of normal enteric organisms, which are susceptible to the antibiotic, and subsequent overgrowth of insensitive organisms. Superinfection of the bowel with yeasts and *Staph. aureus* may occur.

COLLECTION OF SPECIMENS. Stool specimens for bacteriologic study should be sent to the laboratory as soon as possible after collection and the material should be plated promptly to prevent overgrowth of coliform organisms.

DIRECT SMEAR EXAMINATION. There are several instances of enteric infection wherein direct microscopic examination of a portion of stool will yield helpful diagnostic information.

*Moniliasis.* If Gram stain of a stool smear reveals a predominant presence of yeast forms, microscopic examination may confirm a clinical impression of post-antibiotic diarrhea with monilial super-infection.

*Pseudomembranous enterocolitis.* In cases of suspected pseudomembranous enterocolitis, the stool may show, on Gram stain, the exclusive or predominant presence of staphylococci along with many pus cells.

*Amebic dysentery.* All cases of diarrhea should be examined directly for the cysts and trophozoites of *Entamoeba histolytica,* but the frequent existence of the carrier state, which varies in different geographic areas, makes the finding of this organism an associative rather than a diagnostic test in many cases.

*Cholera.* In areas where the disease is endemic, the clinical picture and epidemiology of cholera usually are sufficient to make the diagnosis, but the possibility of an isolated case, especially in an era of jet air transport, may require laboratory diagnosis. The mucous flakes of an infected stool are most apt to contain the organism and microscopic examination can reveal the typical gram-negative vibrio.

CULTURE OF STOOL ON DIFFERENT MEDIUMS. The finding of *Shigella* in bacillary dysentery is most easily achieved during the first 3 or 4 days of acute symptoms. Beyond this period, isolation of enteric pathogens becomes increasingly difficult. Conversely, stool cultures for *Salmonella* in cases of "enteric fever" usually do not become positive until after the first week of symptomatic disease. When many cases of diarrhea occur simultaneously, and an outbreak of food poisoning is suspected, it is also important to attempt culture from the suspicious foods. Such cultures from suspected foods may be carried out in staphylococcal food poisoning, botulism, and *Salmonella* or *Shigella* infections.

*Selective mediums.* The major differentiation achieved by selective enteric me-

diums is to distinguish the nonpathogenic lactose-fermenting organisms, especially *Esch. coli* and *Aerobacter aerogenes,* from the non-lactose-fermenting pathogens. A breakdown of this differentiation may be seen by reference to textbooks and manuals of bacteriology. The selective mediums most commonly used for this classification of gram-negative, non-spore-forming bacteria are Endo's agar, eosin-methylene-blue agar, and SS agar (containing desoxycholate and citrate). A blood-agar plate should be employed if there is a question of infection with *Staph. aureus.* Inoculation of stool into selenite broth as an enrichment medium will permit the growth of species of *Shigella* and *Salmonella* while suppressing the normal enteric flora. Subculture onto selective mediums will then permit identification.

*Fermentation reactions.* After enteric organisms have been classified according to their ability to ferment lactose, further differentiation of species is based on other sugar-fermentation reactions and specific slide agglutinations with antiserums to the various individual types. In general, *Shigella* strains are nonmotile, whereas *Salmonella* strains are motile in hanging-drop preparations.

*Botulism.* Food poisoning due to *Clostridium botulinum* requires laboratory confirmation by isolation of the gram-positive bacillus by anaerobic methods and demonstration of the type-specific toxin in the incriminated food.

*Cholera.* In addition to the direct microscopic search for the vibrio in mucopurulent flakes of the stool, growth in culture is readily achieved at pH 8 in 1-percent peptone water. The peptone-water culture can be tested for the cholera red reaction by the addition of concentrated sulfuric acid.

CEREBROSPINAL FLUID

INTRODUCTION. The clinical diagnosis of suspected meningitis should always be confirmed by examination of the cerebrospinal fluid. The microorganisms that most commonly produce meningitis are *Neisseria intracellularis, Diplococcus pneumoniae, Str. haemolyticus, Micrococcus pyogenes,* and *Mycobacterium tuberculosis.* Among infants, *H. influenzae* is an important etiologic agent. More rarely, the gram-negative bacilli may produce meningitis. In addition, certain fungi, notably *Cryptococcus neoformans* (torula), invade the leptomeninges. The laboratory diagnosis of the various viral meningitides requires animal or tissue-culture inoculation of properly collected specimens of cerebrospinal fluid.

COLLECTION OF THE SPECIMEN. When a free flow of cerebrospinal fluid becomes established, the appearance of the fluid may provide the first indication concerning the causative agent. Pyogenic bacteria will usually produce cloudy fluid by the time symptomatology has become established. A clear fluid may, nevertheless, be infected. Several milliliters of fluid should be collected directly from the spinal needle in a sterile tube and the material transported directly to the laboratory for smear and culture. If there is a suspicion of viral meningitis, a second aliquot of 2 ml should be collected in a sterile tube and promptly frozen for subsequent virus isolation.

A cell count of the cerebrospinal fluid performed prior to bacterial examination will usually prove helpful in the tentative classification of meningitis, but atypical situations may cause confusion. A high white-cell count in the cerebrospinal fluid with a predominance of polymorphonuclear cells is highly suggestive of invasion by the pyogenic bacteria, whereas lymphocytosis is more apt to characterize tuberculous and viral infection. Whenever meningitis is suggested on the basis of the cerebrospinal-fluid cell count, a portion of fluid should

also be analyzed for sugar and chloride content (see Unit 18).

CEREBROSPINAL-FLUID SMEARS. Direct smear of undiluted cerebrospinal fluid or the centrifuged sediment may establish an immediate diagnosis. Gram stain may distinguish the gram-negative intracellular meningococcus from the gram-positive pyogenic cocci, and thereby direct the use of the most appropriate antibiotics. The use of acid-fast stain will establish tuberculous meningitis with a high degree of certainty, but, because the concentration of tubercle bacilli is usually small, diligent and protracted search of the entire acid-fast-stained smear may be necessary to find the organisms.

Fungal infection may be detected with the India-ink stain. A drop of cerebrospinal fluid is mixed with a drop of India ink and viewed microscopically under a coverslip with reduced light. The capsules of the fungus will appear as clear halos around the budding yeast cells.

ROUTINE CULTURE. Final confirmation of the presence of the specific organism in a case of suspected meningitis requires culture of the spinal fluid on appropriate mediums. Meningococci are particularly sensitive to chilling and freezing so that prompt inoculation and incubation of all mediums will give the best results. In general, most pyogenic bacteria (pneumococci, streptococci, staphylococci, and gram-negative bacilli) will grow on the usual laboratory medium—any rich meat infusion, broth, or agar enriched with 5 to 10 percent of blood (rabbit, sheep, or horse). If *H. influenzae* is suspected, horse-blood agar is essential. Primary isolation of meningococci is best achieved by the use of chocolate agar and candle-jar incubation. Growth of the pyogenic bacteria is usually obvious after 18 to 24 hr of incubation at 37.5°C, but an additional 24 hr may be necessary for identifiable growth of small inocula to appear.

ACID-FAST CULTURE. When tuberculous meningitis is suspected, a portion of cerebrospinal fluid should be centrifuged and the sediment inoculated onto specific diagnostic mediums (see Unit 27). Guinea pig inoculation with cerebrospinal-fluid concentrate may also be used as a means of confirming acid-fast invasion of the leptomeninges.

FUNGI. *Cryptococcus neoformans* and the *Candida* yeasts may be cultured at room temperature or at 37°C on all common laboratory mediums. The colony forms are most characteristic when grown on Sabouraud's glucose agar at room temperature. If meningitis due to a fungus infection is suspected, the culture must be kept for at least 7 days because *C. neoformans* may grow very slowly.

### SEROUS-CAVITY TRANSUDATES AND EXUDATES

INTRODUCTION. The pleural, peritoneal, pericardial, and joint spaces may all be the sites of infection, and fluid obtained by aspiration of these cavities should always be examined for microorganisms. Pyogenic bacteria and the tubercle bacillus are the most common etiologic agents of such infections, but rare instances of infection with *Brucella*, fusiform organisms, spirochetes, the *Salmonella* group, and anaerobes are encountered. Since the first aspiration of these cavities is most apt to be free of outside contamination, and since anatomic difficulties may render a second aspiration more difficult or impossible, it is important that possible bacterial disease be considered at the time of the initial entry into the cavity and that suitable examination be made on the fluid obtained.

STAINED SMEARS. Smears for staining with Gram stain, Ziehl-Neelsen stain, India ink, or Wright's stain should be prepared from the fluid directly or from the centrifuged sediment.

CULTURE. Techniques of culture for possible microorganisms in cavity fluids are similar to those for cerebrospinal fluid. Use of concentrates when the fluid obtained seems dilute will enhance favorable identification. Special mediums designed for organisms with fastidious growth requirements (for example, *Brucella*) should be used as indicated.

### EXAMINATION OF PUS AND MATERIAL FROM WOUNDS

No opportunity should ever be lost to obtain material for smear and culture from the drainage of abscess cavities. Serous or purulent exudate from chronic sinus tracts may give valuable data regarding underlying causative organisms or environmental contaminants which may require a change in antimicrobial therapy. Unexplained postoperative febrile responses following "clean surgery" can often be traced to wound sepsis, and the simple procedure of culturing the wound may provide the first step in rational antibiotic therapy. The increasing importance of hospital-acquired infections caused by antibiotic-resistant *Staphylococci* disseminated by professional personnel and contaminated hospital equipment indicates a need for "surface bacteriology." The proper management of the patient with extensive skin burns also requires continuous monitoring of superficial bacterial flora. Material obtained from drainage areas or superficial wounds should be Gram stained. Chronic sinus tracts suggest infection with tuberculosis or actinomycosis. Acid-fast stains should be used and a search for sulfur granules should be carried out. Wound exudate should be cultured aerobically and anaerobically. If there is suspicion of unusual etiologic agents such as *Clostridia* or fungi, the bacteriology laboratory should be alerted so that special procedures may be carried out.

VAGINAL AND PENILE EXUDATES

In the male, gonorrhea and nonspecific urethritis are the chief causes for a penile discharge, whereas gonorrhea, moniliasis, and trichomonal infection are the three most common infections of the female genital tract. Gram stain of a fixed smear will identify the typical gram-negative, intracellular gonococci; cultural confirmation requires inoculation of infusion chocolate agar and incubation for 48 hr in 10-percent carbon dioxide. Yeasts such as *Candida* will generally show up on Gram stain, and may be cultured on special fungus mediums or on blood agar. Wet mounts or hanging-drop preparations will demonstrate trichomonads.

## Serologic Methods for the Diagnosis of Infectious Diseases

### INTRODUCTION

The most precise means by which to establish the etiology of an infectious disease is by the isolation and confirmation of the pathogenicity of the invading organism. There are circumstances, however, when Koch's postulates cannot be satisfied, although the clinical picture is nonetheless suggestive of a particular disease. Observation of the patient late in the course of the disease, previous antimicrobial therapy that has partially suppressed the infecting organism, or diseases associated with small numbers of fastidious microorganisms are all situations that may make it difficult to identify the causative organism. Under such conditions, it is important to be able to detect serum antibodies produced during the infection as a means of indirect diagnosis. The detection of antibodies directed against specific antigens is also used as confirmatory evidence in infections where the etiologic organism has already been isolated. Of greater diagnostic importance than the mere detection of specific antibodies is the demonstration of changes in the antibody titer

during the course of a particular infection. Blood should be obtained during the acute phase of a suspected infectious disease and a second sample should be collected several weeks later. The taking of a single sample late in the course of a disease may have little value if the titer is in a borderline diagnostic range and no base value is available for comparison. It is usually wiser to collect and store frozen serum taken at the onset of a suspected infection and later discard it than to lack this important specimen at a time when the diagnosis rests on a change in antibody titer.

The proper interpretation of the results of serologic tests involves consideration of certain variables that may affect antibody titer at the time of the particular illness. History of previous infection by the same organism, previous vaccination, naturally occurring antibodies, and anamnestic reactions caused by heterologous antigens, may all play a role individually or collectively in the antibody titer observed.

There are a variety of antibodies that can be measured during infectious disease states. Some are specific and arise in direct response to the inciting bacterium, whereas others appear to bear no obviously direct relation to the causative agent. The most commonly measured specific antibody is that which causes in vitro agglutination of microorganisms. Other antibodies are hemolysins, while still others act by fixing complement, thereby inhibiting the lysis of red blood cells. Antibodies against viruses can be measured by in vivo neutralization of the effects of the virus, or by the inhibition of red-blood-cell agglutination.

### AGGLUTINATION REACTIONS

"FEBRILE" AGGLUTINATIONS. Titration of the patient's serum antibody by agglutination of suspensions of known killed bacterial cells ("antigens") is a valuable diagnostic procedure in fevers of unknown origin. This technique aims to de-

453

termine the greatest dilution of the patient's serum that will cause agglutination of a known bacterial antigen. "Significant" agglutination titers vary considerably with the procedures used and the method of preparing the antigen. The laboratory in which the test is performed should be consulted regarding the significance of titers based on the usual "normal" values obtained for particular antigenic solutions.

*Typhoid and other Salmonella infections.* The Widal agglutination test is useful in the diagnosis of typhoid fever and other *Salmonella* infections. *Salmonella* bacteria contain a flagellar or "H" antigen and a somatic "O" antigen. After the second week of *Salmonella* infections, titers of antibodies to these antigens rise to a level that aids in the serologic diagnosis of the disease. High or rising levels of "O" agglutinins are consistent with active disease, whereas high titers of the "H" agglutinins are more consistent with old infection or recent vaccination. Titers of "O" agglutinins of 1 : 80 or higher should be considered to have diagnostic significance, especially when this titer represents a rise from a lower level.

*Brucellosis.* Because of the difficulties which may be encountered in culturing *Brucella,* the agglutination test takes on added importance. The test must be performed carefully with antigen material that has been well standardized. Agglutinin titers above 1 : 100 are suggestive of active brucellosis, although most proved instances of *Brucella* infection are associated with much higher titers. Titers in the vicinity of 1 : 100 may be compatible with past or "subclinical" infection. It is important to obtain blood for *Brucella* agglutinins prior to skin testing with *Brucella* antigen, since such injected antigenic material may produce elevated serum antibody titers. Because of antigenic interrelations, individuals immunized with cholera vaccine may develop *Brucella* agglutinins. There is also some cross-agglutination reaction between *Past. tularensis* and *Br. abortus* and *Br. melitensis.*

*Tularemia.* Agglutination tests are possible with serums of patients suspected of *Pasteurella* infection but antigenic material must be obtained from a reliable standard source. Some cross-reaction with *Brucella* occurs.

*Leptospirosis.* Agglutinating antibodies which may reach extremely high titers are found in leptospiral infections. These antibodies reach a peak late in the course of the disease and are of little help in diagnosing the acute infection.

*Rat-bite fever.* Agglutination tests can be performed against *Streptobacillus moniliformis.* As in most agglutinations, changes in titer over a period of time are of greater significance than a single high titer.

*Rickettsial diseases.* Although rickettsial and proteus organisms are not otherwise closely related, they apparently share certain antigens in common. During the course of many rickettsial infections, antibodies are produced which agglutinate certain strains of *Proteus vulgaris* designated "OX." These differential agglutinations form the basis of the Weil-Felix reaction. The variation in Weil-Felix reaction for the more common rickettsial diseases is shown in Table 76.

Table 76. *The Weil-Felix reaction in the differential diagnosis of rickettsial diseases.*

| Disease | Etiologic agent | Weil-Felix reaction |
|---|---|---|
| Epidemic typhus | *R. prowazeki* | OX–19 |
| Endemic typhus | *R. mooseri* | OX–19 |
| Scrub typhus | *R. tsutsugamushi* | OX–K |
| Rocky Mountain spotted fever | *R. rickettsi* | OX–19 (weakly) OX–2 |
| Mediterranean fever | *R. conori conori* | OX–19 (weakly) OX–2 |
| South African tick fever | *R. pijperi pijperi* | OX–19 (weakly) OX–2 |
| Rickettsial pox | *R. akari* | negative |
| Q fever | *Coxiella burneti* | negative |

HETEROPHILE REACTION (PAUL-BUNNELL TEST). The heterophile agglutination reaction measures the agglutination of sheep red blood cells by the serum of patients suffering from infectious mononucleosis. Elevated titers are more apt to be found during the second or third week of the disease and the value of the test is chiefly as confirmatory evidence. The level at which the titer of sheep-cell agglutinins becomes diagnostic varies with the technique employed and the laboratory should be consulted relative to the significance of a particular titer. Sheep-cell agglutinins may occasionally be present in normal serum or in the serum of patients with serum sickness; these agglutinins must be distinguished from the agglutinin of infectious mononucleosis. Agglutinins of normal serum and serum sickness are adsorbed by guinea pig kidney; the agglutinins of infectious mononucleosis are not. This difference serves to distinguish these antibodies and to preserve the specificity of the heterophile test as evidence of infectious mononucleosis. In some apparently bona fide cases of infectious mononucleosis, sheep-cell agglutinins cannot be demonstrated.

COLD AGGLUTINATION. Positive cold-hemagglutination reactions are demonstrable in the serum of about one-half of the patients with primary atypical pneumonia. The cold agglutinin usually develops in the serum during the second week of the illness. Washed human group O red cells are used in the performance of the test. A titer of 1 : 64 or greater is generally considered significant; a rising titer is more diagnostic.

### ANTISTREPTOLYSIN-O DETERMINATION (ASL-O TITER)

Antistreptolysin-O is an antibody directed against streptolysin-O, a hemolysin produced by group A streptococci. An elevated titer of this antibody in the blood usually reflects a recent group A beta hemolytic streptococcal infection. Since acute rheumatic fever practically always follows group A streptococcal infection of the upper respiratory tract, the antistreptolysin-O titer has value as supporting evidence in the differential diagnosis of acute rheumatic fever. A rise in titer of the antibody is first detectable in the second week after group A streptococcal infection; a maximum is reached in about 4 weeks; in general, a return to the initial antibody level requires several months. Because of the ubiquity of streptococcal infection, it is not uncommon to encounter antistreptolysin-O levels of 100 to 200 Todd units in normal individuals. If only a single serum specimen is available from a suspected case of rheumatic fever, the evaluation of the significance of the test must be made on the absolute magnitude of the titer. The majority of rheumatic-fever patients show vigorous responses to streptolysin-O with an antibody titer of 500 units or higher. Under these conditions, a single determination serves as a valuable diagnostic aid. In the case of levels below 500 units, the usefulness of the test can be extended by demonstrating a change in titer over a period of weeks. Since not every patient with streptococcal infection produces antibody to streptolysin-O, the absence of an antistreptolysin-O response does not eliminate the diagnosis of rheumatic fever.

### SEROLOGIC TESTS FOR SYPHILIS

Serologic tests for syphilis are based on the presence of "reagin" in the patient's blood, appearing during the second or third week of infection. The antigen used in the test is an alcohol-soluble lipid which is obtained from beef heart and reacts with syphilitic reagin in the presence of lecithins and cholesterol. Both flocculation and complement-fixation tests employ the same antigenic material.

FLOCCULATION TESTS (Hinton, Kahn, Kline, Mazzini). These tests depend on the combination of the cardiolipin antigen with reagin to form grossly visible aggregates. Flocculation tests tend to be highly sensitive and are used for rapid screening.

COMPLEMENT-FIXATION TEST (Wassermann). This test depends on the ability of reagin to fix complement in the presence of cardiolipin and thereby inhibit hemolysis of red cells. Anticomplementary serum may destroy complement and result in a falsely positive test when syphilitic reagin is absent.

BIOLOGIC FALSE POSITIVE TESTS. There are a number of clinical states in which positive serologic test results may be found in the absence of syphilitic infection. Included among these are smallpox vaccination and infections such as malaria, leprosy, and measles. Disseminated lupus erythematosus and infectious mononucleosis are other instances in which a falsely positive test result may occur.

TREPONEMA PALLIDUM IMMOBILIZATION TEST (TPI). When a biologic false positive result of a serologic test for syphilis is suspected, confirmation of syphilis can be achieved by demonstrating immobilization of *Treponema pallidum* by specific antibodies in the patient's serum by the third week of infection. Diluted serum is mixed with live *T. pallidum* obtained from a rabbit chancre and the mixture is examined microscopically. If specific antibody is present, the treponemes are immobilized, whereas normal serum or serum from patients with biologic false positive serologic tests has no effect on the motile spirochetes.

### COMPLEMENT-FIXATION TESTS

Complement-fixation tests are often useful in establishing or confirming a clinical diagnosis. Infections that may be associated with specific and measurable complement-fixing antibodies include rickettsial diseases, gonorrhea, glanders, Weil's disease, blastomycosis, amebiasis, malaria, toxoplasmosis, schistosomiasis, trichinosis, and echinococcal disease. The estimation of these antibodies is difficult and should be carried out in laboratories specifically trained in these procedures. Certain state public health laboratories and the Communicable Disease Center of the U. S. Public Health Service in Atlanta, Georgia, may be consulted on such specialized problems. The demonstration of rising antibody titers is most important and requires serum collected during both the acute and the convalescent phases of the disease.

### TESTS FOR THE DETECTION OF ANTIVIRAL ANTIBODIES

Because viruses cannot be cultured by the same simplified techniques as bacteria, measurement of antibodies in viral diseases assumes greater importance. As in other antibody determinations, it is important to secure paired specimens of acute-phase and convalescent-phase serums in order to evaluate changes in titer that may have resulted from the illness. Although specific viral diseases may vary somewhat in the time sequence of antibody production, the first "acute" specimen should be collected at the onset of the illness and the "convalescent" specimen may be taken during the third or fourth week after onset. Serum specimens should be collected with sterile technique and stored in the frozen state. It is wise to measure antibody titers in both specimens simultaneously, using the same stock of antigen. Antibody tests in virus disease include neutralization tests, complement-fixation tests, and hemagglutination-inhibition tests.

NEUTRALIZATION TESTS. Neutralization tests depend on the specific protective properties of virus-neutralizing antibodies which can be measured in susceptible animals or in tissue culture. If neutralizing antibodies are present in the serum, the animals or tissue-culture cells are protected, in comparison to control animals or tissue cultures that are challenged by virus and serum that lacks neutralizing antibody. Serum dilutions can be used to quantitate the titer of these antibodies.

COMPLEMENT-FIXATION TESTS. As in bacterial complement-fixation tests, antiviral serum will often fix complement in the presence of specific antigen. Viral diseases in which complement-fixing antibody may be demonstrated include poliomyelitis, Coxsackie infection, lymphocytic choriomeningitis, psittacosis, and the encephalitides.

HEMAGGLUTINATION-INHIBITION TESTS. Certain viruses agglutinate red cells, and specific antibodies to these viruses may in turn inhibit such hemagglutination. This inhibition reaction may be quantitated by dilution of the antiserums. Changes in titer between acute-phase and convalescent-phase serums form the basis for serologic diagnosis. A fourfold or greater increase in titer is considered to have considerable diagnostic significance. Diseases characterized by measurable hemagglutination inhibition titers include influenza, mumps, dengue, and the encephalitides.

## Skin Tests

A variety of antigens of bacterial, viral, protozoal, and fungal origin have been utilized for skin tests. The purpose of a skin test may be to detect a specific sensitivity or to determine susceptibility to infection by a specific causative agent. Skin tests are of great value in the differential diagnosis of infectious diseases and have also been of use in epidemiologic studies and population surveys. Material for use in skin tests is available from

pharmaceutical companies, from state departments of health, or from the U. S. Public Health Service. The manufacturer's directions should be followed in applying and interpreting skin tests. The usual dosage of vaccine is 0.1 ml and the material is injected intradermally. A positive test reaction is manifested by a wheal or a well-defined area of erythema and induration, usually at least 10 mm in diameter. A central area of necrosis may be present in the more severe reactions. When employed for the differential diagnosis of infectious diseases, a positive reaction may indicate either active disease or a past infection (immunity). Occasionally, there may be a loss of skin sensitivity with overwhelming infection by the specific organism, for example, tuberculosis; this is known as a state of anergy. The interval between the onset of a specific infection and the development of allergy necessary for a positive skin reaction may vary from a few days to several weeks for different diseases. Once established, positivity usually persists for the rest of the patient's life.

There are two types of skin-test reactions. The immediate type appears as a wheal within approximately 15 min after the injection, and disappears within a few hours. In the delayed type, there is no reaction for a number of hours following injection; then erythema and induration appear, reaching a maximum after 24 to 48 hr and persisting for several days. From among a wide variety of antigens available, the following skin tests are of practical clinical importance.

IMMEDIATE TYPE: TRICHINOSIS, ECHINOCOCCOSIS, TOXOPLASMOSIS

There are examples of humoral allergy. Antigens derived from *Trichinella, Echinococcus,* and *Toxoplasma* upon injection unite with specific antibodies at the site of inoculation. Such antigen-antibody reactions lead to a histaminelike reaction to produce a wheal within 5 to

14 min. A delayed reaction to these antigens may also appear.

### DELAYED TYPE

The delayed type of skin test reflects true tissue allergy. The dermal reaction of erythema and induration results from injury of the tissues.

TUBERCULIN TEST. There are two tuberculin preparations, Old Tuberculin (O.T.) and Purified Protein Derivative (P.P.D.). Various dilutions of either preparation may be used, but for screening purposes a 1 : 1000 dilution of O.T. containing 0.1 mg of O.T. or intermediate strength P.P.D. equivalent to 0.0002 mg is generally employed. If the reaction is negative at these dilutions, stronger concentrations are sometimes injected before the patient is labeled a "negative reactor." If active tuberculosis is suspected, a weaker dilution than that ordinarily used should be used initially in order to avoid severe necrotic reactions. Both the O.T. and P.P.D. skin tests are read after 48 hr. A positive reaction is shown by *induration* of at least 5 mm with surrounding erythema. Since dilute solutions of O.T. and P.P.D. deteriorate on standing, freshly prepared dilutions should be used.

BRUCELLOSIS. Brucellergen, a nucleoprotein derived from *Brucella*, is the antigen of choice for this test. Since injection of the antigen may stimulate the production of agglutinins, the skin test must not be performed before blood has been drawn for *Brucella* agglutination tests. In addition, skin tests for brucellosis may be of limited value because there have been reports of negative skin reactions in 6 to 39 percent of cases of proved chronic brucellosis.

TULAREMIA. The Foshay antigen, prepared by treating *Past. tularensis* with nitrous acid, is of value in the early diagnosis of tularemia since skin sensitivity develops before the titer of blood agglutinins rises. Moreover, the Foshay antigen does not stimulate appreciably the production of antibodies.

COCCIDIOIDOMYCOSIS, HISTOPLASMOSIS. Antigens derived from broth cultures of *Coccidioides immitis* and *Histoplasma capsulatum* may be used for skin tests similar to the tuberculin reaction. These skin tests are of value in the differential diagnosis of calcified pulmonary lesions which may be indistinguishable from tuberculosis by x-ray.

BLASTOMYCOSIS. Antigen derived from the culture of *Blastomyces hominis* may be used for a skin test in the diagnosis of both the cutaneous and the systemic forms of blastomycosis.

LYMPHOGRANULOMA INGUINALE. The Frei test employs an antigen, "Lygranum," obtained from the egg-yolk-sac culture of the virus of lymphogranuloma inguinale. There is a specific dermal reaction in patients infected with this virus. Since there may be tissue allergy to chick-embryo material, a control skin test is made on the other arm, using uninfected chick-embryo material. Because of the close antigenic relation between the viruses of lymphogranuloma inguinale and psittacosis, false positive Frei reactions may result from infections with these other viruses.

### SKIN TESTS FOR SUSCEPTIBILITY TO INFECTION

Knowledge of a person's susceptibility to diphtheria or mumps may aid in the management of individuals who have had contact with these infections. In a case of epidemic parotitis, a mumps skin-test reaction may help in the differential diagnosis.

MUMPS. Material from an infected monkey or embryonated egg will produce an inflammatory reaction when injected into the skin of a person who has been previously infected with mumps virus, even if the clinical disease has not been apparent. Control skin tests with uninfected material must be used. The sites of injection are examined after 48 hr. An erythematous skin reaction and induration of more than 10 mm at the site of injection with the antigen is taken as presumptive evidence of immunity.

DIPHTHERIA. The antigen for the Schick test is toxin derived from *C. diphtheriae*. A positive reaction on intradermal injection will result from tissue injury in persons who have insufficient specific neutralizing antitoxin. A control injection, employing heated toxin, is placed on the other forearm. The tests are observed at 2 and 4 days after injection. A negative reaction indicates that the person is probably immune to diphtheria.

## REFERENCES

1. R. J. Dubos, ed., *Bacterial and Mycotic Infections of Man* (ed. 3; Lippincott, Philadelphia, 1958).
2. T. M. Rivers, ed., *Viral and Rickettsial Infections of Man* (ed. 3; Lippincott, Philadelphia, 1959).
3. E. Jawetz, J. L. Melnick, and E. A. Adelberg, *Review of Medical Microbiology* (ed. 3; Lange Medical Publications, Los Altos, California, 1958).
4. Society of American Bacteriologists, M. J. Pelczar, Jr., chairman, *Manual of Microbiological Methods* (McGraw-Hill, New York, 1957).
5. H. S. Willis and M. M. Cummings, *Diagnostic and Experimental Methods in Tuberculosis* (ed. 2; Thomas, Springfield, 1952).

# Unit 27

# Sputum Tests

The examination of the sputum is one of the most valuable procedures in the diagnosis and management of respiratory diseases. Sputum is a fluid composed of the secretions, exudations, and exfoliations of the bronchopulmonary tree. The sputum therefore reflects the pathologic processes within the area from which it came.

The methods involved in the examination of the sputum are usually simple and it is often possible to obtain critical information quickly and inexpensively. The examination of the sputum is therefore a useful procedure that should be well understood by every clinician.[1-6]

## COMPOSITION AND PROPERTIES OF THE SPUTUM

Sputum contains in solution the mucopolysaccharide that has been secreted by the mucus-secreting cells of the bronchial tree. The concentration of mucopolysaccharide is 0.5–3.0 percent. To this is added the water and inorganic salts arising from other bronchial secretory cells. In addition, there may be desquamated cells, products of tissue breakdown, products of bacterial activity, local exudates, and aspirated saliva, as well as other materials from the mouth and pharynx. The content of any of these components may vary greatly, so that the many attempts that have been made to quantitate these in relation to specific diseases have not yielded specific diagnostic findings.

The sputum is ordinarily slightly acid, with pH values between 6.5 and 7.0. When there is chronic inflammation or necrosis within the bronchopulmonary tree, the pH of the sputum may fall. Occasionally urea-splitting bacteria may produce enough ammonia to cause the sputum to become alkaline. This is particularly true if the sputum has been left standing without refrigeration. The specific gravity of sputum is variable, and values from 1.008 to 1.030 have been reported in a variety of disease states.

The protein content is also variable. The mucopolysaccharides of sputum probably are linked with protein, accounting for some of the protein that is found in sputum. In addition, serum proteins may appear in consequence of local inflammation. Nucleoproteins can be demonstrated in direct proportion to the cellular content of the sputum. Various breakdown products of proteins, fats, and carbohydrates may be observed in sputum that has been derived from areas of tissue decomposition. Certain drugs, such as sulfonamides and particularly isoniazid, may appear in saliva and in sputum in sufficient concentrations to induce bacteriostasis.

## DIAGNOSTIC SIGNIFICANCE OF EXAMINATION OF THE SPUTUM

*The amount of mucus* produced under ordinary circumstances is so small that the mucus is readily propelled upward through ciliary action or brought up through mild coughing. It is ordinarily

460

swallowed unless the amounts are large enough to be expectorated. When the bronchial tree is irritated, the amount of mucinous secretion generally is increased. Chronic irritation is a more potent stimulus to secretion of increased amounts of mucus than is acute bronchial irritation. Thus the volume of sputum will ordinarily be small unless there is chronic bronchial irritation or unless the lesion provides an anatomic basis for the pooling of secretions, such as may occur in bronchiectasis and lung abscess.

Although the mucus is colorless, the presence of a large amount of cellular exudate will ordinarily impart a greenish or yellowish color to the sputum. Deep-green and gray streaks of purulent material are often seen when the sputum contains an admixture of secretions from the upper nasopharynx. When the inflammatory process in the bronchopulmonary tree is severe, there may be sufficient capillary damage to cause the sputum to have blood streaks or to be frankly bloody. When the blood cells have entered the sputum shortly before expectoration, the sputum can be expected to be bright red. If, on the other hand, some time has elapsed between the extravasation of blood and the expectoration of the sputum, the sputum will be darker and may assume a rusty or a prune-juice color. In chronic congestive states, the hemoglobin-breakdown products may be discernible only as small amounts of pigment in mononuclear cells. The sputum may be colored because of the inhalation of dusts.

*The odor of sputum* may occasionally offer some insight into the nature of the underlying process. Ordinarily, sputum has no odor. However, in the presence of anaerobic infections within the lung, the sputum may have a characteristic foul odor. The foul odor most often arises from infection due to the fusobacteria and spirochetes that are commonly found in the mouth. Since these organisms are extremely sensitive to penicillin and to other commonly used antibacterial agents, it has become increasingly uncommon to detect the odor of anaerobic infections of the lung. An odor similar to that detected with anaerobic infections of the lung may arise in the presence of chronic atrophic rhinitis, and some confusion in diagnosis may therefore arise.

Formed elements such as bronchial casts, elastic fibers, and sulfur granules, may be detected in the sputum and are of diagnostic value when seen. In prebacteriologic days, the presence of elastic fibers was considered to be strong evidence for underlying tuberculosis.

From the examination of the sputum it is often possible to surmise the nature of the underlying process. For example, in *pneumococcic lobar pneumonia* there is a dense fibrinous exudate within the alveoli and large numbers of pneumococci and polymorphonuclear leukocytes are seen. Some degree of bronchial inflammation is almost always present. It is not surprising, therefore, that the sputum in lobar pneumonia is characteristically scant and mucopurulent and contains large numbers of polymorphonuclear leukocytes as well as gram-positive diplococci. Whether there is manifest blood depends upon the extent of capillary damage. Since the arrival of effective antibacterial therapy, it is relatively uncommon to encounter "prune-juice" sputum, although some blood is frequently seen in the sputum in pneumonia.

In the same manner it can be anticipated that the sputum in *staphylococcic pneumonia* will consist of increased amounts of mucus coming from the bronchial tree and the large amount of pus that is commonly found in staphylococcic abscesses in the lung. The sputum is purulent, abundant, yellow, and mucinous, and contains large numbers of polymorphonuclear leukocytes as well as staphylococci.

In *Hemophilus influenzae* pneumonia, the sputum is frequently mucopurulent and pale green in color. The stained

461

smears contain large numbers of poly-morphonuclear leukocytes and such large numbers of minute coccobacillary forms that these may frequently be over-looked because of the impression that they are a pale pink background to the entire stained specimen. In fact, when it appears that a sputum is singularly lack-ing in bacterial flora on rapid micro-scopic examination, the possibility of *H. influenzae* pneumonia should be con-sidered and the smear reexamined. The organisms may have been missed simply because they are so numerous and form a dense background.

Occasionally it will be observed that the sputum is copious and, if permitted to stand, will form layers. The mucinous layer is the heaviest and therefore is found at the bottom of the container. Over it is the serous portion of the spu-tum which contains the suspended cells and detritus. The formed elements of the serous layer will settle as the sputum is permitted to stand, but will generally set-tle to the interface of the mucinous and serous portions. Thus, three layers may be observed, the lowermost one being mucoid, the intermediate one being cel-lular, and the topmost, the serous layer. The significance of the copious sputum is apparent from the considerations that have been presented above. When there is chronic bronchial irritation, the secre-tion of mucus is stimulated. Similarly, if there is cavitation, bronchial dilatation, or some other means whereby secretions may be pooled and yet have access to the bronchial lumen, the sputum may be copious. A *copious sputum* therefore should suggest the possibility of chronic bronchitis, bronchiectasis, abscess, tuber-culosis, or obstruction in the bronchial tree (the last being most commonly due to neoplasia).

*The cellular content of the sputum* is often of great diagnostic significance. Ordinarily in acute bacterial infections of the bronchi or of the pulmonary pa-renchyma, the cellular exudate will con-sist almost exclusively of polymorphonu-clear leukocytes and these can be readily observed in the stained smears made from the sputum. If mononuclear cells are found in any number exceeding an occasional one, it may be assumed that the acute inflammatory process has been modified. Mononuclear cells will be found in the exudate from the broncho-pulmonary tree under relatively few cir-cumstances: (*a*) healing pneumonia, which may be healing spontaneously or in consequence of antibacterial therapy; (*b*) viral pneumonia; (*c*) chronic inflam-mation such as may occur with gran-ulomatous processes (tuberculosis, my-cosis) or with underlying neoplasia. Mononuclear cells are not expected to be in the sputum unless the inflammatory process is resolving or unless the nature of the stimulus is such that large num-bers of mononuclear cells may be present in the local pathologic lesion. Conversely, in viral pneumonia the appearance of polymorphonuclear leukocytes in the sputum and the disappearance of mono-nuclear cells suggests secondary bacterial invasion.

In *chronic congestive heart failure* it is common to observe in the sputum mono-nuclear cells containing pigment derived from the breakdown of hemoglobin. The sputum is often frothy and consists of a mixture of mucus, air, saliva, and what-ever exudate may be coming from the bronchopulmonary tree.

Eosinophils may be seen in the spu-tum in asthmatic bronchitis and in proc-esses characterized by the infiltration of large numbers of eosinophiles into the lesion. In lipoid pneumonias, mononu-clear cells are frequently seen to contain vacuoles that stain with fat stains such as sudan III.

METHODS OF EXAMINING SPUTUM

Sputum should be freshly obtained whenever possible. The gross description of the sputum should be recorded utiliz-ing the principles stressed above. When the gross examination of the sputum suggests the presence of formed bodies such as sulfur granules, casts, or fungi, the sputum may be examined in the unstained state under the microscope. Generally, unstained smears are not examined unless the gross description of the sputum suggests the presence of bodies that are readily recognized in the unstained state.

PREPARATION AND EXAMINATION OF GRAM-STAINED SMEARS. In the preparation and staining of smears, it is desirable to use only new, clean, and thoroughly flamed slides. Bloody, cheesy, or purulent portions of the specimen should be chosen for smearing and the smear should be as uniform as possible. Should the mucinous quality of the sputum be so great that it is almost impossible to break the mucinous strands in order to make an adequate smear, the presence of encapsulated organisms such as Friedländer's bacilli should be suspected.

When the smears have been made and allowed to dry without heat, they should be fixed by passage through a flame once or twice. The sputum is then stained. For the Gram method, the smear is covered with gentian violet for 1 min, washed, covered with Gram's iodine solution for 1 min, and washed with water. The smear is then decolorized by flooding it with 95-percent alcohol (note that acid alcohol must not be used). The alcohol serves to extract gentian violet from those portions of the smear that are gram-negative. The slide may be rocked back and forth gently to assist the extraction process and the alcohol should be changed two or three times. Decolorization should continue while gentian violet can be seen being extracted into the layer. Approximately 30 sec is an average time for decolorizing, but no precise statement of the time of decolorization can be made because of variations in thickness of smear and content of stainable materials. The decolorized slide is

then counterstained for 14 or 20 sec with safranine.

The slide is examined after drying for its content of cells and bacteria. It is extremely important from the considerations presented above to note the number and nature of cells encountered as well as the relative numbers and varieties of bacteria seen. The pathogens of the pulmonary tree can often be recognized on smear and specific treatment begun promptly.

EXAMINATION FOR ACID-FAST ORGANISMS. In acid-fast staining, the Ziehl-Neelsen method is most commonly used. The slide is prepared as above, dried, and fixed, and the smear is flooded with carbol fuchsin. The carbol fuchsin is heated gently until it steams. This is conveniently done by placing the slide over a cup of boiling water. Steaming should go on for approximately 5 min, after which the carbol fuchsin may be washed away. The slide is decolorized in acid alcohol with repeated floodings of the slide until no more red dye appears in the acid alcohol. It is often necessary to decolorize for from 30 sec to 2 min. After rinsing in water, the slide may be counterstained with methylene blue for 1 min and examined. Alternately the Kinyoun modification of acid-fast staining, which does not require heat, may be used.

If *Nocardia* or *Actinomyces* are being sought, the amount of decolorization should be minimal. These organisms are but weakly acid-fast and will tend to decolorize completely if left in the presence of acid alcohol for more than 10 to 20 sec.

BACKGROUND STAINING WITH INDIA INK. If fungi are being sought, it may be useful to use background staining which will bring into relief the unstained capsules of fungi. India ink is a commonly used reagent for this purpose. It should be remembered, however, that commercially available India inks often have a

463

great variety of microorganisms in them. If sustained need for background staining is anticipated, it is wise to prepare India ink with 0.3-percent tricresol in order to minimize bacterial contamination.

For India-ink staining, a small fleck of the material to be stained is mixed with a drop of water and a drop of India ink is added. A thin film is spread on a slide and allowed to dry. The film is fixed lightly with heat and stained with a common stain such as methylene blue for 1 min. It is washed, dried, and examined. When capsules are present, they appear as clear halos about a stained cell. In this manner it may be possible at times to demonstrate the presence of monilia, blastomyces, and similar organisms that may be found in sputum.

USE OF WRIGHT'S STAIN. Wright's stain is often used when allergic reactions in the respiratory tract, bronchial asthma, Loeffler's syndrome, or similar states are suspected. For Wright's stains, the film of sputum should be extremely thin.

CYTOLOGIC EXAMINATION FOR MALIGNANT CELLS. Papanicolaou stains are frequently made for the purpose of determining the presence of malignant cells in sputum. In most laboratories special fixatives are available so that the sputum can be discharged directly into the fixative and brought to the laboratory for smearing. The cytologic demands for adequate Papanicolaou staining are sufficiently rigorous to make it unwise that these be made by other than specially trained individuals.

### CULTURAL EXAMINATION

Culture of the sputum should not be carried out unless adequate gross and microscopic descriptions have been made. Very often the cultural findings are impossible to interpret without some knowledge concerning the underlying pathologic process. For example, staph-

ylococci are found in approximately 60 percent of sputums. Whether these are of pathogenic importance can frequently be answered only if the nature of the exudate is known. Thus, if large numbers of mononuclear leukocytes are found in the sputum, the presence of staphylococci offers less cause for alarm than if polymorphonuclear leukocytes are the predominant cells.

Sputum should be brought to the laboratory promptly for culture and should not be allowed to remain at room temperature, since many saprophytes will multiply under these conditions.

It is frequently possible to determine the nature of certain bacteria directly. *Diplococcus pneumoneae, H. influenzae,* and Friedländer's bacillus may be identified directly by capsular swelling that occurs after specific antiserums are mixed with the sputum.

Specimens of sputum that are to be cultured or that are inoculated into animals are of two basic types: those that are free from contamination and can therefore be cultured or inoculated directly, and those that are contaminated with a sufficiently mixed flora to make it difficult to seek out certain pathogens such as tubercle bacilli. These latter specimens must therefore be digested or in some other way prepared before being used as inoculums. Since the contamination results in the loss of many of the tubercle bacilli, it is important to avoid such digestion procedures unless they are necessary.

Cultures should consist of implantation on blood agar and inhibitory mediums such as eosin methylene blue as a minimum. In addition, anaerobic mediums may be used if lung abscess, bronchiectasis, putrid empyema, or other anaerobic infection is suspected. The great improvement in methods of cultivation of tubercle bacilli has made it possible to streak sputum or material aspirated through a bronchoscope directly on the culture mediums.

It is important that the material used for culture be raised from the bronchopulmonary tree and not consist of saliva or postnasal discharge. The gross and microscopic examinations of the sputum will often indicate presence of saliva. Frequently, the microscopic examination will show the presence of large numbers of flat epithelial cells that could have arisen only from the buccal mucosa. These will commonly have large numbers of bacteria adherent to them. The organisms found adhering to the squamous cells are virtually never of pathogenic importance and, in fact, often will not grow out except on special mediums.

Occasionally, in the examination of sputum for the presence of tubercle bacilli, it may be desirable to concentrate the specimen or to remove contaminating bacteria. Various methods, none of them entirely satisfactory, have been used for this purpose. A simple method that is commonly used is to add an equal volume of autoclaved 3-percent NaOH to the sputum and allow the mixture to stand for 10 or 15 min. Alternatively, the mixture is agitated in a shaking machine for 10–15 min. The sputum is then neutralized and centrifuged at high speed for 30 min. The sediment is cultured or injected into guinea pigs.

Another simple method is to mix sputum with an equal volume of solution of sodium hypochlorite (household Clorox). This is allowed to stand for 10 to 15 min and then centrifuged at high speed (at least 3000 rev/min for 30 min). The supernatant is then drained off and a smear is made of the sediment. The organisms concentrated by this method are generally nonviable.

Bronchial aspirations may be treated in the same manner. Gastric aspirations should not be stained, since the number of saprophytic acid-fast bacilli ordinarily found in the stomach is so great that misleading results are almost sure to be obtained. Gastric aspirations should simply be neutralized and cultured or injected into guinea pigs.

The methods for the identification of the common pathogens in culture mediums or in the common laboratory animals are specialized procedures and will not be described at length in this unit. The methods that have been described for the demonstration of pathogenic bacteria and the exudates occurring in their presence are equally applicable to body fluids such as cerebrospinal fluid, joint fluids, and pleural, peritoneal, and other exudates and can be applied to urine, feces, and even whole tissues. If thoughtfully applied, they will provide essential diagnostic information promptly and often permit critical clinical action to be taken (see Unit 26).

## REFERENCES

1. F. P. Basch, P. Holinger, and H. G. Poncher, "Physical and chemical properties of sputum," *Amer. J. Dis. Child.* 62, 981, 1149 (1941).
2. H. Clifford, *The Sputum. Its Examination and Clinical Significance* (Macmillan, New York, 1923).
3. M. M. Cummings, "The laboratory diagnosis of tuberculosis," *Amer. J. publ. Hlth.* 39, 361 (1949).
4. J. J. Kinyoun, "A note on Uhlenhuth's method for sputum examinations for tubercle bacilli," *Amer. J. publ. Hlth.* 5, 867 (1915).
5. I. G. Schaub and M. K. Foley, *Diagnostic Bacteriology* (ed. 5; Mosby, St. Louis, 1958).
6. *Tuberculosis Laboratory Methods, VA-Armed Forces cooperative study on the chemotherapy of tuberculosis* (VA Department of Medicine and Surgery Central Office, Washington, 1958).

# Unit 28

# Diseases of Carbohydrate Metabolism

In terms of public health, diabetes mellitus is of far greater importance than all other diseases of metabolism combined. Minimal glycosuria found on a routine urinalysis is often the first hint of the presence of the disease. This finding, however, does not of itself establish the diagnosis. The demonstration of an elevated fasting blood sugar level and, in some instances, of a decreased tolerance to a glucose load are necessary confirmatory measures.

## Interpretation of Glycosuria

Glycosuria is usually a manifestation of diabetes mellitus. Less commonly, it may represent one of a number of conditions, mostly benign, which are summarized below. It is important to stress that before considering glycosuria to be non-diabetic in origin a low renal threshold for glucose must be demonstrated in the presence of otherwise normal carbohydrate metabolism. This can usually be done by performing an oral glucose tolerance test and collecting urine samples at the time of the blood drawings. The normal person does not have glycosuria below blood sugar levels of 150 to 200 mg/100 ml; these figures take into consideration the variation among people, as well as differences in techniques of blood sugar determination. The reasons for the lowered renal threshold are several, usually involving faulty reabsorption of the filtered glucose.[1, 2] These defects may occur singly or in association with other renal functional abnormalities. There may or may not be associated visible structural kidney changes.

TRUE RENAL GLYCOSURIA. In this condition, significant glycosuria is present in all the patient's urine specimens, even those obtained during fasting. There are no other associated abnormalities in renal function, and the patient is usually asymptomatic. Rarely is the urinary loss of glucose great enough to interfere with normal nutrition or to produce symptoms of hypoglycemia. The condition is probably hereditary and is usually present from birth. A later development of diabetes mellitus is considered an unusual occurrence.[3]

NONSPECIFIC RENAL GLYCOSURIA (Nondiabetic Glycosuria). Glycosuria may occur only transiently. It is usually not present in the fasting state, the renal threshold for glucose being higher than in true renal glycosuria. Renal function is otherwise normal. There is evidence that people with this condition have a greater chance of developing diabetes mellitus than normal people.[4] The differentiation between true and nonspecific renal glycosuria is not always a clear-cut one.

PREGNANCY. In at least 10 percent of pregnant women, particularly toward term, glycosuria occurs.[5] Apparently, this results from reduced reabsorption of glucose by the renal tubules, although increased glomerular filtration may also be a factor.[6] Glycosuria may be confused with lactosuria at term. It should not be assumed that glycosuria during pregnancy is always a benign state.[7] Isolated blood sugar determinations or even a glucose tolerance test should be made. There is good evidence that this abnormality is a prediabetic manifestation.[8]

ADRENOCORTICAL HORMONES. Some individuals while taking adrenocorticosteroids will develop glycosuria. Elevations in the blood sugar concentration and increased glomerular filtration, rather than a reduced renal tubular reabsorption of glucose, apparently account for this phenomenon.[9] The abnormality will usually disappear with cessation of drug administration. Increases in adrenal steroid production may be responsible by similar mechanisms for the transient glycosurias seen in such stress conditions as acute bacterial infections, asphyxia, myocardial infarctions, cerebrovascular accidents, and severe emotional upsets.

ACUTE AND CHRONIC RENAL DISEASE. Glycosuria may occur as one of the many manifestations of organic renal disease. It may be seen following acute tubular necrosis accompanied by proteinuria, pyuria, and hematuria.[10] In severe chronic nephritis, and particularly in nephrosclerosis, the capacity of the tubules to reabsorb glucose may be depressed to the point where glycosuria occurs.[11]

A number of instances of renal disease have now been described, including the Fanconi syndrome and its variants, most often occurring in children but also found in adults, in which disturbed function rests primarily in the tubules. In such cases, aminoaciduria, hyperphosphaturia, and the inability to form an acid urine, as well as glycosuria and other defects in renal function, have been detailed.[12, 13] Clinically, the glycosuria is of little significance here, as compared to the other excretory abnormalities.

RENAL GLYCOSURIA IN ASSOCIATION WITH DIABETES MELLITUS. A number of patients with true diabetes mellitus have, as well, a low renal threshold for glucose. It is most important to recognize this association so as not to attribute the glycosuria in such cases to hyperglycemia and poor diabetic control.

### The Blood Sugar

Under ordinary conditions, the concentration of blood sugar is kept within a remarkably narrow range by an elaborate system of homeostatic mechanisms. Among the many factors important in this regulation are the ability of the intestines to absorb glucose, the capacity of the liver to store and break down glycogen, the mass of skeletal muscles, the functional capacity of the pancreatic islet cells to make and release insulin, the presence of circulating hormonal and nonhormonal insulin "antagonists," and the tissue concentration of enzymes capable of destroying insulin. The physician who attempts to interpret single or serial blood sugar values without being aware of this interplay of influences will often arrive at erroneous conclusions.

The range of normal for the blood glucose concentration will vary with the method of determination. There are two methods in general use at this time. The first measures selectively the blood glucose's reducing powers—"true blood sugar method." [14] The second measures the blood's total reducing power and will be affected by glutathione, ascorbic acid, and other reducing substances, as well as by glucose.[15] It is commonly believed that the concentration of non-glucose-reducing substances in the blood is fairly constant in the range of 20 mg/100 ml of whole blood. One study, however, has shown that this fraction in 35 percent of determinations of blood sugar amounted to 35 mg/100 ml or more. Unfortunately, the amounts of these substances varied not only from individual to individual, but within the same individual at different times as well.[16]

Routine blood sugar determinations are made on whole-blood samples. Where plasma or serum is used, the sugar concentration will average approximately 20 mg/100 ml higher, intracellular glucose concentrations being lower than extracellular.[10]

An additional factor to be considered in evaluating a blood sugar level is whether venous or capillary blood has been used in the determination. In the fasting state, these will closely approximate one another as to glucose content. After a glucose load, however, capillary blood glucose concentration rises an average of 40 mg/100 ml higher than that of venous blood.[16] In this country, venous blood is usually tested; occasionally, in children, capillary blood may be used where venepunctures are difficult.

Recently a new method of blood glucose determination has been introduced employing the specific glucose oxidase enzyme system. By this method, values similar to the "true blood sugar" are obtained. It appears to offer considerable promise in terms of simplicity and accuracy.[17–19]

It is most important in evaluating a blood sugar determination to be aware of the method of determination used, as well as the various physiologic influences that might be acting at the time of the venepuncture.

### THE FASTING BLOOD SUGAR (FBS)

The fasting state requires that the patient has not eaten for at least 8 hr. For the "true blood sugar method" using venous blood, the normal range of concentration is from 70 to 100 mg/100 ml. Below 40 mg/100 ml, one may anticipate symptoms of hypoglycemia. If values above 120 mg/100 ml are obtained on several occasions, the diagnosis of diabetes mellitus may be made without the

performance of a glucose tolerance test.

By methods such as the Folin-Wu technique of testing for total reducing substances in the blood, 80 to 120 mg/100 ml is considered the normal fasting range. Below 60 mg/100 ml, one may anticipate symptoms of hypoglycemia and with values above 150 mg/100 ml the diagnosis of diabetes mellitus may be made.

The blood sugar values noted in the remainder of this discussion will be those determined by a true blood sugar method from venous whole-blood samples. The addition of 20 mg/100 ml to such values will give an approximation of the concentration of total venous whole-blood reducing substances.

### THE GLUCOSE-TOLERANCE TEST (GTT)

At times, abnormalities in carbohydrate tolerance may be demonstrated only under conditions of glucose loading with subsequent serial measurements of blood glucose concentration. Such a loading test is referred to as a glucose-tolerance test. The values for the various blood sugar concentrations when expressed graphically with time as the abscissa make up the glucose-tolerance curve. Because such a curve may only rise, fall, or remain horizontal, the precautions necessary for proper interpretation of a single blood sugar value are multiplied manyfold in the evaluation of this more complicated test procedure.

*Indications.* The glucose-tolerance test is indicated: (i) when a patient exhibiting glycosuria is found to have a normal or only slightly elevated fasting blood sugar concentration; (ii) when the fasting blood sugar concentration is found to be more than 100 but less than 120 mg/100 ml; (iii) when in addition a 2-hr postprandial blood sugar determination gives more than 100 but less than 180 mg/100 ml; (iv) when the diagnosis of Cushing's syndrome or acromegaly is suspected; (v) as an aid in differentiating among the various causes of hypoglycemia.

*Preparation.* It is important that the patient consume an adequate diet containing at least 200–250 gm of carbohydrate daily for 3 days before the test. Carbohydrate restriction in itself has been shown to impair the utilization of glucose, presumably through a temporary decrease in pancreatic insulin concentration.[20]

### TYPES OF GLUCOSE-TOLERANCE TESTS

THE POSTPRANDIAL BLOOD SUGAR DETERMINATION. This is a simple screening test in which blood for sugar determination is drawn 2 hr after the patient has begun to eat a meal containing from 50 to 100 gm of carbohydrate. A blood sugar value below the upper limits of normal for fasting excludes a diagnosis of diabetes mellitus. A value above this requires the performance of a formal glucose-tolerance test. As a method for finding new cases of diabetes, this technique has been found to be most informative, being superior to the FBS and certainly to urine testing alone.[5, 21]

THE ORAL GLUCOSE-TOLERANCE TEST. *Method.* Samples of urine and whole blood are obtained from the patient in the fasting state. He then consumes a cooled solution containing 100 gm of glucose dissolved in 500 ml of lemon-flavored water. Some workers use 1.75 gm of glucose per kilogram of ideal body weight in the adult. In pediatric practice, the amount of glucose taken is dependent on age: from 0 to 1½ years, 2.5 gm/kg; from 1½ to 3 years, 2.0 gm/kg; from 3 years to adolescence, 1.75 gm/kg. Blood and urine samples are obtained at 30, 60, 90, 120, and 180 min after beginning glucose ingestion. The patient should not smoke, exercise, or become unduly excited during the test.

*Interpretation.* The criteria upon which a diagnosis of diabetes mellitus is established vary from clinic to clinic. It is the responsibility of the examining physician to decide which standards he will use. The following figures are generally accepted. The FBS should be below 100 mg/100 ml (true blood sugar values), the peak below 160 mg/100 ml (this may occur either at the 30-min or the 60-min sampling), and the 2-hr value below 120 mg/100 ml. If the peak is greater than 160 mg/100 ml and the 2-hr value is above 120 mg/100 ml, in the properly performed test, the diagnosis of diabetes mellitus is made. In curves approaching borderline, 1- and 2-hr values, the level of 140 mg/100 ml at 1½ hr is also required.[16, 21, 22]

For discussion of the various borderline curves, the reader is referred to the standard sources.[3, 5, 10] Almost all agree that to make a diagnosis of diabetes mellitus the blood sugar, following a glucose load, should not only rise abnormally high, but remain high for a prolonged period of time; both the height and the duration of elevation of the curve in the glucose-tolerance test should be abnormal. However, it must be recalled that not all diabetic-like curves mean true or uncomplicated diabetes. Similar curves may be seen in patients with thyrotoxicosis, pheochromocytoma, Cushing's syndrome, and acromegaly. Following cure of the underlying disease, carbohydrate tolerance will often return to normal in patients with these conditions.

So-called flat oral GTT curves, in which the peak value is no more than 20 mg/100 ml above the fasting level, usually have no clinical significance. Many normal people will exhibit such curves. Patients with intestinal malabsorption may behave similarly.[9]

Following carbohydrate restriction and in association with advanced liver disease, diabetic types of curves may be found.[20, 23] These may be distinguished from those seen in true diabetes mellitus in that the FBS will be low normal in starvation and low normal or low with liver disease. With prolongation of the test, the patient with liver disease may develop severe hypoglycemia. Measurement of the serum inorganic phosphorus as a differential aid in these conditions has at times been of value. In normal people, the serum inorganic phosphorus concentration will fall during the course of a GTT, presumably owing to its participation in the processes of glucose utilization. This same fall occurs in patients with liver disease, despite their abnormal GTT curve. In diabetics, the phosphorus concentration falls little, if at all. Unfortunately, the changes are, at times, equivocal ones.[10, 23] Changes in the serum potassium during the course of a GTT have not proved of value in diagnosis.[10]

THE INTRAVENOUS GTT. The intravenous injection of glucose for a test of tolerance is not required for routine diagnosis. It is of value in conditions where poor intestinal absorption or vomiting after glucose ingestion makes the oral test unsatisfactory.

*Method.* Several methods are available.[5] Perhaps the most widely used one requires the infusion into the patient of 0.5 gm glucose per kilogram of body weight as a 20-percent glucose solution over a 30-min period. Fasting 30-, 60-, 90-, and 120-min samples of blood and urine are obtained.

*Interpretation.* The same general statements concerning interpretation apply to the intravenous GTT as to the oral GTT. The 30-min blood sugar level may rise as high as 200 mg/100 ml and glycosuria may accordingly occur at this time. At 120 min, the blood sugar in the normal person will have fallen to 120 mg/100 ml or below.

THE INSULIN-TOLERANCE TEST (ITT)

The insulin-tolerance test is employed to determine the patient's hypoglycemic response to the effects of insulin. The extent and duration of the hypoglycemic

action of intravenously administered insulin are dependent upon a variety of factors—the anti-insulin effects of the anterior pituitary and the adrenal cortical hormones, the presence of other non-hormonal humoral antagonists, the reserve of available liver glycogen, and probably other, as yet unknown, factors.

*Method.* The patient, for the 3 days preceding the test, is maintained on a high-carbohydrate diet, as for the GTT. After a fasting sample of blood is drawn, 0.1 unit of crystalline insulin per kilogram of ideal body weight is injected intravenously. Blood samples for glucose determination are taken at 20, 30, 45, 60, and 120 min. Where increased insulin sensitivity is suspected, the dose should be reduced to 0.05 unit/kg. In all tests, equipment for the intravenous administration of hypertonic glucose should be at hand.[24]

*Interpretation.* In normal subjects, the blood sugar concentration under such a test procedure will fall to approximately 50 percent of the fasting value in between 10 and 30 min; it will have returned to normal by 90 to 120 min. A greater and more prolonged fall, with or without hypoglycemic symptoms, is evidence for abnormal sensitivity to insulin. A lesser fall speaks for insulin resistance.[24]

The test is now used primarily to determine the presence of insulin resistance in patients with suspected Cushing's syndrome or acromegaly. In those states in which an exaggerated hypoglycemic response is anticipated, such as anterior-pituitary or adrenal-cortical insufficiency, less dangerous and more direct laboratory aids should be employed. A 6-min insulin-tolerance test has been suggested for distinguishing between patients with labile and unstable diabetes mellitus.[2]

OTHER TESTS OF CARBOHYDRATE METABOLISM

Combined glucose-insulin-tolerance tests have only very specialized uses;

their discussion is beyond the scope of this manual.[10, 24] Epinephrine- and glucagon-tolerance tests to determine the reserve of available liver glycogen may be of value in liver diseases where glycogen stores are reduced and in glycogen-storage disease (Von Gierke's disease) where there is impaired glycogenolysis.[10]

A tolbutamide-tolerance test has been employed to differentiate between normal and mildly diabetic patients in whom the routine glucose-tolerance test may not be diagnostic. The test makes use of the more rapid fall in blood sugar in the normal as compared to the diabetic when tolbutamide is administered intravenously.[25]

### The Problem of Hypoglycemia

A state of hypoglycemia exists when the blood sugar concentration is 40 mg/ 100 ml or less (true blood sugar value). The concentration at which patients will become symptomatic may be considerably below this. The more rapid the fall in glucose concentration, the more likely the occurrence of symptoms at a given level. The most common cause of hypoglycemia is improper insulin administration in patients with diabetes mellitus. The diagnosis here is usually obvious. There are a number of less common causes which may present difficult diagnostic problems. The usual classification divides the various causes for spontaneous hypoglycemia into organic and functional categories (Table 77). A more practical clinical approach separates the diseases producing hypoglycemia according to the conditions under which the hypoglycemia occurs.[26] The *fasting* hypoglycemias occur only in the postabsorptive state. Here the mechanisms for maintaining fasting normoglycemia, such as decreasing insulin secretion, glycogenolysis, and gluconeogenesis are impaired. The *stimulative* or reactive hypoglycemias follow carbohydrate ingestion and a consequent rise in blood sugar

Table 77. *Spontaneous hypoglycemias* [a]

| | |
|---|---|
| Organic—recognizable anatomic lesion | |
| Pancreatic islet cell tumors | (mixed) [b] |
| Hepatic disease | (fasting) |
| Anterior pituitary insufficiency | (mixed) |
| Adrenal cortical insufficiency | (mixed) |
| Fibromas and sarcomas | (fasting) |
| Central nervous lesions | (fasting) |
| Functional—no recognized anatomic lesion | |
| Functional hyperinsulinism | (stimulative) |
| Alimentary | (stimulative) |
| Idiopathic spontaneous hypoglycemia of infancy | (mixed) |
| Renal glycosuria | (fasting) |
| Lactation | (fasting) |
| Severe continuous muscular exertion | (fasting) |

[a] Modified from Conn and Seltzer.[26]
[b] Classification as to time of occurrence of the hypoglycemia.

concentration. In these conditions, pancreatic islet cells for unknown reasons respond abnormally to rises in blood sugar levels, with excessive insulin release. The *mixed* types of hypoglycemia combine the characteristics of the first two groups.

*Method of differentiation.* In establishing the presence of the fasting-type hypoglycemia, provocative fasts lasting from 5 to 72 hr may be necessary. Two hours of exercise, as on a stationary bicycle, may be used to conclude the fast. The patient must be watched carefully for hypoglycemic symptoms. In the normal person, the blood sugar will not fall below 50 mg/100 ml under such conditions.

Where a stimulative-type hypoglycemia is suspected, the routine GTT is prolonged to 5 hr, blood samples being taken every half hour from the second hour on. Symptoms of hypoglycemia should be carefully watched for and if necessary other specimens taken accordingly. Since in many normals an asymptomatic reactive hypoglycemia may develop with such a procedure, it is well before making the clinical diagnosis to be sure that the complaints suspected of being due to the hypoglycemia are actually produced by this chemical abnormality. In the diagnosis of the mixed types, the performance of a 5-hr GTT followed by a fast of appropriate duration is an efficient approach.

### The Ketone Bodies (Acetone Bodies)

When the body's utilization of glucose is limited by either a reduction in carbohydrate intake or the presence of diabetes mellitus, fat is mobilized and used for production of energy. When the mobilization of fat is excessive, there is an increased accumulation of ketone bodies in the blood. Acetoacetic acid and $\beta$-hydroxybutyric acid are more important in this regard than their decarboxylation product, acetone; it is their increased concentration that contributes so heavily to the development of ketoacidosis in the patient with uncontrolled diabetes mellitus.

As has been discussed in Unit 19, $\beta$-hydroxybutyric acid comprises the bulk of the ketone bodies, acetoacetic acid being present in significant but smaller amounts. Acetone comprises less than 1/20 the total concentration.[27] Though neither nitroprusside nor ferric chloride reagents can demonstrate the presence of $\beta$-hydroxybutyric acid, this deficiency is not a limiting one, since the presence of any one of the ketone bodies has a similar clinical meaning.

The introduction of the nitroprusside tablets ("Acetest") and powder ("Acetone Test-Denco") has simplified considerably the detection of abnormally high levels of ketone bodies in various fluids. Not only are the time and equipment required less, but only drops of the fluid to be tested are needed for the estimation. This is of special importance in estimating blood levels.

In comparing urine and blood ketone-body levels, it is of importance to know that until maximal renal excretion of these substances is exceeded significant amounts are absent from the blood.

Clinically, this is of importance because it is the blood concentration that is primarily responsible for the production of acidosis. Since a 4+ urinary ketone reaction may occur with an insignificant, as well as an extremely high, blood concentration, the use of a serum ketone test (serum acetone test) as a simple guide to the degree of ketosis in diabetic acidosis has become justifiably popular.[28]

*Method for determining plasma ketone levels.* Five milliliters of oxalated blood is centrifuged to separate plasma from cells. A drop of plasma is added to nitroprusside powder (or a nitroprusside tablet), as described for urine in Unit 19. Depending on the development of a purple color, the test is read as 0 to 4+. Contamination with whole blood does not interfere with the reading sufficiently to obscure a 4+ reaction. If a 4+ reaction should occur, 2 drops of plasma and 2 drops of tap water are mixed in a new clean tube, making a 1 : 2 dilution; 1 : 4 and 1 : 8 dilutions of the plasma are similarly made and tested.[28]

*Interpretation.* Because ketone bodies do not accumulate in the blood until they are being maximally excreted in the urine, it is unusual to find ketonemia unless a 4+ ketonuria is present. However, rare cases of diabetic ketoacidosis have been reported in which ketonuria is absent because of renal failure, and the test should be carried out in all cases of unexplained coma. Since a 4+ in the undiluted plasma ketone test indicates a severe degree of ketosis (usually 40 mg/100 ml or more), the serial dilutions are not necessary for making the diagnosis of ketoacidosis. It is of interest that a strongly positive reaction (3+ or more) has not been seen in any condition other than diabetic ketoacidosis.[28]

Serial determinations by the serum-dilution method do have a real value in the treatment of cases of diabetic acidosis. The degree of ketonemia has been found to correlate well with the final prognosis. It has been found very useful, early in therapy, in estimating the degree of insulin resistance to be encountered; and, in following the effects of treatment, it parallels well the serum pH and carbon dioxide levels, but is much simpler to determine.[28]

## REFERENCES

1. G. Mudge, "Clinical patterns of tubular dysfunction," *Amer. J. Med.* 24, 788 (1958).
2. J. V. M. Taggart, "Combined clinic on disorders of renal tubular function," *Amer. J. Med.* 20, 448 (1956).
3. E. P. Joslin, H. F. Root, P. White, and A. Marble, *Treatment of Diabetes Mellitus* (ed. 9; Lea and Febiger, Philadelphia, 1952).
4. I. P. Ackerman, S. F. Fajans, and J. W. Conn, "The development of diabetes mellitus in patients with non-diabetic glycosuria," *Clin. Res. Proc.* 6, 251 (1958).
5. G. G. Duncan, ed., *Diseases of Metabolism* (ed. 3; Saunders, Philadelphia, 1953).
6. G. W. Welsh and E. A. H. Sims, "Renal tubular reabsorption of glucose and the mechanism of glucosuria in pregnancy," *Clin. Rec. Proc.* 6, 287 (1958).
7. H. L. C. Wilkerson and Q. R. Remen, "Studies of abnormal carbohydrate metabolism in pregnancy; the significance of impaired glucose tolerance," *Diabetes* 6, 324 (1957).
8. E. R. Carrington, H. S. Reardon, and C. R. Shuman, "Recognition and management of problems associated with diabetes during pregnancy," *J. Amer. med. Ass.* 166, 245 (1958).
9. E. R. Froesch, A. I. Winegrad, and A. E. Renold, "Mechanism of glucosuria produced by the administration of steroids with glucocorticoid activity," *Prog. 49th Meeting Soc. clin. Invest.* 26, 1957.
10. T. S. Danowski, *Diabetes Mellitus* (Williams & Wilkins, Baltimore, 1957).
11. J. A. Hawkins, E. A. McKay, and D. D. Van Slyke, "Glucose excretion in Bright's disease," *J. clin. Invest.* 1, 247 (1925).
12. H. Bickel *et al.*, "Cystine storage disease with aminoaciduria and dwarfism (Lignac-Fanconi disease)," *Acta Paediat.* (supp. 90), 42, 1 (1952).
13. L. A. Wallis and R. L. Engle, "The adult Fanconi syndrome," *Amer. J. Med.* 22, 13 (1957).
14. N. Nelson, "Photometric adaptation of the Somogyi method for determination of sugar," *J. biol. Chem.* 153, 375 (1944).
15. O. Folin and H. Wu, "System of blood analysis: Simplified and improved method for determination of sugar," *J. biol. Chem.* 41, 367 (1920).
16. H. O. Mosenthal, "Interpretation of glucose tolerance tests," *Med. Clin. N. Amer.* 31, 299 (1947).
17. E. R. Froesh, A. E. Renold, and N. B. McWilliams, "Specific enzymatic determination of glucose in blood and urine using glucose oxidase," *Diabetes* 5, 1 (1956).
18. J. E. Middleton and W. J. Griffiths, "Rapid colorimetric micromethod for estimating glucose in blood and CSF using glucose oxidase," *Brit. med. J.* 2, 1525 (1957).
19. A. Saifer and S. Gerstenfeld, "The photometric microdetermination of blood glucose with glucose oxidase," *J. lab. clin. Med.* 51, 448 (1958).

20. J. W. Conn, "Interpretation of the glucose tolerance test: The necessity for a standard preparatory diet," *Amer. J. med. Sci. 199*, 555 (1940).

21. J. H. Moyer and C. R. Womack, "Glucose tolerance; comparison of 4 types of diagnostic tests in 103 control subjects and 26 patients with diabetes," *Amer. J. med. Sci. 219*, 161 (1950).

22. S. F. Fajans and J. W. Conn, "An approach to the prediction of diabetes mellitus by modification of the glucose tolerance test with cortisone," *Diabetes 3*, 296 (1954).

23. R. H. Williams, ed., *Textbook of Endocrinology* (ed. 2; Saunders, Philadelphia, 1955).

24. R. Fraser, F. Albright, and P. H. Smith, "The value of glucose tolerance tests, insulin tolerance tests, and the glucose insulin tolerance test in the diagnosis of endocrinological disorders," *J. clin. Endocr. 1*, 298 (1941).

25. R. H. Unger and L. L. Madison, "A new diagnostic procedure for mild diabetes mellitus," *Diabetes 7*, 455 (1958).

26. J. W. Conn and H. W. Seltzer, "Spontaneous hypoglycemia," *Amer. J. Med. 19*, 460 (1955).

27. J. Nash, J. Lister, and D. H. Vobes, "Clinical tests for ketonuria," *Lancet 1*, 801 (1954).

28. C. T. Lee and G. G. Duncan, "Diabetic coma: the value of a simple test for acetone in the plasma, an aid to diagnosis and treatment," *Metabolism 5*, 144 (1956).

# Unit 29

# Thyroid-Function Tests

## Thyroid Physiology

An understanding of thyroid physiology is necessary for the interpretation of data derived from the thyroid-function tests commonly employed. A more complete review is available elsewhere.[1]

On the average, 100 $\mu$g of iodide is ingested per day. This is almost totally absorbed from the small intestine and is transported in the plasma in solution or very loosely attached to proteins. Minor amounts of this iodide are secreted by the salivary glands and stomach and recycled through the intestine. Definitive removal from the plasma is achieved by the kidneys, which normally filter and excrete over 50 percent of an ingested iodine load within 24 hr, and the thyroid gland, which collects 20–50 percent of an ingested dose in the same period.

Iodide is concentrated by the thyroid through an energy-dependent transport system. This process can be readily demonstrated by blocking further metabolism of the concentrated iodide through the action of drugs such as propylthiouracil. In the rat, and probably in the human, the normal gradient of iodide concentration in thyroid to iodide concentration in plasma is about 20 : 1. The concentrating mechanism is stimulated by chronic iodine deficiency or administration of thyroid-stimulating hormone, and is greatly diminished in hypopituitary states. Certain anions, including thiocyanate and perchlorate, compete with iodide in the transport system. The latter competes

successfully enough to be used clinically as an antithyroid agent.

Concentrated iodide is normally rapidly metabolized, perhaps by a peroxidase, to some as yet undefined intermediate. The oxidized iodide intermediate then displaces a hydrogen molecule from tyrosine to form monoiodotyrosine, which in turn accepts a second iodine molecule to form diiodotyrosine. The iodinated tyrosines are presumably coupled to form tetraiodothyronine (thyroxine) or triiodothyronine. The iodination of tyrosine and the coupling reaction are believed to take place while the respective amino acids are already in place as units of the thyroglobulin molecule. This process may take place within the follicles rather than in the cells.

Thyroglobulin, the characteristic thyroid protein, of molecular weight about 650,000, is stored as "colloid" in the follicles, usually in sufficient quantity to supply the individual with hormone for a 2-month period if new synthesis is prevented. The organic iodine contained in thyroglobulin is distributed so that 40–50 percent is in diiodotyrosine, 20–30 percent in monoiodotyrosine, 15–20 percent in thyroxine, and less than 5 percent in triiodothyronine. Thyroglobulin eventually undergoes enzymatic hydrolysis and thyroxine and triiodothyronine are liberated into the plasma. The iodotyrosines simultaneously liberated are deiodinated by a specific enzyme within the gland, and their iodine is reutilized.

475

Although this account of thyroid-hormone biogenesis has been amply demonstrated by in vivo and in vitro studies, very little has been established about most of the specific enzymatic steps involved.

Circulating thyroxine and triiodothyronine associate reversibly with certain plasma proteins (thyroxine-binding globulin, albumin, and possibly thyroxine-binding prealbumin). A portion is believed to be free in solution. Almost none is excreted by the kidneys. The two compounds gain access to the cells, where they probably affect energy-supply systems, and secondarily influence the rate of many, if not all, metabolic functions. The specific biochemical actions of the hormones that have been demonstrated include dissociation ("uncoupling") of the normally linked processes of oxygen utilization and high-energy phosphate-bond formation, and the inhibition of certain dehydrogenase reactions. The physiologic locus of these actions has not yet been established. Within cells, the iodothyronines may be enzymatically oxidized and deaminated to form the pyruvic acid analogs, deaminated to form the propionic analog, or deaminated and decarboxylated to form the acetic acid derivatives. It has recently been suggested that the acetic acid derivatives are the molecules that are actually active at the cellular level, since they stimulate certain metabolic reactions without a latent period, in contrast to the iodothyronines. The cells also contain enzymes that deiodinate tetraiodothyronine to triiodothyronine, and that completely deiodinate both iodothyronines.

It is not yet clear whether the metabolism of the hormones described above is related to their stimulating action, or whether these reactions simply represent degradation of excess hormone. The iodide released from the iodothyronines returns to the plasma pool and then is either excreted or reaccumulated by the thyroid once again. In the human liver, thyroxine is conjugated with glucuronate and probably with sulfate and is excreted in the bile. The conjugates are broken down by bacterial enzymes and most of the thyroxine is reabsorbed. This cycle is of minor physiologic importance in the human, although quite active in rodents. Fecal excretion disposes of less than 5 percent of thyroxine produced.

The thyroid gland is directly under the control of the pituitary, which regulates hormone production through a feedback system. In response to alteration of plasma thyroid-hormone levels, or some metabolic effect of the hormone, ventral hypothalamic nuclei are stimulated. The nuclei (hypothetically) secrete a material into the hypophyseal-portal system of blood vessels, which in turn stimulates the adenohypophyseal beta cells to alter production of thyroid-stimulating hormone (TSH). The released TSH stimulates thyroid activity, augmenting the rate of release of iodothyronines, the avidity of the gland for iodide, and the rate of synthesis of thyroid hormone.

### Thyroid-Function Tests

The tests of thyroid function to be described below fall into three distinct categories. Group 1 includes the tests for radioactive iodine ($I^{131}$) uptake, for protein-bound iodine, and for protein-bound iodine[131] and the conversion ratio, which are direct measurements of thyroid-gland metabolism of iodine. From the foregoing discussion on thyroid physiology, it will be apparent that iodine metabolism can be directly equated with thyroid-hormone metabolism. This is especially valid since thyroid hormone, its precursors, and its metabolites are the only iodine-containing substances synthesized in the body. Group 2 includes determinations of serum cholesterol and basal metabolic rate, which measure the effect of secreted thyroid hormone on tissue metabolism throughout the body. Group 3 includes the TSH test and triiodothyronine thyroid suppression test, which involve exogenously induced alterations of the pituitary-thyroid relationship.

Throughout the following discussion, the stable isotope of iodine ($I^{127}$) will be referred to simply as iodide or iodine, and the radioactive isotope ($I^{131}$) will be identified by a superscript.

### RADIOACTIVE-IODINE UPTAKE [2]

In a subject who is in iodine balance, the inorganic iodide accumulated by the thyroid each day is equal to the amount of organic iodine secreted. When ordinary quantities of stable iodide are ingested, then the fraction collected by the thyroid will be directly proportional to the secretion rate of thyroid hormone, or to the "activity" of the gland. Radioactive iodide[131], an easily procurable $\gamma$-emitting isotope with physical half-life of 8 days, can be detected after administration of a tracer dose, and is handled by the gland exactly as is the stable isotope.

PROCEDURE. In the adult, 10 to 20 $\mu$c of $I^{131}$ are administered orally, without regard to food intake. Smaller amounts are used in infants aged 1–4 years (1–2 $\mu$c) and in children aged 5–10 years (2–10 $\mu$c) in an effort to reduce potential radiation-induced carcinogenic effects in the thyroid gland. Many clinicians avoid the test completely in children under 1 year of age. A similar quantity of $I^{131}$ is placed in a flask for use as a reference standard. After the desired time interval, usually 24 hr, the radioactivity in the patient's thyroid gland is measured by a scintillation crystal detector. The standard is measured at the same time, and net counts are derived by subtracting background radiation. From this the percentage uptake can be determined. Several commercial units are available and are satisfactory for this work.

TECHNICAL CONSIDERATIONS. The geometry of patient-to-crystal and standard-to-crystal distances must be standardized. Use of a simultaneously measured standard corrects for physical decay of the isotope occurring after administration of the tracer dose. Correction must be made for absorption of radiation by neck tissue overlying the gland, and for back-scatter $\gamma$-rays. Most laboratories put the standard for counting in a large beaker of water or plastic phantom neck simulating the normal location of the thyroid gland. In addition, a 3-mm lead shield is placed over the scintillation crystal to absorb weak back-scatter $\gamma$-rays from patients and standard. Neck counts due to tissue and blood inorganic $I^{131}$ can be estimated by determining radioactivity over some remote body region, such as the low thigh, but can usually be disregarded in determinations made 24 hr after administration of the tracer dose. In a typical calculation, thigh counts per minute (CPM) are subtracted from observed neck CPM. The net neck CPM is then expressed as a percentage of the net standard CPM, obtained by subtracting room background from observed CPM with the standard in water or a plastic phantom.

VARIANTS OF THE $I^{131}$ UPTAKE PROCEDURE. Many other techniques have been devised to measure the avidity of the thyroid for iodine. Since urinary excretion is the only significant pathway of iodide metabolism other than thyroidal collection, cumulative urinary $I^{131}$ excretion at 24 and 48 hr after administration of a tracer dose will be reciprocally related to thyroidal uptake at these time periods.[3] The difficulties involved in securing complete timed urine specimens make estimation of thyroidal uptake by this technique less desirable than counting over the gland. The technique is useful when the subject cannot be brought to the radioactivity-detecting apparatus. Thyroidal $I^{131}$ clearance,[4] determined by

measuring changes in thyroidal and serum I[131] content over a 1–2-hr period, is
a precise measurement of thyroid avidity
for the iodide ion. In practice, it is much
more cumbersome and of no greater
clinical value than the uptake test described above. Another variant is measurement of I[131] uptake at 8 and 48 hr, and
quantitation of the change during the
interval.[5] The normal gland continues to
collect I[131] during this period, whereas
the thyrotoxic gland usually contains less
I[131] at 48 hr than at 8.

SOURCES OF ERROR, LIMITATIONS, AND IN-
TERPRETATION.[6] Thyroidal collection of
the I[131] and secretion of organified I[131]
go on simultaneously. The amount of the
tracer dose in the thyroid gland at a particular time represents the summation of
these two activities. In the normal gland
with adequate thyroidal iodine stores,
radioactivity builds up over 24–48 hr and
then gradually decreases, describing a
curve as shown in Fig. 45. The hyperplastic gland, with small iodine stores,
typically has an accelerated uptake of
I[131] and begins to release hormonal I[131]
within 2–12 hr. I[131] content at 24 hr may
be less than at 6 or 8 hr. Radioactive-
iodide uptake is best quantitated by
measurements taken at 2, 8, 24, and pos-

sibly 48 hr after administration of the
trace dose. In practice, it is usually possible to derive sufficient information
from one determination at 24 hr.

Hypothyroidism is associated with thyroidal uptake at 24 hr of 2–20 percent,
euthyroidism with 20–50 percent, and
hyperthyroidism with 50–100 percent.
Elevation of plasma iodide due to absorption of iodine in any form lowers I[131]
uptake by dilution of the tracer dose and
saturation of the gland. The effect of one
episode of excess ingestion of inorganic
iodine is generally dissipated within 2
days to a month, depending on the
amount absorbed. The problem is important, however, because of the innu-
merable iodine-containing cough syrups
and vitamin, mineral, and tonic preparations in common use, and the frequent
use of iodine for skin antisepsis. Long-
term excessive intake of iodine results in
depression of uptake for over a month,
roughly equal to the period during which
the preparation was taken. Lipid-soluble,
iodinated-radiographic contrast mediums
(Lipiodol, Telopaque) are retained by
the body for a considerable period and
depress I[131] uptake for up to 12 months
after administration. Water-soluble
agents, such as Diodrast, usually are totally excreted within 1 or 4 weeks. In

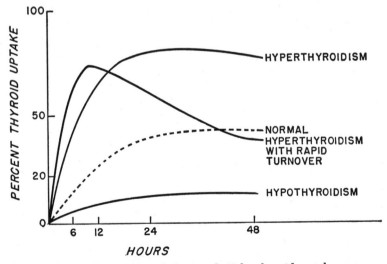

Fig. 45. Typical normal and abnormal 48-hr thyroid uptake curves.

478

each instance, the time necessary for removal of the excess iodine from the body is greatest in hypothyroidism and least in hyperthyroidism. Decreased urinary clearance of $I^{131}$ in patients with renal disease may augment thyroid uptake during the early phase of the disease, but eventually a new equilibrium is obtained, and the $I^{131}$ uptake should return to normal. Quantitation of uptake at but one time interval may not provide a true picture of the uptake curve. This difficulty is frequently observed in thyrotoxicosis, where the measured uptake is above normal at 6–12 hr but, because of the rapid hormonal $I^{131}$ secretion, may be in the normal range at 24 hr.

LOCALIZATION OF ACCUMULATED $I^{131}$. Malignant thyroid tissue, cysts, and areas of inflammation or fibrosis almost invariably accumulate $I^{131}$ less actively than normal tissue. If a particular area in a thyroid gland is under suspicion, use of a movable, well-collimated (aperture about 1 cm) scintillation detector will permit manual comparison counting over normal and abnormal tissue. Refinement of this technique has been achieved by several commercially available scanning devices which automatically pass a focused scintillation crystal detector back and forth over the thyroid and graphically register the intensity of radiation. In general, an area of decreased uptake associated with the position of a firm nodule is taken to suggest malignant disease, but, as above, may be due to an adenoma, an area of fibrosis, inflammation, or a cyst. Malignant tissue may be hidden under a layer of active normal tissue and thus not identified. In practice, manual or automatic scanning has as yet provided very little improvement in management of thyroid disease, although it has considerable promise if improved, and great academic interest. Whole-body scanning also has been used to locate extrathyroidal thyroid-tumor metastases that collect iodide[131].

PROTEIN-BOUND IODINE (SERUM PRECIPITABLE IODINE)

Thyroid hormone (thyroxine, triiodothyronine) circulates in the plasma loosely attached to proteins and is precipitated with them by a variety of protein-denaturing agents. In general, the level of hormone in the plasma is proportional to the rate of secretion by the thyroid gland.

METHOD.[7] The plasma proteins of an aliquot of serum are precipitated by Somogyi's reagents and washed free of iodide by distilled water. The organic material is then ashed under conditions preventing vaporization of iodine. The residual iodine present is estimated colorimetrically by its catalytic effect on the decolorization of ceric ion by arsenite ion. A useful variant of this procedure (butanol extractable iodine[8]) involves (1) extraction of serum iodide, iodotyrosines, and thyroid hormone into acid butanol, (2) removal of iodide and iodotyrosines by an alkaline wash, and (3) subsequent iodine estimation on the residue, as above.

SOURCES OF ERROR, LIMITATIONS, AND INTERPRETATION. This test is perhaps the most accurate index of thyroid hormone activity available. In most laboratories, hypothyroidism is associated with values of 0–3.5 $\mu$g/100 ml of protein-bound iodine (PBI), euthyroidism with 3.5–8 $\mu$g/100 ml, and hyperthyroidism with higher values. Determination of total plasma iodine is a useful check on results of the test for protein-bound iodine. If the total plasma iodine exceeds the protein-bound iodine by 4–6 $\mu$g/100 ml, the test should be interpreted with caution. The usual washing procedure may not rid the precipitated proteins of iodide if this ion is present in high concentrations following ingestion of iodine or its use for antisepsis. This contamination will elevate the apparent "PBI." Many useful iodinated roentgen contrast mediums (Telopaque, Lipiodol) are precipitated with protein and appear as PBI.[9] Administration of triiodothyronine, which is not firmly bound to plasma proteins and therefore rapidly leaves the plasma, results in a low serum PBI. The patient remains euthyroid nevertheless, since tissue supplies of hormone are adequate. For the reasons given above, the test is not valid within 3–4 days after a single ingestion of excessive iodide, within 1–2 months after long-term administration of iodide preparations, within 1 or 2 weeks following intravenous pyelogram examination, within 2 months to 2 years following administration of lipid-soluble iodinated contrast mediums, or while triiodothyronine is being given.

*Hyperestrogenism,* as in pregnancy, increases the specific plasma thyroxine-binding sites, thereby elevating PBI levels. This elevation, to 8–10 µg/100 ml, is not associated with hyperthyroidism, since the thyroid hormone is apparently not available to the tissues in increased amount. An opposite effect is produced by administration of testosterone. *Mercury,* when present in plasma as a diuretic agent, causes precipitation of iodine during the PBI determination. A false depression of PBI may be seen for 2–3 days following therapeutic use of this compound. The *nephrotic syndrome* is associated with a depression of PBI, which is usually stated not to correlate with cellular hypothyroidism. *Severe malnutrition* is frequently the cause of a depressed PBI, perhaps representing both diminished thyroxine-binding protein and true thyroidal hypofunction. Iodinated proteins present in serum in certain unusual conditions (Hashimoto's thyroiditis, thyroid carcinoma, congenital metabolic defects in hormone synthesis) may elevate PBI but are probably metabolically inactive. Use of the butanol extractable iodine procedure circumvents the latter error, since it does not measure iodoprotein content of plasma. The error of the determination of PBI when done by skilled technicians is usually from 0.5–1.0 µg/100 ml on duplicate samples. The test requires much effort and meticulous laboratory technique if it is to be trustworthy.

PROTEIN-BOUND IODINE[131] AND CONVERSION RATIO [10]

Radioactive iodine[131] collected by the thyroid is oxidized, formed into thyroid hormone, and stored as thyroglobulin. Thyroglobulin is hydrolyzed, and the thyroxine and triiodothyronine contained are subsequently secreted into the plasma. During the first 72 hr after administration of I[131], the radioactive material in the plasma consists of iodide[131], representing largely I[131] not yet collected by the thyroid or excreted by the kidney, and I[131]-labeled hormone, secreted by the thyroid and bound to plasma protein. The absolute amount of protein-bound hormonal I[131] present and the proportion of total plasma radioactive material present as hormonal I[131] vary directly with the rate of production and secretion of hormone by the gland, and inversely with thyroidal iodine stores.

METHOD. Forty-eight hours after administration of 50 µc of I[131], an aliquot of serum is obtained. Total radioactivity is quantitated by counting 2 ml of serum in a well scintillation counter. Comparison is made with a suitable dilution of a standard. Serum radioactivity is expressed as percentage of administered dose per liter of plasma. An equal volume of serum is mixed with 4 volumes of 20-percent trichloracetic acid and the protein precipitate collected by centrifugation. This precipitate is washed twice with 5-percent trichloracetic acid. Residual radioactivity is measured, compared with a standard, and expressed as percentage of dose per liter of protein-bound I[131]. The ratio of protein-bound I[131] to total I[131], representing the proportion already metabolized by the gland, is known as the conversion ratio.

480

SOURCES OF ERROR, LIMITATION, AND INTERPRETATION. The percentage of PBI[131] per liter and conversion ratio measure the same biochemical phenomena and thus vary coordinately. Both are decreased by dilution if plasma iodide level is elevated owing to recent iodine ingestion, since a smaller amount of I[131] will enter the thyroid with each microgram of iodide. Both are augmented in the presence of small thyroid iodine stores occasioned by iodine-deficient diet, compensatory hyperplasia of a remnant of tissue left after surgical or radiation-induced partial thyroidectomy, or defect in thyroglobulin storage. Elevation of PBI[131] and conversion ratio due to a hyperplastic gland remnant can be inferred if the PBI is concommitantly low and I[131] uptake accelerated. Administration of exogenous thyroid hormone will decrease pituitary stimulation of the thyroid and thus depress PBI[131] and conversion ratio. With these limitations, it will be found that these tests vary directly with the level of thyroid function. Commonly accepted values at 48 hr are:

|  | PBI[131] (percent/L) | Conversion ratio (percent) |
|---|---|---|
| Hypothyroidism | Below 0.02 | Below 10 |
| Euthyroidism | 0.02–0.2 | 10–40 |
| Hyperthyroidism | 0.1–3.0 | Above 40 |

### SERUM CHOLESTEROL

PRINCIPLE, SOURCES OF ERROR, AND LIMITATIONS. The serum cholesterol level represents the balance of absorption, synthesis, and degradation (see Unit 24). In hyperthyroidism, degradation and synthesis are both augmented, and the plasma cholesterol level stabilizes usually at a level lower than normal.[11] The reverse is true in hypothyroidism. Variation of cholesterol is large, both among individuals and over a period of time in the same individual, limiting the usefulness of the test. Cholesterol levels are influenced by many factors. Elevation of serum cholesterol in hypothyroidism is relatively con-

sistent, and is very unusual in thyrotoxicosis. Serum cholesterol depression in hyperthyroidism is so inconstant as to make the test nearly valueless. Serum cholesterol levels are sometimes under 150 mg/100 ml in hyperthyroidism and are usually above 280 mg/100 ml in hypothyroidism. The test is not recommended as a useful parameter of thyroid function.

### BASAL METABOLIC RATE

Although the exact mechanism is unknown, administration of thyroid hormone augments utilization of energy and production of heat by the body. When corrected for age, sex, body shape, and body size, and standardized for activity and temperature, caloric production varies directly but not closely with the amount of hormone being secreted by the thyroid gland.

METHOD.[12] The resting, fasted subject respires oxygen-enriched air in a spirometer containing an apparatus for absorbing exhaled water vapor and carbon dioxide (see Unit 34). The decrease of oxygen in the system is graphically recorded. The quantity of oxygen used is corrected to standard temperature and pressure and, by means of an assumed respiratory quotient, expressed as calories produced per unit surface area (calculated from standard height-weight tables). This figure is then expressed as a percentage of "normal" calorie production per surface area obtained experimentally on a large series of healthy people.

SOURCES OF ERROR, LIMITATION, AND INTERPRETATION. Lack of sleep, activity, eating, smoking, anxiety, and dyspnea due to heart failure or pulmonary disease increase the basal metabolic rate (BMR). Gas leaks in the apparatus will falsely elevate the determination, as can a perforated ear drum. Normal values do not hold for very obese or extremely thin sub-

481

jects. Certain neoplastic diseases (for example, leukemia) are associated with a high BMR, which does not represent hyperthyroidism. Pyrexia elevates the BMR.

A value of the BMR below minus 20 percent suggests hypothyroidism, although numerous normal individuals have such a metabolic rate. Values above plus 20 percent suggest hyperthyroidism and are of strong supporting diagnostic value when above plus 30 percent if the test was done at truly basal conditions.

The test has major value when repeated determinations are used to assess the clinical status of a patient receiving exogenous thyroid hormone or an anti-thyroid drug. In these instances, one or both of the more exact determinations (PBI, $I^{131}$) may be invalidated by the therapy.

THYROID-STIMULATING HORMONE TEST [13]

In primary myxedema, the residual thyroid tissue, if present at all, is unable to respond to administration of thyroid-stimulating hormone (TSH) with an increase in $I^{131}$ uptake. In pituitary myxedema, the hypofunctioning thyroid tissue can usually be stimulated by administration of TSH.

METHOD. Uptake of $I^{131}$ is determined before and after the administration of 20 units of TSH daily for 3 days.

SOURCES OF ERROR, LIMITATIONS, AND INTERPRETATION. The TSH preparation must be potent. The $I^{131}$ determinations must be accurate. Elevation of the $I^{131}$ uptake to near normal level (20 percent) following TSH is strong evidence of secondary myxedema, since false positive results are quite unusual. Lack of response is not so useful a result, since after atrophy secondary to prolonged hypopituitarism the thyroid may fail to respond to the standard period of TSH stimulation.

TRIIODOTHYRONINE THYROID SUPPRESSION TEST [14]

Difficulty may arise in interpretation of the $I^{131}$-uptake test if the result is in the area of overlap (40–60 percent) between euthyroidism and hyperthyroidism. It has been shown that administration of thyroid hormone, by inhibiting pituitary TSH release, will cause a decrease in $I^{131}$ uptake in a normal gland or one with compensatory hyperplasia. Contrariwise, administration of thyroid hormone to a patient with Graves's disease will not significantly alter the thyroidal $I^{131}$ uptake. This fact is empirically true, although whether this is due to decreased sensitivity of the hypothalamic-pituitary complex or to the functional autonomy of the thyroid gland in Graves's disease is not known. It is also held that a similar lack of responsiveness to suppression is characteristic of the thyroid gland in Graves's disease in the prethyrotoxic state, when eye signs alone are present. Usually *l*-triiodothyronine, which has a rapid onset of action, is administered.

METHOD. A test of $I^{131}$ uptake is performed in the usual manner. Following this, 75 $\mu$g of *l*-triiodothyronine is administered orally each day for 7 days, and the uptake is then repeated. The patient should be observed for signs of thyroid-hormone excess.

SOURCES OF ERROR, LIMITATIONS, AND INTERPRETATION. Depression of the uptake to the hypothyroid level (under 20 percent) is strong evidence for a normal pituitary-thyroid relation. As in all biologic phenomena, results vary, but the thyrotoxic gland will rarely respond with a reduction in uptake of more than a few percent.

MISCELLANEOUS TESTS

*Urinary iodide* determination is a useful check on the absorption of excess quantities of iodine. The normal value varies geographically but is commonly about 100 $\mu$g/24 hr. *Plasma gamma globulin* is frequently elevated in Hashimoto's thyroiditis and can be detected by alterations of A/G ratio, protein electrophoresis, or the cephalin flocculation test. *Autologous antithyroglobulin antibodies* have recently been discovered in the serum of patients with Hashimoto's thyroiditis and a variety of other thyroid lesions. At present, studies for such antibodies are not generally available.

The *uptake of I*[131]*-labeled thyroxine or triiodothyronine* [15] by heterologous red cells incubated in vitro in patients' serum has been proposed as a thyroid-function test that is free of the artifacts due to ingestion of iodine. The percentage uptake under standard conditions varies directly with the metabolic state of the individual. This test probably measures the relative saturation of plasma thyroxine-binding sites by endogenous thyroid hormone. It is not generally available as a clinical procedure.

## Interpretation of Thyroid-Function Tests in Disease

Characteristic changes in the thyroid-function tests in disease are shown in Table 78. In each of the tests, considerable overlap is found between normal and pathologic states. For example, on

Table 78. *Thyroid-function tests in various states.*

| Condition | I[131] uptake (percent) | PBI ($\mu$g/100 ml) | PBI[131] 48 hr (percent/L) | Conversion ratio, 48 hr (percent) | Serum cholesterol concentration (mg/100 ml) | BMR (percent) | TSH test | Triiodothyronine test |
|---|---|---|---|---|---|---|---|---|
| Primary hypothyroidism | 0–20 | 0–3 | 0–0.02 | <10 | Elevated | <−20 | No response | |
| Secondary (pituitary) hypothyroidism | 10–20 | 1–4 | Depressed | <10 | Normal | <−20 | Increased uptake | |
| Euthyroidism | 20–50 | 3.5–8 | 0.02–0.2 | 10–40 | Normal, 150–280 | −20 to +20 | | Decreased I[131] uptake |
| Thyrotoxicosis | 50–100 | >8 | 0.1–3 | 40–90 | Normal or depressed | >+20 | | No change in I[131] uptake |
| Adenomatous colloid goiter | 20–50 | 3.5–8 | 0.02–0.2 | Normal | Normal | Normal | | |
| Active subacute thyroiditis | Depressed | Normal | Depressed | Depressed | Normal | Normal or elevated | | |
| Recovery subacute thyroiditis | Normal or elevated | Normal | Normal or elevated | Normal or elevated | Normal | Normal | | |
| Hashimoto's thyroiditis | Normal, depressed, or elevated | Low, normal, or elevated | Low, normal, or elevated | Low, normal, or elevated | Normal | Normal or low | | |
| Iodine-deficiency functional hyperplasia | Elevated or normal | Depressed or normal | Elevated or normal | Elevated or normal | Normal | Normal or low | | Decreased I[131] uptake |
| Thyrotoxicosis factitia | Depressed | Elevated | Depressed | Depressed | Normal or depressed | Normal or elevated | Increased uptake | |
| Primary or metastatic thyroid neoplasia | Normal | Normal | Normal | Normal | Normal | Normal | | |

$I^{131}$ uptake of 55 percent after 24 hr does not make the diagnosis of thyrotoxicosis certain, nor does the use of radioisotopes and fancy machinery necessarily make the procedure exact. In every instance, the thyroid-function tests should be considered carefully in the light of the clinical problem. Usually, an apparent contradiction can be resolved by repetition of the test or further observation of the patient. Since a thyroid problem that is difficult to diagnose rarely constitutes a medical emergency, observation can be of great value. Needle biopsy of the gland can be done if facilities are available, and may rapidly resolve a problem not settled by more indirect methods of study.

In *subacute thyroiditis,* the inflammatory process prevents the normal uptake of $I^{131}$ and hormone synthesis and destroys the integrity of the follicles. Large amounts of thyroglobulin may be released into the plasma, with elevation of PBI, and even transitory thyrotoxicosis. During the recovery phase, the thyroid avidly collects iodide, so that $I^{131}$ uptake may be above normal. Also, stored thyroidal iodine is diminished, so accumulated $I^{131}$ is rapidly passed through the gland, resulting in a high $PBI^{131}$ and conversion ratio.

*Hashimoto's thyroiditis* is a more chronic process, which may interfere little with thyroid function, destroy the gland almost entirely, or leave a small portion of intact tissue. In this condition, the follicles may be unable to store hormone normally, and iodoprotein is often released from the thyroid in addition to thyroxine.

The function tests give extremely variable results, ranging from values characteristic of glandular hypofunction (low $I^{131}$, low PBI, low $PBI^{131}$, low BMR) through euthyroidism associated with normal $I^{131}$ uptake, normal BMR, and elevated PBI, to results suggestive of hyperfunction (elevated $I^{131}$ uptake, elevated $PBI^{131}$).

In *chronic iodine deficiency,* the adult usually achieves iodine balance through growth of a goiter and coincident increase in plasma iodide clearance by the thyroid gland. Thus the fractional uptake of $I^{131}$ will be augmented, but if compensation has been achieved, PBI, BMR, and cholesterol are normal. $PBI^{131}$ may be elevated if there is a small amount of stored iodine, or normal, if there is a larger pool of organic iodide with which the tracer mixes, as in some large nodular glands.

In *functional hyperplasia* of the thyroid after subtotal thyroidectomy, the uptake is usually normal, but turnover of thyroidal iodine may be accelerated, with high $PBI^{131}$. After $I^{131}$ therapy, perhaps because of radiation-induced damage in the remaining thyroid cells, elevated uptake and rapid conversion of $iodide^{131}$ to $PBI^{131}$ are sometimes found associated with normal or low PBI levels. Infants under 1 year are reported to have elevated $I^{131}$ uptake and $PBI^{131}$ with normal PBI, because environment is said to elevate $I^{131}$ uptake, without change in PBI. Unfortunately, thyroid carcinoma usually does not alter the results of any of the known thyroid-function tests.

## REFERENCES

1. J. Wolff and R. C. Goldberg, *Biochemical Disorders in Human Disease* (Academic Press, New York, 1957), p. 289.
2. E. H. Quimby, S. Feitelberg, and S. Silver, *Radioactive Isotopes in Clinical Practice* (Lea and Febiger, Philadelphia, 1958).
3. F. R. Keating, Jr., M. H. Power, J. Berkson, and S. F. Haines, "The urinary excretion of radioiodine in various thyroid states," *J. clin. Invest. 36,* 1138 (1947).

4. N. B. Myant, E. E. Pochin, and E. A. G. Goldie, "The plasma iodide clearance rate of the human subject," *Clin. Sci. 8,* 135 (1949).

5. D. D. Adams and H. D. Purves, "The change in thyroidal $I^{131}$ content between 8 and 48 hours as an index of thyroid activity," *J. clin. Endocr. 17,* 127 (1957).

6. S. C. Werner, H. B. Hamilton, E. Leifer, and L. D. Goodwin, "An appraisal of the radioiodine tracer techniques as a clinical procedure in the diagnosis of thyroid disorders," *J. clin. Endocr. 10,* 1054 (1950).

7. S. B. Barker, M. U. Humphrey, and M. H. Soley, "The clinical determination of protein-bound iodide," *J. clin. Invest. 30,* 55 (1951).

8. E. B. Man, D. M. Kydd, and U. B. Peters, "Butanol extractable iodine of serum," *J. clin. Invest. 30,* 531 (1951).

9. R. L. Rapport and G. M. Curtis, "The clinical significance of the blood iodine: A review," *J. clin. Endocr. 10,* 753 (1950).

10. D. E. Clark, R. H. Moe, and E. E. Adams, "The rate of conversion of administered radioactive iodine into protein-bound iodine of the plasma as an aid in the evaluation of thyroid function," *Surgery 26,* 331 (1949).

11. J. P. Peters and E. B. Man, "The significance of serum cholesterol in thyroid disease," *J. clin. Invest. 29,* 1 (1950).

12. S. C. Werner, *The Thyroid* (Hoeber-Harper, New York, 1955), p. 125.

13. A. Querido and J. B. Stanbury, "The response of the thyroid gland to thyrotropic hormone as an aid in the differential diagnosis of primary and secondary myxedema," *J. clin. Endocr. 10,* 1192 (1950).

14. S. C. Werner, "A new and simple test for hyperthyroidism employing l-triiodothyronine and the 24 hours $I^{131}$ uptake method," *Bull. N. Y. Acad. Med. 31,* 137 (1955).

15. M. W. Hamolsky, A. Goloditz, and A. S. Freedberg, "Further studies on use of *in vitro* RBC uptake of 1-triiodothyronine[131] as a diagnostic test of thyroid function," *J. clin. Endocr. 19,* 103 (1959).

# Unit 30

## Tests of Ovarian and Testicular Function

URINARY GONADOTROPIN ASSAYS

Although the nature of the actual secretions of the anterior pituitary is unknown, it is generally believed that the cells of this gland produce three hormones that regulate gonadal function. These gonadotropins are: (i) the follicle-stimulating hormone (FSH); (ii) the luteinizing hormone (LH), or interstitial-cell-stimulating hormone (ICSH); and (iii) prolactin or the lactogenic hormone, also referred to as luteotropin (LTH). FSH and LH are separable, with relative ease, from extracts of pituitaries of slaughterhouse animals.[1] Therefore, they are regarded as distinct hormones, despite the close interrelation of their actions. The chemical properties of the gonadotropins have been reviewed elsewhere.[2]

Stimulation of growth of the granulosa cells and formation of the theca folliculi are functions of FSH in the female, but development of the ovum is not. In the male, FSH regulates growth of the seminiferous tubules and spermatogenic activity. In females, LH acts in concert with FSH to promote follicular maturation and especially to stimulate estrogen secretion [3] and, of course, produces luteinization. In addition, LH will repair atrophic ovarian interstitial tissue. In males, LH stimulates androgen secretion by the Leydig cells, and consequently growth of the accessory structures. The exact function of prolactin in the human is not clear. In laboratory animals, at least, it governs secretion of progesterone by the corpus luteum.[4]

In nonpregnant humans, gonadotropic material is excreted in the urine. Although this material exhibits both the FSH and LH activity associated with pituitary extracts, its biologic and chemical nature has thus far eluded precise characterization. For example, it is uncertain whether the gonadotropin in urine is a single molecular species possessing both FSH and LH activity or whether two different molecules are present. Pending resolution of this problem, the generic term *human pituitary gonadotropin* (HPG) is used to refer to gonadotropin of pituitary origin.[5] The use of the term FSH to refer to HPG is inaccurate. Prolactin has not as yet been detected in human urine by reliable methods.[6]

There are two kinds of bioassay methods for gonadotropic activity: differential assays, which respond specifically to either FSH or LH, and nondifferential assays, which respond to both FSH and LH.

On the basis of studies on pituitary extracts, several assays are thought to be specific for FSH. These assays are based on:

(1) Follicular growth in hypophysectomized immature female rats; [7]

(2) Increase in ovarian weight in intact immature rats treated with human chorionic gonadotropin (HCG); [8]

(3) Increase in ovarian weight in intact immature mice treated with HCG.[9]

486

Assays thought to be specific for LH (ICSH) are based on:

(1) Repair of the interstitial tissue in the ovaries of hypophysectomized immature female rats; [7]

(2) Enlargement of the prostate in hypophysectomized immature male rats; [10]

(3) Enlargement of the seminal vesicles in hypophysectomized immature male rats; [11]

(4) Pigment deposition in the feathers of the weaver finch; [12]

(5) Depletion of ascorbic acid from the ovaries of intact pseudopregnant rats.[13]

Of these differential bioassays, only the ovarian-weight method in intact mice treated with HCG and the ventral-prostate method in hypophysectomized rats have been widely applied to the bioassay of urine. These methods have served chiefly as experimental tools. For example, it has been possible to demonstrate the existence of LH activity as measured by the ventral-prostate assay in the urine of normal women throughout the menstrual cycle and of normal men. Highest titers of this LH activity are found in postmenopausal urine. In normal women there occurs a mid-cycle peak of excretion of LH activity, associated with the time of ovulation.[14, 15]

The nondifferential methods of measuring pituitary gonadotropin are based on enlargement of the ovaries of immature intact rats and enlargement of the uterus of immature intact mice. These methods are simpler and less expensive than the differential assays and are therefore employed for clinical purposes. Since none of the methods in current use is sufficiently sensitive to permit routine measurement of HPG in blood, assays are performed with urine after extracting and concentrating the hormonally active material.

METHODS OF MEASURING HPG. Several satisfactory methods for estimating HPG in urine are available.[16, 17] One widely used procedure devised by Albert [5, 18] involves extraction of the gonadotropin from urine by adsorption onto kaolin, followed by elution with alkali and precipitation with acetone. The precipitate is dissolved in water and assayed by the ovarian-weight method in intact rats. One half of the extract is injected into each of two immature rats (21 to 23 days old) in divided doses over a period of 4 days. The animals are autopsied on the fifth day and the ovaries are weighed. By applying the mean weight of the ovaries of the two animals to a previously prepared dose-response curve, which relates mean ovarian weight to dose, one obtains the titer of HPG per 24 hr of excretion. Results are expressed in rat units. Five rat units are defined as an increase in ovarian weight of 150 percent over noninjected controls. When the titer of HPG is less than 5 rat units per 24 hr, it cannot be detected by the ovarian-weight response. However, the uterus of the immature rat responds to smaller quantities of HPG. By preparing a suitable dose-response curve, uterine weight may be used as a measure of HPG activity within the range of 2.5 to 5.0 rat units.

When the Albert method is used, a 24- or 48-hr specimen of urine is collected at refrigerator temperature without addition of preservatives. Since the entire specimen must be extracted, an aliquot is insufficient. If a low or subnormal titer of HPG is anticipated, a 48-hr specimen should be obtained. The urine should be extracted promptly after collection. Where delay is unavoidable, the specimen may be frozen.

### INTERPRETATIONS AND LIMITATIONS

The clinical application of HPG assay has been the subject of several excellent reviews.[5, 18–20]

Because of variations in sensitivity of test animals, results of HPG assays expressed in rat units cannot be regarded as quantitatively reliable, and minor changes in the excretion of HPG may not be significant. Optimally, urine extracts should be tested in parallel with a reference standard and results expressed in terms of the reference material. A universally available reference standard would also permit comparison of results between laboratories. At present, no such material is available. Standard dose-response curves are therefore usually based on extracts of postmenopausal urine prepared by each individual laboratory. In normal men and women during reproductive life, HPG is present in the urine in low titers. When the Albert method is used, 5–10 rat units per 24 hr is the normal range. Occasionally, absence of gonadotropic activity is encountered, perhaps more often in normally menstruating women than in men.[18] The amount of active material excreted by women before the menopause is slightly lower than that excreted by men, except during the mid-cycle period. Little or no HPG is excreted by children before puberty. HPG excretion becomes greatly elevated in women at the menopause (greater than 25 rat units per 24 hr), remaining high even after cessation of symptoms. No comparable increase occurs in men, although high titers are encountered in castrated males. HPG assays are especially useful in distinguishing between amenorrhea due to gonadal failure, where HPG excretion is elevated, and that resulting from pituitary deficiency, where HPG activity may not be detectable. In *Turner's syndrome*, HPG titers are sometimes as elevated as those found in menopausal individuals. Titers are usually elevated in *Klinefelter's syndrome*. Individuals with *testicular insufficiency* may be classified according to whether HPG excretion is normal, elevated, or low. In *panhypopituitarism*, HPG is minimal or not detectable. Starvation, debility, and administration of estrogens in sufficient dosage also result in a subnormal excretion of HPG.

## HUMAN CHORIONIC GONADOTROPIN (HCG)

Chorionic gonadotropin is a hormone of pregnancy produced by the chorionic villi of the placenta. Its principal function in primates is to prolong the secretory life of the corpus luteum of the menstrual cycle until placental production of estrogens and gestagens is sufficient to satisfy the needs of pregnancy.[21] Although HCG is a luteotropic hormone in primates, it exhibits many different kinds of gonad-stimulating activity in lower mammals and all other classes of vertebrates. Thus, in both intact and hypophysectomized male rats, HCG stimulates testicular androgen secretion and, consequently, enlargement of the accessory sexual structures. In intact female rats, acting together with circulating FSH, HCG stimulates follicular development, luteinization, and estrogen secretion. In all its biologic effects in lower mammals, the action of HCG resembles that of pituitary LH, although these two hormones are dissimilar chemically.

Detection of HCG in body fluids is important for diagnosis of pregnancy. An activity similar to HCG is present also in abnormal states, including chorionepithelioma, hydatidiform mole, and certain testicular neoplasms. As in the case of HPG, there is no chemical method for detection of HCG. Therefore biologic assays are relied on. Bioassay methods used for measurement of HCG are responsive to HPG as well, and therefore are nonspecific. However, specificity is achieved by taking advantage of the fact that enormous quantities of HCG are produced during pregnancy. Aliquots of body fluids, usually urine, to be tested for HCG activity are diluted to so low a concentration that HPG, if present, would not be detected.

Assays for HCG are of two kinds, qualitative and quantitative. Qualitative tests, useful in pregnancy diagnosis, are designed to detect only a certain level of

488

HCG. Assays that are truly quantitative must be carried out on the test material and a reference standard simultaneously. The result of a quantitative assay, properly designed, is based on a comparison of the responses to both the test extract and the reference material. An international standard for HCG has been available for many years. Results of quantitative assays should be expressed in international units.

The classical tests for pregnancy diagnosis, the Aschheim-Zondek (A–Z) [22] and Friedman [23] rabbit tests, although very sensitive, are being replaced by the less sensitive but much more rapid and convenient amphibian-spermiation tests. Use of amphibian spermiation as an end point was introduced by Galli-Mannini in 1947.[24] The material to be tested is injected into the dorsal or ventral lymph sac of any one of a number of amphibian species.[25–27] Two to 3 hr later, urine is taken up with a small glass pipette inserted a few millimeters into the cloaca and a drop is placed on a glass slide. The presence of sperm in the urine is taken as a positive response. Each animal may

be used repeatedly, a week's rest after a test being sufficient. For pregnancy tests, a sample of morning urine, collected no sooner than 2 weeks following the first missed period, is best. Urine should be kept refrigerated prior to use. Because of the relative insensitivity of the amphibia and the need for a large dose of urine, it is sometimes desirable to extract the urine, lest toxic materials present injure the test animals.

Although suitable for pregnancy diagnosis, amphibian-spermiation tests, because of their insensitivity, are unsatisfactory for quantitative assays. Here the methods of choice are ovarian hyperemia in intact rats [28, 29] and prostatic enlargement in intact rats.[30]

The bioassay of human chorionic gonadotropin has been the subject of a comprehensive review.[19]

### INTERPRETATIONS AND LIMITATIONS

Figure 46 indicates the concentration of HCG in urine and serum during pregnancy, in international units.

A high excretion of HCG in pregnancy after the first trimester "peak period" is

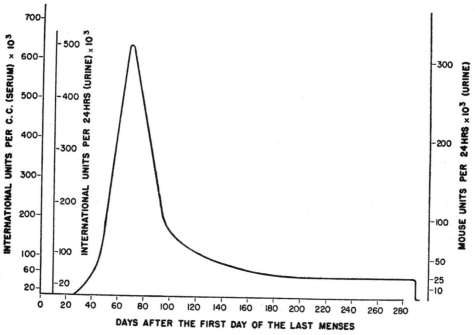

Fig. 46. Concentration of chorionic gonadotropin in serum and urine during pregnancy.[28]

suggestive of hydatidiform mole. However, the finding of a high HCG titer is not diagnostic (unless pregnancy has been ruled out), since there is an overlap of values among individuals experiencing normal pregnancy and those with a hydatidiform mole. Tests for HCG are useful in gauging the success of removal of a mole, since the titer should fall rapidly and not be detectable 2 months later. Monthly tests for 6 months following removal of a mole will guard against the possibility of secondary growths, which can in this way be detected before they are clinically evident.

The presence of HCG in males is diagnostic of neoplastic testicular disease such as chorionepithelioma, since males do not normally excrete this hormone.

### SEMEN ANALYSIS

Analysis of semen is most commonly performed in connection with problems of infertility.[31] However, considerable variability is evident among normal males, and in the individual case it is difficult to set any lower limit to the sperm count, percentage of motile sperm, or percentage of abnormal forms consistent with fertility. In severe eunuchoidism and in eunuchism, no semen is produced. Average normal values are as follows: volume, 2.5 ml or more; consistency, viscid; sperm count, 60 million or more per milliliter; more than 60 percent normally formed; and 60 percent or more motile after 6 hr.

### VAGINAL SMEAR IN ENDOCRINE DIAGNOSIS

Information of clinical value concerning the level of ovarian function can be secured by any physician willing to familiarize himself with those aspects of the smear which reflect endocrine activity.[32-34] The technique depends upon the fact that the vaginal epithelium, like all the epithelia of the female reproductive tract, undergoes cyclic proliferation and involution in response to rhythmic changes in the secretion of the ovarian hormones. The cells present in vaginal secretion, having been shed from that layer of the epithelium which is superficial at the moment of sampling, reveal by the extent of their differentiation the hormonal influences exerted upon them in the immediate past. The vaginal smear thus constitutes a direct bioassay of ovarian hormone secretion in the patient under study. Moreover, it permits a continuous, rather than an episodic, evaluation of ovarian function and is simple, painless, and inexpensive.

During each cycle, secretion of estrogen stimulates proliferation of the epithelium and progressive cornification of the superficial layers. The addition of progesterone causes the most superficial cells to expand as the result of a curious vacuolization of the cytoplasm, which can be seen to clear and lose its affinity for stains. The corresponding cell types that are of the greatest importance in the endocrine evaluation of the smear may be conveniently divided, according to their staining properties, into two large groups: (1) *cornified cells,* which are large, thin, and polygonal, their nuclei being small and pyknotic, and their cytoplasm staining orange-red with the Shorr trichrome technique; (2) *noncornified cells,* which may be further divided, according to their level of origin from the vaginal epithelium, into basal and precornified cells. The *basal* cells, which are derived from the deep layer, are small to medium in size, but larger than leukocytes. They are round or oval, and have well-defined edges. Their nuclei are large and vesicular, and their cytoplasm generally stains clear blue or violet. The *precornified* cells, which are the type most frequently encountered in vaginal smears, are thought to be derived from the middle layer. In size, they are intermediate between the basal and superficial cornified cells. Their nuclei, which vary in size from small to medium, are round and vesicular. Their cytoplasm stains clear blue, light green, or light violet. Folding of the edges ("envelope folding") is sometimes observed; curling may result in the formation of the so-called "navicular" cells.

PREPARATION OF VAGINAL SMEARS. Smears should be taken before bimanual examination of the vagina has been performed, since lubricating jellies interfere with the staining characteristics of the cells. The secretion is aspirated into a glass pipette attached to a strong-walled rubber bulb of approximately 1-oz capacity. With the bulb compressed, the pipette is inserted into the posterior fornix. The bulb is then released and the pipette slowly withdrawn. The aspirated secretion is expelled onto a clean glass slide and fixed *immediately* for 1–2 min in a solution of 95-percent ethyl alcohol. Prompt fixation is essential, since drying leads to distortion of the cells and their staining characteristics.

If more than one smear is to be fixed in a single jar of alcohol, it is essential to attach a metal paper clip to each slide to prevent contact with adjacent slides. Although single slides can be stored indefinitely in alcohol before staining, a series should be kept no longer than 2 weeks because rusting of the clips will alter the staining characteristics of the smear. Smears of grossly bloody secretions should be spread as thinly as possible and the red cells hemolyzed by preliminary fixation in a 10-percent acetic acid–alcohol solution before transfer to the standard fixative. The staining time of such slides should be increased to 5 min.

STAINING OF VAGINAL SMEARS. The single differential stain of Shorr (S–3, obtainable from E. F. Mahady & Co., Boston) is applied by dropper, left on for 1 min, and the slide dehydrated by carrying it through 80-percent, 95-percent, and absolute alcohol, the slide being dipped 10 times in each solution. After blotting and thorough clearing in xylol, it is mounted as a permanent preparation and examined microscopically. Reliance should be placed only on the appearance presented by the thin areas of the slide. Smears stained by the Shorr technique are not satisfactory for chromosomal sexing, which is described separately. The percentage of cornified squamous cells varies in proportion to the amount of estrogen being secreted. Conversely, the percentage of basal cells varies with the degree of atrophy of the vaginal epithelium. A minimum of 400 cells distributed through 7 fields should be counted.

INTERPRETATION. Because the relative proportions of the different epithelial-cell types vary during the menstrual cycle, a single smear taken during active reproductive life is most informative when it indicates a subnormal level of estrogen secretion. On the other hand, a highly cornified smear obtained from a prepubertal child or a postmenopausal woman may possess great diagnostic value. In sexually immature or senile patients, in whom estrogen secretion is normally minimal, a high percentage of cornified cells suggests the action of exogenous estrogen or, less commonly, the presence of an estrogen-secreting tumor. The fact that the vagina atrophies only gradually after the natural menopause and that the basal cells may not attain predominance until 10–20 years have elapsed must, of course, be taken into account.

URINARY SEDIMENT IN ENDOCRINE DIAGNOSIS. In such patients as prepubertal children, in whom the taking of a vaginal smear may be inexpedient, information concerning the level of estrogen secretion can be secured by examination of the urinary sediment. The lower two-thirds of the urethra, like the vagina, is a derivative of the urogenital sinus and its epithelium exhibits parallel cycles of growth in response to estrogenic stimulation.[85]

491

The rounded urethral basal cells may be readily distinguished from the more polygonal precornified and cornified cells by microscopic examination of a hanging-drop preparation of the unstained sediment obtained from a clean voided urine specimen. For more precise appraisal of the degree of cornification, a 25-ml sample of freshly voided urine is centrifuged at 1500 rev/min for 15 min, the supernatant carefully decanted, and the sediment spread on a glass slide that has been coated with albumin. The slide is fixed immediately in 95-percent alcohol for at least 20 min and stained by the Shorr technique.

### CHROMOSOMAL SEXING

The sexual dimorphism in the resting nuclei of human tissues has proved of diagnostic value in the study of hermaphroditism and of hypogonadal syndromes. In suitably prepared smears of epithelial surfaces, a small plano-convex body, the so-called "chromatin corpuscle," can be demonstrated in a large proportion of the epithelial cells of normal females and in only a small proportion of male cells. Circumstantial evidence suggests that this body, which is approximately $1\mu$ in diameter, results from the fusion of the heterochromatic portions of the two X chromosomes. In general, buccal smears are more satisfactory for chromosomal sexing than are vaginal smears [36] because of the higher percentage of cells with vesicular nuclei in the former.

METHOD OF OBTAINING BUCCAL SMEARS. In adults, the buccal mucosa may be scraped with a clean microscope slide and smeared with a second slide. In infants, a narrow metal spatula is employed to scrape the oral mucosa. The slide should be fixed *immediately* in 95-percent ethanol.

THE FEULGEN STAIN FOR CHROMOSOMAL SEXING. Because of their high content of desoxyribonucleic acid, the chromatin corpuscles take the Feulgen stain. The following method is a modification of that described by Lillie.[37]

*Reagents.* (1) *Schiff's Reagent.* Dissolve 1.0 gm of fuchsin and 1.9 gm of sodium metabisulfite ($Na_2S_2O_5$) in 100 ml of 0.15$N$ hydrochloric acid. Shake the solution at intervals or in a mechanical shaker for 2 hr. The solution is now yellow to light brown in color. Add 500 mg of fresh activated charcoal and shake 1–2 min. Filter into a graduated cylinder, washing the residue with enough distilled water to restore the original 100-ml volume. The solution should now be colorless. If yellow color remains, charcoal decolorization should be repeated. Store at 0–5°C.

(2) *Light Green Stain.* Mix 5 parts of 0.05-percent aqueous light green and 95 parts of 80-percent ethanol.

(3) *Bisulfite Solution.* Mix 5 ml of 10-percent potassium metabisulfite and 5 ml of 1$N$ hydrochloric acid. Add 100 ml of distilled water (total volume 110 ml). Prepare immediately before use and discard each time.

*Staining Procedure.* (1) Transfer buccal smears from 95-percent ethanol to 1$N$ hydrochloric acid that has been preheated to 60°C. Leave for 10 min. Then immerse the slides in Schiff's reagent for 10 min.

(2) Wash for 1, 2, and 2 min in three successive baths of bisulfite solution; wash for 5 min in running water.

(3) Counterstain the slides by dipping them once, briefly, in light green stain.

(4) Complete the dehydration by dipping slides 10 times in 95-percent ethanol and then immersing them in absolute ethanol for 7 or 8 min. Clear by immersing in xylol for 4–5 min.

(5) Mount with 1 drop of Harleco or other synthetic resin.

INTERPRETATION. The nuclear chromatin takes a clear purplish color. The proportion of nuclei containing chromatin corpuscles is ascertained under oil immersion, a total of 100 cells being examined. The chromatin corpuscle is demonstrable in approximately 30–50 percent of the epithelial nuclei of normal females and 0–4 percent of those of normal males. In the majority of cases of gonadal dysgenesis (Turner's syndrome), the chromosomal sex is male, and in the true Klinefelter's syndrome it is female. Patients with true hermaphroditism can be demonstrated to have a distinct chromosomal sex; patients with pseudohermaphroditism have a chromosomal sex in harmony with their gonadal sex.[38]

### CYTOLOGIC EXAMINATION FOR MALIGNANT CELLS

The cytologic diagnosis of genital cancer from the study of the vaginal smear is an undertaking beyond the competence of the "occasional microscopist."

The method has proved of great value as a case-finding technique,[39] but staining and interpretation must be done by personnel specializing in this technique.

METHOD OF OBTAINING SPECIMENS FOR CYTOLOGIC EXAMINATION. Material for cytologic examination should be obtained before bimanual examination to prevent contamination with lubricating jellies. A dry, sterile pipette equipped with a strong rubber suction bulb is introduced into the posterior fornix, with the bulb compressed. Pressure on the bulb is released and the vaginal contents are aspirated. The material is then forcibly blown upon a clean slide. The slide is immediately dropped into a solution of equal parts of ether and 95-percent ethanol. The slide should remain in the fixative solution until it is processed in the laboratory.

## REFERENCES

1. H. L. Fevold and F. L. Hisaw, "Interactions of gonad-stimulating hormones in ovarian development," *Amer. J. Physiol. 109*, 655 (1934).
2. C. H. Li and H. M. Evans, "Chemistry of anterior pituitary hormones," in G. Pincus and K. V. Thimann, ed., *The Hormones* (Academic Press, New York, 1948), vol. 1, chap. 14, p. 631.
3. R. O. Greep, H. B. van Dyke, and B. F. Chow, "Gonadotropins of the swine pituitary. I. Various biological effects of purified FSH and pure ICSH," *Endocrinology 30*, 635 (1942).
4. E. B. Astwood, "The regulation of corpus luteum function by hypophysial luteotrophin," *Endocrinology 28*, 309 (1941).
5. A. Albert, "Gonadotropins," *Fertility and Sterility 10*, 60 (1959).
6. R. C. Bahn and R. W. Bates, "Histologic criteria for detection of prolactin: lack of prolactin in blood and urine of human subjects," *J. clin. Endocr. 16*, 1337 (1956).
7. H. M. Evans, M. E. Simpson, S. Tolksdorf, and H. Jensen, "Biological studies of the gonadotropic principles in sheep pituitary substance," *Endocrinology 25*, 529 (1939).
8. S. L. Steelman and F. M. Pohley, "Assay of the follicle-stimulating hormone based on the augmentation with H. C. G.," *Endocrinology 53*, 604 (1953).
9. P. S. Brown, "Experimental examination of an assay for urinary follicle-stimulating hormone," *J. Endocr. 14*, 257 (1956).
10. R. O. Greep, H. B. van Dyke, and B. F. Chow, "Use of the anterior lobe of the prostate gland in the assay of ICSH," *Proc. Soc. exp. Biol. (N. Y.) 46*, 644 (1941).

11. J. W. McArthur, "The identification of pituitary interstitial cell stimulating hormone in human urine," *Endocrinology 50*, 304 (1952).

12. S. Segal, "Response of the weaver finch to chorionic gonadotropin and hypophysial luteinizing hormone," *Science 126*, 1242 (1957).

13. A. F. Parlow, "Bioassay of pituitary luteinizing hormone by the ovarian ascorbic acid depletion method," in A. Albert, ed., *Human Pituitary Gonadotropin*, in press.

14. J. W. McArthur, F. M. Ingersoll, and J. Worcester, "Urinary excretion of interstitial cell stimulating hormone by normal males and females of various ages," *J. clin. Endocr. 18*, 460 (1958).

15. J. W. McArthur, J. Worcester, and F. M. Ingersoll, "Urinary excretion of interstitial cell and follicle-stimulating hormone activity during the normal menstrual cycle," *J. clin. Endocr. 18*, 1186 (1958).

16. J. A. Loraine and J. B. Brown, "A method for the quantitative determination of gonadotropins in the urine of non-pregnant human subjects," *J. Endocr. 18*, 77 (1959).

17. S. G. Johnsen, "A clinical routine method for the quantitative determination of gonadotropins in 24 hour urine samples," *Acta endocr. (Kbh.) 31*, 209 (1959).

18. A. Albert, "Human urinary gonadotropin," *Recent Progr. Hormone Res. 12*, 227 (1956).

19. J. A. Loraine, "The Clinical Application of Hormone Assay," (Livingstone, Edinburgh, 1958).

20. J. C. Loraine, "Bioassay of pituitary and placental gonadotropins in relation to clinical problems in man," *Vitamins and Hormones 14*, 305 (1956).

21. F. L. Hisaw, "The placental gonadotrophin and luteal function in monkeys (*Macaca mulatta*)," *Yale J. Biol. Med 17*, 119 (1944).

22. B. Zondek, "Uber die Hormone des Hypophysen vorder lappens. IV. Darstellung des Folliklerefenshormons (Prolan A). Methodik der klinischen Harnanalyse zum Nachuris des Prolan," *Klin. Wschr. 91*, 1207 (1930).

23. M. D. Friedman, "On the mechanism of ovulation in the rabbit. IV. Quantitative observations on the action of extracts of urine of pregnancy," *J. Pharmacol. exp. Ther. 45*, 7 (1932).

24. C. Galli-Mannini, "Pregnancy test using the male toad," *J. clin. Endocr. 7*, 653 (1947).

25. G. L. Haskins, Jr., and A. I. Sherman, "The quantitative assay of serum chorionic gonadotropin in pregnancy, using the modified male frog technique," *J. clin. Endocr. 12*, 385 (1952).

26. J. V. Thorborg and K. Hansen, "The use of *Xenopus laevis, Bufo bufo*, and *Rana esculenta* as test animals for gonadotropic hormones," *Acta endocr. (Kbh.) 6*, 51 (1951).

27. B. M. Hobson, "Conditions modifying the release of spermatozoa in male *Xenopus laevis* in response to chorionic gonadotrophin," *Quart. J. exp. Physiol. 37*, 191 (1952).

28. A. Albert and J. Berkson, "A clinical bioassay for chorionic gonadotropin," *J. clin. Endocr. 11*, 805 (1951).

29. R. Borth, B. Lunenfeld, and H. de Watteville, "Effect of serum used as vehicle on the quantal assay of human chorionic gonadotropin by the ovarian hyperemia response in rats," *Acta endocr. (Kbh.) 24*, 119 (1957).

30. J. A. Loraine, "The estimation of chorionic gonadotropin in the urine of pregnant women," *J. Endocr. 6,* 319 (1950).

31. R. S. Hotchkiss, *Etiology and Diagnosis in the Treatment of Infertility in Men* (Thomas, Springfield, 1952).

32. I. L. C. De Allende and O. Orias, *Cytology of the Human Vagina* (Hoeber, New York, 1950).

33. I. L. C. De Allende, E. Shorr, and C. G. Hartman, "A comparative study of the vaginal smear cycle of the rhesus monkey and the human," *Contr. Embryol. Carneg. Instn. 31,* 3 (1943).

34. E. Shorr, "An evaluation of the clinical applications of the vaginal smear method," *J. Mt. Sinai Hosp. 12,* 667 (1945).

35. L. O. Vincze, P. D. Taft, and J. W. McArthur, "A study of cornification in vaginal, buccal, and urinary sediment smears," *J. clin. Endocr. 19,* 281 (1959).

36. E. Marberger, R. A. Boccabella, and W. O. Nelson, "Oral smear as a method of chromosomal sex detection," *Proc. Soc. exp. Biol. (N. Y)* 89, 488 (1955).

37. R. D. Lillie, *Histopathologic Technique and Practical Histochemistry* (Blakiston, New York, 1954).

38. M. L. Barr, "Sex chromatin and phenotype in man," *Science 130,* 679 (1959).

39. P. Calabresi and N. V. Arvald, "Cytological screening for uterine cancer through physicians' offices," *J. Amer. med. Ass. 168,* 243 (1958).

# Unit 31

# The Adrenal Cortex

## Physiologic Considerations

The two human adrenal glands form a triangular cap over both kidneys in the retroperitoneal space. Although embryologically distinct, the cortex and the medulla of each gland form a single anatomic unit, despite separate hormonal and nervous control. The adrenal is concerned with facilitating adaptation to change in the internal and external environment. Thus the medulla secretes epinephrine and norepinephrine as the immediate response to potentially damaging circumstances; the cortex responds more slowly and more specifically to the ancient demands of sodium and potassium metabolism, to stresses that require more prolonged mobilization of energy for adaptation, and finally to the varying demands for stimulation and inhibition of general anabolism.

Cortisol (hydrocortisone) is secreted from the fasciculata-reticularis zone of the cortex in response to stimulation by adrenocorticotropic hormone (ACTH). Cortisol is antianabolic, stimulates gluconeogenesis, has minor effects on sodium and potassium metabolism, and probably acts upon some cellular system in response to a need for adaptation to change. While current assay procedures are not sensitive enough to detect circulating ACTH in normal man, there is considerable evidence that anterior-pituitary secretion of ACTH is elicited by falling blood levels of cortisol and by stimuli from higher nervous centers, per-

haps acting through a hypothalamic ACTH-releasing hormone. ACTH is probably secreted at a constant slow rate, can be increased within 1 min under stimulation, and is inhibited by high blood levels of cortisol (or its congeners). This inhibition is brief after short periods of exogenous hypercortisolism but may extend for as long as a year after prolonged adrenal overactivity. The half-life of ACTH in the serum is approximately 5 min.

Farrell and co-workers [1] indicate that aldosterone is secreted from the zona glomerulosa of the adrenal cortex in response to "glomerulotropin" secretion from the midbrain. Bartter [2] suggests there is probably a "tonic" rate of secretion of aldosterone which is increased following decrease in effective blood volume (or carotid pulse pressure) and decreased following increase in blood volume. Volume receptors in the atrial walls and carotid arteries transmit inhibitory signals via the vagus nerve and stimulatory signals via the cardio-accelerator nerve which result in appropriate change in the rate of glomerulotropin secretion. Aldosterone itself acts primarily to accelerate exchange of potassium for sodium in the renal tubule and elsewhere.

Despite adult blood levels of cortisol, children excrete very small quantities of androgen and 17-ketosteroids in the urine. At puberty, the adrenal secretion becomes qualitatively altered in that androgen secretion appears, urinary 17-

496

ketosteroid excretion increases, and the body responds with growth of axillary and pubic hair and increased sebaceous activity of the skin. These observations led Albright to postulate a third type of adrenocortical secretion which is androgenic and anabolic. However, the exact site of secretion, the control, and the chemical nature of the adrenal androgen have eluded definition to date. Despite lack of corroboration, it is generally suspected that pituitary gonadotropins may join with ACTH in the control of adrenal androgen secretion.

### Chemical Considerations

The hormones of the adrenal cortex are 19-carbon and 21-carbon steroids with a basic structure (and nomenclature) as shown in Fig. 47. Biosynthetic pathways of the major steroids are illustrated in Fig. 48.

The term 17-ketosteroid (17-KS) is used for steroids with a ketone group at

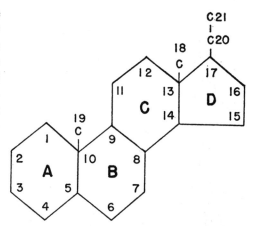

Fig. 47. Basic structure of adrenal steroids.

carbon 17, derived from adrenal and testicular androgen and cortisol. The term 17-hydroxycorticosteroid (17-OHCS) is used for cortisol and other 21-carbon steroids possessing a dihydroxy acetone group at carbon 17.

Cortisol and other 17-OHCS are largely reduced in ring A (Fig. 47) by the liver, and conjugated to form water-

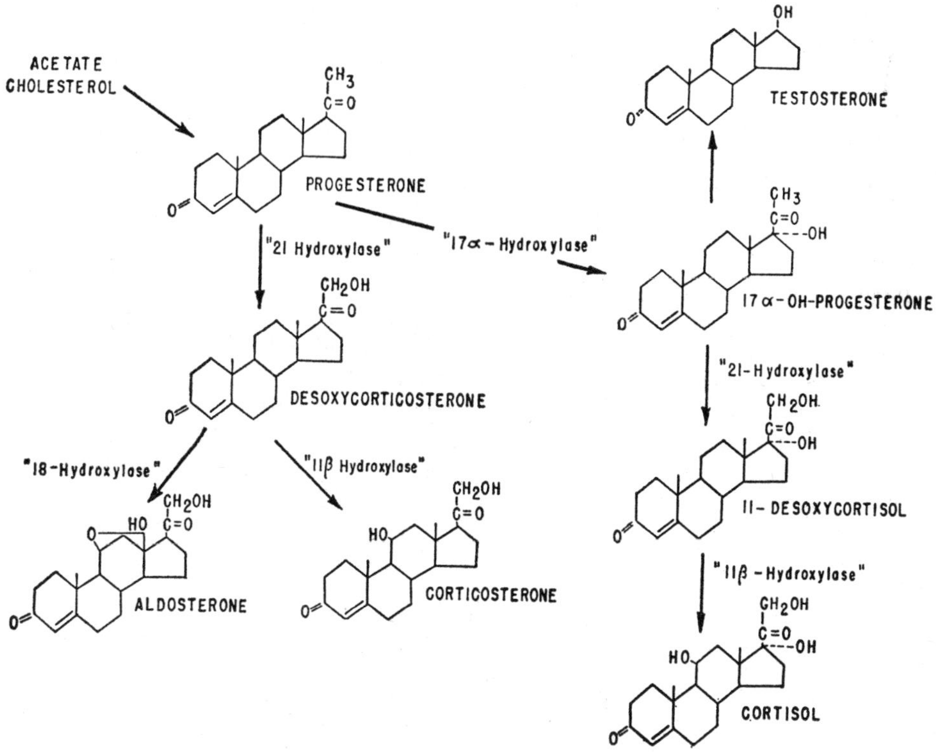

Fig. 48. Biosynthetic pathways of the major steroids.

soluble glucuronides and sulfates which are subsequently excreted in the urine. In addition to reduction, a part of the 17-hydroxycorticosteroids are cleared at carbon 17 to form 17-KS. These are also excreted in the urine, predominantly as water-soluble glucuronides and sulfates.

The dihydroxyacetone grouping of the 17-OHCS reacts with sulfuric acid and phenylhydrazine to form a yellow color in the Porter-Silber reaction. This reaction can be carried out in plasma (Nelson-Samuels),[3] in urine after hydrolysis and extraction with methylene chloride,[4, 5] and in urine following butanol extraction.[6] The 17-ketosteroids are measured by any of several procedures all utilizing the *m*-dinitrobenzene reaction of Zimmermann. This reaction is also used to quantitate the 17-OHCS following the cleavage of the dihydroxyacetone side chain to a 17-KS.[7, 8]

ADRENOCORTICAL DISEASES. A summary of abnormalities seen in diseases of the adrenal cortex is given in Table 79.

*Addison's disease* [9] or hypoadrenocorticism, is an uncommon disorder characterized by weakness, hypotension, increased pigmentation, and sensitivity to stress due to lack of adrenocortical function. Adrenocortical failure is usually unexplained, even by the findings at autopsy, although some cases are due to tuberculosis or to other infections or neoplastic processes. Adrenocortical insufficiency may be mild or complete and rarely may consist of selective lack of aldosterone or cortisol secretion.

*Cushing's syndrome* [10] is hyperadrenocorticism predominantly with respect to cortisol secretion and may be due to bilateral adrenal hyperplasia, unilateral adenoma, or carcinoma. In the fully developed clinical picture, the patient presents mild obesity with muscle atrophy, thin skin with bruising and striae, osteoporosis, and hypertension.

The *adrenogenital syndrome* is associated with a marked increase in urinary 17-KS excretion and a deficiency in 17-OHCS. It may be due to carcinoma, adenoma, or bilateral adrenal hyperplasia.[11] In the congenital cases due to bilateral adrenal hyperplasia, precocious genital development (male) or pseudohermaphroditism (female) are identifying features. The underlying defect in the adrenogenital syndrome is due in some cases to deficiency of 21-hydroxylase. In other cases, both 21-hydroxylase and 11-$\beta$-hydroxylase are deficient. Precursors of cortisol (17-hydroxyprogesterone, 11,17-dihydroxyprogesterone) accumulate and are excreted in the urine as pregnanediol and pregnanetriol (see Fig. 48).

Primary aldosteronism [12] is usually associated with marked increases in urinary aldosterone excretion. Clinically, it may

Table 79. *Representative abnormalities in adrenal diseases.*

| Test | Addison's disease | Cushing's syndrome | Adrenogenital syndrome | Primary aldosteronism |
|---|---|---|---|---|
| Hct. | ↓ | ↑ | ↑ | |
| Percentage of lymphocytes | ↑ | ↓ | | |
| Serum: | | | | |
| Na | ↓ | | May be | ↑ |
| K | ↑ | ↓ | "salt | ↓ |
| $CO_2$ | ↓ | ↑ | losers" | ↑ |
| Glucose-tolerance test | ↓ FBS | Diabetic GTT | | Diabetic |
| Bone age | | | ↑ | |

produce hypertension with hypokalemic alkalosis and may be due to adenoma or to bilateral hyperplasia.

### Tests of Adrenal Cortical Function

DETERMINATION OF THE NUMBER OF CIRCULATING EOSINOPHILS

PRINCIPLE. An inverse relation exists between adrenal cortical activity and the circulating blood eosinophils. The number of circulating eosinophils is low in Cushing's syndrome [13] and normal to slightly increased in Addison's disease.[14] Following the administration of a single dose of 25 mg of ACTH intramuscularly to subjects with essentially normal adrenal cortical function, a marked drop in circulating eosinophils ensues.[15, 16] The maximum eosinopenic effect occurs within 4 hr following the administration of ACTH. Patients with Addison's disease show no change or a slight decrease in circulating eosinophils following the administration of ACTH.[17, 18] However, following the administration of cortisone, the Addisonian subjects show a normal response, that is, a decrease in eosinophils.[19] The mechanism underlying the eosinopenia induced by ACTH and cortisol is still unknown.

METHOD. Samples of venous blood are obtained with balanced oxalate or ethylene diamine tetraacetic acid (EDTA) as anticoagulant prior to and 4 hr after an intravenous injection of 25 mg of standard ACTH. The subject is continued in a fasting condition during the 4-hr period. The samples of venous blood may be stored at 4°C for several hours. Capillary blood may be used, in which case the blood is diluted immediately with the eosin diluting fluid.

The eosin diluting fluid consists of either a hypotonic solution of eosin (Dunger's solution)[20] or phloxine-methylene blue in water and propylene glycol (Randolph's stain).[21] Following the dilution and staining of the eosinophils, the cells are counted directly in a Fuchs-Rosenthal counting chamber which is 0.2 mm deep and has a ruled area of 16 mm².

*Preparation of Dunger's hypotonic solution of eosin.*[15] Five milliliters of a 2-percent eosin solution [2 gm of eosin A (pentabromofluorescein) per 100 ml] is mixed with 5 ml of acetone and 90 ml of distilled water. The solution is stored at 4°C, is filtered prior to use, and should be prepared fresh every 2 weeks. The blood is mixed by gentle shaking, drawn up in a white-cell pipette to the 0.5 mark if the eosinophil count is normal or high and to the 1.0 mark if the count is low, and finally diluted with the eosin fluid to the 11 mark. The pipettes are shaken gently for 30 sec, following which a Fuchs-Rosenthal counting chamber is filled and allowed to sit for approximately 3 min. Using the low-power magnification, the eosinophils are identified by their rounded granules taking a light-pink stain. They are swollen and in some instances may show disruption of the membrane. Rupture may be held to a minimum by gentle shaking. In the hypotonic solution, the red blood cells are lysed, and the majority of the white blood cells are ruptured. The eosinophils are counted in 16 squares of each of 4 chambers.

The calculation is made as follows. The total number of eosinophils per square millimeter is calculated by counting all cells in 16 squares of each of 4 chambers and dividing by 64. Multiplication by the factor 100 in the instance in which the blood was drawn to the 0.5 mark gives the number of eosinophils per cubic millimeter. If the blood is drawn to the 1.0 mark, the factor 50 instead of 100 is used in the final calculation.

INTERPRETATIONS AND LIMITATIONS. The normal eosinophil count is between 100 and 300 cells/mm³.[22] The absolute eosinophil count is of value only in certain circumstances because of the wide variations in the normal range. In Cushing's syndrome, the number of circulating eosinophils is low—between 0 and 30/mm³.[23] In Addison's disease, the eosinophil levels are usually at the upper limits of normal and on occasions higher. In subjects with essentially normal adrenal cortical function, following the injection of corticotropin, there occurs a decrease in the number of circulating eosinophils (range: −49- to −98-percent decrease). In subjects with Addison's disease, there is usually no decrease (range: +26 to −38 percent).[15, 16]

### THE WATER-LOAD TEST

The water-load test represents an indirect test of adrenal cortical deficiency based upon the resultant metabolic changes of hormonal deficiency. Subjects with adrenal cortical insufficiency (Addison's disease and hypopituitarism) are unable to excrete large volumes of a dilute urine in response to a water load in a normal manner.

PROCEDURE. At 6 p.m. the patient is given dinner without fluids and fluids are omitted thereafter. The subsequent program is as follows:

| | |
|---|---|
| 10:30 p.m. | Patient voids and discards |
| 10:30 p.m.– 7.30 a.m. | Overnight urine volume recorded |
| 8:30 a.m. | Patient voids and discards. Patient drinks water, 20 ml/kg, slowly over 20 min |

| | |
|---|---|
| 8:30 a.m.– 9:30 a.m. | |
| 9:30 a.m.–10:30 a.m. | Hourly urine volume recorded |
| 10:30 a.m.–11:30 a.m. | |
| 11:30 a.m.–12:30 a.m. | |

INTERPRETATIONS AND LIMITATIONS. Normally at least one of the hourly day urines following hydration is larger in volume and lower in specific gravity than the overnight urine. The reverse relation obtains in patients with Addison's disease. The test is nonspecific in that it may give a positive result in a variety of disorders, including malabsorption syndromes, edematous states, renal insufficiency, and severe electrolyte depletion. The test carries the risk of water intoxication in patients with untreated adrenal insufficiency.

### DETERMINATION OF URINARY 17-KETOSTEROIDS

PRINCIPLE. Steroids possessing a ketone group at carbon 17 of the steroid nucleus are designated 17-ketosteroids. A colorimetric test for these steroids is based upon the Zimmermann reaction. This reaction itself is a general reaction for a $CH_2CO$ grouping (that is, an active methylene group adjacent to a ketone group) which reacts with *m*-dinitrobenzene in the presence of alkali to produce a red color. With steroids, the transient color produced depends upon the position of the ketone group. Steroids with a ketone group at carbon 17 react with *m*-dinitrobenzene in alkaline solution to produce an intense, broad absorption band with a maximum at about 520 m$\mu$ whereas steroids with a $\Delta^4$-unsaturated 3-ketone group show a maximum of comparable density at 380 m$\mu$. Steroids with a ketone group at carbon 20 show very weak absorption at 520 m$\mu$. Estrone is a 17-ketosteroid; however, since it is a weak phenolic substance, it is removed in the alkaline wash and is not included in the colorimetric determination for neutral 17-ketosteroids. The urinary 17-ketosteroids are metabolites of: (1) adrenal cortical steroids such as cortisol; (2) adrenal androgens; and (3) gonadal androgens. They therefore represent an index of the activity of the adrenal cortex and the gonads in the male and an approximation of the activity of the adrenal cortex in the female.

A number of methods for the determination of neutral urinary 17-ketosteroids have been described. All are based on the Zimmermann reaction. One of these, a micromodification, is recommended.[24]

INTERPRETATIONS AND LIMITATIONS. The 17-ketosteroid excretions are conditioned by a number of variables: completeness of collection of urine; artifacts introduced during the hydrolysis step; age; sex; interfering substances such as urinary pigments, ketosteroids other than the neutral 17-ketosteroids, and nonketonic chromogenic substances; stress to which the subject is exposed; and, finally, the specific endocrine disorder.

The 17-ketosteroid values are highest during the early morning hours and lowest during sleep, with intermediate values during the day. In normal subjects there is a moderate variation in the 17-ketosteroid excretion in a 24-hr period. These fluctuations are probably the result of emotional status and physical activity.

The urinary 17-ketosteroid values for normal subjects are higher in men than in women, the difference representing the contribution of the male gonads. The 17-ketosteroid levels in various conditions are shown in Table 80. Differentiation among adrenal hyperplasia and adrenal benign and malignant tumors on the basis of the levels of 17-ketosteroids is frequently impossible because of the considerable overlapping of the range of values. In such instances, other diagnostic tests must be resorted to.

Ingestion of Benemid [p-(di-n-propyl-sulfamyl)-benzoic acid] in doses of 2 gm/day causes a 50-percent reduction in the excretion of 17-ketosteroids.[25] Meprobamate (2-methyl-2n-propyl-1,3-propanediol dicarbamate) reacts with m-dinitrobenzene in the Zimmermann reaction, producing a colored complex with an absorption maximum at 395 m$\mu$.[26] Ingested meprobamate is excreted in urine and is present in the final urinary extract subjected to the Zimmermann reaction for

Table 80. *Urinary levels of 17-ketosteroids in various conditions.*

| Condition | Urinary 17-ketosteroids (mg/24 hr) |
|---|---|
| Normal adult males (30 yr) | 8–25 |
| Normal adult females (30 yr) | 4–14 |
| Addison's disease | Low (decreased 70–80% in males and 75–95% in females) |
| Cushing's disease: | |
| Adrenal hyperplasia | High (average 18.1) |
| Adrenal benign tumor | Normal (average 5.7) |
| Adrenal malignant tumor | Very high (average 124.4) |
| Adrenogenital syndrome | May be very high (6–123); highest values in older age group |
| Panhypopituitarism | Low |
| Idiopathic hirsutism | Upper limit of normal and occasionally higher |
| Primary ovarian agenesis | Low (decreased 50%) |
| Menopausal women | Normal |
| Eunuchoid men | Low (decreased 30–50%) |
| Myxedema | Low |
| Thyrotoxicosis | Normal |
| Starvation | Low (decreased 50%) |

the determination of urinary 17-ketosteroids and 17-ketogenic steroids. Unless the Allen correction (readings at 470, 520, and 570 m$\mu$) is used, false high values for 17-ketosteroids will result. A history of medications administered to subjects should accompany urine specimens sent to the laboratory for steroid analysis.

THE DETERMINATION OF ADRENAL CORTICAL STEROIDS AND STEROID METABOLITES IN URINE

PRINCIPLE. To date, 40 steroids have been isolated from bovine adrenal glands. A number of these have also been identified in the adrenal-vein blood and the adrenal gland of human subjects. These steroids are metabolized largely in the liver to water-soluble sulfate and glucuronide conjugates and in unknown conjugated forms. The determination of these metabolites involves the hydrolysis of the conjugates either by acid, which results in some destruction and loss of steroids and the production of artifacts, or by enzymatic hydrolysis, which may be incomplete.

Determination by the Porter-Silber reaction depends upon the formation of a chromogen following reaction of the steroid with phenylhydrazine and sulfuric acid. The steroid metabolites reduced at carbon 20 are not measured by the Porter-Silber reaction although they comprise 30 percent or more of the metabolic products of cortisone and cortisol. A second chemical determination depends on the conversion of the 21-carbon adrenal steroids to 19-carbon 17-ketosteroids, followed by estimation of the formed 17-ketosteroids by the Zimmermann reaction. This procedure (the Norymberski method)[27] for measuring steroid metabolites includes those which are reduced at carbon 20. The basis of the Reddy-Jenkins-Thorn method[4, 6, 28] is similar to the Porter-Silber reaction.

INTERPRETATIONS AND LIMITATIONS. The excretion values for normal subjects vary, depending on the procedure employed. The influence of age on the urinary levels of steroids is greater for 17-KS than that for 17-OHCS, while the influence of body weight and height is more pronounced for 17-OHCS than that for 17-KS. The influence of sex on the excretion values for 17-OHCS is ascribed entirely to the sex difference in body weight and height.

The excretion of the 17-hydroxycorticoids and 17-OHCS is highest in the morning and lowest during the night. A similar diurnal rhythm has been demonstrated for the plasma level of corticosteroids and for the 17-ketosteroids. The diurnal rhythm for the urinary 17-hydroxycorticoids is not changed by night work, forced rest in bed, four-hourly feedings, or starvation. The 17-hydroxycorticoid excretion is enhanced in individuals subjected to emotional stimuli and surgical procedures. The excretion levels remain unaltered in individuals exposed to cold, anoxia, or physical exercise and exertion.

The high background colorimetric absorption in the Reddy-Jenkins-Thorn procedure has been a disturbing difficulty with this method. The application of the Allen color correction increases the sensitivity and reproducibility of the method.

A number of substances interfere with the specificity of the phenylhydrazine–sulfuric acid reaction. These substances are paraldehyde, quinine and colchicine, iodine and iodides, and sulfamerazine and chlorpromazine. The Norymberski procedure measures more 17-hydroxycorticosteroids than does the Reddy-Jenkins-Thorn procedure, in particular the metabolites reduced at carbon 20. Therefore it is to be expected that the values obtained by the Norymberski procedure will be greater than those obtained with the Reddy-Jenkins-Thorn procedure. Urinary glucose, in large quantities, may interfere with the Norymberski methods by utilizing the bismuth reagent; in such instances, pituitary-suppression tests with administered corticosteroids may be of considerable help.

THE DETERMINATION OF ADRENAL
CORTICAL STEROIDS AND STEROID
METABOLITES IN BLOOD

PRINCIPLE. The color reactions used for the estimation of adrenal cortical hormones and their metabolites in blood are the same as those used for the determination of these steroids in urine. To date, the most widely used reaction has been the one with phenylhydrazine and sulfuric acid (Porter-Silber reaction) for the dihydroxyacetone side chain at carbon 17. The most extensively applied procedure has been described by Nelson and Samuels.[3, 27] Usually cortisol is the only steroid measured in plasma with this procedure. Both cortisol and corticosterone have been isolated from human adrenal venous blood[29, 30] in a ratio of 5–10 parts

502

of cortisol to one part of corticosterone.

Over 90 percent of the steroid measured by the phenylhydrazine–sulfuric acid reaction is normally found in the plasma. On standing, the steroids penetrate the red blood cells. Therefore plasma should be separated from cells quickly. The plasma can be stored in the frozen state for several weeks.

There is a high background absorption in the colorimetric procedure in the Nelson and Samuels method which varies between aliquots of the same plasma. Differences between duplicate determinations vary from 0.0 to 5.1 μg/100 ml.[31]

INTERPRETATIONS AND LIMITATIONS. *Levels of free corticosteroids in peripheral blood of normal subjects.* Considerable variations in steroid levels occur in the same individual from day to day. The spread may be from 6 to 18/μg. The plasma levels are highest in the morning and lowest in the evening. This same diurnal rhythm holds for night workers and blind subjects. The pronounced hourly variations in adrenal cortical activity render the evaluation of the status of adrenal function by determination of single plasma levels less reliable than that by 24-hr urinary determinations. A number of drugs interfere with the specificity of the phenylhydrazine–sulfuric acid reaction (see above).

*Levels of free corticosteroids in peripheral blood under conditions of stress and disease.* The concentrations of the adrenal cortical steroids in plasma represent the summations of: (i) the adrenal cortical secretion rate; (ii) the binding and utilization by tissues; (iii) the metabolism of the steroid, especially by the liver; and (iv) the excretion in urine and feces. It is apparent, therefore, that there are severe limitations to the use of the absolute levels of plasma corticosteroids as an index of adrenal cortical activity. Plasma levels are elevated by anesthesia, surgical procedures, or administration of typhoid vaccine, and in the presence of

hepatocellular damage. Modest increases occur during periods of emotional stress, and brief increases may follow intense physical exercise. Plasma values are high in Cushing's syndrome and low in Addison's disease. Low to absent values are found in adrenogenital syndrome and low to moderate values occur in hypopituitarism.

SUPPRESSION TESTS BY ADMINISTRATION OF EXOGENOUS CORTICOIDS

These tests depend upon the inhibition of ACTH by administration of corticoids such as prednisone, dexamethazone, 9-α-fluorocortisol, and 9-α-fluoroprednisolone.[32]

*9 F F Suppression test.* The administration of 0.5 mg of 9-α-fluorocortisol (9 F F) every 6 hr for 2 days will produce at least a 50-percent depression of the urinary 17-KS and 17-OHCS of normal subjects and at least a 50-percent depression of the increased 17-KS excretion in the adrenogenital syndrome due to bilateral adrenal hyperplasia. The increase in 17-OHCS in Cushing's syndrome is not similarly depressed by this dose but is depressed 50 percent by 2 mg of 9 F F given every 6 hr for 2 days when bilateral adrenal hyperplasia, but not when tumor, is the cause of the Cushing's syndrome.

*Test of pituitary ACTH response by inhibition of 11-oxygenation.*[33] A nonsteroid compound, SU-4885 [2-methyl-1,2-bis-(3-pyridyl)-1-propanone], inhibits 11-β-hydroxylase, thereby resulting in reduced blood levels of cortisol and eliciting a secondary increase in ACTH production. This, in turn, stimulates increased secretion of 17-hydroxy,11-desoxycorticosterone. The increment in 17-OHCS gives a measure of ACTH stimulation.

ACTH-STIMULATION TEST (THORN TEST)

A measure of adrenal cortical reserve is provided by the Thorn ACTH test.[8] Twenty-five to 50 U.S.P. units of ACTH of known potency dissolved in 500 ml of 0.9-percent sodium chloride solution is infused intravenously over an 8-hr period on each of 2 successive days. Twenty-four-hour urine specimens are collected on 2 days preceding the infusion and on the 2 days of the ACTH infusion. Blood samples may also be drawn in the morning of these 4 days for direct eosinophil counts. In adult hospitalized subjects without endocrine disease, there is an eosinopenia of 80–100 percent on both days of ACTH infusion, a mean increased excretion of 17-ketosteroids of 4 mg/ 24 hr over the control values, and a mean increased excretion of 14 mg/24 hr for the 17-hydroxycorticoids. The Addisonian subject may be protected from an untoward reaction to ACTH by the oral administration of 100–250 $\mu$g/24 hr of 9-$\alpha$-fluorocortisol, which itself does not contribute appreciably to the urinary 17-ketosteroids or 17-hydroxycorticoids. Subjects with panhypopituitarism usually show a less than normal response to ACTH infusion. The magnitude of the response is in proportion to the extent and duration of the secondary adrenal atrophy. Nevertheless, the increased excretion of 17-hydroxycorticoids or 17-OHCS following the administration of ACTH over a 3–4-day period is of sufficient magnitude to enable one to differentiate primary from secondary adrenal insufficiency. The response of subjects with Cushing's disease to the ACTH-stimulation test is greater than normal in patients with adrenal hyperplasia, minimal in patients with adenoma, and *usually* absent in patients with adrenal carcinoma. In subjects with the adrenogenital syndrome, the administration of ACTH induces a normal response in the urinary levels of 17-hydroxycorticoids and an excessive response in the levels of 17-ketosteroids, pregnanetriols, 17-ketogenic steroids, and 17-OHCS. In subjects with "idiopathic hirsutism," the excretion of 17-ketosteroids, 17-ketogenic steroids,

and pregnanetriols are usually within the normal range, even after the administration of ACTH.

A number of modifications of the original Thorn ACTH-infusion test have been described utilizing intramuscular injections of ACTH gel. Essentially the same responses as outlined above are obtained with these modifications. The ACTH-stimulation test may be carried out utilizing the measurement of plasma corticoids as an index of adrenal cortical response. In such instances, the responses are comparable to those obtained utilizing the measurement of urinary corticoids.

## THE DETERMINATION OF URINARY ALDOSTERONE

PRINCIPLE. Urinary aldosterone may be estimated by a bioassay method based on the change in the urinary sodium-potassium ratio in adrenalectomized rats or dogs following the intravenous injection of the extract containing aldosterone.[34, 35] The reliability and the sensitivity of the assay are enhanced by prior chromatographic purification of the crude extracts.

Urinary aldosterone may be determined by a chemical method that depends on the quantitative separation of aldosterone by at least two successive paper chromatographic fractionations [36, 37] and colorimetric determination of the eluted aldosterone spot, or by a chemical method in which the aldosterone is quantitatively separated by two column chromatographic fractionations, acetylation with $C^{14}$ acetic anhydride, followed by further column and paper chromatographic fractionations, and, finally, quantitative determination of the spot on the paper chromatogram by counting and determination by alkali fluorescence.[38]

INTERPRETATIONS AND LIMITATIONS. Variations in excretion of aldosterone are normally governed by changes in the volume of body fluids (see Unit 21). A marked increase in excretion is usually found in primary aldosteronism and variable increases are found in edematous states such as congestive heart failure, nephrotic syndrome, and toxemia of pregnancy, and in liver disease with ascites. A physiologic increase is found in conditions characterized by a contraction of body fluids and in normal subjects on low-sodium diets. Aldosterone excretion may be normal or increased in Cushing's syndrome, and normal or decreased in hypopituitarism. In adrenogenital syndrome, it is usually normal except in those patients who have a "salt-losing" form of the disease, in whom an increase in aldosterone may occur. In Addison's disease, aldosterone excretion is decreased.

## REFERENCES

1. G. Farrell, "The physiological factors which influence the secretion of aldosterone," *Recent Progr. Hormone Res. 15,* 275 (1958).
2. F. C. Bartter, I. H. Mills, E. G. Biglieri, and C. S. Delea, "Studies on the control and physiologic action of aldosterone," *Recent Progr. Hormone Res. 15,* 311 (1958).
3. D. H. Nelson and L. T. Samuels, "A method for the determination of 17-hydroxycorticosterone in the peripheral circulation," *J. clin. Endocr. 12,* 519 (1952).
4. R. H. Silber and C. C. Porter, "The determination of 17, 21-dihydroxy-20 ketosteroids in urine and plasma," *J. biol. Chem. 210,* 923 (1954).
5. R. E. Peterson, A. Darrer, and S. L. Guerra, "Evaluation of the Silber-Porter procedure for determination of plasma hydrocortisone," *Analyt. Chem. 29,* 144 (1957).
6. W. J. Reddy, D. Jenkins, and G. W. Thorn, "Estimation of 17-hydroxycorticoids in urine," *Metabolism 1,* 511 (1952).
7. J. I. Appleby, G. Gibson, J. K. Norymberski, and R. D. Stubbs, "Indirect analysis of corticosteroids. I. The determination of 17-hydroxycorticosteroids," *Biochem. J. 60,* 453 (1955).
8. G. Birke, E. Diczfalusy, and L. O. Plantin, "Assessment of the functional capacity of the adrenal cortex. I. Establishment of normal values," *J. clin. Endocr. 18,* 736 (1958).
9. G. W. Thorn, P. Forsham, and K. Emerson, Jr., *The Diagnosis and Treatment of Adrenal Insufficiency* (Thomas, Springfield, 1949).
10. F. Albright, "Cushing's syndrome, its pathological physiology, its relationship to the adrenogenital syndrome, and its connection with the problem of the reaction of the body to injurious agents (alarm reaction of Selye)," *Harvey Lect. 38,* 123 (1942–1943).
11. L. Wilkins, *The Diagnosis and Treatment of Endocrine Disorders in Childhood and Adolescence* (Thomas, Springfield, 1950), chap. 13.
12. J. W. Conn, "Presidential address: Painting background: Primary aldosteronism, new clinical syndrome," *J. lab. clin. Med. 45,* 3 (1955).
13. C. M. Plotz, A. I. Knowlton, and C. Ragan, "The natural history of Cushing's syndrome," *Amer. J. Med. 13,* 597 (1952).
14. G. W. Thorn, P. H. Forsham, T. F. Frawley, D. L. Wilson, A. E. Renold, D. S. Fredrickson, and D. Jenkins, "Advances in the diagnosis and treatment of adrenal insufficiency," *Amer. J. Med. 10,* 595 (1951).

15. A. G. Hills, P. H. Forsham, and C. A. Finch, "Changes in circulating leukocytes induced by the administration of pituitary adrenocorticotrophic hormone (ACTH) in man," *Blood 3*, 755 (1948).

16. G. W. Thorn, P. H. Forsham, F. T. G. Prunty, and A. G. Hills, "Test for adrenal cortical insufficiency; response to pituitary adrenocorticotrophic hormone," *J. Amer. med. Ass. 137*, 1005 (1948).

17. A. G. Hills, G. D. Webster, Jr., O. Rosenthal, F. C. Dohan, E. M. Richardson, H. A. Zintel, and W. A. Jeffers, "Quantitative evaluation of primary adrenal cortical deficiency in man," *Amer. J. Med. 16*, 328 (1954).

18. P. H. Forsham, G. W. Thorn, F. T. G. Prunty, and A. G. Hills, "Clinical studies with pituitary adrenocorticotropin," *J. clin. Endocr. 8*, 15 (1948).

19. G. W. Thorn, A. E. Renold, D. L. Wilson, T. F. Frawley, D. Jenkins, J. Garcia-Reyes, and P. H. Forsham, "Clinical studies on the activity of orally administered cortisone," *New Engl. J. Med. 245*, 549 (1951).

20. R. Dunger, "Eine einfache Methode der Zählung der eosinophilen Leukozyten und der praktische Wert dieser Untersuchung," *Münch. med. Wschr. 57*, 1942 (1910).

21. T. G. Randolph, "Blood studies in allergy. I. The direct counting chamber determination of eosinophils in propylene glycol aqueous stains," *J. Allergy 15*, 89 (1944).

22. B. F. Fisher and E. R. Fisher, "Observations on the eosinophil count in man; a proposed test of adrenal cortical function," *Amer. J. med. Sci. 221*, 121 (1951).

23. L. Recant, D. M. Hume, P. H. Forsham, and G. W. Thorn, "Studies on the effect of epinephrine on the pituitary-adrenocortical system," *J. clin. Endocr. 10*, 187 (1950).

24. P. Vestergaard, "Rapid micro-modification of the Zimmermann/Callow procedure for the determination of 17-ketosteroids in urine," *Acta Endocr. 8*, 193 (1951).

25. L. I. Gardner, J. F. Crigler, and C. J. Migeon, "Inhibition of urinary 17-ketosteroid excretion produced by 'Benemid,'" *Proc. Soc. exp. Biol. (N. Y.) 78*, 460 (1951).

26. S. Salvesen and R. Nissen-Meyer, "Influence of meprobamate therapy on the estimation of 17-ketosteroids and 17-ketogenic steroids," *J. clin. Endocr. 17*, 914 (1957).

27. K. Eik-Nes, D. H. Nelson, and L. T. Samuels, "Determination of 17, 21-hydroxycorticosteroids in plasma," *J. clin. Endocr. 13*, 1280 (1953).

28. W. J. Reddy, "Modification of the Reddy-Jenkins-Thorn method for the estimation of 17-hydroxycorticoids in urine," *Metabolism 3*, 489 (1954).

29. E. B. Romanoff, P. Hudson, and G. Pincus, "Isolation of hydrocortisone and corticosterone from human adrenal vein blood," *J. clin. Endocr. 13*, 1546 (1953).

30. D. Jenkins, P. H. Forsham, J. C. Laidlaw, W. J. Reddy, and G. W. Thorn, "Use of ACTH in the diagnosis of adrenal cortical insufficiency," *Amer. J. Med. 18*, 3 (1955).

31. C. A. Gemzell, "Methods of estimating corticosteroids in plasma," *Acta Endocr. (Kbh.) 18*, 342 (1955).

32. G. W. Liddle, "ACTH suppression tests in patients with Cushing's syndrome," Paper 17. 41st Meet. Endocrine Soc., June 1959.

33. G. W. Liddle, D. Island, E. M. Lance, and A. P. Harris, "Alterations of adrenal

steroid patterns in man resulting from treatment with a chemical inhibitor of 11 β hydroxylation," *J. clin. Endocr. 18*, 906 (1958).

34. S. A. Simpson and J. F. Tait, "A quantitative method for the bioassay of the effect of adrenal cortical steroids on mineral metabolism," *Endocrinology 50*, 150 (1952).

35. G. W. Liddle, J. Cornfield, A. G. T. Casper, and F. C. Bartter, "The physiological basis for a method of assaying aldosterone in extracts of human urine," *J. clin. Invest. 30*, 1410 (1955).

36. R. Neher and A. Wettstein, "Physicochemical estimation of aldosterone in urine," *J. clin. Invest. 35*, 800 (1956).

37. L. Hernando-Avendano, J. Crabbé, E. J. Ross, W. J. Reddy, A. E. Renold, D. H. Nelson, and G. W. Thorn, "Clinical experience with physicochemical method for estimation of aldosterone in urine," *Metabolism 6*, 518 (1957).

38. P. J. Ayres, O. Garrod, S. A. Simpson, J. F. Tait, "A method for the determination of aldosterone, cortisol and corticosterone in biological extracts, particularly applied to human urine," *Biochem. J. 65*, 639 (1957).

# Unit 32

# Calcium, Phosphorus, and Bone Metabolism

METABOLIC CONSIDERATIONS

Phosphorus occurs in abundance in virtually all foodstuffs and hence a low phosphorus intake is difficult to maintain. The normal daily intake is 0.5–2.0 gm. Essentially all dietary phosphorus is absorbed except that which is bound to unabsorbed calcium and magnesium and excreted in the stool. In adults, urinary phosphorus reflects intake. Measurement of urinary phosphorus is of little clinical value. The total inorganic phosphorus of serum is decreased following feeding. Fasting levels of serum phosphorus are affected by and are a useful guide to endocrine status (see Table 81).

Calcium occurs in most foodstuffs and daily intakes less than 150 mg are difficult to maintain. The usual American diet contains 400–800 mg of calcium, plus

Table 81. *Relation of serum total inorganic phosphorus to hormonal status.*

| Condition | Serum phosphorus [a] (mg/100 ml) |
|---|---|
| Hypoparathyroidism | 6.0–12.0 |
| Growth in childhood; acromegaly | 4.5–6.0 |
| Postmenopausal female | 4.0–5.0 |
| Young adult | 3.0–4.0 |
| Hyperparathyroidism | 2.0–3.0 |
| Osteomalacia (with secondary hyperparathyroidism) | 1.0–3.0 |

[a] Since the relative concentrations of $HPO_4^-$ and $H_2PO_4^-$ depend on the pH of the medium, it is awkward to express the phosphorus content of biologic fluids as milliequivalents per liter and is more convenient to use milligrams per 100 ml or millimoles per liter [= 10(mg/100 ml)/31].

the calcium of milk and milk products (1200 mg/quart). All calcium is unabsorbed except that which is absorbed under the influence of vitamin D and of parathyroid, growth, and sex hormones. Urinary calcium bears a rough relation to intake (see Table 82) and the previ-

Table 82. *Relation of urinary calcium to calcium intake.*

| Diet | Calcium content (mg/day) | Usual range of urinary calcium (mg/day) [a] |
|---|---|---|
| Bauer-Aub low-calcium diet [1] | 150 | 40–100 |
| Milk- and cheese-free diet | 400–800 | 80–150 |
| Normal diet | 800–2000 | 100–200 |
| Plus milk | 2000–3000 | 150–300 |

[a] The range is given for adults; children excrete roughly 2 mg/kg body weight. Whereas the Sulkowitch qualitative reaction for calcium in the urine may be useful in excluding hyper- or hypoparathyroidism, it has been generally replaced by the more accurate quantitative measurement of 24-hr urinary calcium.

ous level of a patient's calcium intake should influence evaluation of urinary calcium excretion.

Measurement of urinary calcium following 3 days on a low-calcium intake (such as the Bauer-Aub diet [1]) permits evaluation of endogenous factors in calcium metabolism. In some patients (for example, those with renal stones) it may be more informative to continue the patient's customary calcium intake and to judge the urinary calcium accordingly.

508

The normal level of total serum calcium is 8.5–10.5 mg/100 ml (4.3–5.3 mEq/L, 2.1–2.6 mM/L) and may be subdivided as in Figure 49.[2] The level of serum calcium is determined by:

1. The level of *serum protein*[3] (each decrease of 1.0 gm/100 ml in serum albumin is accompanied by a decrease of 0.5–1.0 mg/100 ml in total serum calcium);

2. The level of *serum phosphorus* (in general, serum calcium varies inversely with serum phosphorus according to the equations

$$Ca + P \rightleftharpoons \text{Calcium phosphate},$$
$$K_{sp} = (Ca) \times (P),$$

where the concentrations of calcium and phosphorus refer to their chemical activities and where calcium phosphate refers to hydroxyapatite of bone);

3. The level of parathyroid-hormone activity (parathyroid hormone controls serum calcium levels by affecting renal phosphate excretion[4] and bone resorption;[5] see Fig. 50). The major stimulus to parathyroid activity is the level of ionized serum calcium.

CHEMICAL CONSIDERATIONS

Calcium is difficult to measure in biologic fluids with either oxalate precipitation[6] or ethylene diamine tetraacetic acid (EDTA) titration[7] techniques. Normal levels vary from laboratory to laboratory. Erroneous reports of high serum calcium levels are not uncommon. All laboratory reports of calcium levels must be viewed with healthy skepticism. In general, multiple determinations increase the accuracy of diagnosis. Quantitative 24-hr urinary calcium measurements usually follow aberrations in serum calcium, and the degree of deviation of calcium level is usually greater in urine than in blood. Thus, in mild hyperparathyroidism, the calcium in the serum might be 11.5 mg/100 ml and the calcium in the urine, 20 mg/100 ml, when the 24-hr urine volume was 1000 ml.

The measurement[8] of serum phosphorus is easy and is reliable in most laboratories. Since red cells are rich in phosphorus, hemolysis of specimens must be avoided. Alkaline phosphatase is measured by several reliable techniques. Phosphatase activity may increase and later decrease in stored serum. Since limited substrate is present in the standard techniques, serums suspected of having high phosphatase values should be retested at shorter intervals of incubation (for example, 10, 15, 30, and 60 min in

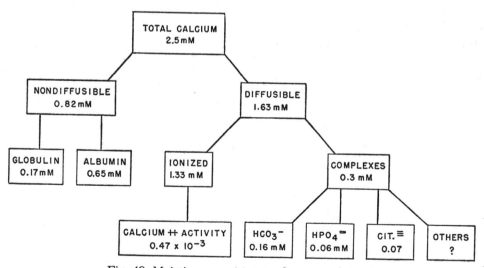

Fig. 49. Moieties comprising total serum calcium.[2]

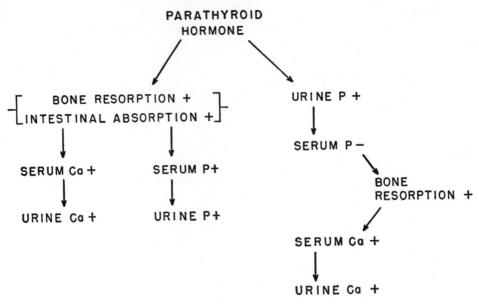

Fig. 50. Actions of parathyroid hormone.

the Bodansky procedure) and appropriate corrections [9] used to express the true total phosphatase activity.

### BONE PHYSIOLOGY

Since bones (plus teeth) contain 99 percent of total body calcium, calcium and phosphorus metabolism are closely related to bone metabolism. Albright [4] has suggested that bone may be thought of in terms of three surfaces (see Fig. 51).

On the first type of surface, specialized connective-tissue cells (osteoblasts) deposit a protein matrix (osteoid). Osteoblastic activity depends upon stress and strain and upon stimulation of sex and growth hormones, and is inhibited by 17-hydroxycorticosteroids. Osteoid is a specialized tissue composed primarily of oriented collagen fibers in ground substance, and probably is specially calcifiable [10] because of its intramolecular orientation.

On the second type of surface, bone resorption proceeds by unknown mechanisms which may include pH, local citrate concentration, and parathyroid-hormone activity. Where resorption is active,

one may observe ragged resorption lacunae with multinucleated osteoclasts.

The third type of surface is represented by the top and bottom margins of the bone rectangle in Fig. 51. This type of surface is devoid of metabolic activity. The proportion of metabolically inactive bone increases with age.

The process of calcification converts osteoid to bone. Intra- and intermolecular rearrangements of collagen according to lines of stress and strain, formation of larger collagen bundles, loss of water, and increasing calcium content characterize the maturation of bone. The lack of calcification in hypophosphatasia [11] is associated with the absence of alkaline phosphatase from bone. This correlation suggests that alkaline phosphatase and related enzymes are essential to the calcification process.

In addition to numerous localized bone diseases, there are three main classes of metabolic generalized bone disease whose characteristics are listed in Table 83. The common causes of these metabolic bone diseases are listed in Table 84. A valuable atlas of rare bone diseases is that of Fairbanks.[12]

## NORMAL

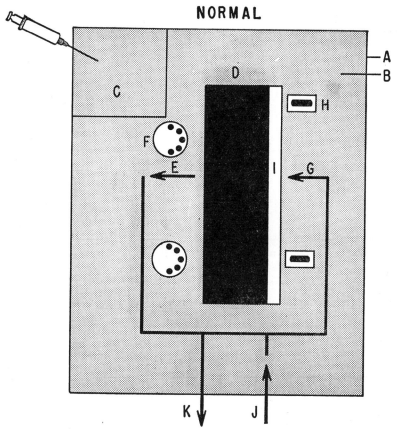

Fig. 51. Albright scheme of bone metabolism: *A*, skin; *B*, extracellular fluid; *C*, serum; *D*, calcified osteoid—mature bone; *E*, net Ca and P flux from bone; *F*, osteoclast; *G*, net Ca and P flux into bone; *H*, osteoblast; *I*, osteoid; *J*, Ca and P absorption; *K*, Ca and P excretion.

LABORATORY TESTS

The clinical indications for study of calcium metabolism are as follows: (1) signs and symptoms referable to the skeleton, such as pain, tenderness, deformity, and fracture; (2) signs and symptoms suggestive of hypercalcemia, such as nausea, vomiting, weight loss, constipation, polyuria, polydipsia, muscle weakness, and hypotonicity; (3) presence of calcium-containing kidney stones; (4) metastatic calcification; and

Table 83. *The metabolic bone diseases.*[a]

| Name | Defect | Serum | | | Histologic features | Prominent Roentgen changes |
|------|--------|----|---|-------|---------------------|----------------------------|
| | | Ca | P | P'tase | | |
| Osteoporosis | Deficient matrix formation | N | N | N | Thin cortex; thin trabeculae | Collapsed vertebrae |
| Osteomalacia | Deficient calcification | N | ↓ | ↑ | Osteoid seams increased; osteoblastic activity | Symmetric pseudofractures |
| Osteitis | Excess resorption | ↑ | ↓ | ↑ | Increased osteoclasts; increased osteoblasts; fibrous marrow | Skull, cysts, subperiosteal resorption in phalanges |

[a] The more common causes for these metabolic bone diseases are listed in Table 84.

Table 84. *Causes of metabolic bone disease.*

| Osteoporosis | Osteomalacia | Osteitis |
|---|---|---|
| Immobilization | Calcium lack | Primary hyper- |
| Postmenopausal | Vitamin D lack | parathyroid- |
| state | Malabsorption | ism |
| Cushing's syn- | Vitamin D re- | Chronic acido- |
| drome | sistance | sis |
| ACTH, corti- | Hypophospha- | |
| coid therapy | tasia | |
| Thyrotoxicosis | Hypercalcuria in | |
| Acromegaly | renal tubular | |
| Vitamin C defi- | acidosis and | |
| ciency | Fanconi syn- | |
| | drome | |

(5) the presence of a condition in which calcium metabolism is known to be frequently abnormal. Tables 85–91 are concerned with the interpretation of disturbances of calcium metabolism.

Table 85. *Major causes of hypocalcemia.*

Hypoparathyroidism
  Postoperative
  Idiopathic
  Pseudo
Hypoproteinemia
Acute pancreatitis
Renal failure
Malabsorption syndrome

Table 86. *Major causes of hypercalcemia.*

Primary hyperparathyroidism due to—
  Adenoma
  Multiple adenomata
  Primary hypertrophy and hyperplasia
  Multiple endocrine adenomata
  Primary hyperplasia
Milk-alkali syndrome [13]
Vitamin D intoxication
Acute osteoporosis
Metastatic malignant disease
Multiple myeloma
Sarcoidosis [14]
Berylliosis
Idiopathic hypercalcemia with failure to thrive (in infants) [15]

Table 87. *Major causes of hyperphosphatemia.*

Childhood
Acromegaly
Renal failure (creatinine clearance < 10%) [16]
Vitamin D intoxication

Table 88. *Major causes of hypophosphatasemia.*

Hypophosphatasia
Milk-alkali syndrome
Vitamin D intoxication
Scurvy
Hypothyroidism
Other growth defects

Table 89. *Major causes of hyperphosphatasemia.*

Liver disease
Metabolic bone disease: osteomalacia, osteitis
Local bone disease
Paget's disease [4]
Following fractures
Polyostotic fibrous dysplasia [4]
  (phosphatase occasionally elevated)
Bone tumors
  Primary, especially osteogenic sarcoma
  Secondary, especially carcinoma of prostate

Table 90. *Major causes of hypocalciuria.*

Hypoparathyroidism
Renal failure, nephrosis
Rickets, osteomalacia
Metastatic cancer of the prostate

Table 91. *Causes of hypercalciuria.*

Primary hyperparathyroidism
Immobilization, especially in children and in Paget's disease
Idiopathic hypercalciuria [17]
Renal tubular acidosis [18]
Fanconi syndrome (renal stones rare)
Excess milk intake
Vitamin D intoxication
Metastatic malignancy
Multiple myeloma (renal stones rare)
Hyperthyroidism (renal stones rare)
Following mercurial diuretics, magnesium or $NH_4Cl$ therapy

OTHER STUDIES

The serum acid phosphatase is elevated in carcinoma of the prostate with spread beyond the prostatic capsule. The serum total proteins and serum protein electrophoretic pattern may reveal hyperglobulinemia in sarcoid or the "M" protein in myeloma, and may explain hypocalcemia without tetany in nephritis, nephrosis, liver disease, malabsorption syndrome, and idiopathic panhypoproteinemia.

Recent attempts to sharpen the diagnosis of disorders of calcium metabolism with calcium infusions,[19] phosphate deprivation,[20] and determination of the relative rate of phosphate and creatinine clearance [21] have not proved of clinical value in the mild forms of calcium or bone disorder or in patients with complicating renal disease. Reliance is better placed on accurate and repeated measurement of serum calcium, phosphorus, phosphatase, and 24-hr urinary calcium.

Study of radioactive calcium metabolism [22] has been useful in current research on bone metabolism, but is not practical for clinical use in its present form.

Bone biopsy may be useful in disorders of bone metabolism, particularly if microradiography, polarizing microscopy, and autoradiography can also be carried out. Unfortunately, few pathology departments today have the skill, time, and experience to produce useful microscopic bone specimens.

Measurement of fecal calcium (over a 3-day period) may provide useful information regarding increased or decreased calcium absorption. In actual practice, this procedure often gives misleading information, owing to variation in bowel function, inaccurate control of calcium intake, and an inadequate period of prior accommodation to diet. If such a study is indicated, a full balance study is probably the only reliable means.

## REFERENCES

1. W. Bauer and J. C. Aub, "Studies of inorganic salt metabolism. I. The ward routine and methods," *J. Amer. diet. Ass.* 3, 106 (1927).
2. W. F. Neuman and M. W. Neuman, *The Chemical Dynamics of Bone Mineral* (University of Chicago Press, Chicago; copyright 1958 by the University of Chicago).
3. F. C. McLean and A. B. Hastings, "Clinical estimation and significance of calcium-ion concentrations in the blood," *Amer. J. med. Sci.* 189, 601 (1935).
4. F. Albright and E. C. Reifenstein, Jr., *Parathyroid Glands and Metabolic Bone Disease* (Williams and Wilkins, Baltimore, 1947).
5. N. A. Barnicot, "The local action of the parathyroid and other tissues on bone in intracerebral grafts," *J. Anat.* 82, 233 (1948).
6. C. H. Fiske and M. A. Logan, "Determination of calcium by alkalimetric titration; precipitation of calcium in the presence of magnesium, phosphate, and sulfate, with applications to analysis of urine," *J. biol. Chem.* 93, 211 (1931).
7. J. Lehmann, "A photoelectric micro-method for the direct titration of calcium in serum with ethylenediaminetetracetate," *Scand. J. clin. lab. Invest.* 5, 203 (1953).
8. C. H. Fiske and Y. SubbaRow, "The colorimetric determination of phosphorus," *J. biol. Chem.* 66, 375 (1925).
9. A. Bodansky, "Phosphatase studies; determinations of serum phosphatase. Factors influencing accuracy of determination," *J. biol. Chem.* 101, 93 (1933).
10. M. J. Glimcher, A. J. Hodge, and F. O. Schmitt, "Macromolecular aggregation states in relation to mineralization: The Collagen: Hydroxyapatite system as studied in vitro," *Proc. nat. Acad. Sci.* 43, 860 (1957).
11. J. C. Rathbun, "Hypophosphatasia," *Amer. J. Dis. Child.* 75, 822 (1948).
12. T. Fairbanks, *An Atlas of General Affections of the Skeleton* (Livingstone, Edinburgh and London, 1951).

13. C. H. Burnett, R. R. Commons, F. Albright, and J. E. Howard, "Hypercalciuria without hypercalcemia or hypophosphatemia, calcinosis, and renal insufficiency. A syndrome following prolonged intake of milk and alkali," *New Engl. J. Med.* 240, 787 (1949).

14. P. H. Henneman, E. F. Dempsey, E. L. Carroll, and F. Albright, "The cause of hypercalciuria in sarcoid and its treatment with cortisone and sodium phytate," *J. clin. Invest.* 35, 1229 (1956).

15. R. Lightwood, "Idiopathic hypercalcemia with failure to thrive: Nephrocalcinosis," *Proc. roy. Soc. Med.* 45, 401 (1952).

16. R. Goldman and S. Bassett, "Phosphorus excretion in renal failure," *J. clin. Invest.* 33, 1623 (1954).

17. P. H. Henneman, P. H. Benedict, A. P. Forbes, and H. R. Dudley, "Idiopathic hypercalciuria," *New Engl. J. Med.* 259, 802 (1958).

18. F. Albright, C. H. Burnett, W. Parson, E. C. Reifenstein, Jr., and A. Roos, "Osteomalacia and late rickets. The various etiologies met in the United States with emphasis on that resulting from a specific form of renal acidosis, the therapeutic indications for each etiological sub-group, and the relationship between osteomalacia and milkman's syndrome," *Medicine* 25, 399 (1946).

19. J. E. Howard, T. R. Hopkins, and T. B. Connor, "On certain physiologic responses in intravenous injection of calcium salts into normal, hyperparathyroid and hypoparathyroid persons," *J. clin. Endocr.* 13, 1 (1953).

20. E. L. Chambers, Jr., G. S. Gordan, and E. C. Reifenstein, Jr., "Tests for hyperparathyroidism: Tubular resorption of phosphate, phosphate deprivation and calcium infusion," *J. clin. Endocr.* 16, 1507 (1956).

21. B. E. C. Nordin and R. Fraser, "The effect of intravenous calcium on phosphate excretion," *Clin. Sci.* 13, 477 (1954).

22. G. C. H. Bauer, A. Carlsson, and B. Lindquist, "Evaluation of accretion, resorption and exchange reactions in the skeleton," *Kungl. Fysiograf. Sällskap. Lund Forhand.* 25, 1 (1955).

## Unit 33

# Cardiac Catheterization and Other Tests Related to the Cardiovascular System

Catheterization of the right side of the human heart was first done by Forsmann[1] and later developed by Cournand[2] into a useful clinical method. It is helpful in the evaluation of selected patients with valvular heart disease, constrictive pericarditis, cor pulmonale, and heart failure of obscure cause. In the field of congenital heart disease it has provided the clinician with a precise way of defining abnormalities both of anatomy and of function. Perhaps most important, it has given everyday cardiology a solid backbone of hemodynamics. Recently, catheterization of the left side of the heart has been done and found useful in the evaluation of lesions of the mitral and aortic valves.

The catheter may be used: (1) to record pressures in various locations; (2) to obtain blood from these areas for determination of its oxygen or dye content; (3) as an exploratory tool to probe through abnormal communications and hence to help to localize them; (4) to allow the injection of indicator substances or radiopaque material directly into selected areas of the circulation. From the data thus obtained one may calculate: (1) by the Fick or dye-injection method, cardiac output and the volume of the abnormal shunts of congenital heart disease; (2) by the Poiseuille equation, the resistance of a vascular bed to flow and the area of a stenotic valve orifice.

## Indications for Cardiac Catheterization

CONGENITAL HEART DISEASE.[3] In general, catheterization is of use when the diagnosis is in doubt; when the severity of a known lesion is the basis of deciding whether surgery is needed; or when there is reason to suspect a complicating factor that would make the planned operation difficult or unsatisfactory.

VALVULAR HEART DISEASE. With catheterization one can localize stenotic lesions and estimate their severity.[4, 5] Methods for the evaluation of valvular insufficiency are not as yet perfected.

OTHER FORMS OF HEART DISEASE. Generally, catheterization does not supply an etiologic diagnosis but may be useful in excluding treatable valvular or congenital heart disease. It is also occasionally useful as an objective physiologic index for evaluating a patient's course or the results of therapy.

Even when catheterization is most useful, the diagnostic information that it gives may be incomplete or equivocal. Data must always be weighed with other clinical evidence.

## Methods

Details of technique vary in different laboratories, but certain principles are important. For ordinary diagnostic work one needs a trained team of at least four persons: the operator, who inserts and manipulates the catheter; a radiologist, who performs the fluoroscopy needed for the procedure and supervises angiocardiography; [6, 7] an assistant, who attends to the recording of pressures and monitors the electrocardiogram; a laboratory technician, to perform blood analyses for oxygen or dye. Pressures are recorded through the catheter by connecting it with a manometer. The catheter used for the right side of the heart is radiopaque. Therefore chambers from which blood samples are drawn may be identified both by fluoroscopy and by their characteristic pressure records. For study of the right side of the heart,[5, 8] the catheter is usually inserted into an antecubital vein and threaded into the heart and pulmonary arteries. In small children it may be necessary to use a femoral vein. Arterial blood samples are obtained from an indwelling needle left in the radial or brachial artery. Left-atrial pressure may be satisfactorily measured during catheterization of the right side of the heart by wedging the catheter as far as possible out a pulmonary artery. This maneuver occludes the vessel so that the only pressures acting at the tip of the catheter are those transmitted from the left atrium. This is called "pulmonary capillary" or "wedge" pressure.[9, 10] The measurement may be falsely high unless the catheter is firmly stuck in place.[5]

There are several approaches to the left side of the heart.[11, 12] (1) With a bronchoscope one may insert a needle into the left atrium from the left main-stem bronchus; a small plastic catheter is then threaded through the needle and pushed into the ventricle. (2) The atrium may be entered with a needle inserted from the back. (3) A needle may be introduced behind the suprasternal notch and directed downward into the atrium.[13] (4) The left ventricle has been punctured directly through the anterior chest wall.[14] (5) A catheter may be inserted into the left ventricle in retrograde fash-

ion via the femoral artery and aorta.

Opinions vary as to the comparative safety and effectiveness of these methods. The posterior and bronchoscopic approaches are the ones most commonly used. Recently a long flexible needle guided by a catheter in the right atrium has been inserted through the interatrial septum.[15] This appears to be a promising method.

Measurement of oxygen consumption is necessary if one wishes to calculate rates of flow by the Fick method.

## Risk and Contraindications

Deaths from catheterization of the right side of the heart were found to occur in 0.1 percent of a large series.[16, 17] There is an increased risk in patients with coronary disease, Ebstein's abnormality, severe pulmonary vascular disease, and complete heart block. The usual cause of death is ventricular fibrillation or standstill. Pulmonary infarction has occurred as a result of the catheter's being left too long in the wedge position and from injections of contrast material into the pulmonary artery for angiocardiograms. Transient neurologic disturbances attributed to air embolization have occurred in patients with right-to-left shunts. Rarely, knotting of the catheter necessitates surgical removal. Ventricular ectopic beats are almost the rule during the insertion of the catheter, but they usually disappear when the position of the tip is changed. Occasionally forceful contraction of a segment of vein around the catheter may occur, causing the patient pain and often making further manipulation impossible. Local phlebitis at the site of insertion of the catheter is common but not usually a major problem.

None of the methods for study of the left side of the heart has had sufficient trial for its safety to be finally assessed.[12] With the transthoracic approach, small pneumothorax and hemopericardium are very common. Sudden death from ventricular fibrillation has been reported; facilities for opening the chest and treatment of such emergencies should always be immediately available. Death has also resulted from tears in the great vessels. The average patient, premedicated with opiates, experiences moderate discomfort and has mild pleuritic chest pain for 12–24 hr after the test. All patients should be observed for at least 24 hr after the procedure because of the occasional occurrence of later cardiac tamponade and sizable hemo- or pneumothorax. In general, since the risk of catheterization of the left side of the heart appears appreciable, it should be done only to answer very specific questions when surgery of the aortic or mitral valve is being considered.

## The Study of Pressure Records

Each part of the heart has a distinctive pressure pattern by which it can usually be recognized.[5, 18] There are three basic types of curves—arterial, ventricular, and atrial (or venous). Simultaneously recorded pressure tracings from the right side of the heart are shown in Fig. 52. At times it is of interest to know the average level of pressure throughout the cardiac cycle. Such mean pressures may be obtained with an electronic damping device. Various reference points for pressure measurements have been used.[19] The zero point in our description will be 5 cm posterior to the angle of Louis in the supine patient. This is a rough approximation of the level of the right atrium.

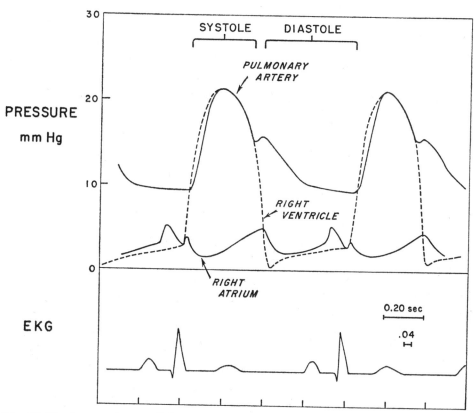

Fig. 52. Simultaneously recorded pressure tracings from right atrium, right ventricle, and pulmonary artery of a normal person. Ejection of blood from the ventricle into the pulmonary artery occurs during systole. A "dicrotic" notch in the downstroke of the arterial tracing signals the closure of the semilunar valve. In the diastolic period between contractions, the ventricular pressure falls lower than that in the atrium. Opening of the tricuspid valve and filling of the ventricular cavity result.

NORMAL PRESSURE CURVES.[20] The *ventricular curve* is characterized by wide swings of pressure from diastole to the peak of systole. The arterial tracing coincides with it during the period of ventricular ejection. But in diastole, closure of the semilunar valves prevents the arterial pressure from falling to ventricular levels. The ejection (systolic) pressure must be higher in the left than in the right ventricle because the resistance to flow is greater in the peripheral vascular bed than in the lung. The higher filling pressure of the left ventricle is probably due to the fact that more force is needed to distend the thicker-walled cavity.

In general, the *atrial pressure* is governed by the filling pressure of the corresponding ventricle. The atrial tracing usually consists of three positive deflections with valleys in between: the *A wave* is due to atrial contraction; the *C wave* (often only a notch on the downstroke of the *A*) signals the impact of the first part of ventricular systole; the *V wave* shows the effect of continued closure of the mitral or tricuspid valve as blood accumulates in the atrium during the latter part of ventricular contraction.

ARTIFACTS.[21, 22] Various artifacts can deform pressure tracings. Excessive damping due to air in the recording system or to obstruction of the catheter can cut off both the peaks and the valleys in the record. Motion of the catheter in the heart may superimpose jagged oscillations on a pressure tracing. Inertia of the recording system can cause overshooting, especially in records with wide swings of pressure. Records that appear unusual should be interpreted with care and repeated if possible.

### The Estimation of Blood Flow

THE CARDIAC OUTPUT: SYSTEMIC
BLOOD FLOW [2, 23]

The essence of the Fick principle is most easily expressed in terms of a simple problem from grade-school arithmetic. If each one of a string of coal cars passing a station delivers ⅓ of a load, then, in order to deliver 2 loads, 6 cars must pass. Similarly, if one knows the amount of oxygen extracted by the tissues from each liter of blood (the difference between the concentration of the gas in arterial and venous samples) and the actual amount of oxygen delivered per minute (in the resting patient the same as the oxygen uptake by the lungs), then it is easy to calculate how many liters of blood must go round the circulation every minute in order to deliver the measured quantity of oxygen:

$$\text{Systemic blood flow (L/min)} \qquad (1)$$
$$= \frac{\text{oxygen consumption (ml/min)}}{\text{arterial oxygen content} - \text{venous oxygen content (ml/L)}}.$$

In practice, one obtains samples from a peripheral artery and from the right side of the heart for a period of 1 or 2 min while oxygen consumption is being measured. Venous blood is obtained from the heart itself because specimens from different parts of the body differ widely in their content of oxygen. For measurement of flow it is necessary to have mixed venous blood, representative of all areas. It is also important that none of the variables involved should change during the period of measurement. Absence of a steady state [24] lessens the accuracy of measurements made on patients beginning to exercise or recovering from exertion.

NORMAL VALUES.[25, 26] Since normal blood flow is closely related to body size, it is best expressed as an "index" corrected for surface area. The normal cardiac index at rest is 2.5–4.5 L/min m². While the error of the method should be about 10 percent, the cardiac output is not a fixed quantity. With moderate exercise the average person raises his resting level usually by about 0.6 L/min m² for each 100-ml/min m² increase in his oxygen consumption.[5, 26, 27] Emotion also has an important effect, so that measurements made at the beginning of a study when the patient is frightened and excited are often higher than "normal." [25]

VALUES IN DISEASE. Because of difficulties in obtaining a truly basal cardiac output, a high value is often of no diagnostic significance. Elevated resting outputs,[28, 29] however, are characteristic of thyrotoxicosis, beriberi, and severe anemia (less than 7 gm/100 ml of hemoglobin). The cardiac index tends to be low in cases of congestive cardiac failure [30] and in clinically severe mitral-valve disease.[31] When the high-output states lead to congestive failure, the rate of flow falls, but sometimes remains greater than normal. The low-output states often may be distin-

guished only by the failure of a normal resting flow to increase with exercise.[30] When cardiac output is inappropriately low for oxygen consumption, the extraction of oxygen from each liter of flow increases, and venous oxygen may fall so low that clinical cyanosis of the extremities results.[32]

### THE ESTIMATION OF SHUNTS

In a left-to-right shunt, some of the oxygenated blood from the left side of the heart passes through an abnormal communication and reenters the pulmonary circuit (see Fig. 53). In a right-to-left shunt, some of the returning peripheral blood fails to reach the lungs but instead flows through a defect into

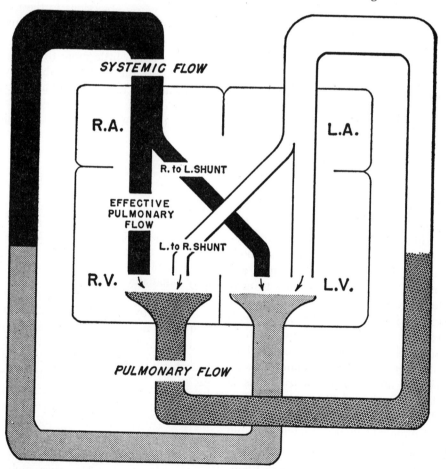

Fig. 53. Diagram of the circulation in a large septal defect with bidirectional shunting:
Systemic flow = effective pulmonary flow + right-to-left shunt flow,
Pulmonary flow = effective pulmonary flow + left-to-right shunt flow.

the left side of the heart or the aorta. Shunts are estimated by comparison of the systemic, total pulmonary, and "effective pulmonary" flows.[5] Effective pulmonary flow is the volume of mixed venous blood from the systemic circulation that actually reaches the lungs and is oxygenated. From Fig. 53 it is evident that:

$$\text{Right-to-left shunt flow} = \text{systemic flow} - \text{effective pulmonary flow}, \quad (2)$$

$$\text{Left-to-right shunt flow} = \text{pulmonary flow} - \text{effective pulmonary flow}. \quad (3)$$

To calculate pulmonary flows by the Fick method one needs for the denominator, the change in the oxygen content of the blood whose flow is to be measured, and for the numerator, the rate at which oxygen was taken up by this blood in the lungs. No significant amount of oxygen is added to fully oxygenated blood reentering the lungs from a left-to-right shunt. Therefore the measured oxygen uptake is the numerator for both equations of pulmonary flow:

$$\text{Total pulmonary flow (L/min)}$$
$$= \frac{\text{oxygen consumption (ml/min)}}{\substack{\text{pulmonary venous oxygen} \\ - \text{ pulmonary arterial oxygen (ml/L)}}}, \quad (4)$$

$$\text{Effective pulmonary flow (L/min)}$$
$$= \frac{\text{oxygen consumption (ml/min)}}{\substack{\text{pulmonary venous oxygen} \\ - \text{mixed venous blood oxygen (ml/L)}}}. \quad (5)$$

All the terms in these equations are obtainable from catheterization of the right side of the heart except for the oxygen content of pulmonary venous blood. Assuming, however, that the lungs are normal, it is usually reasonable to estimate this as being 97 percent of the oxygen capacity of the patient's blood. "Mixed venous blood" must be obtained from the chamber just peripheral to that involved in a left-to-right shunt. The accuracy of any of these calculations is far less than that of the cardiac output. All flows are best expressed as indices: (liters/minute)/square meter (L/min m²).

### The Calculation of Resistance to Flow

It is important to correlate a rate of flow with the head of pressure needed to maintain it.[5, 27, 32] Any local impedance to flow produces a pressure difference over the involved area. This fall in pressure represents the loss of energy that is expended in overcoming frictional resistance. Such pressure differences occur not only with local constrictions, such as valvular stenosis, but also in the peripheral or pulmonary vascular bed largely as a result of relative narrowing at the arteriolar level.

A simplified form of Poiseuille's equation may be used to describe the resistance to flow of any segment of the circulation:

$$\text{Resistance} = \frac{\text{pressure drop}}{\text{rate of flow}}.$$

There are many objections to the use of such a simplified formula in the human circulation.[33, 34] But the calculated resistance, though little more than a mnemonic, offers the best available way of measuring the narrowing of a vascular bed which may occur in disease states. Among the more convenient equations are:

$$\text{Pulmonary resistance (Wood units)}$$
$$= \frac{\substack{\text{mean pulmonary arterial pressure} \\ - \text{ pulmonary capillary pressure (mm Hg)}}}{\text{pulmonary flow (L/min)}}, \quad (6)$$

$$\text{Pulmonary resistance (author's units)}$$
$$= \frac{\substack{\text{mean pulmonary arterial pressure} \\ - \text{ pulmonary capillary pressure (mm Hg)}}}{\text{pulmonary index (L/min m²)}}. \quad (7)$$

The systemic resistance may be similarly calculated.

The normal pulmonary resistance as calculated by Eq. (6) is higher in infants than in adults. Taking surface area into account, as in Eq. (7), however, makes values similar for patients of all ages and sizes. This is particularly useful in the study of pulmonary resistance in congenital heart disease. Using a numerical conversion factor, one may also express resistance, as calculated from Eq. (6), in absolute units: dynes · seconds · centimeters⁻⁵. However, such units are unnecessarily cumbersome and add no clinically useful information.

VALUES. The normal pressure drop across the pulmonary circuit is 6–10 mm Hg. The normal pulmonary flow is 2.5–4.5 L/min m² or 5–7 L/min in the average adult. The upper limit of normal values for pulmonary vascular resistance is:

by Eq. (6), 3 units (for adults),

by Eq. (7), 5 units (for all ages).

Levels over 5 units from Eq. (7) indicate abnormally high pulmonary vascular resistance. Normally, with exercise and higher rates of flow, the pulmonary pressure rises only slightly and the calculated resistance therefore falls. In disease states, pressure and flow may increase *pari passu*.[35] The normal systemic resistance is 16–22 Wood units or 22–30 of the units used by the author.

CLINICAL APPLICATIONS. Pulmonary-artery pressures greater than 30/15 (mean = 20 mm Hg) are defined as pulmonary hypertension.[5, 32, 36] Calculation of the pulmonary resistance helps to distinguish in a general way among three distinct causes, which may, however, be additive:[5, 32] abnormally increased pulmonary flow; abnormally elevated left atrial pressure; increased resistance to flow in the lungs. (1) *Pulmonary hypertension due to increased flow* is generally mild and associated with large left-to-right shunts. The mean pressure in the pulmonary artery may rise to 40–50 mm Hg when the pulmonary index is 10–15 L/min. (2) *Pulmonary hypertension purely secondary to increased left atrial pressure* is likewise mild. If mean left atrial pressure is 25 mm Hg and the normal pulmonary-artery pressure difference of 6–10 mm Hg is maintained, the mean pulmonary-artery pressure may be 35 mm Hg simply on this account. (3) Pressures over 40–50 mm Hg, however, are almost always due at least in part to *increased pulmonary vascular resistance*, which commonly augments pulmonary hypertension from the first and second causes.

## Catheterization Findings in Heart and Lung Disease

### VENTRICULAR FAILURE [30, 37]

The failing ventricle does not empty normally with systole, and there is an increase in its residual volume at the beginning of diastole. The cardiac output is usually lowered, but this is too variable to be included in a useful definition. The ventricles may fail independently, but left-ventricular decompensation may eventually cause the right also to fail.

*The failing right ventricle* has a mean diastolic pressure greater than 6 mm Hg. *The failing left ventricle* has a mean diastolic pressure greater than 12 mm Hg. It is obvious that atrial and venous pressures must also be elevated to match the increase in ventricular filling pressure. Functional mitral or tricuspid regurgitation resulting from dilatation of the failing left or right ventricle may also produce C–V waves in the corresponding atrial-pressure tracing.[38]

ROLE OF CATHETER STUDY. Catheterization may be useful in making a diagnosis of early decompensation. To diagnose right-ventricular failure, however, catheterization is seldom needed because distention or abnormal pulsation of the neck veins often faithfully mirrors the abnormal behavior of the ventricle. An increase in ventricular diastolic pressure is also seen in constrictive pericarditis and in severe ventricular hypertrophy, both of which may interfere with ventricular diastolic filling by making the walls of the chamber less distensible.[5, 39] In ventricular hypertrophy the elevation is usually only in the *end* diastolic pressure, probably as the result of the impact of atrial systole on the more rigid ventricular wall.[39, 40]

### LUNG DISEASE

Cor pulmonale is characterized by increased pulmonary-artery pressure, which is largely or entirely due to an elevated pulmonary vascular resistance.[36, 41] Cardiac output is often elevated but may be normal or low. The increased demands on the heart may contribute to the development of right-ventricular failure. Arterial unsaturation may occur as the result of pulmonary disease. Examples are chronic idiopathic pulmonary fibrosis and emphysema, the pneumoconioses, idiopathic pulmonary hypertension,[42] and the syndrome of repeated pulmonary embolization. Many cases of clinically severe emphysema, however, show no pulmonary hypertension or only temporary increases of pressure during periods of respiratory decompensation.[41]

### CONSTRICTIVE PERICARDITIS

The chief disadvantage of the rigid constricting envelope in this disease is the limit it sets on ventricular filling in diastole.[43] This puts an absolute ceiling on the stroke output of the heart. In most cases, both ventricles are constricted. Venous blood is dammed at a high pressure in the atria and in the veins. Since the defect is not primarily in ventricular emptying, the early diastolic pressure of the ventricle is normal, but rises to the high atrial level very soon after the mitral and tricuspid valves open. The brief period of relatively normal pressure is called the "early diastolic dip."[44] Although the combination of a marked dip and a virtually normal right-ventricular systolic pressure is characteristic of constrictive pericarditis, it also occurs in other conditions interfering with normal diastolic filling. Occasionally, in severe cases, a markedly flattened right-ventricular pressure curve is obtained.[45]

USES OF CATHETER STUDY. When the diagnosis is in doubt, catheterization can supplement the clinical data. When the result of surgery is unsatisfactory, catheterization may help one to decide whether there is still constriction of the left ventricle.[46]

LIMITATIONS. Similar catheterization findings have been reported in amyloidosis of the heart, subendocardial fibrosis, and the diffuse myocardial fibrosis that may complicate constrictive pericarditis.[47, 48] There is no adequate way by catheter study to distinguish these conditions from pericardial disease, which is the only one that can be helped by surgery.

### EVALUATION OF SHUNTS

LEFT-TO-RIGHT SHUNTS. When there is communication between similar chambers of the right and left sides of the heart, left-to-right flow occurs through the defect because resistances are higher in the systemic than in the pulmonary circuit.[49] The wasteful rerouting of oxygenated blood back to the lungs augments pulmonary flow. The commonest examples are interatrial septal defect, patent ductus arteriosus, and interventricular septal defect. Because the shunt is predominantly from left to right, the patient does not ordinarily have arterial unsaturation or cyanosis. Very large shunts, however, may lead to heart failure, often during childhood.[3] When a defect is large, the pressures in the two communicating chambers tend to become identical.[49, 50]

*Pulmonary Vascular Obstruction.* An increase in pulmonary resistance radically alters the effect of a simple communication between the left and the right sides of the heart. The condition may be congenital or acquired and is due to obliterative and vasoconstrictive changes in the vessels of the lung.[50] When pulmonary resistance approaches systemic levels,[3] there is said to be pulmonary vascular obstruction. The shunt may practically cease, or there may be equal flow in both directions. Sizable right-to-left shunts cause arterial unsaturation and cynanosis.

*Role of Cardiac Catheterization.* Cath-

Table 92. *Representative data from catheter study of congenital and acquired heart disease.*

| Condition | Vena cava O₂ (vol %) ±1.5 vol %ᵃ | Right atrium Pressure (mm Hg) | Right atrium O₂ (vol %) ±1.0 vol %ᵃ | Right ventricle Pressure (mm Hg) | Right ventricle O₂ (vol %) ±0.5 vol %ᵃ | Pulmonary artery Pressure (mm Hg) | Pulmonary artery O₂ (vol %) | Pulmonary "capillary" pressure (mm Hg) | Radial artery Pressure (mm Hg) | Radial artery O₂ (vol %) | Oxygen capacity (vol %) |
|---|---|---|---|---|---|---|---|---|---|---|---|
| Normal | 12.7 | 0–3 | 13.8 | 15–30 / 0–3 | 13.4 | 15–30 / 8–15 | 13.7 | 3–10 | 100–140 / 70–90 | 17.6 | 18.0 |
| Atrial septal defect | 13.0 | 3 | 18.5 | 55 / 3 | 18.2 | 40 / 10 | 17.9 | 4 | 100 / 70 | 20.0 | 20.6 |
| Ventricular septal defect | 14.0 | 3 | 14.8 | 35 / 3 | 17.5 | 35 / 15 | 17.8 | 10 | 100 / 70 | 19.0 | 19.5 |
| Eisenmenger's syndrome | 16.0 | 8 | 16.8 | 110 / 8 | 18.5 | 110 / 80 | 18.5 | 6 | 110 / 80 | 20.8 | 24.1 |
| Tetralogy of Fallot | 14.0 | 4 | 14.3 | 110 / 4 | 15.3 | 10 / 4 | 15.5 | 4 | 110 / 80 | 19.0 | 26.0 |
| Pulmonic stenosis | 15.0 | 6 | 15.5 | 150 / 6 | 15.8 | 12 / 6 | 15.6 | 5 | 100 / 70 | 20.0 | 20.6 |
| Mitral stenosis | 10.8 | 10 | 11.0 | 45 / 10 | 11.1 | 55 / 33 | 11.1 | 21 | 105 / 80 | 19.4 | 20.6 |

ᵃ The absolute values for oxygen content of samples taken from the vena cava and right heart chambers depend on hemoglobin content as well as saturation with oxygen. Owing to differences in oxygen content of blood in SVC, IVC, and coronary sinus, and because mixing of venous blood entering the right atrium is incomplete until it reaches the pulmonary artery, the normal range of variation in oxygen content of blood samples taken consecutively from venae cavae to pulmonary artery is appreciable, but diminishes with each successive chamber. The values given are the upper limits of these variations in normals.

eterization helps in the selection of patients for corrective surgery. It gives authoritative answers to three important questions in such cases.

*The location of the defect* [51] is accomplished by passage of the catheter through the communication into the left side of the heart and the detection of a sudden increase in the oxygen content of blood in the right side of the heart. One can often diagnose a simple lesion without catheterization. It is not needed for typical cases of patent ductus arteriosus.

*The size of the shunt* [52] may be estimated by the method already described. Fortunately, the calculation is exact enough for clinical purposes, though grossly inaccurate in the presence of large shunts.

*The pulmonary resistance* [53, 54] must always be taken into account in evaluating a left-to-right shunt. A small or moderate flow may be due either to a small defect or to a large one with a high pulmonary resistance. Pulmonary vascular obstruction increases the risk of surgery and makes the result less satisfactory. However, the available data do not allow any rigid correlation between calculated resistance and operability.[55]

*Example 1.* In a typical case of atrial septal defect, the foregoing questions may be answered from the data in Table 92. If the measured oxygen consumption is 210 ml/min, the body surface area is 1.5 m², and the calculated pulmonary venous oxygen content is $0.97 \times 20.6 = 20.0$ ml/100 ml, the following values are obtained:

from Eq. (1),

$$\text{Systemic flow} = \frac{210 \text{ ml/min}}{200 \text{ ml/L} - 130 \text{ ml/L}}$$

$$= 3 \text{ L/min},$$

and

$$\text{Systemic index} = \frac{3 \text{ l./min}}{1.5 \text{ m}^2}$$

$$= 2.0 \text{ L/min m}^2;$$

from Eq. (4),

$$\text{Pulmonary flow} = \frac{210 \text{ ml/min}}{200 \text{ ml/L} - 179 \text{ ml/L}}$$

$$= 10.0 \text{ L/min},$$

and

$$\text{Pulmonary index} = \frac{10 \text{ L/min}}{1.5 \text{ m}^2}$$

$$= 6.7 \text{ L/min m}^2;$$

from Eq. (5),

Effective pulmonary flow

$$= \frac{210 \text{ ml/min}}{200 \text{ ml/L} - 130 \text{ ml/L}} = 3.0 \text{ L/min},$$

and

Effective pulmonary index

$$= \frac{3 \text{ L/min}}{1.5 \text{ m}^2} = 2.0 \text{ L/min m}^2;$$

from Eq. (3),

Left-to-right shunt flow

$$= 10 \text{ L/min} - 3 \text{ L/min} = 7 \text{ L/min},$$

and

$$\text{Left-to-right shunt index} = \frac{7 \text{ L/min}}{1.5 \text{ m}^2}$$

$$= 4.7 \text{ L/min m}^2;$$

from Eq. (2),

Right-to-left shunt flow

$$= 3 \text{ L/min} - 3 \text{ L/min} = 0 \text{ L/min};$$

and from Eq. (7),

Pulmonary resistance

$$= \frac{25 \text{ mm Hg} - 6 \text{ mm Hg}}{4.7 \text{ L/min m}^2}$$

$$= 4 \text{ author's units.}$$

The jump in blood oxygen content occurs in the right atrium. The slight discrepancies between the oxygen content of samples from the right atrium, the right ventricle, and the pulmonary artery are within normal limits and probably due to incomplete mixing.[56]

Therefore we know that the shunt is at the atrial level, that it is large, and that the pulmonary resistance is normal, in spite of the somewhat increased pulmonary-artery pressure. Such a case at present is considered favorable for closure of the defect.

*Example 2.* A similar evaluation can be made of the case of Eisenmenger's syndrome from Table 92. If oxygen consumption is 200 ml/min, the body surface area is 1.6 m², and the calculated pulmonary venous oxygen content is $0.97 \times 24.1 = 23.5$ ml/100 ml, the following values are obtained:

from Eq. (1),

$$\text{Systemic flow} = \frac{200 \text{ ml/min}}{208 \text{ ml/L} - 168 \text{ ml/L}}$$

$$= 5.0 \text{ L/min},$$

and

$$\text{Systemic index} = \frac{5.0 \text{ L/min}}{1.6 \text{ m}^2}$$

$$= 3.1 \text{ L/min m}^2;$$

from Eq. (4),

Pulmonary flow $= \dfrac{200 \text{ ml/min}}{235 \text{ ml/L} - 185 \text{ ml/L}}$

$= 4.0$ L/min,

and

Pulmonary index $= \dfrac{4.0 \text{ L/min}}{1.6 \text{ m}^2}$

$= 2.5$ L/min m$^2$;

from Eq. (5),

Effective pulmonary flow

$= \dfrac{200 \text{ ml/min}}{235 \text{ ml/L} - 168 \text{ ml/L}}$

$= 3.0$ L/min,

and

Effective pulmonary index

$= \dfrac{3.0 \text{ L/min}}{1.6 \text{ m}^2} = 1.9$ L/min m$^2$;

from Eq. (3),

Left-to-right shunt flow
$= 4.0$ L/min $- 3.0$ L/min $= 1.0$ L/min,
and

Left-to-right shunt index

$= \dfrac{1.0 \text{ L/min}}{1.6 \text{ m}^2} = 0.6$ L/min m$^2$;

from Eq. (2),

Right-to-left shunt flow
$= 5.0$ L/min $- 3.0$ L/min $= 2.0$ L/min,
and

Right-to-left shunt index $= \dfrac{2.0 \text{ L/min}}{1.6 \text{ m}^2}$

$= 1.3$ L/min m$^2$;

and from Eq. (7),

Pulmonary resistance

$= \dfrac{90 \text{ mm Hg} - 6 \text{ mm Hg}}{2.5 \text{ L/min m}^2}$

$= 34$ author's units,

which is greater than the systemic resistance. The left-to-right shunt occurs at the ventricular level and hence, by inference, this is also likely to be the site of the right-to-left shunt. Here both shunts are small and the right-to-left predominates. The pulmonary resistance is grossly elevated. At present it is felt that the gain from the closure of such a defect usually does not warrant the risk of surgery. In cases of pulmonary vascular obstruction, operation may be performed if technically feasible provided there is still a predominant left-to-right shunt.[54, 55]

*Limitations.* Because of poor mixing of blood involved in shunts and the mathematical structure of the Fick equa-

tion, the accuracy of such blood-flow calculations is far less than that of the cardiac output in ordinary individuals. Calculating flows to the first decimal place in Examples 1 and 2 has been done only for clarity of presentation and is really not mathematically justifiable. Absurdly high values for pulmonary flow may result from small errors in measuring the arteriovenous differences. Reference to Table 92 will show that consecutive samples from normal hearts may vary slightly in oxygen content because of incomplete mixing of venous blood.[52, 56] Since one must ignore variations within this range, shunts involving less than one-third of the cardiac output may be missed. The localization of even a large shunt by oxygen data alone may be inaccurate.[57] Ordinary catheterization also frequently fails to distinguish between single and multiple sites of shunting.

SHUNTS WITH ARTERIAL UNSATURATION.[3] Some blood returning from the periphery bypasses the lungs and reaches the systemic arteries without being oxygenated. If the hemoglobin is normal, a fall in arterial saturation to 85 percent produces cyanosis that is obvious to most observers.[32] Such cyanosis usually involves the lips, whereas that due to a low output often affects only the extremities. At catheter study the presence of a right-to-left shunt is suggested by unsaturation of an arterial blood sample. The diagnosis is confirmed and the defect is located if the catheter happens to pass through it.

*Right-to-left shunt* (little or no left-to-right flow). A typical tetralogy of Fallot is the commonest example.[3] Here, pulmonic stenosis is severe enough to necessitate a rise in right ventricular pressure to systemic levels. This results in right-to-left shunting through a ventricular septal defect, which robs the lungs of part of their blood flow. The problem is that an inadequate amount of returning venous blood reaches the lungs and becomes oxygenated. Pulmonic stenosis with an atrial defect or patent foramen ovale may also be associated with a pure right-to-left shunt. At catheterization, identical systolic pressures in the right ventricle and brachial artery suggest that the septal defect is at the ventricular rather than the atrial level.[60]

*Mixed shunts.*[3, 61] Flow occurs in both directions through a defect or a group of defects. The anatomy of such cases is varied. Bidirectional shunting can occur in a simple septal defect or patent ductus arteriosus, especially if it is large or associated with severe pulmonary vascular obstruction, in the tetralogy of Fallot when the pulmonary stenosis is mild and the ventricular defect large, and in many other more complex conditions.

*Limitations.* (1) Arterial unsaturation may be due to pulmonary disease as well as to a right-to-left shunt. The distinction may be clinically apparent in patients without heart disease. But the pulmonary changes of severe mitral disease or left-ventricular failure may also produce a considerable fall in arterial oxygen saturation.[62] (2) The site of a large right-to-left shunt may not be located conclusively unless the catheter happens to pass through it. On the other hand, passage of the catheter through a patent foramen ovale does not prove that this is the site of a shunt. If the right-to-left shunt happens to be small, the arterial oxygen may not be definitely low and the presence of an important defect may be missed.

*Role of Catheterization.* The place of catheterization in the diagnosis of such lesions is limited. Its chief uses are: to tell whether the factor that tends to produce the shunt is pulmonic stenosis or an increased resistance to flow in the lungs; to help locate the site of the shunt; and to estimate the size of the shunt. Often these questions must be answered by angiocardiography. Angiocardiography in fact may replace catheterization altogether in suspected cases of transposition of the great vessels and in tricuspid or pulmonary atresia.[63]

### VALVULAR DISEASE

Valvular stenosis results in a rise of pressure proximal to the site of narrowing and produces a pressure difference over the affected area. The difference is increased by decreasing the size of the stenotic orifice or by increasing the flow through it. At ordinary rates of flow in the resting patient, a valve orifice must be reduced by more than one-half before a significant pressure difference occurs.[4] The presence of a characteristic murmur on physical examination suggests only that a certain type of deformity exists. Catheterization or other clinical data are needed in order to estimate the severity of the condition.[64] Even so, the relation of estimated valve areas to symptoms or disability is far from quantitative.

In valvular insufficiency,[18, 65] because of the reflux of blood through the leak, the ventricle must pump a greater volume of blood than normal: total ventricular output is equal to the sum of the volume effectively moved forward and the volume regurgitated. In order to accommodate the larger amount of blood that must be handled, the ventricle must increase its diastolic volume. The extra load leads to hypertrophy and ultimately to myocardial failure.

MITRAL-VALVE DISEASE.[66, 67] The price of maintaining flow through the stenotic valve is a rise in left-atrial pressure. A sustained atrial pressure of 35 mm Hg may cause pulmonary edema because it is transmitted directly to the pulmonary capillary bed. This ceiling on left-atrial pressure also imposes a limit on the rate of mitral flow. The cardiac output is often lowered. The atrium can discharge only during ventricular diastole. Therefore tachycardia (for example, uncontrolled atrial fibrillation), which reduces the fraction of time the ventricle is in diastole, can further aggravate the problem of atrial emptying. Secondary pulmonary vascular disease may compound the injury to the heart by increasing the pulmonary resistance against which the right ventricle must work. These pulmonary vascular changes are usually partly reversible after successful mitral valvulotomy.

In mitral insufficiency,[65] the left ventricle must deliver an excessive stroke output, much of it backward into the left atrium. The systolic gush of blood tends to elevate the left-atrial pressure even before left-ventricular failure begins.

*Role of Cardiac Catheterization.* Mitral stenosis is diagnosed at cardiac catheterization by finding a pressure difference over the mitral valve during the filling period of the left ventricle.[4] The area of a stenotic valve may be calculated by the Gorlin formula, Eq. (8). This is an empirical modification of Poiseulle's equation, based on the assumption that the valve area is directly proportional to the rate of flow it allows, and inversely proportional to the square root of the pressure difference it necessitates. The formula allows for the fact that blood can flow only during ventricular diastole and therefore must flow at a considerably faster rate than the overall cardiac output. The Gorlin formula is:

Mitral-valve area (cm²)

$$= \frac{\text{mitral flow (ml/sec of diastole)}}{31 \times \sqrt{\text{(mean left atrial press.} - \text{mean left ventr. dias. press.)}}}. \quad (8)$$

The ratio of ventricular filling time to the duration of a complete cardiac cycle is called the "percentage diastole." It may be estimated by inspection of either the arterial or the ventricular pressure record. For example, in Fig. 51 the percentage diastole of the *right* ventricle is about 55 percent or, expressed as a decimal, 0.55. Mitral flow is calculated as follows:

Mitral flow (ml/sec of diastole)

$$= \frac{\text{cardiac output (ml/sec)}}{\text{fractional diastole of left ventricle}}. \quad (9)$$
$$\text{(expressed as a decimal)}$$

The left-ventricular diastolic pressure is generally normal in patients with no lesion except mitral stenosis. In such cases, the mitral-valve area may be calculated from data obtained from study of the right side of the heart, with an assumed left-ventricular diastolic pressure of 5 mm Hg.

*Example 3.* In the case of mitral stenosis from Table 92, by inspection of a radial-artery pressure tracing, the fraction of diastole was found to be 0.50. The oxygen consumption was 200 ml/min. Then, from Eq. (1),

Cardiac output = 2.4 L/min
                = 40 ml/sec;

from Eq. (9),

$$\text{Mitral flow} = \frac{40}{0.50}$$
$$= 80 \text{ ml/sec of diastole;}$$

from Eq. (8),

$$\text{Mitral-valve area} = \frac{80}{31\sqrt{(21 - 5)}}$$
$$= 0.65 \text{ cm}^2,$$

which represents tight stenosis.

*Evaluation.* The Gorlin formula is only an estimate. Because of inherent errors, any calculated mitral area in excess of 2 cm² must be considered possibly normal, in spite of the fact that the actual area of the normal valve is probably 4 cm² or more. On the other hand, any calculated valve area less than 1.0 cm² is usually associated with significant stenosis at operation.[63] Two important reservations apply: [4, 67] (i) the formula is not valid if there is any mitral insufficiency; (ii) in the presence of left-ventricular failure, the formula can be used only if the true ventricular diastolic pressure is measured by study of the left side of the heart.[68] Ignoring these restrictions will result in erroneous diagnoses of tight mitral stenosis. Therefore the use of the formula is limited to those cases in which only the *degree* of mitral stenosis is in question, and those few cases without murmurs that present as primary pulmonary hypertension.[69]

*Differentiation of Mitral Stenosis and Mitral Regurgitation.* Rheumatic deformity of the mitral valve may produce varying combinations of stenosis and insufficiency. Diagnosing the *predominant* lesion is of importance, since at present operations for mitral stenosis are considerably safer and more satisfactory than those for insufficiency. There are many clinical and laboratory criteria that help to distinguish the two conditions, though unfortunately they are not always reliable.[69] Study of the right side of the heart is probably of little use. Even study of the left side seems to give misleading results at times.[65] An important advantage, however, is that it allows accurate measurement of the left-ventricular diastolic pressure and the fluctuations of the mitral pressure difference throughout the cardiac cycle. With this knowledge one can often make a more accurate prediction of the valvular defect.[70]

AORTIC-VALVE DISEASE.[64] In aortic stenosis[71] there is obstruction to the outflow from the left ventricle, which is nevertheless capable of generating very high pressures and maintaining flow. The systolic pressure difference over the valve is often 80–100 mm Hg and may occasionally rise as high as 200 mm Hg (left-ventricular systolic pressure of about 300 mm Hg). But peripheral arterial pressure, pulse pressure, and cardiac output are often normal.[39, 71] The arterial pulse in severe cases usually shows a delay in its upstroke time with an "anacrotic notch" on the rising pressure wave. Such a pulse contour, however, sometimes is seen in patients with no aortic disease.[72] The Gorlin formula may also be used as in mitral disease to estimate the severity of aortic stenosis, with the same reservations.[71] The left side of the heart should be studied in most cases being considered for surgery. Without catheterization, severe aortic stenosis may be very difficult to distinguish from inconsequential thickening and stiffness of the aortic leaflets, which is common-

ly seen in older people. Limited experience to date suggests that it is unwarranted to ascribe angina pectoris, heart failure, or fainting to isolated aortic stenosis unless the calculated valve area is 0.8 cm² or less. Severe left-ventricular hypertrophy such as may occur in certain cases of systemic hypertension and idiopathic myocardial hypertrophy can produce marked physiologic subvalvular aortic stenosis[73] and must be distinguished clinically from cases of anatomic stenosis.

For assessing the severity of aortic regurgitation, present standard laboratory techniques offer little advantage over ordinary clinical methods such as measurement of the blood pressure. With combined aortic stenosis and insufficiency, a radial-artery pulse tracing may be of some use in deciding whether the aortic insufficiency is functionally important.[39, 74, 75]

*Cardiac Catheterization in Pulmonic Stenosis.*[3, 76] When the ventricular septum is intact, the entire cardiac output must be forced through the pulmonic valve by the right ventricle. Pulmonary-artery pressure tends to fall, but flow is not usually greatly reduced until myocardial failure supervenes. In general, the degree of stenosis can be satisfactorily estimated from the systolic pressure difference over the valve. The difference is usually greater than 50 mm Hg in clinically significant cases and 80 mm Hg or more in the severe ones in which surgery appears definitely indicated. There are two exceptions: (1) in severe stenosis when the cardiac output falls as the result of right-ventricular failure, the pressure difference may decrease moderately; (2) conversely, in atrial septal defect, because of increased flow, a difference as high as 50 mm Hg may be recorded in the presence of a normal valve.[77] Infundibular pulmonic stenosis may be suggested if the catheter locates a small area beneath the valve with pressure midway between those of the right ventricle and the pulmonary artery.[76] This method of diagnosing infundibular stenosis is not always reliable. Angiocardiography may give further information. An important function of catheterization is to diagnose associated septal defects that are surgically important but may be missed by other clinical methods.

### The Dye-Dilution Method [58]

This technique has recently provided a new source of information from catheter study.

PRINCIPLE.[78] The instantaneous injection of a small amount of dye into the inflow of the heart allows the substance to circulate through the cardiovascular system as a "bolus," the shape of which is influenced by the anatomy and flow characteristics of the human circulation. These produce a characteristic dispersal of indicator particles. As the dye passes a sampling site in any peripheral artery, its varying concentrations in the labeled blood may be recorded as a function of

time (Fig. 54). The graph obtained resembles the statistician's "normal frequency distribution curve," except that its descending limb is somewhat skewed, and its latter part is deformed by reappearance of dye the second time round the circulation. The cardiac output can be calculated from such a record. In general, the area under the curve is inversely proportional to the rate of flow. Rapid flow produces a brief contact of the bolus with the sampling site and a high, narrow "Gothic" curve. With lesser rates of flow, a slow-motion picture of the bolus, and hence a broader curve, is recorded. When correction is made for recirculation, the basic flow equation is

$$\text{Rate of flow} = \frac{q}{ct},$$

where $q$ is the amount of indicator injected, $c$ is its average concentration during the passage of the bolus, and $t$ is the time required for the bolus to pass a given point. It will be seen that the denominator of the right-hand member

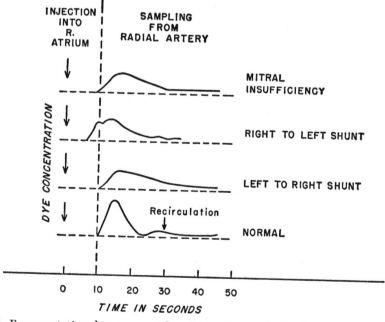

Fig. 54. Representative dye curves. This illustration is idealized: cardiac outputs and central volumes are similar in all four of these cases. In actual practice, a large central volume and a low forward cardiac output further distort (flatten) the curves of valvular insufficiency and left-to-right shunts.

of this equation is equal to the area under the dye curve.

The central circulatory volume also importantly affects the shape of the dye curve and, with certain important reservations, can be calculated from it. Here, the dye bolus is used simply as a marker. The volume it traverses is directly proportional to its mean circulation time, assuming a uniform rate of flow in all areas. (This assumption is not always justified.) High volumes also cause greater dispersal of dye particles, with broadening and flattening of the curve.

CLINICAL USES. The dye technique can be used to measure cardiac output with the same accuracy as the Fick method (10-percent error). But its chief use has been in the study of a group of conditions that separate one portion of blood flow from another.

*Right-to-left shunts.* Part of the bolus short-circuits the lungs, causing a premature appearance of the dye and an early hump superimposed on the dye curve.

*Left-to-right shunts and valvular insufficiency.* Part of the bolus is trapped in the central circulation: (*a*) by the back-and-forth flow past the leaking valve; (*b*) in the merry-go-round of a left-to-right shunt. In either case, the trapped blood is more gradually released from the central circulation than normally. This causes a delay in the disappearance time of the dye, and a rather characteristic shape of the dye curve. Attempts to quantitate abnormalities of this type have been disappointing, probably because increased residual volumes of the heart chambers can produce similar changes.[79] In order to localize defects or valvular regurgitation, several injections into different chambers are made. The method is especially useful when shunting through more than one defect is present. It can also distinguish between the arterial unsaturation of shunts and that of pulmonary disease. Because

injections into the right and left sides of the heart produce somewhat different curves, the method can be used to verify the position of the tip of the catheter. Newer indicators and methods of injection and sampling have recently broadened the usefulness of the technique.[80–82] In detecting and measuring shunts these newer methods can be superior to the Fick method.

### The Venous Pressure

PRINCIPLE. The peripheral venous pressure often reflects the right-atrial pressure and the right-ventricular diastolic pressure. Hence it can be a valuable index of cardiac function. Pressure in an antecubital vein[83] is usually 0–5 mm Hg higher than that in the right atrium.

METHOD. The patient lies supine, his arm slightly abducted and flat on the bed. A No. 20 or larger needle is inserted into an antecubital vein. A small amount of sodium citrate or heparin is injected through the needle to prevent clotting and the needle is connected with a saline-filled manometer such as is used for measuring cerebrospinal-fluid pressure (preferably one of greater than 2-mm bore, in order to minimize effects of capillarity). A preliminary check of the patency of the system is made by applying pressure to the upper arm. This should cause a prompt response in the manometer. Readings should be taken during quiet breathing. The zero point is along an imaginary line 5 cm posterior to the sternum when the patient is lying flat, or 4 cm if he is sitting at 45 degrees.[84] Since the arm is usually at a lower level than this, the number of centimeters difference must be noted with a ruler and subtracted from the observed reading.

RESULTS. Normal values are 20–110 mm $H_2O$ (1–8 mm Hg) but the extremes are uncommon. In children and in patients with thick chests (antero-posterior diameter greater than 20 cm) the use of the conventional zero point will give misleading results.[19] In such cases, it is best to refer pressures to a point midway between the front and back of the chest. Whenever the measurement is made in the latter way, the normal range of pressure is 50–150 mm $H_2O$. Elevation occurs in:

(1) Conditions that elevate the filling pressure of the right ventricle: right-ventricular failure; and constrictive pericarditis; [19]

(2) Tricuspid-valve disease;

(3) Local venous obstruction, as by a substernal thyroid tumor or blockage of the superior vena cava; [83]

(4) Increased intrathoracic pressure: (*a*) during cough or the Valsalva maneuver; (*b*) during expiration when there is partial bronchial obstruction, as in acute bronchial asthma;

(5) Certain high-output conditions, where, presumably because of unusually rapid flow, the peripheral venous pressure is considerable higher than that of the right atrium.[29]

CLINICAL APPLICATIONS. The formal measurement of venous pressure is necessary only when there are no discernible neck veins. Usually, increased venous pressure and abnormal venous flow may be diagnosed clinically by distention of the superficial neck veins in the sitting position, or systolic pulsation of the deep veins due to abnormally large V waves. The latter may be prominent even in cases without visible superficial distention. Elevation of venous pressure due to right-ventricular failure is often not fixed.[30, 83] It may appear only after exercise. When present, it can disappear rapidly with rest or treatment. The manometric method is often not suitable for diagnosing slight phasic elevations due to an abnormal V wave in mild or moderate right-ventricular failure. The damping of the system may obliterate such an abnormal wave altogether.[85]

## The Circulation Time [86]

PRINCIPLE. The appearance time of an injected substance was first used as a means of studying the circulation by Blumgart and Weiss. The only clinically important test measures the "arm-to-tongue" time and depends on the patient's recognizing the taste of an injected substance. The three most commonly used agents are decholin, saccharin, and magnesium sulfate. Although the data obtained are crude,[87] the test has a limited clinical usefulness. The most important variables affecting the circulation time are the cardiac output and the central volume. The behavior of the injected material is probably exactly the same as that described in the section on the dye-dilution method.[88]

METHOD. The patient must be alert. He is warned that he will experience a bitter, sweet, or burning taste, and that he must give an immediate signal when he does. Five milliliters (1 gm) of sodium dehydrocholate is injected through a No. 18 or No. 19 needle into an antecubital vein. Alternatively, 4 ml (2.5 gm) of saccharin or 6 ml of 10-percent magnesium sulfate may be used. The injection must be completed in about 1 sec. The arm should be positioned so that there is no local obstruction to venous flow. The time from the moment of injection until the patient's signal is measured, preferably with a stop watch and by an assistant.

RESULTS. Normally the arm-to-tongue time is 8–18 sec. Prolongation occurs in congestive failure (20–50 sec) and in mitral stenosis, even without failure, and cardiac dilatation (20–30 sec). In general, anything that decreases cardiac output or increases the central blood volume may prolong the circulation times. These same factors may produce a diffuse or absent end point, probably because the indicator is so dispersed that it never reaches the tongue in a high enough concentration to be tasted. Shortening occurs in large right-to-left shunts, and in high-output states, such as thyrotoxicosis, beriberi, anemia, and fever, especially when there is not yet severe congestive failure.

RISK. A few deaths have occurred after the intravenous injection of decholin or magnesium sulfate, especially in very ill patients or when repeated or large doses have been used.[89] If the injection is performed rapidly and the patient is alert, a diffuse or absent end point usually implies heart disease, and the test ought not to be repeated. No deaths have been reported after the use of saccharin, which, however, can cause local venous thrombosis and probably does not give as accurate results as decholin.[87]

CLINICAL APPLICATIONS. The test is largely outmoded. It has two chief uses.

*The emergency diagnosis of acute dyspnea.* Occasionally on physical examination it is not possible to distinguish acute lung disease, such as bronchial asthma or pneumonia, from the pulmonary edema of heart failure.

*The diagnosis of high-output states.* A normal circulation time in a patient with clinical evidence of congestive failure suggests the diagnosis, but a long circulation time in the presence of failure does not exclude these conditions.

## REFERENCES

1. W. Forssmann, "Die Sondierung des rechten Herzens," *Klin. Wschr.* 8, 2085 (1929).
2. A. Cournand, R. L. Riley, E. S. Breed, E. deF. Baldwin, D. W. Richards, Jr., "Measurement of cardiac output in man using the technique of catheterization of the right auricle or ventricle," *J. clin. Invest.* 24, 106 (1945).
3. A. S. Nadas, *Pediatric Cardiology* (Saunders, Philadelphia, 1957).
4. R. Gorlin and S. G. Gorlin, "Hydraulic formula for calculating area of stenotic mitral valve, other cardiac valves, and central circulatory shunts," *Amer. Heart J.* 41, 1 (1951).
5. A. Selzer, F. M. Willett, D. J. McCaughley, and T. V. Feichtmeir, "Uses of cardiac catheterization in acquired heart disease," *New Engl. J. Med.* 257, 66, 121 (1957).
6. H. L. Abrams and H. S. Kaplan, *Angiocardiography of Congenital Heart Disease* (Thomas, Springfield, 1956).
7. C. T. Dotter and I. Steinberg, "Angiocardiography in congenital heart disease," *Amer. J. Med.* 12, 219 (1952).
8. R. J. Bing, "Catheterization of the heart," *Advanc. intern. Med.* 5, 59 (1952).
9. H. K. Hellems, F. W. Haynes, J. F. Gowdney, and L. Dexter, "The pulmonary capillary pressure in man," *J. clin. Invest.* 27, 540 (1948).
10. D. C. Connolly, J. W. Kirklin, and E. H. Wood, "Relationship between pulmonary artery wedge pressure and left atrial pressure in man," *Circulat. Res.* 2, 434 (1954).
11. H. B. Burchell, "Symposium on the diagnostic value of simultaneous catheterization of the aorta and the right and left sides of the heart," *Proc. Mayo Clin.* 31, 105 (1956).
12. A. G. Morrow, E. Brunwald, J. A. Haller, and E. H. Sharp, "Left heart catheterization by the transbronchial route: Technic and applications in physiologic and diagnostic investigations," *Circulation* 16, 1032 (1957).
13. S. Radner, "Suprasternal puncture of the left atrium for flow studies," *Acta med. scand.* 148, 57 (1954).

14. R. Brock, B. B. Milstein, and D. N. Ross, "Percutaneous left ventricular puncture in assessment of aortic stenosis," *Thorax 11*, 163 (1956).

15. I. Ross, E. Braunwald, and A. G. Morrow, "New technique for the measurement of left atrial pressure in man," *Amer. J. Cardiol. 3*, 653 (1959).

16. A. Cournand, R. J. Bing, L. Dexter, C. Dotter, L. N. Katz, J. V. Warren, and E. Wood, "Report of the committee on cardiac catheterization and angiocardiography of the American Heart Association," *Circulation 7*, 769 (1953).

17. M. Bagger, G. Biörck, V. O. Björk, B. Brodén, L. E. Carlgren, A. Carlsten, I. Edler, B. Ejrup, H. Eliasch, A. Gustafson, A. Gyllenswärd, H. A. Hanson, A. Holmgren, H. Idbohrn, S. R. Johnsson, B. Johnsson, G. Jönsson, J. Karnell, S. R. Kjellberg, H. Krook, H. Larsson, L. Lindén, E. Linder, H. Linderholm, H. Lodin, G. Malmström, E. Mannheimer, T. Möller, J. Philipsson, S. Radner, U. Rudhe, G. Ström, B. Söderholm, F. Ulfsparre, L. Werkö, "On methods and complications in catheterization of heart and large vessels with and without contrast injection," *Amer. Heart J. 54*, 766 (1957).

18. C. S. Wiggers, *Physiology in Health and Disease* (Lea & Febiger, Philadelphia, 1949).

19. R. H. Lyons, J. A. Kennedy, and C. S. Burwell, "The measurement of venous pressures by the direct method," *Amer. Heart J. 16*, 675 (1938).

20. R. Bloomfield, H. Lauson, A. Cournand, E. Breed, and D. Richards, "Recording of right heart pressures in normal subjects and various types of cardiocirculatory disease," *J. clin. Invest. 25*, 639 (1946).

21. E. H. Wood and I. R. Leuson, "Measurement of pressure in man by cardiac catheters," *Circulat. Res. 2*, 294 (1954).

22. N. O. Fowler, E. P. Mannix, Jr., and W. Noble, "Difficulties in interpretation of right heart catheterization data," *Amer. Heart J. 53*, 343 (1957).

23. W. F. Hamilton, "The physiology of the cardiac output," *Circulation 8*, 527 (1953).

24. A. P. Fishman, J. McClement, A. Himmelstein, and A. Cournand, "Effects of acute anoxia on the circulation and respiration in patients with chronic pulmonary disease studied during the 'steady state,'" *J. clin. Invest. 31*, 770 (1952).

25. E. A. Stead, J. V. Warren, A. J. Merrill, and E. S. Brannon, "The cardiac output in male subjects as measured by the technique of right atrial catheterization. Normal values with observations on the effect of anxiety and tilting," *J. clin. Invest. 24*, 326 (1945).

26. K. W. Donald, J. M. Bishop, G. Cumming, and O. L. Wade, "Effect of exercise on cardiac output and circulatory dynamics of normal subjects," *Clin. Sci. 14*, 37 (1955).

27. L. Dexter, J. L. Whittenberger, F. W. Haynes, W. T. Goodale, R. Gorlin, and C. G. Sawyer, "Effect of exercise on the circulatory dynamics of normal individuals," *J. appl. Physiol. 3*, 439 (1951).

28. J. M. Bishop, K. W. Donald, and O. L. Wade, "Circulatory dynamics at rest and on exercise in hyperkinetic states," *Clin. Sci. 14*, 329 (1955).

29. W. J. Lahey, D. B. Arst, M. Silver, Lt. G. R. Kleeman, and P. Kunkel, "Physiologic observations on a case of beriberi heart disease with a note on the acute effects of thiamine," *Amer. J. Med. 14*, 248 (1953).

30. B. M. Lewis, H. E. J. Houssay, F. W. Haynes, and L. Dexter, "The dynamics of both right and left ventricles at rest and during exercise in patients with heart failure," *Circulat. Res. 1*, 312 (1953).

31. R. Gorlin, F. W. Haynes, W. T. Goodale, C. G. Sawyer, J. W. Dow, and L. Dexter, "Studies of the circulatory dynamics in mitral stenosis. II. Altered dynamics at rest," *Amer. Heart J. 41*, 30 (1951).

32. P. Wood, *Diseases of the Heart and Circulation* (Lippincott, Philadelphia, 1956).

33. J. R. Pappenheimer and J. P. Maes, "A quantitative measure of the vasomotor tone in the hind limb muscles of the dog," *Amer. J. Physiol. 137*, 187 (1942).

34. H. G. Borst, M. McGregor, J. L. Whittenberger, and E. Berglund, "Influence of pulmonary arterial and left atrial pressures on pulmonary vascular resistance," *Circulat. Res. 4*, 393 (1956).

35. R. L. Riley, A. Himmelstein, H. L. Motley, H. M. Weiner, and A. Cournand, "Studies of the pulmonary circulation at rest and during exercise in normal individuals and in patients with chronic pulmonary disease," *Amer. J. Physiol. 152*, 372 (1948).

36. A. Cournand, "Some aspects of the pulmonary circulation in normal man and in chronic cardio-pulmonary disease," *Circulation 2*, 641 (1950).

37. A. Cournand, "A discussion of the concept of cardiac failure in the light of recent physiologic studies in man," *Amer. J. Med. 37*, 649 (1952).

38. J. McMichael and J. P. Shillingford, "The role of valvular incompetence in heart failure," *Brit. med. J. 1*, 537 (1957).

39. P. Wood, "Aortic stenosis," *Amer. J. Cardiol. 1*, 553 (1958).

40. M. C. McCord, S. Komesu, S. B. Blount, "The characteristics of the right atrial pressure wave associated with right ventricular hypertrophy," *Amer. Heart J. 45*, 706 (1953).

41. J. P. D. Mounsey, L. W. Ritzmann, N. J. Selverstone, W. A. Briscoe, and G. A. McLemore, "Circulatory changes in severe pulmonary emphysema," *Brit. Heart J. 14*, 153 (1952).

42. H. Kuida, G. J. Dammin, F. W. Haynes, E. Rapaport, and L. Dexter, "Primary pulmonary hypertension," *Circulation 23*, 166 (1957).

43. C. G. Sawyer, C. S. Burwell, and L. Dexter, "Chronic constrictive pericarditis. Further consideration of the pathologic physiology of the disease," *Amer. Heart J. 44*, 207 (1952).

44. A. T. Hansen and P. Eskildsen, "Pressure curves from the right auricle and the right ventricle in chronic constrictive pericarditis," *Circulation 3*, 881 (1951).

45. T. K. Lin and M. Anache, "Right heart pressure patterns in constrictive pericarditis," *Amer. Heart J. 51*, 340 (1956).

46. J. G. Scannell, G. S. Myers, and A. L. Friedlich, "Significance of pulmonary hypertension in constrictive pericarditis," *Surgery 32*, 184 (1952).

47. R. M. Gunnar and R. F. Dillon, "The physiologic and clinical similarity between primary amyloid of the heart and constrictive pericarditis," *Circulation 12*, 833 (1955).

48. E. D. Robin and C. S. Burwell, "Hemodynamic aspects of diffuse myocardial fibrosis," *Circulation 16*, 730 (1957).

49. L. Dexter, "Atrial septal defect," *Brit. Heart J. 18*, 209 (1956).

50. J. F. Dammon, Jr., and C. Ferencz, "The significance of the pulmonary vascular bed in congenital heart disease. III. Defects between the ventricles or great vessels in which both increased pressure and blood flow may act upon the lungs and in which there is a common ejectile force," *Amer. Heart J. 52*, 210 (1956).

51. L. Dexter, F. W. Haynes, C. S. Burwell, E. C. Eppinger, M. C. Sosman, and J. M. Evans, "Studies of congenital heart disease. III. Venous catheterization as a diagnostic aid in patent ductus stenosis. Tetralogy of Fallot, ventricular septal defect and auricular septal defect," *J. clin. Invest. 26,* 561 (1947).

52. J. B. Hickam, "Atrial septal defect. A study of intracardiac shunts, ventricular outputs, and pulmonary pressure gradient," *Amer. Heart J. 38,* 801 (1949).

53. J. W. Dushane, J. W. Kirklin, R. T. Patrick, *et al.,* "Ventricular septal defects with pulmonary hypertension," *J. Amer. med. Ass. 160,* 950 (1956).

54. F. H. Ellis, J. W. Kirklin, J. A. Callahan, and E. H. Wood, "Patent ductus arteriosus with pulmonary hypertension. An analysis of cases treated surgically," *J. thorac. Surg. 31,* 268 (1956).

55. O. Heath, H. F. Helmholz, H. B. Burchell, J. W. Dushane, and J. E. Edwards, "Graded pulmonary vascular changes and hemodynamic findings in cases of atrial and ventricular septal defect and patent ductus arteriosus," *Circulation 18,* 1155, 1167 (1958).

56. L. Dexter, F. W. Haynes, C. S. Burwell, E. C. Eppinger, R. P. Sagerson, and J. M. Evans, "Studies of congenital heart disease. II. The pressure and oxygen content of blood in the right auricle, right ventricle, and pulmonary artery in control patients with observations on the oxygen saturation and source of pulmonary capillary blood," *J. clin. Invest. 26,* 554 (1947).

57. D. Bowers, H. B. Burchell, and E. H. Wood, "Difficulty in the precise localization by cardiac catheterization of left-to-right shunts near the pulmonary valve," *Proc. Mayo Clin. 30,* 261 (1955).

58. J. W. Kirklin, "Symposium on diagnostic applications of indicator dilution technics," *Proc. Mayo Clin. 32,* 463 (1957).

59. C. S. Wakai, H. J. C. Swan, and E. H. Wood, "Hemodynamic data and findings of diagnostic value in nine proved cases of persistent common atrio-ventricular canal," *Proc. Mayo Clin. 31,* 487 (1956).

60. H. B. Burchell and E. H. Wood, "Remarks on the technic and diagnostic applications of cardiac catheterization," *Proc. Mayo Clin. 25,* 41 (1950).

61. M. C. McCord, J. van Elk, and S. G. Blount, Jr., "Tetralogy of Fallot: Clinical and hemodynamic spectrum of combined pulmonary stenosis and ventricular-septal defect," *Circulation 16,* 736 (1957).

62. D. Carroll, J. E. Cohn, R. L. Riley, "Pulmonary function in mitral valvular disease. Distribution and diffusion characteristics in resting patients," *J. clin. Invest. 32,* 510 (1953).

63. S. R. Kjelberg, E. Mannheimer, U. Rudhe, and B. Jonsson, *Diagnosis of Congenital Heart Disease* (Year Book Publishers, Chicago, 1955).

64. E. W. Hancock, W. M. Madison, M. H. Proctor, W. H. Abelman, and G. W. B. Starkey, "Aortic stenosis of no physiologic significance," *New Engl. J. Med. 258,* 305 (1958).

65. H. W. Marshall, E. Woodward, and E. H. Wood, "Hemodynamic methods for differentiation of mitral stenosis and regurgitation," *Amer. J. Cardiol. 2,* 24 (1958).

66. B. M. Lewis, R. Gorlin, H. E. J. Houssey, F. W. Haynes, and L. Dexter, "Clinical and physiological correlations in patients with mitral stenosis, V," *Amer. Heart J. 43,* 2 (1952).

67. D. S. Lukas, and C. T. Dotter, "Modification of pulmonary circulation in mitral stenosis," *Amer. J. Med. 12,* 639 (1952).

68. H. Goldberg, J. Dickens, G. Raber, and E. Hayes, "Simultaneous (combined)

catheterization of the left and right heart," *Amer. Heart J. 53,* 579 (1957).

69. D. P. Schilder and W. P. Harvey, "Confusion of tricuspid incompetence with mitral insufficiency. A pitfall in the selection of patients for mitral surgery," *Amer. Heart J. 54,* 352 (1957).

70. J. C. Davila, "Hemodynamics of mitral insufficiency," *Amer. J. Cardiol. 2,* 135 (1958).

71. L. Dexter, D. E. Harken, L. A. Cobb, Jr., P. Novack, R. C. Sehlant, A. O. Phinney, Jr., and F. W. Haynes, "Aortic stenosis," *Arch. intern. Med. 101,* 254 (1958).

72. E. W. Hancock and W. Abelman, "A clinical study of the brachial arterial pulse form: with special reference to the diagnosis of aortic valvular disease," *Circulation 16,* 572 (1957).

73. B. A. Bercu, G. A. Diettert, W. H. Danforth, E. E. Pund, R. C. Ahlvin, and R. R. Belliveau, "Pseudoaortic stenosis produced by ventricular hypertrophy," *Amer. J. Med. 25,* 814 (1958).

74. H. Goldberg, A. A. Bakst, C. P. Bailey, "The dynamics of aortic valvular disease," *Amer. Heart J. 47,* 527 (1954).

75. P. R. Fleming, "The mechanism of the pulsus bisferiens," *Brit. Heart J. 19,* 519 (1957).

76. J. W. Kirklin, D. C. Connolly, H. Ellis, H. B. Burchell, J. Edwards, and E. H. Wood, "Problems in the diagnosis and surgical treatment of pulmonic stenosis with intact ventricular system," *Circulation 8,* 849 (1953).

77. L. McDonald, "The significance of a pressure gradient across the pulmonary valve in atrial defect," *Brit. Heart J. 20,* 268 (1958).

78. P. Meier and K. L. Zierler, "On the theory of the indicator-dilution method for measurement of blood flow and volume," *J. appl. Physiol. 6,* 731 (1954).

79. J. I. E. Hoffman and G. G. Rowe, "Some factors affecting indicator dilution curves in the presence and absence of valvular incompetence," *J. clin. Invest.* 38, 138 (1959).

80. "Symposium on the diagnostic applications of indicator dilution curves recorded from the right and left sides of the heart," *Proc. Mayo Clin. 33,* 535 (1958).

81. H. R. Warner and A. F. Toronto, "Quantitation of backflow in patients with aortic insufficiency using an indicator technic," *Circulat. Res. 6,* 29 (1958).

82. E. Braunwald and A. G. Morrow, "A method for the dilution and estimation of aortic regurgitant flow in man," *Circulation 17,* 505 (1958).

83. H. H. Hussey and H. Jeghers, "Practical considerations of venous pressure," *New Engl. J. Med. 237,* 776 (1947).

84. S. Gitelson, "Determination of the venous pressure in the sitting posture," *Brit. Heart J. 16,* 147 (1954).

85. G. A. Brecher, *Venous Return* (Grune and Stratton, New York, 1956).

86. L. E. Morris and H. L. Blumgart, "Velocity of blood flow in health and disease," *Circulation 15,* 448 (1957).

87. M. M. Mahl and K. Lange, "Reliability of subjective circulation time determinations," *Circulation 17,* 922 (1958).

88. D. F. Heiman, H. L. Conn, and C. R. Joyner, "Estimation of cardiac output, mean circulation time and central blood volume by means of multiple graded dose sodium dehydrocholate," *Circulation 15,* 245 (1957).

89. G. C. Sanchez and L. E. Morris, "Four untoward reactions to sodium dehydrocholate," *New Engl J. Med. 251,* 646 (1954).

# Unit 34

# Pulmonary-Function Tests

For clinical purposes, the student and physician should be able to carry out and interpret the results of the following determinations: (1) vital capacity, tidal volume, and minute ventilation, as well as analysis of the form of the spirographic tracing; (2) maximal breathing capacity (MBC); (3) timed vital capacity (TVC); and (4) arterial blood gases under various conditions. Other tests, such as diffusing capacity, work of breathing, residual lung volume, distribution of inspired air, and dead-space determinations are not generally available to the clinician in his everyday problems and will not be discussed here. The interested reader is referred to several texts for information on these points.[1-4]

## Pulmonary Ventilation and Gas Exchange

### PRINCIPLE

The primary function of the lung is gas exchange—the oxygenation of venous blood and the elimination of the carbon dioxide added as a result of tissue metabolism. A normal arterial oxygen saturation of 95 percent or greater, an arterial blood carbon dioxide pressure of 40 mm Hg, and a pH of 7.40 are maintained in relatively narrow ranges by a remarkably sensitive respiratory center, which rapidly adjusts the rate and depth of respiration in response to the neurogenic and humoral influences that govern its activity.[5] The amount of air respired, ex- pressed in liters per minute, is termed the minute volume of pulmonary ventilation. The minute volume of pulmonary ventilation as recorded at the mouth does *not* reflect the final volume of air that participates in gas exchange, however, since part of each tidal volume is expended on the so-called dead space of the respiratory passages. That fraction of the minute ventilation which participates in gas exchange is termed the alveolar ventilation. In order to calculate this, the volume of the dead space must be known.

METHOD.[2, 6] There are two methods for measuring ventilation: closed-circuit and open-circuit spirometry.

CLOSED-CIRCUIT, REBREATHING SPIROMETRY. The Benedict-Roth metabolism apparatus is the spirometer most commonly used for measurements of ventilation. A permanent record is obtained which allows direct reading of tidal volume, respiratory frequency, minute ventilation, vital capacity, oxygen consumption, maximal breathing capacity, and analysis of the spirogram for breathing patterns during various states (rest, determination of the MBC, and so forth). There are two main disadvantages of closed-circuit systems. (1) Because the subject rebreathes the spirometer gas, the composition of the inspired gas is constantly changing during the test run. The spirometer must be filled initially with a high-oxygen mixture so as to avoid hypoxia as oxygen is

537

consumed by the subject. Oxygen alters tidal volume and minute ventilation, not only in normal individuals but, most importantly, in patients with chronic pulmonary insufficiency, which may lead to inaccuracies and false conclusions as regards these measurements. (2) Variable resistance to air flow as a result of differences in the size of tubing, the presence of the soda-lime canister, and the inertia of the bell causes inaccuracies in the measurement of the tests requiring maximal flow rates (MBC, TVC).

Certain modifications in the standard apparatus for determining the BMR have resulted in a more useful instrument for the measurement of ventilation (the Respirometer). The capacity of the bell has been enlarged, wider-bore rubber tubing and inlet attachments are used, and a two-speed kymograph and an attachment to reduce inspiratory excursions by a ratio of 25 : 1 have been added.

OPEN-CIRCUIT SPIROMETRY. In open-circuit systems, air (or other gas mixture) is inspired through an inspiratory valve and expired through an expiratory valve into a collecting system, either a Tissot spirometer or a Douglas bag. The contents of the bag can then be measured with a portable gas meter or the Tissot spirometer. Open-circuit systems avoid the disadvantages of changing composition of inspired gas, but the problem of variable resistance to air flow is still present.[6]

The basal state is not absolutely necessary, but a 15-min rest period before spirometry and quiet, comfortable surroundings during the test are necessary. With the nose clip and mouthpiece securely in place, there being no leaks in the system, a 3- to 5-min period of resting ventilation is obtained. The slope of the end-expiratory base line should be smooth; it measures oxygen consumption so long as the system is air tight.

All lung volumes and ventilation measurements should be expressed at body temperature (37°C), prevailing barometric pressure, and saturated with water vapor (BTPS). The factors in Table 93 have been calculated for a barometric

Table 93. *Factors to convert gas volumes from room (spirometer) temperature saturated to 37°C saturated (BTPS). Factor × gas volume at temperature of collection (ATPS) = gas volume (BTPS).*

| Gas temperature (°C) | Factor | Gas temperature (°C) | Factor |
|---|---|---|---|
| 20 | 1.102 | 29 | 1.051 |
| 21 | 1.096 | 30 | 1.045 |
| 22 | 1.091 | 31 | 1.039 |
| 23 | 1.085 | 32 | 1.032 |
| 24 | 1.080 | 33 | 1.026 |
| 25 | 1.075 | 34 | 1.020 |
| 26 | 1.068 | 35 | 1.014 |
| 27 | 1.063 | 36 | 1.007 |
| 28 | 1.057 | 37 | 1.000 |

pressure of 760 mm Hg. Small differences in the prevailing pressure make negligible differences in the values of the factor.[3] It is customary to express oxygen consumption and the blood gases in terms of the dry gas at standard temperature and pressure (STPD).

## MINUTE VENTILATION, RESPIRATORY DEAD SPACE, ALVEOLAR VENTILATION

MINUTE VENTILATION. The minute ventilation is the product of tidal volume and the number of breaths per minute (respiratory frequency). It is usually expressed in liters per minute or liters per minute per square meter of body surface area. The normal range is 5.90–7.84 L/min,[7] or 2.5–5.0 L/min m².[3] Minute ventilation increases moderately in elderly individuals.[8]

RESPIRATORY DEAD SPACE. There are two types of respiratory dead space, the anatomic and the physiologic dead space.

*Anatomic dead space* refers to the conducting airways, namely, mouth, nose, pharynx, larynx, trachea, bronchi, and bronchioles. At the level of the respiratory bronchioles, alveoli first make their appearance, and this is the zone of transition from anatomic dead space to the distalmost areas of the lung (that is, the alveoli) where gas exchange takes place. The anatomic dead space in males is between 150 and 220 ml, and in females, between 100 and 150 ml.[9] A useful rule of thumb for clinical use is that the anatomic dead space in milliliters is roughly equal to the subject's weight in pounds. This obviously does not hold for individuals who deviate markedly from predicted normal weight for their age and sex.

*Physiologic dead space* consists of the anatomic dead space *plus* the volume of alveoli that are ventilated out of proportion to their blood flow or indeed are not perfused at all with blood. Thus, a lung deprived of its blood flow by pulmonary-artery thrombosis, though still ventilated, exchanges no gas and therefore behaves like anatomic dead space. The physiologic dead space is equal to the anatomic dead space in normal individuals.

The amount by which the physiologic dead space exceeds the anatomic dead space represents that portion of the respiratory system normally functioning in gas exchange which now receives ventilation in excess of blood flow, resulting in a "dead-space effect." Therefore, an increased physiologic dead space can be demonstrated with pulmonary emboli, pulmonary-artery or arteriolar thrombosis, and overventilation, as with $CO_2$ inhalation or anxiety states. In obstructive emphysema and bronchospastic conditions, the anatomic dead space is increased in proportion to the degree of hyperinflation of the lung, and the physiologic dead space may be increased by overventilation of areas that can still be well ventilated because, in part, of the exclusion of occluded regions. In addition, obliteration of the pulmonary capillary bed increases the physiologic dead space in obstructive emphysema. Dead space is increased in the presence of pulmonary cysts with patent bronchial communication, and in some cases of bronchiectasis. There is an increase in the

volume of the physiologic dead space in the aged.[8]

ALVEOLAR VENTILATION. That portion of each tidal volume which reaches the alveoli to participate in gas exchange is equal to the tidal volume $V_T$ minus the volume expended in the dead space $V_{DS}$, and this difference $V_T - V_{DS}$ multiplied by the respiratory frequency is equal to the minute alveolar ventilation. Normal figures are not available for the volume of alveolar ventilation, but 1.5–3.5 L/min m² for resting adults is probably satisfactory. The prime criterion for normality of alveolar ventilation in any individual is maintenance of normal blood gases. For this purpose, the partial pressure of carbon dioxide in the arterial blood is the most sensitive indicator. Normally, the respiratory center is exquisitely sensitive to changes in the carbon dioxide pressure and rapidly adjusts alveolar ventilation to maintain the pressure in a normal range of 35 to 47 mm Hg. Values above or below this range indicate alveolar hypoventilation or hyperventilation respectively.

One can estimate the volume of alveolar ventilation by subtracting the appropriate figures for anatomic dead space for males and females given above from the determined tidal volume. The normal ratio of dead space to tidal volume is 0.3 or less, that is, normally 30 percent or less of the tidal volume is expended in the dead space.[10]

*Alveolar hypoventilation.* The term alveolar hypoventilation indicates that the volume of inspired air reaching the alveoli is insufficient to oxygenate pulmonary capillary blood adequately and rid it of its carbon dioxide. This can result from uncompensated decreases of tidal volume or respiratory frequency, increased dead-space effect, or abnormalities of the distribution of inspired air. The result is unsaturation of arterial blood and carbon dioxide retention with respiratory acidosis. The causes and significance of alveolar hypoventilation are discussed in the section on blood gases.

*Alveolar hyperventilation.* This term indicates excessive alveolar ventilation. This results in lowering of the carbon dioxide pressure of the blood and a nearly proportional loss of carbon dioxide, which results in respiratory alkalosis. The oxygen pressure of the alveoli and arterial blood is increased, but the flatness of the oxygen dissociation curve at high saturation (Fig. 10, Unit 11) explains why very little extra oxygen is added to the blood as a result of hyperventilation, in contradistinction to the loss of carbon dioxide.[10]

Alveolar hyperventilation with respiratory alkalosis is seen commonly in anxiety states (the hyperventilation syndrome) and during artificial respiration, for instance, in poliomyelitis or during anesthesia, where the patient may be "overbreathed." Occasionally, prolonged hyperventilation is seen as a sequel to encephalitis, head injuries, or intracranial operations. Alveolar hyperventilation is the most important feature of successful acclimatization to high altitude.

### OXYGEN CONSUMPTION

The basal oxygen consumption varies between 105 and 186 ml/min m$^2$ (STPD) in adults of various age groups,[4] decreasing with age, and is closely related to the body surface area. Oxygen consumption is a function of the metabolic needs of the body and has no necessary correlation with the type or severity of pulmonary disease.

Attempts to characterize the efficiency of pulmonary ventilation by relating ventilation to oxygen consumption have yielded interesting information. The ventilatory equivalent of Anthony [11] is the number of liters of ventilation per 100 ml of oxygen consumed. Normally, this is about 2.5, with a very wide range of normal values (1.68 − 3.7). In "metabolic hyperpnea" (exercise, hyperthyroidism, fever) oxygen consumption is increased

proportionally to the increase in ventilation, and the ventilatory equivalent remains normal. "Compensatory hyperpnea" is "wasted ventilation" with an increase in pulmonary ventilation out of proportion to oxygen consumption, resulting in an increased ventilatory equivalent.[7] The commonest cause is hysterical hyperventilation. The commonest iatrogenic cause is seen during the subject's initial anxious experience with the spirometer. An increased ventilatory equivalent is seen in heart failure, in conditions associated with excessive dead-space ventilation, in pulmonary diseases associated with the diffusion block syndrome, and during the latter part of pregnancy.[12]

## The Maximal Breathing Capacity

### PRINCIPLE

The maximal breathing capacity (better termed the maximal voluntary ventilation or voluntary ventilatory capacity) measures the greatest volume of gas that an individual is capable of breathing voluntarily per unit time. This is usually measured during a 15-sec period of effort and the result expressed in liters per minute. The determination of it is the one single test that evaluates the over-all, integrated function of the ventilatory apparatus.

### METHOD

It is remarkable and unfortunate that a test which was originated in 1933, and has been considered invaluable in the study of pulmonary disease, remains nonstandardized to the present time. There are two methods used commonly at present.

RECORDING SPIROMETER. Ideally, the improved Benedict-Roth spirometer should be used. The rubber connecting tubing should be noncorrugated and approximately 1.5 in. in diameter. The soda-lime canister and rubber valves must be removed to reduce resistance to air flow.

Removal of the soda-lime canister also prevents hypocapnia which may result in decreased ventilatory ability toward the end of the test period. The bell should be only one-quarter filled with water for performance of the test. The main advantage of spirometric determinations is that a permanent record of the effort is obtained. The disadvantages are that spirometer inertia and varying resistance to air flow may give variable results.

DOUGLAS BAG — LOW-RESISTANCE VALVE. The expired air can be collected in a Douglas bag and the contents measured with a gas meter. The patient breathes through a low-resistance valve attached to the Douglas bag by rubber tubing similar to that described above. This has the advantage of being portable and allows the same apparatus to be used for determination of walking and exercise ventilation. Comparison of these values with the MBC should require that apparatus with the same resistance to air flow be used.[2] It has the disadvantage of not providing a permanent record of the effort.

PERFORMANCE OF THE TEST. The test is explained carefully to the subject and a complete trial run is demonstrated by the examiner, stressing maximal effort with a "do or die" attitude. A competitive spirit is fostered to better previous attempts. The examiner emphasizes as great a rate and depth of breathing as possible, but should allow the patient to control these variables himself. Normal individuals usually select a frequency of 50 to 60 breaths/min, utilizing 40 to 50 percent of their vital capacity for stroke (tidal) volume. A nose clip is applied, and, with the subject seated expectantly on the edge of a chair, or standing, he is exhorted to "GO! GO! GO!" After several breaths of "warm-up" to give him a running start, a 15-sec period is timed with constant, encouraging shouts of "Faster! Deeper!" The 15-sec volume is corrected to BTPS and multiplied by 4 to give the result in liters per minute.

The test is repeated with 5-min rest periods between efforts, until a stable, maximal value is obtained. Most of the learning is accomplished with the first or second repeat. Rarely does the procedure have to be repeated more than three times to obtain duplicate determinations agreeing within 5 to 10 L/min. The highest value is recorded as the MBC.

CONTRAINDICATIONS

Recent pulmonary hemorrhage has been considered a contraindication a priori. The possibility of promoting respiratory paralysis in incipient or early cases of poliomyelitis due to exhausting exercise has been mentioned by Whittenberger. Because of the rapid, violent deformation of the lung occurring during the MBC test, it has been suggested that aspiration of infected material from diseased to healthy areas of lung might occur. Occasionally, bronchial asthma may be aggravated or an attack precipitated by the performance of the test. Acutely ill or debilitated individuals cannot be expected to perform maximal voluntary effort nor should they be driven to it. In such instances, the test period can be shortened to 3 or 4 sec and the results extrapolated to 1 min. Multiplying the first second's expiratory volume (liters) of the timed vital capacity by 35 gives a reasonable approximation of the MBC.

NORMAL VALUES

Because of the differences in methods employed and the difficulties inherent in obtaining standardized voluntary effort in different subjects, there is a wide range of normal values for the MBC published in the literature. The usual practice is to consider ±20 percent of the normal predicted value as the normal range. Therefore, reduction in the MBC must be large to be considered significant.

The normal values and prediction formulas of Baldwin [4] are most commonly used in this country (Table 94). The

Table 94. *Prediction formulas for maximal breathing capacity and vital capacity.*

| | |
|---|---|
| *Maximal breathing capacity (L/min)* | |
| Males: | $\{86.5 - [0.522 \times$ age (yr)$]\}$ $\times$ BSA (m²) |
| Females: | $\{71.3 - [0.474 \times$ age (yr)$]\}$ $\times$ BSA (m²) |
| Bedside calculation: | 35 × expiratory volume (L) during first second of TVC |
| *Vital capacity, supine (ml)* | |
| Males: | $\{27.63 - [0.112 \times$ age (yr)$]\}$ $\times$ height (cm) |
| Females: | $\{21.78 - [0.101 \times$ age (yr)$]\}$ $\times$ height (cm) |
| Bedside calculation: | |
| Adults—Males: | 2.5 L/BSA (m²) or 25 ml/height (cm) |
| Females: | 2.0 L/BSA (m²) or 20 ml/height (cm) |
| Children—Males: | 250 ml/age (yr) |
| Females: | 200 ml/age (yr) |

MBC increases with age until the third decade, and then progressively decreases. The MBC is less in females than males of comparable stature. In children, normal values should be correlated with age, sex, height, weight, and body surface area, and for this purpose Ferris's tables [13] should be consulted.

### LIMITATIONS

The usefulness of the test is limited by the following factors.

(1) In addition to nonstandardization of the procedure, which makes valid comparison of published results difficult, the wide range of normal values precludes its use as a sensitive test in the detection of minimal abnormalities. For an isolated determination to be considered significant, the reduction must be large.

(2) A significant change in the MBC from day to day or over prolonged periods may be due not only to amelioration or worsening of the disease process, but also to a variety of other hard-to-define factors that enter into any voluntary effort (attitude and motivation of patient as well as of examiner, state of training, emotional factors). Bed rest *per se* usually results in a significant reduction in the MBC.

(3) The test is exhausting (if done properly) and time-consuming, and requires special, relatively expensive equipment. It may be replaced in the future by analysis of fast vital-capacity tracings using a single breath.

(4) Erroneous figures may result with the use of the spirometer at high respiratory rates where the inertia of the moving parts and the development of resonance in the water jacket prevent faithful recording of the actual volume ventilated.[14, 15]

### INTERPRETATIONS

The MBC test is the one test that evaluates the over-all, integrated function of the ventilatory apparatus. The finding of a normal MBC is strong evidence against pulmonary disease as the cause of dyspnea. The exception to this statement is found in the alveolar-capillary block syndrome and in diffuse pulmonary vascular disease, where, in the face of severe dyspnea with the slightest exertion, the MBC more often than not is maintained at normal or near-normal levels. The normal MBC depends on freely mobile thoracic structures, normally functioning respiratory muscles, patency of the tracheobronchial tree offering the least resistance to air flow, ability of the lung tissue to be stretched and deformed rapidly with the least work, delivery of a maximal stroke volume (tidal volume per breath) equal to at least one-half of the predicted normal vital capacity, and coordinated activity of the neuromuscular forces. Assuming maximal cooperation and voluntary effort, and the absence of severe debility or other disease, the MBC may be reduced in the following conditions (with representative examples):

(1) Immobility of the skeletal system (rheumatoid spondylitis, senile emphysema, kyphoscoliosis).

(2) Loss of respiratory-muscle force (poliomyelitis, myositis, myasthenia gravis).

(3) Obstruction to air flow (bronchial asthma, obstructive emphysema, bronchitis with bronchospasm, tracheal or bronchial tumor). In this connection, it is important to note that not only is the MBC reduced, but a progressive rise in the end-expiratory base line with performance of the test is corollary evidence of obstruction to air flow.[16]

(4) Stiff or immobile lung tissue (diffuse, parenchymal fibrotic processes, massive pleural effusion).

(5) Extreme reduction in vital capacity from any cause such that an increase in respiratory frequency cannot compensate for reduction in stroke volume.

(6) Uncoordinated neuromuscular forces; these are not commonly recognized as such, but are sometimes found in obstructive emphysema and bulbar poliomyelitis.

The test finds its greatest use in diagnosing and following the course of obstructive emphysema and in preoperative evaluation for thoracic surgery. In the latter connection, an MBC of less than 40 L/min in the male patient usually indicates a poor operative risk for thoracic surgery.

### RELATION TO DYSPNEA

Dyspnea, like pain, is a subjective sensation, and as such is impossible to define in quantitative terms. Simply stated, dyspnea will occur whenever the individual's ventilatory requirements cannot be easily supplied by his ventilatory capacity.[17] Therefore, dyspnea may occur from increased ventilatory requirements (for example, exercise), reduced ventilatory capacity (for example, obstructive emphysema), or both (for example, fever in the patient with emphysema).

The maximal ventilatory capacity and ventilatory requirements during mild exercise have been related to the sensation of dyspnea by Cournand and Richards.[18] The breathing reserve is equal to the MBC minus the minute ventilation (L/ min, BTPS). Expressed as a percentage of the MBC, it is $(MBC - MV)/MBC$. It was found that dyspnea was experienced when the breathing reserve fell to 60–70 percent of the MBC during standardized exercise (described in the section on blood gases). When the breathing reserve was above 93 percent at rest, there was no dyspnea with the step test; when it was below 80 percent at rest, all patients experienced dyspnea with mild exercise.

## Vital Capacity, Timed Vital Capacity, and the Spirogram

### VITAL CAPACITY

PRINCIPLE. The determination of lung volumes yields much useful information once values have been established in a given individual for future comparison. The volume of air contained in the lungs and the relation of the various subdivisions is affected by many disease processes. With the patient serving as his own control, the subsequent determination of the vital capacity represents a convenient method for the evaluation of therapy and for following the course of a disease process.

DEFINITIONS. Most investigators have adopted the terminology for lung volumes recommended by a group of American physiologists in 1950,[19] and these are presented below and in Fig. 55. Some of the terms formerly used for lung volumes are indicated in parentheses.

The resting end-expiratory or end-tidal position is the usual point of reference for the measurement of lung volumes, since it is the least variable on a respiratory tracing and involves no conscious effort on the part of the patient. A line

543

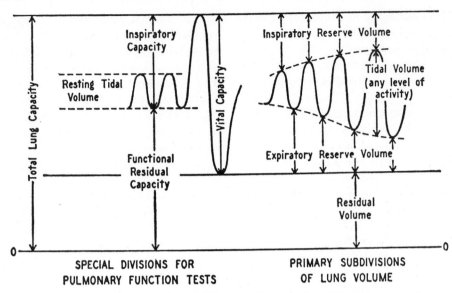

Fig. 55. The subdivisions of lung volume.[19]

joining the end-expiratory points of resting tidal volumes defines the resting expiratory base line.

*Vital capacity* is the maximal volume of air that can be expired after a maximal inspiration. It is the sum of inspiratory capacity and expiratory reserve volume.

*Inspiratory capacity* (complemental or complementary air) is the maximal volume that can be inspired from the end-expiratory level. It can also be thought of as the sum of inspiratory reserve and tidal volume.

*Inspiratory reserve volume* is the volume that can be inspired from an end-tidal inspiratory position.

*Expiratory reserve volume* (supplemental or supplementary air) is the maximal volume of air that can be expired from the end-tidal expiratory level.

*Residual volume* is the volume of air remaining in the lungs (including the dead space) after maximal expiration.

*Functional residual capacity* (mid-capacity) is the volume of air in the lungs at the end-expiratory level. It is the sum of expiratory reserve and residual volume.

*Total lung capacity* is the volume of air contained in the lungs at maximal inspiration. It is the sum of residual volume and vital capacity.

METHOD. The subject is allowed to rest quietly for about 15 min prior to the test. It is not necessary to have the patient in the completely basal state. The surroundings should be quiet. Lung volumes and resting minute ventilation may be determined in the recumbent or seated position and this same position used for subsequent studies. A nose clip is applied and a suitable mouthpiece inserted. When it is certain that there are no leaks in the system, the kymograph is started at low speed. Several minutes may be required for the subject to become accustomed to this new state. When the tidal excursions have become constant, so that a linear end-expiratory base line can be visualized, and several minutes of quiet breathing are available for analysis, the subject is instructed to take in as deep a breath as possible beginning at the end of a quiet expiration. This is the inspiratory capacity. He then expires passively and resumes quiet breathing. When the base line has once again become steady, he is instructed to blow out as much air as possible, again from his resting end-expiratory position.

This is the expiratory reserve volume. The above maneuvers are repeated until maximal values are obtained. This usually requires several efforts. Finally, he is exhorted to take in as deep a breath as possible and then maximally expire. The maximal expiratory effort should take about 5 sec to complete to make certain that the best effort is being obtained. It is important that the vital capacity maneuver be performed slowly, similar instructions being used for each subject.

NORMAL VALUES. Normal individuals of similar age, sex, and stature may deviate as much as ±20 percent from their predicted values. The prediction formula of Baldwin [4] (Table 94) generally yields normal values that are slightly lower than other published series. They are the most commonly used in this country for predicting adult values. For children, the prediction formulas listed in Table 94 may be used where applicable. For greatest accuracy, the tables of Ferris [13] relating the vital capacity to four variables (age, height, weight, and body surface area) should be consulted.

NORMAL VARIATIONS. The vital capacity correlates best with the height of the individual, increasing with height. It normally constitutes about 80 percent of the total lung volume in the third decade, decreasing gradually to approximately 68 percent of the total lung volume in the eighth decade. The inspiratory capacity is also reduced in the older age groups, probably owing to decreased chest expansion. Certain maneuvers that presumably alter pulmonary blood volume, such as change from the supine to the standing position, the Valsalva maneuver, application of positive pulmonary pressure, and application of tourniquets to the thighs in the standing position, will increase the vital capacity by 100 to 300 ml.

LIMITATIONS. Owing to the wide range of normal values (normal range = predicted ±20 percent of the predicted value), reduction in vital capacity must be large to be considered significant. Thus, its measurement cannot be of aid in the detection of subtle or moderate changes as an isolated, single determination. Once the vital capacity of an individual has been determined, however, the reproducibility of the value in health and disease is extremely good and this greatly enhances the value of the determination. The variation in vital capacity repeatedly determined over long periods of time in the same healthy individual does not usually exceed 200 ml.[20, 21]

The absolute value of the vital capacity correlates poorly with the degree of disability in pulmonary disease and has little functional significance when considered alone. Thus, the patient severely disabled with obstructive emphysema may have only a mild reduction in vital capacity, whereas the patient with a 50-percent reduction in vital capacity following pneumonectomy may be perfectly comfortable at rest and on moderate exertion. The value of the test has been greatly increased by introducing the element of time into its determination (see timed vital capacity).

USE AND INTERPRETATION. Reduction in vital capacity as an isolated finding is termed a "restrictive ventilatory defect." The causes of reduction in this lung volume can be categorized broadly, with a few representative examples, as follows: (1) replacement, obliteration, compression, or collapse of lung tissue by tumor, fluid, inflammation, or fibrosis (bronchogenic carcinoma, pleural effusion, interstitial fibrosis, heart failure, thoracoplasty, bronchiectasis); (2) expiratory air trapping (lung cysts with poor bronchial communications, asthma, obstructive emphysema); (3) loss of mobility (rheumatoid spondylitis) or muscular force of the respiratory apparatus, preventing expansion or contraction of the thorax (poliomyelitis, kyphoscoliosis).

Comparison of the vital capacity determined as a single maneuver ("actual" vital capacity) with that obtained by separate determination and addition of the inspiratory capacity and expiratory reserve volume ("combined" vital capacity) yields useful information. Normally, the "actual" and "combined" vital capacities are the same. When the combined vital capacity exceeds the actual capacity, air trapping is certainly present. The discrepancy, which may be as great as 1 L, represents the volume of air trapped. The phenomenon is seen in obstructive emphysema, and may be of aid in the early diagnosis of this disease. It can also be seen with bronchospasm or bronchial secretions from any cause (bronchial asthma, bronchitis). Poor cooperation or malingering should be suspected if the actual exceeds the combined vital capacity in significant amount.

The degree of reversible air trapping due to bronchospasm (bronchial asthma) and that due to irreversible causes (elastic tissue degeneration in obstructive emphysema) may be measured by determining the increase in vital capacity after the administration of bronchodilator drugs.

Analysis of the components of the vital capacity is only occasionally profitable. They vary rather frequently because of normal changes in the resting end-expiratory level, which may amount to as much as 500 ml from time to time, with resultant changes in the inspiratory capacity and expiratory reserve volume.[21] Normally, the expiratory reserve volume in the sitting position is about 25 percent and the inspiratory capacity 75 percent of the vital capacity. The expiratory reserve decreases with paralysis of muscles used in expiration (abdominal muscles and diaphragm). An increase in expiratory reserve and a decrease in inspiratory capacity may be seen with hyperinflation of the lung (bronchial asthma, obstructive emphysema).

The chief value of the vital-capacity determination is to be found in evaluating therapy and following the course of disease. As an isolated determination, the vital capacity is of little value unless the reduction is marked. In view of the excellent reproducibility of the test, however, serial determinations can be of extreme value. As stated above, changes greater than 200 ml on repeated determinations can be considered significant. Thus, changes in the state of cardiac compensation over prolonged periods of stress and therapy can be defined, the effectiveness of bronchodilator therapy assessed, the progressive deterioration (or improvement) of respiratory muscle paralysis in poliomyelitis evaluated, and the course of ankylosing spondylitis followed by serial determinations of the vital capacity.

### TIMED VITAL CAPACITY (TVC)

PRINCIPLE. The maximal ventilatory capacity of the lung depends not only on the size of the bellows as indicated by the vital capacity, which determines the maximal stroke volume, but on the speed with which the volume can be delivered. This is determined mainly by the resistance to air flow in the respiratory passages. Thus, vital-capacity determinations without respect to time give little information as regards the presence of obstructive ventilatory defects. Given enough time, the patient with incapacitating asthma or emphysema may deliver a normal vital capacity. Timing the vital capacity recognizes the fact that the cyclical process of respiration is limited by time.

METHOD. The subject (fitted with nose clip) is instructed to inspire maximally, then expire as *fast* and as *much* as he can. The portions of the total capacity that are delivered in the first, second, and third seconds of expiration are determined and expressed as percentages of the total volume expired. Two methods are available for doing this. (1) The Respirometer kymograph is set to high speed (160 mm/min) and the entire maneuver recorded. With the aid of a special ruler,[22] the expiratory slope is analyzed for the volume of air expired in the first, second, and third seconds. (2) An electronically controlled timing device attached to the wheel of a 6-L spirometer (the Vitalometer) is actuated by the subject's expiration. Two pointers on the wheel record, respectively, the total vital capacity and the fraction delivered in 1, 2, and 3 sec (depending on the time setting).[23] This apparatus is much less expensive than improved spirometers, occupies little space, and is suitable for office as well as hospital determinations.

NORMAL VALUES. Thirty-five young, normal individuals were able to deliver a mean value of 82.7 percent of the vital capacity in the first second of expiration. The lowest value recorded was 72 percent in the first second.[23] The test is highly reproducible in normal subjects. There is an apparent reduction in the older age groups. Pemberton[24] found a mean value of 79.1 ± 7.2 percent for the 1-sec vital capacity in 428 men ranging in age from 40 to 88, which means that the lower limit of normal for 95 percent of this age range is 64.7 percent.

INTERPRETATIONS AND LIMITATIONS. (1) A normal vital capacity, over 83 percent of which is expired in the first second of expiration, indicates normal ventilatory apparatus. Dyspnea on a pulmonary basis is highly unlikely and the MBC can usually be predicted to be normal. This does not apply to the dyspnea of heart failure or the diffusion block syndrome.

(2) Patients with a restrictive ventilatory insufficiency (reduced lung volume) are still capable of delivering the normal timed fractions in the absence of obstruction to air flow. If lung volume is greatly reduced, however, reduction in stroke volume used during the MBC occurs, and the MBC may be reduced.

(3) A reduced TVC (less than 75 percent of vital capacity in the first second) indicates obstruction to air flow, the commonest causes of which are obstructive emphysema and bronchial asthma. A reduced TVC correlates well with reduction in MBC when the latter is due to obstruction to air flow ("obstructive ventilatory defect").

(4) Administration of bronchodilator drugs will result in an improved TVC in the presence of reversible obstructive ventilatory defects.

Thus, with a single maneuver, one can determine the presence or absence of restrictive (total vital capacity) or obstructive ventilatory defects (timed vital capacity). The apparatus is inexpensive by comparison with other ventilatory-function equipment. The test is easily carried out and can be used as a highly reliable screening procedure. It is one of the simplest and most useful tests for the detection of *early* obstructive emphysema.[25]

ANALYSIS OF THE SPIROGRAPH TRACING

Examination of the form of the spirogram can yield useful information. A summary of the possible information obtainable follows.

(1) Air trapping is characteristic of obstructive respiratory diseases (asthma, obstructive emphysema). Its presence is detected by: (*a*) alteration of the end-expiratory base line upward with performance of the MBC,[26] the base line normally being unchanged during the MBC from its resting level; (*b*) inability to return immediately to the end-expiratory base line after performance of the inspiratory-capacity test, with a steplike return to the base line over several respiratory cycles; and (*c*) the discrepancy between the expiratory reserve volume measured alone from the resting end-expiratory level and that determined as part of the vital capacity delivered as a single maneuver. Christie's paper[27] con-

tains excellent graphic examples of the last two phenomena.

(2) So-called "respiratory neuroses" can be detected easily.[16, 27] Patients with anxiety neuroses may display an irregular, shallow type of respiration, with frequent changes in resting end-expiratory position.[27] Subjects with conversion hysteria are noted for their frequent deep, sighing respirations, and, in severe cases, may hyperventilate to the point of alkalotic tetany during their initial experience with spirometry. It must be remembered that transient hyperventilation occurs in the patient anxious about his diagnosis and fearful of the strange apparatus used in pulmonary-function tests. Reassurance and repeated efforts will smooth out the irregular tracing of the (justifiably) nervous individual.

(3) Determinations of expiratory flow rate give much the same information as the TVC, but are probably more accurate in detecting subtle changes.[28] The time required to expire the middle 50 percent of a fast vital capacity maneuver is measured. Mean flow-rate values of 4.5 L/sec in men and 3.7 L/sec in women have been obtained.[28] Normally, the flow rate should be greater than 100 L/min. Values less than this indicate obstruction to air flow.

## Arterial-Blood Studies

### PRINCIPLES

Assessment of respiratory function is not complete without a determination of the end result of the various processes that constitute the primary function of the lung, namely the oxygenation of venous blood and the elimination of its carbon dioxide. This necessitates gas analysis of arterial blood.

### METHOD

#### OBTAINING THE ARTERIAL-BLOOD SAMPLE

Although the radial or the femoral artery can be used, the brachial artery is preferable. It is easier to puncture than the radial, and more convenient than the femoral artery. Riley or Cournand needles are provided with a blunt stylet to insert in the needle so that it may be left in place once the artery has been entered, permitting multiple samples to be drawn.

Complications of arterial puncture are almost unheard of except for occasional formation of a small hematoma. Occasionally, minor degrees of arteriospasm give rise to transient paresthesias in the hand. The site of puncture may be tender for a day or two following the procedure. Conceivably, arteriovenous fistula, tearing of the vessel, and bacterial endarteritis could occur, but the author is not aware of any reports of such results. Upon withdrawal of the needle, enough pressure to obliterate the radial pulse is applied over the puncture site for at least 3 and preferably 5 min.

### ANALYSIS OF THE BLOOD GASES

PRINCIPLE. Blood gases are freed by hemolysis and vacuum extraction. The gases thus liberated are then measured at the same volume as specific reagents are added to absorb the gases separately. The change in pressure as each gas is absorbed is proportional to the volume the gas occupied. The original method as described in 1924 by Van Slyke and Neill [29] is essentially unchanged today, and the interested reader should consult the original paper for details of technique. The determination can be extremely accurate. Duplicate analyses on a 1-ml sample of blood should agree within 0.2 volume percent for both oxygen and carbon dioxide.

OXYHEMOGLOBIN SATURATION. The equation for the saturation of hemoglobin with oxygen is

$$\text{Oxyhemoglobin saturation (percent)} = \frac{O_2 \text{ content (vol. percent)}}{O_2 \text{ capacity (vol. percent)}} \times 100.$$

Until relatively recently, the normal oxyhemoglobin saturation was considered to be 95 percent (range 93–97 percent). Roughton [30] pointed out that this figure was falsely low owing to errors in the determination of the oxygen capacity. If the original technique of Van Slyke and Neill is used, in which blood is rotated for 15 min in a tonometer exposed to room air and ambient temperature, the final oxygen capacity will be falsely high (resulting in lower saturation) because of evaporation of water vapor, conversion in vitro of met- and carboxyhemoglobin to hemoglobin, and failure to correct properly for the amount of dissolved oxygen in the plasma.

Correcting for all three of these variables results in a normal mean saturation of 97 percent. [30] The most accurate method, using spectrophotometric determination, gives a normal saturation of 98.6 percent, with a very narrow range of 98.0–99.3 percent. [31] One has to determine for oneself what to consider normal values from one's own laboratory. If none of the above factors are taken into account, and the errors are consistent, then "normal" oxyhemoglobin saturation will be 95 percent, with a range of 93–97 percent.

It should be noted that one cannot use the resting oxygen-capacity value for the determination of saturation during exercise. Because of hemoconcentration during exercise, a new capacity must be determined for exercise values. With the breathing of 100-percent oxygen for 15 min, one should subtract 2.04 volume percent from the oxyhemoglobin content determination to correct for dissolved oxygen.

ARTERIAL CARBON DIOXIDE CONTENT. Whole-blood carbon dioxide is determined along with oxygen on a 1-ml sample of blood with the Van Slyke manometric apparatus [29] (see Unit 21). If the pH, the oxygen capacity, and the hematocrit are known, suitable nomograms can be used to read off the carbon dioxide content of the plasma and the carbon dioxide pressure. The carbon dioxide content can be obtained directly by centrifuging blood to obtain plasma. [32]

DETERMINATION OF PH. The pH of the blood is determined by means of a closed glass electrode whose voltage output at a given temperature and pH is read directly from the scale of the pH meter. The glass electrode consists of a thin membrane of soft glass that is permeable to hydrogen ions. The potential difference across this membrane is a function of the difference in hydrogen-ion concentration between the serum, which is in contact with one surface, and a solution of standard hydrogen-ion concentration on the opposite side. The potential difference is amplified and measured with a potentiometer calibrated to read directly in pH units. pH meters tend to drift and must be standardized with a buffered solution of known pH immediately prior to use. Blood is introduced into the electrode with only momentary contact with air and the pH is read within a minute, as soon as the reading is stable. Readings are recorded to the nearest $\frac{1}{100}$ of a pH unit. If the electrode is not surrounded by a constant-temperature water jacket, readings of pH must be corrected to body temperature from the (room) temperature at which they are recorded by subtracting 0.014 pH units/C deg of difference. [33]

There are many difficulties in the accurate determination of the pH of the blood. [34] These are all of sufficient magnitude to be of practical importance in evaluating clinical disorders of acid-base balance (Unit 21) and are especially important when knowledge of carbon dioxide pressure is required, since an error of 0.02 pH units results in an error of 1.8 mm Hg in the calculated carbon dioxide pressure. [34] The pH of venous blood is usually 0.02 to 0.04 pH units lower than arterial or "arterialized" blood. Heparin may be used if an anticoagulant is desired. Oxalate and fluoride cannot be used since they lower the pK of bicarbonate. The glycolytic enzymes of blood cells produce lactic acid which causes rapid lowering of pH on standing. pH determinations should therefore be done *within 10 min* after the blood is drawn. Correction for the change due to glycolysis over this period can be made, if desired, by adding 0.001 pH unit per minute of elapsed time.[34] With longer periods of standing, the error due to glycolysis is variable and the correction uncertain. Placing the sample in ice partially inhibits glycolysis and is satisfactory for most clinical purposes if a delay of up to an hour is unavoidable. However, when calculation of the carbon dioxide pressure is required, rapid measurement of pH with correction for glycolysis is preferable. Loss of carbon dioxide from the sample, resulting in increasing alkalinity, is prevented by keeping the blood in the capped syringe into which it was drawn. Various other difficulties inherent in the method may also lead to inaccuracies.[34]

DETERMINATION OF THE CARBON DIOXIDE PRESSURE OF THE BLOOD. The pressure of carbon dioxide in the arterial blood may be determined directly by the bubble-equilibration technique of Riley, but, despite improvements in method,[35] the indirect calculation of the pressure of carbon dioxide from a nomogram based on the Henderson-Hasselbach equation remains as accurate a method as is available at the present time. The three unknowns of the Henderson-Hasselbach equation are: the pH of the blood, pressure of carbon dioxide in the blood, and the plasma bicarbonate concentration. If two of these are known, the third may be calculated. The nomogram of Van Slyke and Sendroy[36] expresses this relation and allows the pressure of carbon dioxide to be read off without the need for calculation (see Fig. 56). An error of 0.02 unit in the pH reading results in an error of approximately 1.8 mm Hg in the calculation of the carbon dioxide pressure.

## NORMAL VALUES FOR ARTERIAL-BLOOD GASES

Table 95 presents averages of mean determinations and the ranges represent the highest and lowest figures reported. The ranges given in the table represent the limits of normal for 95 percent of the population.

ARTERIAL OXYHEMOGLOBIN SATURATION. The normal range has been discussed above. The saturation is lower in elderly individuals without apparent abnormality of the cardiopulmonary system. Tenney[8] reports a range of 87–94 percent in 18 normal male subjects varying in age from 68 to 89. Others[38] have reported the saturation lower by 1–2 percent when compared with young adults.

Saturation does not change with moderate exercise, but may decrease by 1–2 percent with the severest exertion.[36] It rises to 100 percent with oxygen breathing. It may increase by 1 or 2 percent with voluntary hyperventilation.

FACTORS INFLUENCING PH AND CARBON DIOXIDE CONTENT AND PRESSURE IN ARTERIAL BLOOD. Variations within the entire range of pH and carbon dioxide content and pressure in arterial blood occur in some individuals, whereas others show little fluctuation.[39]

The pressure of carbon dioxide in arterial blood should not be considered static, with a normal value of 40 mm Hg. It is determined by the ratio of carbon dioxide production to alveolar ventilation and can change immediately with changes in either one of these variables. A variety of conditions result in normal fluctuations over a wide range.[40] Thus, it increases with sleep (to as much as 52 mm Hg)[41] and breath-holding, and rises postprandially. It is decreased by about 4 mm Hg premenstrually, being highest in women at the time of ovulation.[42] It

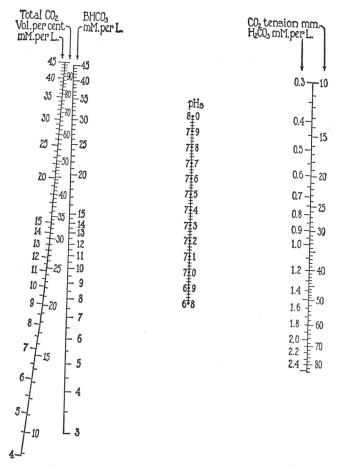

Fig. 56. Nomogram of Van Slyke and Sendroy,[36] based on the Henderson-Hasselbach equation for the graphic calculation of the blood carbon dioxide pressure.

decreases by an average of 5 mm Hg with change in posture from supine to standing.[40] It decreases with severe exercise.[43] It can be reduced by about 20 to 25 mm Hg with a short period of voluntary hyperventilation.[44] It decreases with

Table 95. *Arterial blood (brachial artery) adult values.*[36]

| Characteristic | Mean | Range |
|---|---|---|
| Oxygen— | | |
| pressure (mm Hg) | 95.2 | 80–104.0 |
| content (vol. percent) | 19.4 | 17.3–22.3 |
| capacity (vol. percent) | 20.2 | 16.8–23.1 |
| saturation (percent) | 96.4 | 90.5–101.0 |
| pH | 7.426 | 7.37–7.49 |
| Carbon dioxide— | | |
| pressure (mm Hg) | 41.0 | 35.0–47.0 |
| content (vol. percent) | 48.9 | 42.8–57.1 |

anxiety, in proportion to the degree of increased ventilation—an important consideration when drawing blood samples. It increases as a manifestation of the attempted respiratory compensation for metabolic alkalosis (hypoventilation) and a decrease in metabolic acidosis (hyperventilation or Kussmaul breathing). These fluctuations must be kept securely in mind when evaluating the results of arterial blood studies in cardiopulmonary diseases.

### Exercise Tests

PRINCIPLE. By subjecting the patient to the stress of mild exercise, the integrated behavior of the cardiopulmonary system can be evaluated under conditions which simulate the usual activities of everyday living such as walking and stair-climbing. During exercise, the increased oxygen requirement and carbon dioxide production of the muscles necessitate increased alveolar ventilation. Increased oxygen consumption is achieved in part by increased diffusion of oxygen from alveoli to pulmonary capillary blood and augmentation of cardiac output. The many factors involved in the cardiopulmonary adjustments to the demands of exercise are still not completely elucidated,[43] but for practical purposes it is sufficient to realize that inability to increase ventilation and oxygen consumption in proportion to the increase in work will be reflected in abnormalities of the blood gases. Thus exercise, by creating a stress on the respiratory apparatus, allows objective as well as subjective evaluation of disability (manifested by dyspnea and fatigue). There may be accompanying deviations in the blood gases from pre-exercise levels.

METHOD. For clinical purposes, the step test [4] is used most commonly; it consists of stepping up and down on a platform 20 cm high, 30 times over a period of 1 min. An arterial blood sample is drawn through the indwelling arterial needle at the end of 1 min for analysis of its oxygen saturation, carbon dioxide content, and pH. An even simpler method is to have the patient in the supine position perform straight leg-raising at the rate of 60 times/min for 2 min. Blood is drawn at the end of this time while the subject continues the exercise until the sample is obtained. This usually requires 30 sec to 1 min. Determination of oxygen consumption, ventilation, gas-exchange ratio, oxygen debt, and ventilatory equivalent during and after the exercise are probably not worth the effort expended.

During these maneuvers, the patient should be carefully observed for objective evidence of dyspnea (distress; labored, heaving respiration), and his subjective sensations should be noted as well.

INTERPRETATIONS AND LIMITATIONS. The main disadvantages of the step test (or leg-raising) are that the duration of the test prevents the development of the steady state, and the mild degree of exercise is not sufficient for the detection of abnormalities except in those obviously handicapped by cardiopulmonary disease.[4]

The main advantages of the exercise tests described are that no special equipment, such as a treadmill or a stationary bicycle, is needed, and the duration and mildness of the exercise makes it suitable for most patients, except those who are completely bedridden, in whom the test would serve no useful purpose anyway.[4]

In normal individuals, there is no change in arterial oxygen saturation or carbon dioxide pressure with mild to moderate exercise. Desaturation of arterial blood upon mild exercise in patients with chronic pulmonary disease is considered a sign of far-advanced disease.[4] Desaturation (or increased unsaturation from control values) of arterial blood with exercise can occur in the following situations:

(a) In the presence of anatomic shunts (right-to-left intracardiac shunts, pulmonary hemangioma) the saturation decreases for two reasons: (i) the volume of unsaturated mixed venous blood flowing through the shunt may increase during exercise, and (ii) the shunted venous blood contains less oxygen than at rest because of increased extraction of oxygen by exercising muscles.

(b) For the same reasons, pulmonary diseases associated with "physiologic shunting" (hypoventilated alveoli—those with ventilation reduced out of proportion to blood flow) frequently show a drop in saturation with exercise (emphysema). When demonstrated, this is usually a sign of far-advanced disease.

(*c*) Any process that limits the ventilatory response to exercise may result in a state of hypoventilation relative to the increased demands of work, and desaturation will occur. Obstructive pulmonary disease (bronchial asthma, obstructive emphysema), afflictions of the neuromuscular apparatus of the chest (poliomyelitis and myasthenia gravis), and thoracic deformity (kyphoscoliosis) are representative examples.

(*d*) Diseases with a primary reduction in oxygen-diffusing capacity of the lung ("alveolar-capillary block syndrome") are characterized by the presence of normal saturation at rest which falls precipitously with mild exertion. The block to the diffusion of oxygen is demonstrated by creating an increased need for oxygen with exercise.

(*e*) Occasionally, oxyhemoglobin saturation may *increase* from an abnormal level during mild exercise in patients with pulmonary disease. This has been noted in bronchiectasis and obstructive emphysema. Presumably, the hyperinflated state of the lung during exercise promotes increased ventilation of poorly ventilated areas by increase in diameter of the obstructed airways.

## Causes of Decreased Arterial Oxygen Saturation in Cardiopulmonary Disease

Clinically, a diminished arterial oxygen saturation is detected as cyanosis. When the arterial oxygen saturation is decreased to the extent that most observers would agree on its presence, it is usually around 80 percent or below.[45] Thus, to detect slight to moderate degrees of hypoxemia, arterial blood must be analyzed (or an ear oximeter used). Indeed, this is the only way to discover mild degrees of unsaturation early in the course of pulmonary disease.

Although the magnitude of unsaturation is directly related to the magnitude of the defect causing it, there is a poor correlation between the degree of unsaturation and the amount of disability associated with it. Thus, the patient with "cyanotic" congenital heart disease may be relatively comfortable with a saturation of 80 percent, whereas the patient with emphysema may obtain a near-normal arterial saturation but only at the expense of a near-maximal amount of respiratory work. He is thus incapacitated for any activity greater than rest, being unable to increase his ventilation any further. He is using his entire breathing reserve to maintain near-normal blood gases.

There are four general causes of abnormality in arterial oxygen saturation and carbon dioxide pressure in cardiopulmonary disease (see Table 96).

UNEVEN VENTILATION-PERFUSION RELATION. Any process that causes uneven distribution of inspired air will lead to a decrease in the amount of oxygen the arterial blood carries away from the lung, provided the blood flow to the poorly ventilated areas is always relatively greater in amount than ventilation (or is not reduced proportionally). Blood perfusing these poorly aerated or "hypoventilated" areas extracts insufficient oxygen and rids itself of little carbon dioxide, and is mixed with blood from well-ventilated alveoli in the pulmonary veins. This is called the "venous-admixture" effect.[10] It always results in hypoxemia and ultimately with increasing abnormality in carbon dioxide retention. Early in the course of chronic pulmonary disease, hyperventilation of relatively normal areas of lung is able to maintain a normal carbon dioxide pressure but unable to add sufficient oxygen to pulmonary capillary blood to achieve normal saturation. This is explainable by the difference in the dissociation curves for oxygen and carbon dioxide.[10] Diseases associated with poor ventilation of well-perfused areas of lung are those which lead to uneven distribution of inspired air, such as bronchial asthma or

Table 96. *Causes of cyanosis and the alterations in the blood gas pressures in pulmonary disease.*

| Cause of cyanosis | Example | Rest [a] | | Exercise [b] | | Hyper-ventilation [c] | | Breathing pure O₂ [d] | |
|---|---|---|---|---|---|---|---|---|---|
| | | $P(O_2)$ | $P(CO_2)$ | $P(O_2)$ | $P(CO_2)$ | $P(O_2)$ | $P(CO_2)$ | O₂ saturation (percent) | $P(CO_2)$ |
| Normal | | → | | → | | ↑ +23 mm Hg | ↓ −20 mm Hg | 100 | → |
| Decreased ventilation-to-perfusion ratio | Emphysema: Mod. severe | → or ↓ | → | → or ↑ | → | Mod. ↑ | Mod. ↓ | 100 | → |
| | Severe | ↓ ↓ | ↑ | ↓ ↓ ↓ | ↑ ↑ | → or ↓ | → or ↑ | 100 | may ↑ |
| Impairment of diffusion | Beryllium poisoning | → | → or ↓ | ↓ ↓ ↓ | ↓ | → | ↓ | 100 | → |
| Alveolar hypoventilation (primary) | Morphine poisoning | ↓ | ↑ | Depends on etiology | | Depends on etiology | | 100 | → or ↑ |
| Veno-arterial shunts | Pulmonary hemangioma | ↓ | → | ↓ ↓ | → | → | ↓ | <100 | → |

$P(O_2)$, $P(CO_2)$ = partial pressure of blood gases; ↑ = increase; ↓ = decrease; → = normal or no change. The oxygen pressure and oxyhemoglobin saturation vary in the same direction. The oxygen pressure determination is a more sensitive indication of altered blood gas on the flat portion of the oxygen dissociation curve.

[a] Rest: sufficient time should be allowed to allay the initial anxiety and consequent hyperventilation attendant upon arterial puncture.

[b] Exercise: 30-step test [4] or straight leg raising with sample drawn when dyspnea first noted or experienced, or for 2 min.

[c] Hyperventilation: 30 sec to 1 min of maximal voluntary overbreathing. Sample then drawn with subject continuing hyperventilation until sample obtained.

[d] Breathing pure oxygen: patient breathes for 15 min. Patients with chronic carbon dioxide retention must be watched closely for signs of decreasing ventilation. The saturation will reach 105 to 108 percent in normal individuals. Subtraction of dissolved oxygen (2.04 vol. percent) from content as determined gives the true value for oxyhemoglobin saturation.

obstructive emphysema. The behavior of the blood gases under various conditions is outlined in Table 96.

ALVEOLAR HYPOVENTILATION. Any process that results in an uncompensated decrease in tidal volume or respiratory rate, or an increase in dead space, will result in alveolar hypoventilation which leads to hypoxemia and hypercapnia. Determination of the arterial carbon dioxide pressure is the most sensitive indicator of small changes in alveolar ventilation because, owing to the character of the oxygen dissociation curve, small changes in ventilation are not reflected by changes in oxygen saturation. The commonest causes of alveolar hypoventilation are: (1) depression of the respiratory center's responsiveness to the arterial pressure of carbon dioxide by anesthetic agents, morphine, and barbiturate intoxication, and head injury with or without increased intracranial pressure; (2) neuromuscular-skeletal disease or defect where the ventilatory apparatus is incapable of providing sufficient alveolar ventilation (poliomyelitis, myasthenia gravis, crushed chest injury, thoracic deformities), and (3) pulmonary diseases that reduce functioning lung tissue severely (bilateral pleural effusion), or so increase the work of breathing that normal alveolar ventilation is impossible (obstructive emphysema). Recently, "idiopathic" alveolar hypoventilation has been described in patients, many of whom are massively obese, who hypoventilate chronically without demonstrable cause.[46] Oxygen therapy will increase the oxygen saturation to normal in patients with alveolar hypoventilation, but will not rid the blood of carbon dioxide, which can be accomplished only by increasing alveolar ventilation. This may necessitate artificial respiration.

DIMINISHED DIFFUSION OF OXYGEN. A number of diseases with diffuse pulmonary involvement have been described whose primary effect on pulmonary function

may be a block to the diffusion of oxygen across the alveolar-capillary septae —the "alveolar-capillary block" syndrome.[47, 48] These include sarcoidosis and other diffuse granulomatous disease of unknown etiology, scleroderma, beryllosis, asbestosis, the Hamman-Rich syndrome (progressive interstitial fibrosis), miliary tuberculosis, pulmonary lymphangitic carcinomatosis, histiocytosis X, and sulfur dioxide poisoning. The arterial blood picture is characteristic. The ar-

Table 97. *Physiologic patterns of pulmonary insufficiency.*

| Pattern | Type of disturbance | Chief symptom | Example | Pulmonary-function changes |
|---|---|---|---|---|
| **Ventilatory** | | | | |
| Restrictive | Reduction in functioning lung tissue | Dyspnea | Pleural fibrosis | Reduced vital capacity |
| Obstructive | Obstruction to air flow in bronchial tree | Dyspnea | Bronchial asthma | Reduced MBC and TVC |
| **Alveolar-respiratory (respiratory gas exchange)** | | | | |
| Ventilation-perfusion abnormalities in pure form (distribution defect) | | | | |
| Increased dead-space ventilation | Ventilation of poorly perfused lung tissue | Dyspnea | Lung cyst freely communicating with bronchial tree | Hyperventilation at rest; increased ventilatory equivalent; characteristic x-ray picture |
| Increased venous admixture | Shunting of venous blood from right to left, bypassing alveolar surfaces | Cyanosis and effects of secondary polycythemia | Pulmonary hemangioma | Arterial blood studies under various conditions (Table 96) |
| Diffusion defect (primary) | Decrease in oxygen diffusing capacity | Dyspnea and cyanosis with exertion | Pulmonary beryllosis | Decreased vital capacity, normal MBC, increased minute ventilation and characteristics of arterial blood (Table 96) |
| Combined ventilatory and alveolar-respiratory insufficiency | Nonspecific fibrosis of lung parenchyma, obstruction to air flow, and obliteration of pulmonary capillary bed | Dyspnea; cyanosis and cor pulmonale in severe cases | Obstructive emphysema and fibrotic processes usually localizing at level of respiratory bronchiole | Decreased vital capacity, reduced MBC and TVC; hypoxemia and respiratory acidosis in severe cases |

Table 98. *Changes in and uses of pulmonary-function tests in various conditions.*

| Condition | VC | TVC | MBC | Arterial blood | Use of pulmonary-function tests |
|---|---|---|---|---|---|
| Obstructive emphysema | Decreased | Decreased | Decreased | Early, no changes in blood gases; later, mild hypoxemia, and finally, obvious unsaturation (cyanosis) and respiratory acidosis | 1. Obstruction of air flow must be demonstrated (TVC) to justify diagnosis<br>2. Reduction in MBC correlates well with degree of dyspnea and disability<br>3. Use MBC and TVC to follow course and evaluate therapy<br>4. Use TVC to quantify obstructive defect potentially reversible with bronchodilator therapy<br>5. Arterial blood gases and pH to define immediate status of patient, e.g., hypoventilation, acute respiratory acidosis |
| Bronchial asthma | Decreased | Decreased | Decreased | Blood gases usually normally maintained except for occasional mild oxyhemoglobin unsaturation. In status asthmaticus, alveolar hypoventilation may occur with respiratory acidosis | 1. Assessment of bronchodilator and steroid therapy by noting increase in VC, MBC, and/or TVC; TVC and maximal mid-expiratory flow rate determination are simplest<br>2. Measure arterial $P(CO_2)$ in acute asthma and status asthmaticus to detect onset of alveolar hypoventilation<br>3. Deterioration of MBC and TVC and changes in blood gases may indicate development of irreversible obstructive emphysema |
| Heart failure and mitral stenosis | Decreased | Normal unless cardiac asthma present | Decreased but not to same degree as in obstructive respiratory disease | Variable changes in oxyhemoglobin saturation—may be surprisingly severe unsaturation or normal saturation. Normal $P(CO_2)$; occasionally respiratory alkalosis may exist | 1. Vital capacity reduction correlates best with dyspnea and disability in heart disease as compared with MBC in pulmonary disease<br>2. Evaluate therapy and chart course and degree of compensation with serial VC determination<br>3. Arterial $P(CO_2)$ may be normal or low, with heart failure in contradistinction to respiratory acidosis in primary obstructive lung disease; this may be a differential point |

| Condition | | | | | Comments |
|---|---|---|---|---|---|
| Respiratory muscle paralysis (e.g., poliomyelitis) | Decreased | Normal | Decreased (hazardous to perform) | With acute anxiety, respiratory alkalosis; with progression of the disease, respiratory acidosis and hypoxemia | 1. Reduction in VC parallels severity of respiratory-muscle paralysis 2. Arterial $P(CO_2)$ to determine level of alveolar ventilation during acute and convalescent stage 3. When VC falls to 50 percent of predicted, give trial in respirator; when less than 33 percent of predicted, more extensive use of respirator |
| Alveolar-capillary (diffusion) block syndrome | Decreased | Normal | Normal or slightly reduced | Normal or near normal saturation at rest; drops precipitously with exercise; $P(CO_2)$ normal or low (respiratory alkalosis) | 1. Evaluate therapy by serial determinations of minute ventilation, ventilatory equivalent, vital capacity, and arterial blood gas changes with exercise |
| Idiopathic alveolar hypoventilation (Pickwickian syndrome) | Decreased (particularly expiratory reserve volume) | Normal | Normal or reduced slightly | Increased $P(CO_2)$ diagnoses hypoventilation with certainty | 1. Follow arterial blood $P(CO_2)$, tidal volume, and minute ventilation to detect change in alveolar ventilation with therapy (e.g., weight reduction) |
| Polycythemia vera | Normal | Normal | Normal | Normal blood gases although saturation may be at lowest limits of normal e.g., 90 percent | 1. To differentiate primary from secondary polycythemia, do arterial blood studies and simple pulmonary-function tests |
| Pneumonectomy | Reduced to ½ normal | Normal unless obstructive emphysema is present or develops postoperatively | Reduction is less than that seen in VC—usually 60–70 percent of normal predicted for two lungs | Normal if remaining lung normal | 1. MBC best for preoperative assessment; value less than 40 L/min indicates poor operative risk and possibility of dyspnea postoperatively 2. Reduction in TVC postoperatively may indicate development of obstructive emphysema in remaining lung |
| Pregnancy | Normal (loss of expiratory reserve volume equaled by increase in inspiratory capacity) | Normal | Normal | Normal | 1. Serial determination of vital capacity to follow state of compensation in cardiac conditions 2. Increase in minute ventilation (plus 40 percent of control values) may lead to dyspnea during pregnancy in patients with pulmonary disease; MBC and VC normally maintained |

terial oxygen saturation is usually within normal limits at rest until the terminal stages of the disease. The arterial carbon dioxide pressure is normal or low. With even mild exercise, the oxygen saturation drops precipitously and the carbon dioxide pressure may be further reduced (respiratory alkalosis). With 100-percent oxygen breathing at rest, the oxygen saturation reaches 100 percent. These characteristics, coupled with the findings of tachypnea at rest and marked hyperventilation on exercise, an increased ventilatory equivalent, reduction in vital capacity, and a normal or near-normal MBC in the face of distressing dyspnea with the slightest exertion, allow a strong presumptive diagnosis of the diffusion-block syndrome to be made.

ANATOMIC SHUNTS. Intrapulmonic, venoarterial shunts (pulmonary hemangioma or arteriovenous fistula) and intracardiac "right-to-left" shunts (tetralogy of Fallot, or reversal of flow with atrial septal defect) present a characteristic picture. The carbon dioxide pressure is usually within normal limits because the respiratory apparatus is still capable of increasing alveolar ventilation to eliminate the shunted, venous carbon dioxide. With exercise, the saturation decreases further because less oxygen is carried in the venous blood owing to increased oxygen transfer in the muscles. Therefore, the venous-admixture effect is increased. A greater volume of blood may also be shunted during exercise, owing to intravascular and intracardiac pressure changes. Breathing 100-percent oxygen fails to achieve 100-percent saturation and is a key difference in helping to distinguish the decreased saturation of anatomic shunting from that due to the other causes listed in Table 96.

MIXED DEFECT. It should be noted that combinations of the defects described above frequently exist in the same pa-

tient. In severe obstructive emphysema, there may be a diffusion defect secondary to reduction in vascular bed in addition to altered ventilation-perfusion relation and alveolar hypoventilation. In scleroderma with a primary diffusion defect, heart failure may be superimposed owing to cardiac involvement by the disease. This will result in further alterations in the blood gases. It is useful to remember that oxygen unsaturation of arterial blood at rest is due to the venous-admixture effect of blood from poorly ventilated areas of lung in the absence of anatomic shunts or obvious hypoventilation. It is not usually due to diffusion defect, where unsaturation is characteristically precipitated by exercise. The simple tests available to the clinician do not always allow the separation or quantitation of these defects. Marshaling all the clinical information available, however, will frequently allow one to make valid assumptions as to the nature of the underlying disease.

### Abnormal Physiology in Pulmonary Disease

Many investigators follow the categorization of physiologic defects in pulmonary disease as developed by Cournand.[4, 18] This is presented in Table 97 with certain additions and modifications. One should not be misled by this table into thinking that all forms of pulmonary insufficiency group themselves into isolated physiologic defects. Indeed, one of the commonest chronically disabling pulmonary diseases—obstructive emphysema—is characterized by ventilatory and alveolar-respiratory insufficiency. Also, certain diseases may present with pure ventilatory defect, but with progression of the disease or superimposition of recurrent respiratory infections the pattern of alveolar-respiratory insufficiency will be added. Pure alveolar-respiratory insufficiency probably never exists. Even in the alveolar-capillary block syndrome there is usually an associated restrictive ventilatory defect.

Changes in vital capacity, timed vital capacity, maximal breathing capacity, and arterial blood gases have been listed in Table 98 in various diseases and conditions affecting the respiratory apparatus. Some of the uses of these simple, readily available determinations are listed in the last column.

## REFERENCES

1. J. H. Knowles, *Respiratory Physiology and Its Clinical Application* (Harvard University Press, Cambridge, 1959).
2. J. H. Comroe, Jr., "Pulmonary function tests" in J. H. Comroe, Jr., ed. *Methods in Medical Research* (Year Book Publishers, Chicago, 1950), vol. 2, p. 74.
3. J. H. Comroe, Jr., R. E. Forster, A. G. DuBois, W. A. Briscoe, and E. Carlsen, *The Lung. Clinical Physiology and Pulmonary Function Tests* (Year Book Publishers, Chicago, 1955).
4. E. de F. Baldwin, A. Cournand, and D. W. Richards, Jr., "Pulmonary insufficiency; physiological classification, clinical methods of analysis, standard values in normal subjects," *Medicine* 27, 243 (1948).
5. J. S. Gray, *Pulmonary Ventilation and Its Physiological Regulation* (American Lecture Series 63; Thomas, Springfield, 1950).
6. E. A. Gaensler and I. Lindgren, "Open circuit techniques for the measurement of ventilation. A review," *Scand. J. clin. lab. Invest.* (Supplement 20), 7, 19 (1955).
7. H. W. Matheson and J. S. Gray, "Ventilatory function tests. III. Resting ventilation, metabolism and derived measures," *J. clin. Invest.* 29, 688 (1950).
8. S. M. Tenney and R. M. Miller, "Dead space ventilation in old age," *J. appl. Physiol.* 9, 321 (1956).
9. P. H. Rossier and A. Bühlmann, "The respiratory dead space," *Physiol. Rev.* 35, 860 (1955).
10. R. L. Riley and A. Cournand, "'Ideal' alveolar air and the analysis of ventilation-perfusion relationships in the lungs," *J. appl. Physiol.* 1, 825 (1949).
11. H. W. Knipping and A. Moncrieff, "The ventilatory equivalent for oxygen," *Quart. J. Med.* 1, 17 (1932).
12. D. W. Cugell, N. R. Frank, E. A. Gaensler, and T. L. Badger, "Pulmonary function in pregnancy. I. Serial observations in normal women," *Amer. Rev. Tuberc.* 67, 568 (1953).
13. B. C. Ferris, J. L. Whittenberger, J. R. Gallagher, and C. W. Smith, "Maximum breathing capacity and vital capacity in male and female children and adolescents," *Pediatrics* 9, 659 (1952); 12, 341 (1953).
14. R. J. Shephard, "Some factors affecting the open-circuit determination of maximum breathing capacity," *J. Physiol.* 135, 98 (1957).
15. L. Bernstein and D. Mendel, "The accuracy of spirographic recording at high respiratory rates," *Thorax* 6, 297 (1951).
16. A. Cournand, D. W. Richards, Jr., and R. D. Darling, "Graphic tracings of respiration in the study of pulmonary disease," *Amer. Rev. Tuberc.* 40, 487 (1939).
17. D. W. Richards, Jr., "The nature of cardiac and of pulmonary dyspnea," *Circulation* 7, 15 (1953).

18. A. Cournand and D. W. Richards, Jr., "Pulmonary insufficiency: I. Discussion of physiological classification and presentation of clinical tests," *Amer. Rev. Tuberc.* 44, 26 (1941).

19. J. Pappenheimer *et al.*, "Standardization of definitions and symbols in respiratory physiology," *Fed. Proc.* 9, 602 (1950).

20. H. Rahn, W. O. Fenn, and A. B. Otis, "Daily variations of vital capacity, residual air and expiratory reserve including a study of the residual air method," *J. appl. Physiol. 1*, 725 (1949).

21. A. G. W. Whitfield, J. A. H. Waterhouse, and W. M. Arnott, "The total lung volume and its subdivisions. A study in physiological norms. I. Basic data," *Brit. J. soc. Med. 4*, 1 (1950).

22. M. S. Segal, J. A. Herschfus, and M. J. Dulfano, "A simple method for the determination of vital capacity-time relationships," *Dis. Chest 22*, 123 (1952).

23. E. A. Gaensler, "Analysis of the ventilatory deficit by timed capacity measurements," *Amer. Rev. Tuberc. 64*, 256 (1951).

24. J. Pemberton and E. G. Flanagan, "Vital capacity and timed vital capacity in normal men over forty," *J. appl. Physiol. 9*, 291 (1956).

25. J. K. Curtis, H. K. Rasmussen, and J. T. Mendenhall, "Detection of early pulmonary emphysema," *Amer. Rev. Tuberc. 72*, 569 (1955).

26. R. V. Christie, "The elastic properties of the emphysematous lung and their clinical significance," *J. clin. Invest. 13*, 295 (1934).

27. R. V. Christie, "Some types of respiration in the neuroses," *Quart. J. Med. 4*, 427 (1935).

28. E. C. Leuallen and W. S. Fowler, "Maximal mid-expiratory flow," *Amer. Rev. Tuberc. 72*, 783 (1955).

29. D. D. Van Slyke and J. M. Neill, "Determination of gases in blood and other solutions by vacuum extraction and manometric measurements," *J. biol. Chem. 61*, 523 (1924).

30. F. J. W. Roughton, R. D. Darling, and W. S. Root, "Factors affecting the determination of oxygen capacity, content and pressure in human arterial blood," *Amer. J. Physiol. 142*, 708 (1944).

31. D. S. Drabkin and C. F. Schmidt, "Spectrophotometric studies; observation of circulating blood in vivo and the direct determination of the saturation of hemoglobin in arterial blood," *J. biol. Chem. 157*, 69 (1945).

32. R. B. Singer and A. B. Hastings, "Improved clinical method for estimation of disturbances of acid base balance of human blood," *Medicine 27*, 223 (1948).

33. T. B. Rosenthal, "Effect of temperature on pH of blood and plasma in vitro," *J. biol. Chem. 173*, 25 (1948).

34. J. W. Severinghaus, M. Stupfel, and A. F. Bradley, "Accuracy of blood pH and $pCO_2$ determinations," *J. appl. Physiol. 9*, 189 (1956).

35. G. L. Brinkman, C. J. Johns, H. Donoso, and R. L. Riley, "A modification of the method of Riley, Proemmel and Franke for determination of oxygen and carbon dioxide tension in blood," *J. appl. Physiol. 7*, 340 (1954).

36. D. D. Van Slyke and J. Sendroy, Jr., "Studies of gas and electrolyte equilibria in blood. XV. Line charts for graphic calculations by the Henderson-Hasselbach equation, and for calculating plasma $CO_2$ content from whole blood content," *J. biol. Chem. 79*, 781 (1928).

37. W. S. Spector, ed., *Handbook of Biological Data* (Saunders, Philadelphia, 1956), p. 272.

38. F. E. Greifenstein, R. M. King, S. S. Latch, and J. H. Comroe, Jr., "Pulmonary

function studies in healthy men and women 50 years and older," *J. appl. Physiol. 4,* 641 (1952).

39. N. W. Shock and A. B. Hastings, "Studies of acid-base balance of the blood in normal individuals," *J. biol. Chem. 104,* 585 (1934).

40. H. Rahn, "The sampling of alveolar gas," in W. M. Boothby, ed., *Handbook of Respiratory Physiology* (Air University, USAF School of Aviation Medicine, Randolph Field, Texas, 1954).

41. E. D. Robin, R. D. Whaley, C. H. Crump, and D. M. Travis, "The nature of the respiratory acidosis of sleep and of the respiratory alkalosis of hepatic coma" (abstract), *J. clin. Invest. 36,* 924 (1957).

42. R. L. Goodland and W. T. Pommerenke, "Cyclic fluctuations of the alveolar carbon dioxide tension during the normal menstrual cycle," *Fertil. and Steril. 3,* 394 (1952).

43. C. F. Schmidt, "The respiration," in P. Bard, ed., *Medical Physiology* (ed. 10; Mosby, St. Louis, 1956).

44. V. O. Bjork and H. J. Hilty, "The changes in the arterial oxygen and carbon dioxide tension during voluntary hyperventilation as a test of lung function," *J. thorac. Surg. 27,* 541 (1954).

45. J. H. Comroe, Jr., and S. Botelho, "The unreliability of cyanosis in the recognition of arterial anoxemia," *Amer. J. med. Sci. 214,* 1 (1947).

46. J. H. Auchincloss, Jr., and R. Gilbert, "The cardiorespiratory syndrome related to obesity: Clinical manifestations and pathologic physiology," *Progr. cardiovas. Dis. 1,* 423 (1959).

47. A. Cournand, "The syndrome of 'alveolar-capillary block.' Clinical, physiologic, pathologic, and therapeutic considerations," *Proc. roy. Coll. Phys. Surg. Canada 34* (1952).

48. R. Austrian, J. H. McClement, A. D. Renzetti, K. W. Donald, R. L. Riley, and A. Cournand, "Clinical and physiologic features of some types of pulmonary disease with impairment of alveolar-capillary diffusion. The syndrome of 'alveolar-capillary block,'" *Amer. J. Med. 11,* 667 (1951).

*Additional References for the Interested Reader*

K. W. Donald, "The definition and assessment of respiratory function," *Brit. med. J., 1,* 1068 (1953).

A. Cournand, "Cardiopulmonary function in chronic pulmonary disease," *Harvey Lect. 46,* 68 (1950–51).

L. J. Henderson, *Blood, A Study in General Physiology* (Yale University Press, New Haven, 1928).

J. C. Gilson and P. Hugh-Jones, *Lung Function in Coalworker's Pneumoconiosis* (Med. Res. Council, Special Report Series, No. 290; Her Majesty's Stationery Office, London, 1955).

A. L. Barach and H. A. Bickerman, eds., *Pulmonary Emphysema* (Williams and Wilkins, Baltimore, 1956).

J. L. Lilienthal and R. L. Riley, "Circulation through the lung and diffusion of gases," *Ann. Rev. Med. 5,* 237 (1954).

Seminars in pulmonary physiology, *Amer. J. Med. 10,* 77, 210, 356, 375, 481, 642, 719 (1951).

B. L. Gordon, ed., *Clinical Cardiopulmonary Physiology* (Grune and Stratton, New York, 1957).

# Index

Amino acids, contributions to nonprotein nitrogen, 345

Aminoaciduria, 318, 322–323

Ammonia: in blood, normal values, 5; excretion, in acid-base balance, 369; intoxication, 408; metabolism, 408; in urine, tests, 295; in urine, normal values, 9

Amphibian-spermiation tests, 489

Amylase: in ascitic fluid, 274; in urine, 437–438; pancreatic, 433; pancreatic, normal values after secretin stimulation, 439; serum, determination of, 435–436; serum, normal values, 5

Amyloidosis, Congo-red test for. See Congo-red test

Anaphylactoid purpura, 195

Androgen, physiology, 496–497

Anemia: and acute blood loss, 115–116; and anemic anoxia, 106–107; definition, 100, 108; etiologic classifications, 109; and examination of bone marrow, 91; functional classification, 110; in leukemia, 173; leukemoid reactions, 169; due to pyridoxine deficiency, 111; red-cell count in, 33–34; reticulocytosis in, 111

hemolytic, 138, 139; acid-serum reactions, 137–138; associated with methemoglobinemia and Heinz-body formation, 149–150; due to extrinsic defects of red cells, 140–149; due to intrinsic defects of red cells, 118–125; in porphyria, 330; tests, 116–118, 141–149

hypochromic, 108–111; osmotic fragility in, 123

iron-deficiency, 108–111

macrocytic, 112–114, 168

normocytic normochromic, 115

pernicious: gastric secretion in, 382; hemosiderin in bone marrow in, 95; leukopenia in, 168; pathologic physiology, 112; Schilling test, 113–114; see also Vitamin $B_{12}$, deficiency

sickle-cell: differentiation from sickle-cell trait, 132–133; pathologic physiology, 129, 131; tests, 131–132, 136; urine concentrating ability in, 354; variants, 133

Anergy, 457

Angiocardiography, 526, 529

Anisocytosis, 75, 76, 132; in iron-deficiency anemia, 109

Anisotropic droplets in urine sediment, 312

Anoxia: anoxic, 106; anemic, 106–107; histotoxic, 107–108; stagnant, 107; tissue, 106

Anterior urethritis, two-glass test in, 311

Antibiotics, effect on urobilinogen, 414

Antibodies: in blood groups, 219–224; complete, 217; immune, 217; in infants, 217; nature of, 216–217; in paroxysmal nocturnal hemoglobinuria, 136; production, 163; spontaneous, 216

incomplete, 217; detection with trypsinized cells, 146; see also Agglutinins, incomplete

Antibody titers, in infectious diseases, 453–457

Anticoagulants: choice for eosinophil count, 499; choice for erythrocyte sedimentation rate, 251; in collecting blood samples, 22–23; detection in blood stream, 197; effect on thromboplastin generation, 207; in hematocrit

determination, 54–55; preservative mixtures, 24; use in collecting fluid from serous effusions, 269; use in obtaining synovial fluid, 286

Antidiuretic hormone (ADH), 353, 358, 359, 365, 366

Antifibrinolysins in vitro, 201

Antigen-antibody reaction: in immunoelectrophoresis, 243; nature, 217–218

Antiglobulin test. See Coombs test

Antihemophilic factor (AHF), 188; normal values in plasma, 11; preparation for thromboplastin-generation studies, 205

Antihemophilic globulin. See Antihemophilic factor

Antisphering factor, 84

Antistreptolysin-O determination, 455

Antithrombins, 192

Antithromboplastin, 191, 192

Aortic-valve disease, cardiac catheterization, 528

Arterial puncture, 548

Arthritis, synovial fluid in, 287. See also Rheumatoid arthritis

Aschheim-Zondek test, 489

Ascites, pathologic physiology, 266, 268. See also Serous effusions

Ascitic fluid: amylase in, 274; bilirubin in, 274; characteristics in cirrhosis, 268; culture, 452; exudative type, causes, 268; protein content, 270. See also Chylous effusions

Ascorbic acid, normal values in blood, 5

Ascorbic acid load test, normal values, 14

Atrial pressure, 518

Atrial septal defect, sample calculation of shunt, 524

Autoagglutination, 141, 142, 231

Autoagglutinins in blood typing, 227

Ayer manometer, 279

Azobilirubin, 410

Bacteremia, 447

Bacteria in urine sediment, 318

*Bacteroides*, 448

Barium sulfate adsorption, of plasma, 198, 205

Basal metabolic rate (BMR), 481–482

Basket cells, 77

Basophilic stippling in Heinz-body anemias, 149

Basophils, properties, 176

Bauer-Aub diet, 508

Beer's law, 40, 47

Bence-Jones proteins, 246, 298, 299; analytic method for identification, 301–302; identification by electrophoresis of urine proteins, 302; pathologic physiology and clinical significance of, 300–301

Benedict-Roth spirometer, 537, 540

Benedict's qualitative test, 306, 308

Benedict's reaction, effect of phenolic acids on, 326

Benemid, effect on 17-ketosteroids, 501

Benzidine-nitroprusside stain, preparation and use with urine sediment, 312

Benzidine test for hemoglobinuria, 323. See also Hemoglobin

Beta-hydroxybutyric acid, 309, 472

Bial's test, 307

Sputum (*cont.*)
pneumonias, 461–462; preparation and staining of smears, 463–464
Stable factor. *See* Proconvertin
Standard deviation: calculation, 16; of differential white-cell count, 80–81; of duplicate determinations, 18; and frequency distribution, 4; for white-cell and red-cell counts, 20
*Staphylococcus albus,* 448
*Staphylococcus aureus,* 445, 448, 452; in stool, 450
Starvation, glucose-tolerance test in, 469
Statistical concepts, 16–17
Steatorrhea, 375, 379
Sternheimer-Malbin stain, 312, 314–315, 317
Sternum, aspiration of marrow from, 94
Stipple cells, 85
Stomal ulcer, 390
Stool: calcium in, 513; chemical tests for blood in, 377–378; culture of, 449–450; fat, 375, 378–379, 440; fat, normal values, 14; macroscopic examination and characteristics, 374–377; microscopic examination, 378–379; muscle fibers in, 379; nitrogen, normal values, 14; pancreatic enzymes in, 440; in pancreatic insufficiency, 440–441; physiology, 374–375
*Streptococcus,* beta hemolytic, 445, 446; anti-streptolysin-O titers and, 455
Stuart factor, 188–189; deficiency, test for, 209–210; normal values in plasma, 11; preparation for coagulation studies, 207
Subacute bacterial endocarditis, urine in, 320
Subarachnoid hemorrhage, 281
Subarachnoid space, block in, 280
Sudan III: method for stool fat, 378; stain, 274
Sugar, blood. *See* Glucose, in blood
Sulfates, normal values in serum, 7
Sulfhemoglobin, 48–51
Sulfhemoglobinemia, 49
Suppression tests of adrenal cortical function, 503
Supravital stains, 86, 95
Synovial cavity, histology, 285
Synovial fluid: blood in, 287; cell counts, 286; characteristics of, 285, 288; clotting, 286; culture of, 452; glucose concentration in, 287; mucin in, 286–287; in normal and in disease of joints, 288; normal values, 14; obtaining and examining, 285–288
Syphilis: biologic false positive test, 456; complement-fixation test, 456; flocculation tests, 456; paroxysmal cold hemoglobinuria in, 149; serologic tests, 284, 455–456

Tactoids, 129
Tapeworm, fish, macrocytic anemia due to, 112
Target cells, 131, 134
Tart cells, 184
"Tes-Tape," 305
Testicular insufficiency, HPG excretion in, 488
Testosterone: effect on protein-bound iodine, 480; polycythemia due to, 152
Tetralogy of Fallot, 525
Thalassemia: compared with iron-deficiency anemia, 110; osmotic fragility in, 123; special tests for, 135; types described, 134–135
Thiocyanate, 475

Thirst center, 358
Thormählen test for melanuria, 325
Thorn test, 503–504
Three-glass test, 310–311
Throat, culture of, technique, 446
Thrombasthenia, 66, 194, 196, 200, 207; clot retraction in, 202
Thrombin, 191
Thrombocyte. *See* Platelets
Thrombocytopathia. *See* Thrombasthenia
Thrombocytopenia, 194, 195, 196; and bone-marrow examination, 93; clot retraction in, 65, 70, 202; in paroxysmal nocturnal hemoglobinuria, 137
Thrombocytopenic purpura, 115
Thrombocytosis, 196; in polycythemia vera, 153. *See also* Platelets
Thromboplastin: and coagulation, 191–192; plasma, formation, 190–191; plasma, defects in formation, 194; tissue, 190. *See also* Plasma thromboplastin antecedent; Plasma thromboplastin component; Platelet thromboplastic factor
Thromboplastin generation: cross-correction studies, 204; modified prothrombin-consumption test, 204–206; studies, 206–207
Thromboplastin-generation test, 194, 204; effect of Stuart-factor deficiency on, 210; normal values, 11
Thymol flocculation: normal values, 8; test, method for, 420–421
Thymol turbidity: normal values, 8; test, principle and method, 420
Thyroglobulin, 475
Thyroid: biopsy of, 484; functional hyperplasia, 484; localization of $I^{131}$, 479; physiology, 475–476
Thyroid disease: basal metabolic rate in, 481–482; protein-bound iodine in, 480; serum cholesterol in, 481
Thyroid-function tests: categories, 476–477; in disease, 483–484
Thyroid hormone, actions, 476
Thyroid-stimulating hormone (TSH), 476; test, 482
Thyroiditis: Hashimoto's, 483, 484; subacute, 484
Thyroxine, 475; $I^{131}$-labeled, 483
Timed vital capacity: principle and method, 546–547; normal values, 547
Tissot spirometer, 538
$Tj^a$ factor, 222
Tobey-Ayer test, 280
Tocantins-O'Neill-Jones needle, 94
Tolbutamide-tolerance test, 471
Tollen's test, 307
Toluol, use as preservative for urine, 293
Töpfer's reagent, 112, 387, 388
Total fatty acids, normal values in serum, 6
Total lung capacity, definition, 544
Tourniquet test, 194, 195
Toxic granulation, 175
Toxoplasmosis, skin test, 457
Transaminase, serum glutamic oxaloacetic (SGOT), 258–259, 423; normal values, 8
Transaminase, serum glutamic pyruvic, 423
Transferrin, 108, 244